D1076290

)Y

E

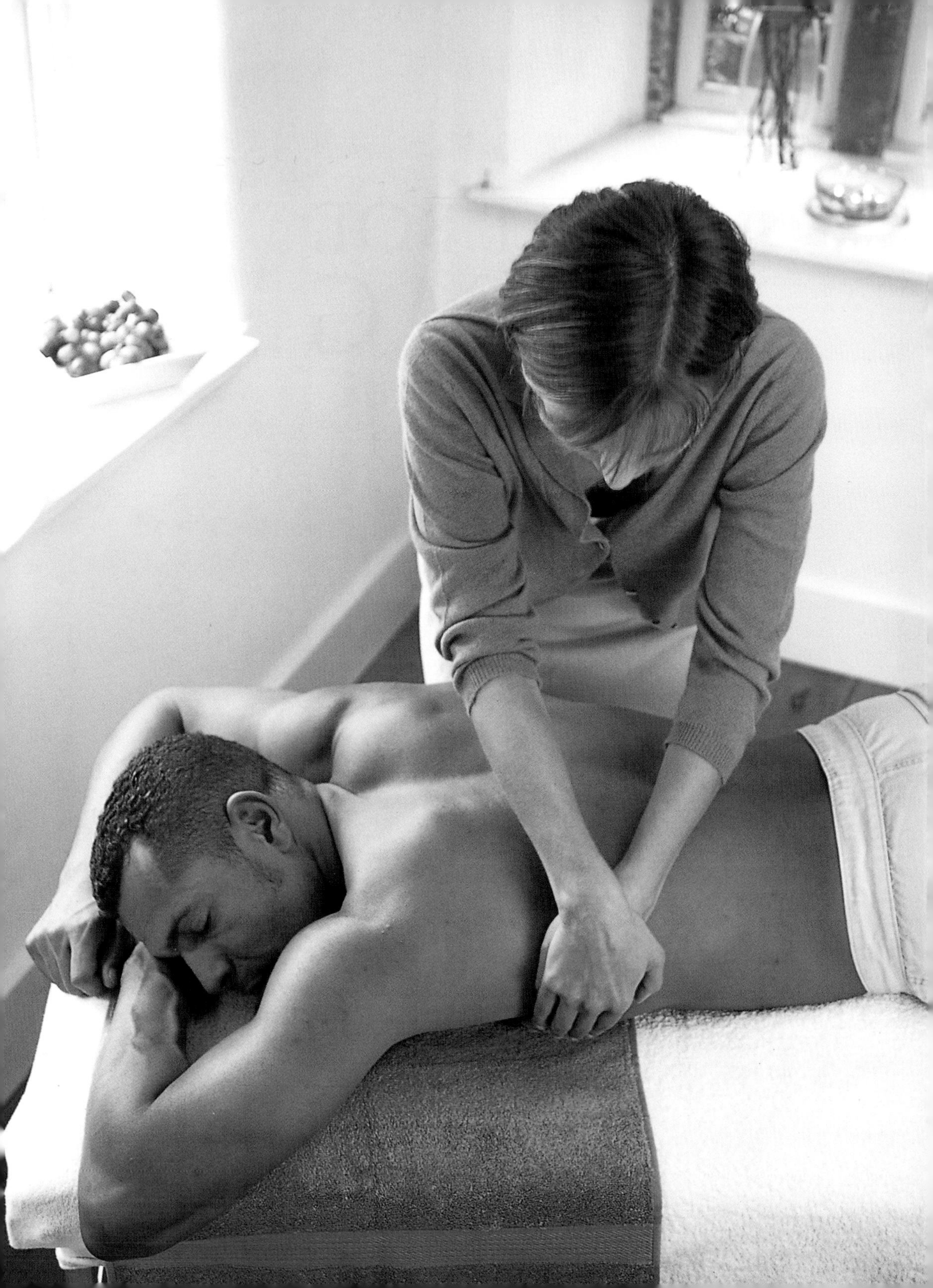

WHOLE BODY MASSAGE

THE ULTIMATE PRACTICAL MANUAL OF HEAD, FACE, BODY AND FOOT MASSAGE TECHNIQUES

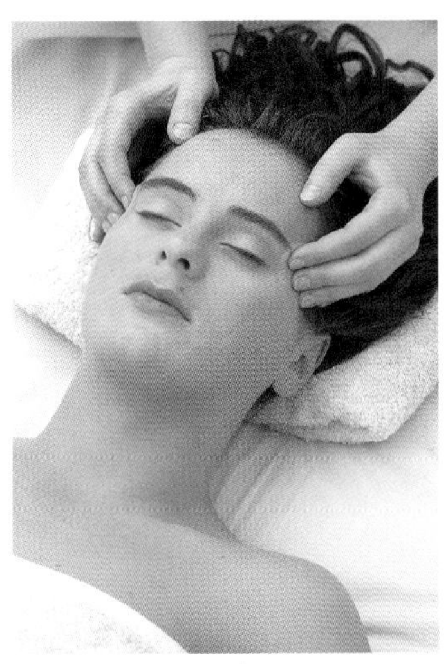

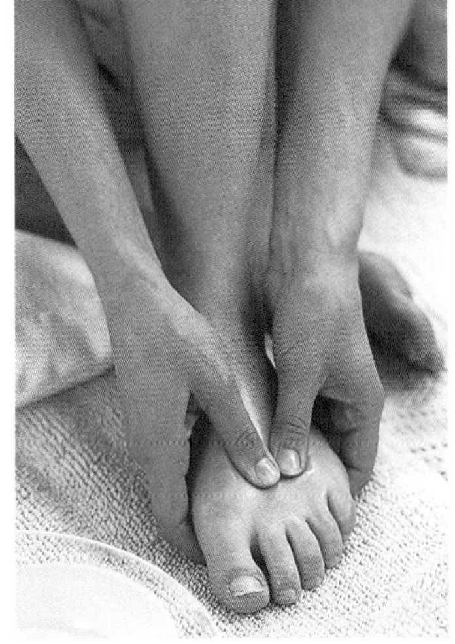

NITYA LACROIX
FRANCESCA RINALDI
SHARON SEAGER
RENÉE TANNER

PHOTOGRAPHS BY
MICHELLE GARRETT & ALISTAIR HUGHES

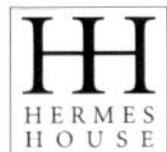

This edition is published by Hermes House,
an imprint of Anness Publishing Ltd,
Blaby Road, Wigston, Leicestershire LE18 4SE

Email: info@anness.com

Web: www.hermeshouse.com; www.annesspublishing.com

If you like the images in this book and would like to investigate using them for publishing, promotions or advertising, please visit our website www.practicalpictures.com for more information.

Publisher: Joanna Lorenz
Editorial Director: Helen Sudell
Senior Editor: Joanne Rippin
Project Editor: Ann Kay
Designers: Nigel Partridge, Design Principals
Photographers: Michelle Garrett, Alistair Hughes
Editorial Reader: Lindsay Zamponi
Production Controller: Stephen Lang

ETHICAL TRADING POLICY
Because of our ongoing ecological investment programme, you, as our customer, can have the pleasure and reassurance of knowing that a tree is being cultivated on your behalf to naturally replace the materials used to make the book you are holding. For further information about this scheme, go to www.annesspublishing.com/trees

A CIP catalogue record for this book is available from the British Library.

Previously published in three separate volumes: *Mind-Blowing Head Massage*, *Mind-Blowing Foot Massage*, *The Book of Massage & Aromatherapy*

PUBLISHER'S NOTE
The author and publishers have made every effort to ensure that all instructions contained within this book are accurate and safe, and cannot accept liability for any resulting injury, damage or loss to persons or property, however it may arise. If you do have any special needs or problems, consult your doctor or another health professional. This book cannot replace medical consultation and should be used in conjunction with professional advice.

The reader should not regard the recommendations, ideas and techniques expressed and described in this book as substitutes for the advice of a qualified medical practitioner or other qualified professional. Any use to which the recommendations, ideas and techniques are put is at the reader's sole discretion and risk.

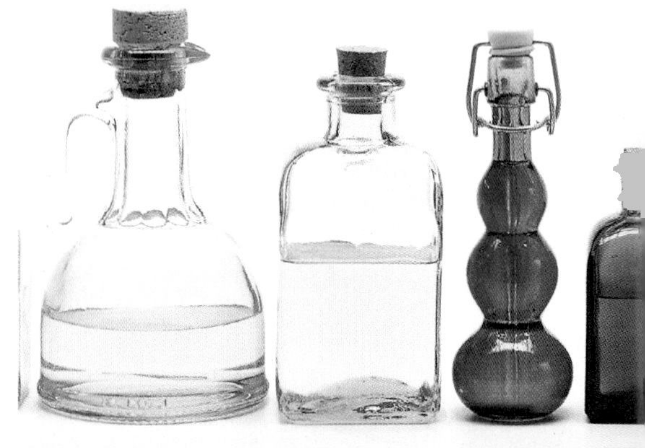

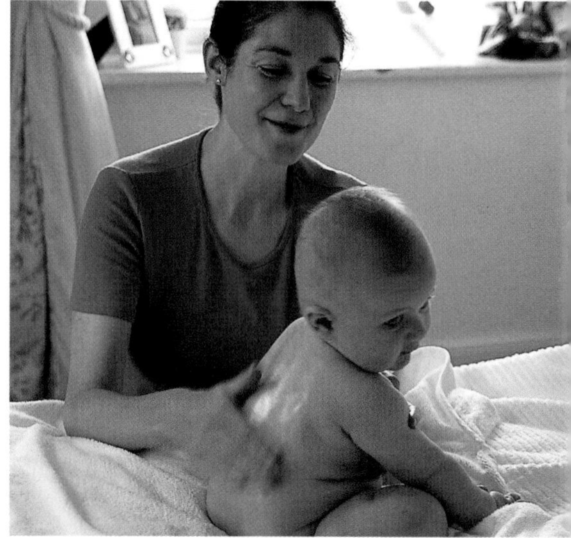

Contents

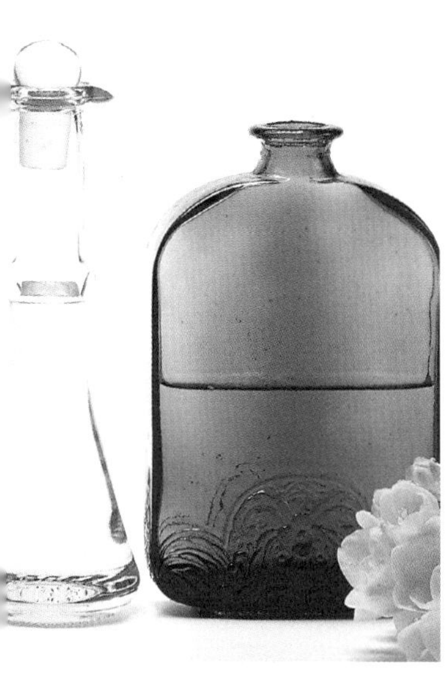

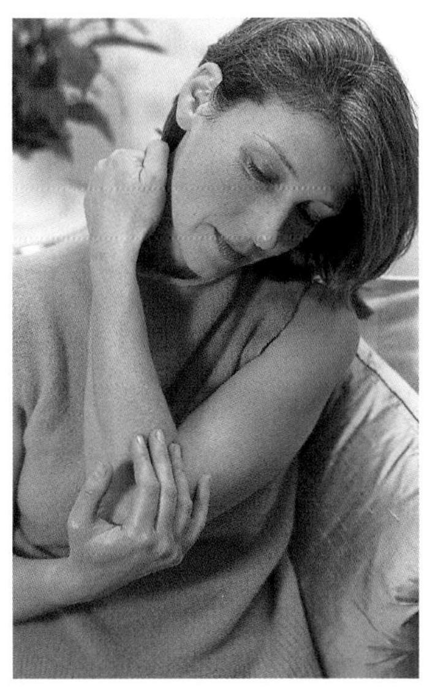

Preface

Massage is a touch therapy that is not only a wonderfully pleasurable and relaxing experience, but also brings countless health benefits. A massage treatment can relieve tension in the body, calm the mind, and nourish the soul, bringing healing on a number of different levels simultaneously.

approaches to massage

In general terms there are two main approaches in massage: those that are "energy"-based, and those that are more concerned with muscular physiology, though the trend is towards increasing integration. Energy-based approaches are influenced by ideas from the East, where it is widely believed that a universal life force enters and leaves the body at energy centres known as "chakras" and runs through the body along special channels, or "meridians". If this vital flow of energy is blocked through tension or injury, then pain or illness will result. Energy-based techniques use thumb or finger pressure at points along the meridians to help release blocked energy, enabling it to flow freely again through the body. They also focus on realigning the body's subtle energies through the chakra system to bring harmony and balance.

In the West, we come from a tradition of muscular-based massage. This approach is more concerned with physiology and focuses on the muscular-skeletal system. It is generally a fairly firm style of massage, and sports massage has grown out of this tradition. Increasingly, essential plant oils are used in massage for specific therapeutic effects. Known as aromatherapy, this is a lighter style of massage and focuses on introducing the aromatic oils into the body via the skin. This type of massage is popular for its "feel-good" factor, as well as being particularly effective in treating emotional or mental problems.

head massage

With its origins in India, head massage is a relatively new addition to the different types of massage therapy available in the West, yet it is a newcomer that has very rapidly gained popularity – perhaps because it captures the spirit of the modern age so well.

Head massage is quick to receive, and does not involve undressing or necessarily using oils. It is mess free, convenient and possible to do almost anywhere. Head massage is also effective in dealing with a range of physical and emotional complaints, especially those that are stress related, while it can also form an essential part of body-care routines.

body massage

The fast pace of modern life, combined with a sedentary lifestyle and an emphasis on mental activity, puts the whole body under a great strain. Body massage involves a flowing sequence of soothing and stimulating strokes combined to bring a harmonious state of relaxation and invigoration. Massaging much larger areas of the body can bring greater relief to body systems, and can be used to work on specific problems and stresses, as well as improving energy levels.

foot massage

A foot massage can be highly therapeutic, particularly as many of us spend much of our lives on our feet and they tend to take a huge amount of stress. Massage techniques for the feet are similar to those used elsewhere on the body, but need to be adapted for maximum effectiveness. Massage is equally good for relaxing and invigorating feet, especially when specific aromatherapy oils are used, while there are also routines for the feet and legs that improve circulation and general well-being. For a complete foot work-out, massage may be used alongside reflexology and acupressure, which aim to free blockages in vital energy pathways, easing everything from a headache to a sluggish immune system.

about this book

This book begins with an overview of the history of massage. It goes on to explain the importance of the power of touch and how massage affects our body systems. It shows how massage can be used to treat the symptoms of stress – both at home and at work – or to alleviate common conditions such as asthma, insomnia and headaches, as well as body tension and aches and pains from driving or computer work.

Clear information is given on the basic massage strokes, and by following the step-by-step instructions you are guided through massages for every part of your body from head to toe.

Each section is divided into chapters on techniques, the massages and therapeutic treatments. Some step-by-step sequences are also included for self-massage routines, as well as shorter, quick-fix, stress-busting treatments that can be used throughout the day.

This book makes massage accessible and easy to integrate into your everyday life. By working on the body with sensitivity and awareness, changes can be effected through the body's systems, encouraging relaxation and peace of mind, and harmonizing body and soul. Massage combined with the healing properties of essential oils can improve overall health and harmony – of mind, body and spirit – rather than simply easing tired muscles and aching limbs. It is a truly holistic therapy.

▷ While the hands relax and soothe the body and mind, the oils work their intrinsic aromatic magic, to uplift the spirits, and balance the whole system.

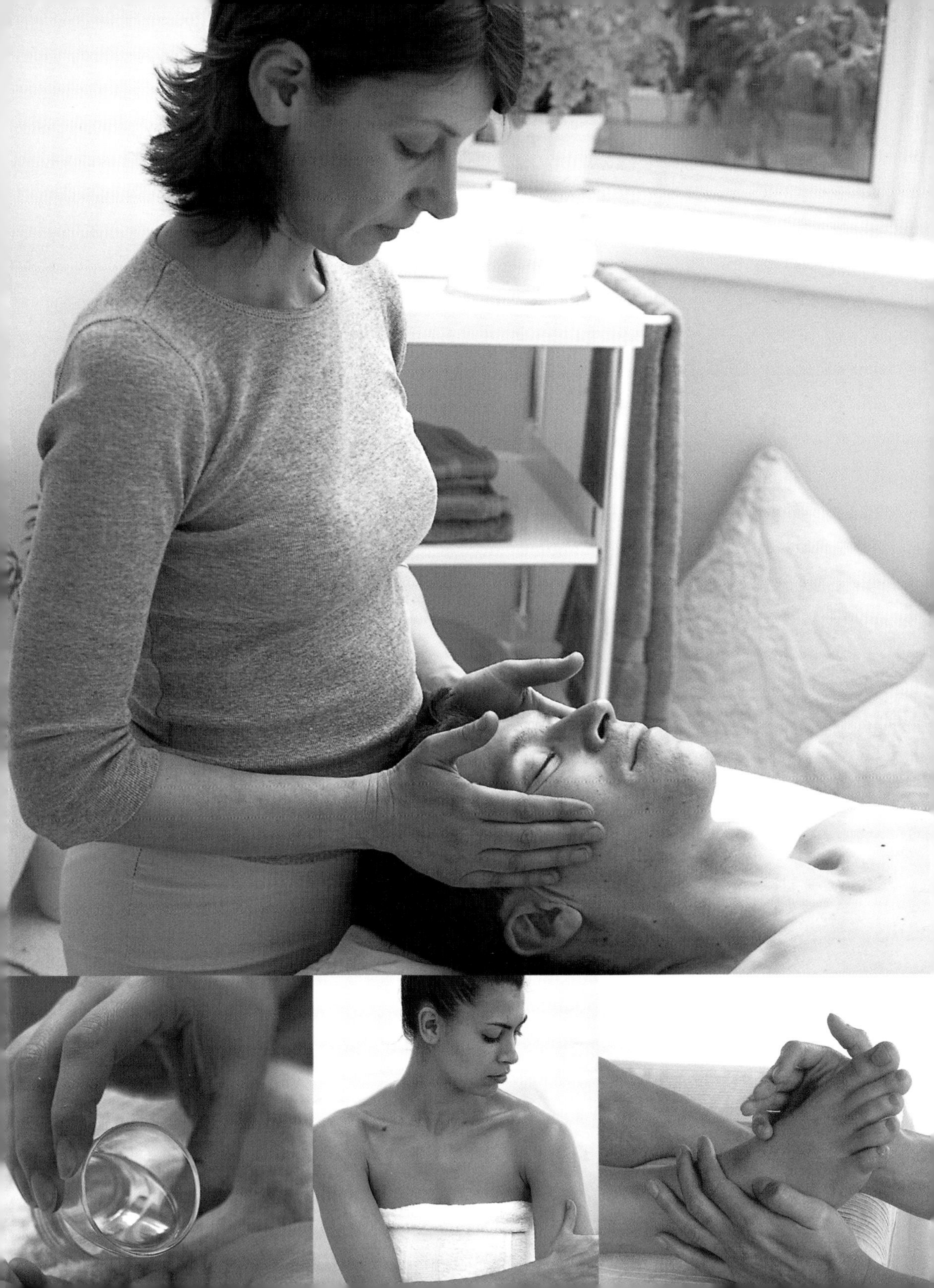

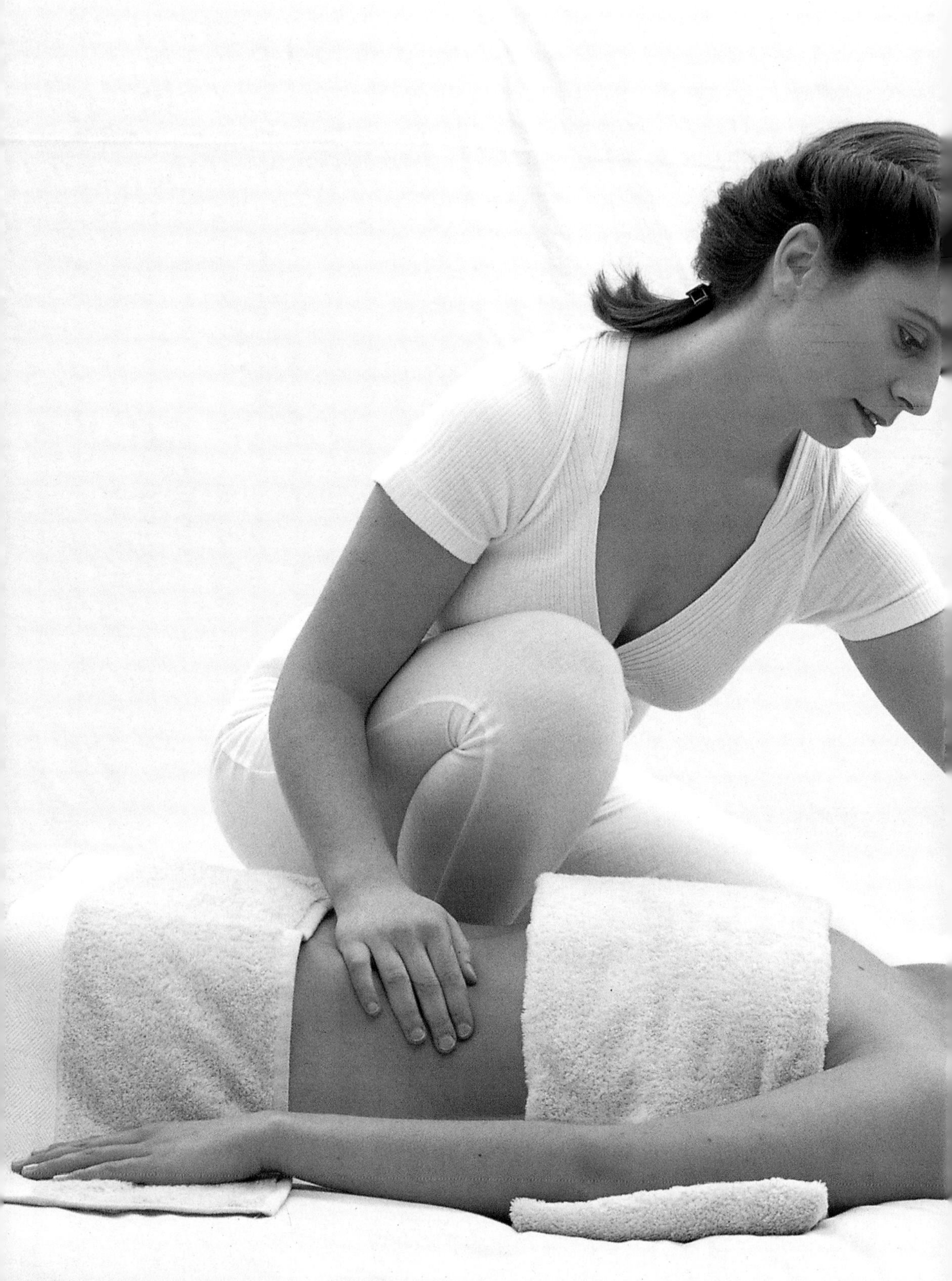

Part One
Holistic Massage

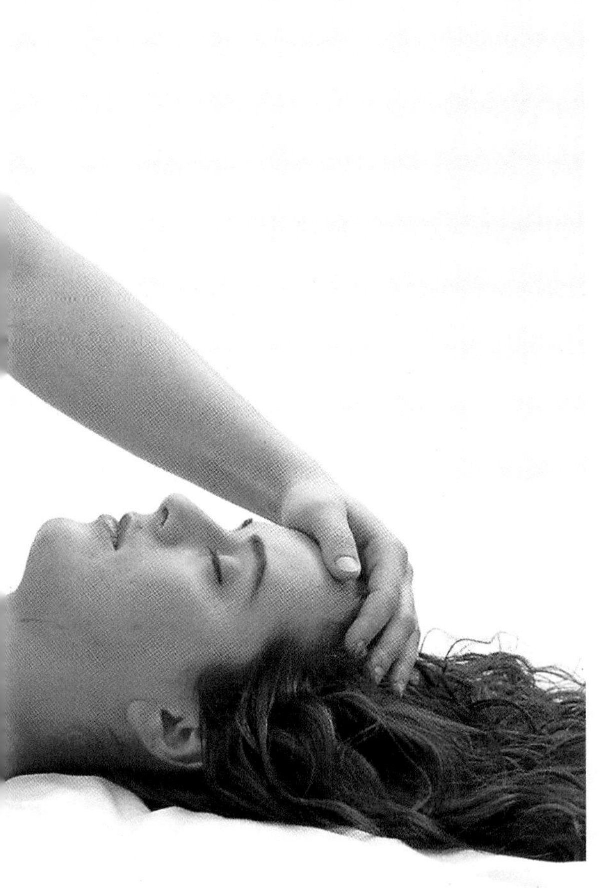

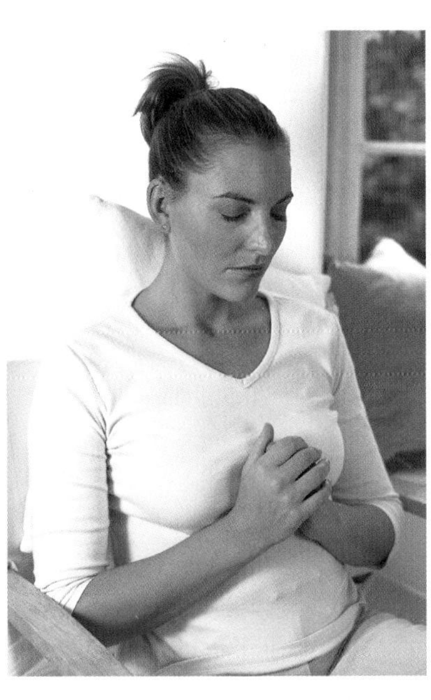

Massage in history

Massage is one of the oldest therapies in the world, and to discover its precise origins is almost impossible. The use of touch for grooming, stroking and rubbing is a behaviour that we share with many animals. Touch is instinctive, and from here it is a small step to develop this natural ability into a healing art. There is evidence that every culture throughout the world has used massage in some form or other, and every language, ancient or modern, has a word for massage. In the East the tradition of massage has always been unbroken, although its practice has been more staggered and erratic in Western cultures.

the ancient and classical world

Ancient Chinese medical texts, dating back some 5000 years, advocate stroking the body to "protect against colds, keep the organs supple and prevent minor ailments". Another text contains information that is akin to the passive limb movements used in modern Swedish massage. In India, Ayurvedic scripts from around 4000 years ago also recommend rubbing the body to treat and prevent disease. Since then massage has been inextricably linked with Indian culture. For instance, it is customary for a bride and groom to receive a massage before their wedding day, and most Indian mothers are taught how to massage their newborn babies and young children.

In ancient Egypt, *bas-relief* carvings dating back more than 4000 years show Pharaoh Ptah-Hotep receiving a leg massage from a male servant, while centuries later, Queen Cleopatra is recorded as enjoying a foot massage during dinner parties. However, enjoyment of massage was not restricted to the wealthy. Ancient records show that even the lowliest Egyptian workers were paid in wages of body oil sufficient for daily use.

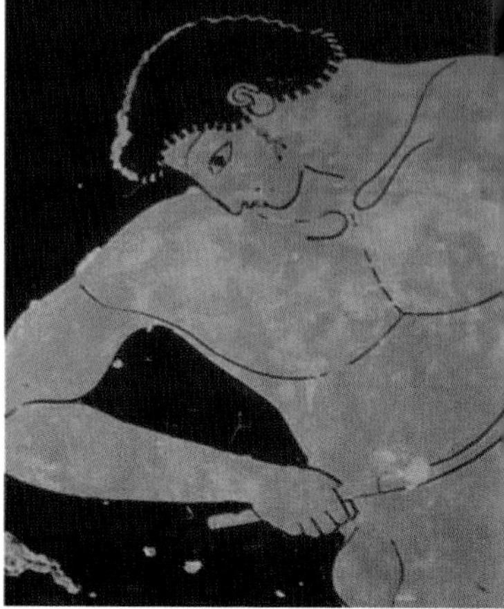

△ The Greeks used oil to cleanse themselves before bathing and massage. Here an athlete in a gymnasium removes the oil from his body.

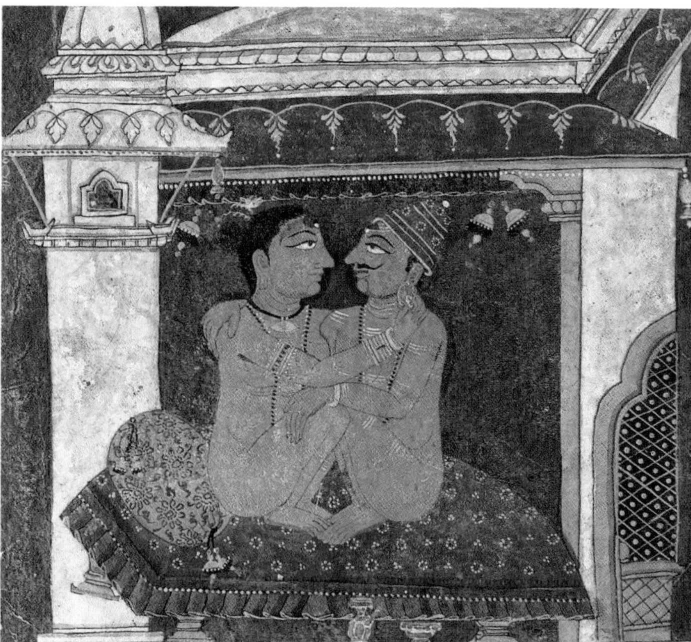

▽ The Kama Sutra and ancient Ayurvedic scripts contain many references to sensual massage, which was used for pleasure, spiritual practice and general health and well-being.

For the ancient Greeks, the pursuit of physical excellence was paramount, and massage played an intrinsic part in their exaltation of the body. Their famous medical centres, or gymnasia, contained open-air training rooms, sports grounds and massage rooms. In ancient Greece, massage was highly recommended for treating fatigue, sports or war injuries, as well as illness. Writing in the 5th century BC, Hippocrates, the reputed "father of modern medicine", stated that a successful physician must be experienced in the art of "rubbing", and prescribed a scented bath followed by a daily massage with oils as the pathway to good health and fitness.

The Romans were equally fond of massage and incorporated it into their bathing rituals. For the wealthy, it was

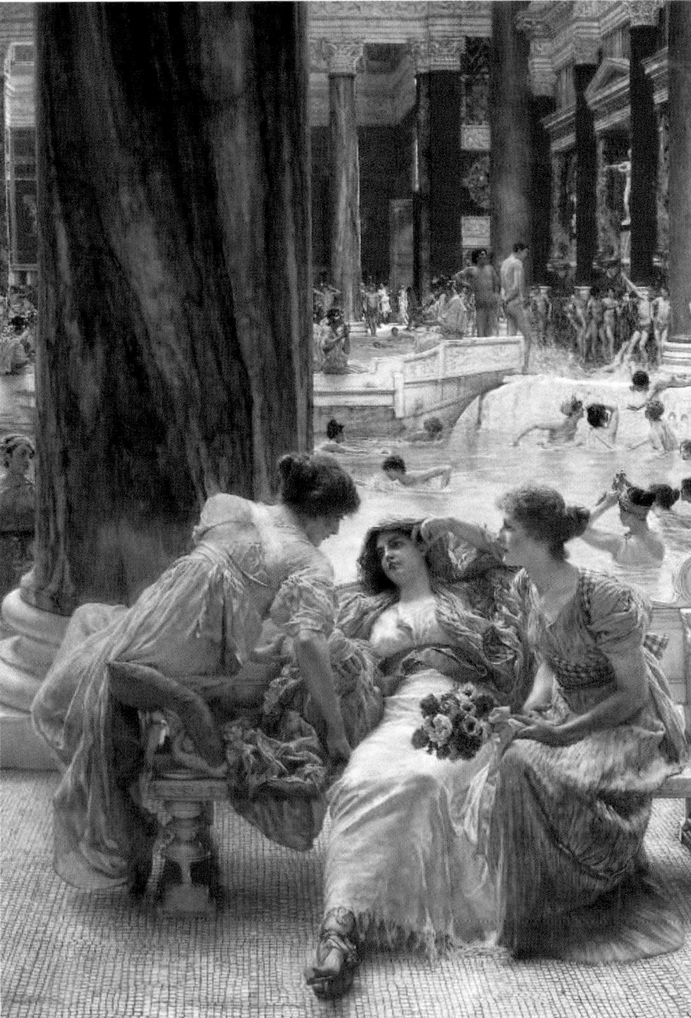

▷ **The Roman Empire placed great value on bodily pleasures and rituals, including massage and cleansing, which were practised in the ubiquitous Roman baths.**

customary to attend the baths and have stiff muscles rubbed with warm vegetable oil. This was followed by a full body massage to awaken the nerves, get the circulation going and mobilize the joints. The routine was completed as fine oil was liberally applied all over the body to nourish the skin and keep it fine and smooth. Physicians also promoted the therapeutic benefits of massage. One of the most famous of these was Galen (AD130–201), who wrote books on massage, exercise and health. He also classified different massage strokes, and used massage in the treatment of many diseases.

the Middle Ages and beyond

After the decline of the Roman Empire, the Arab world became the centre of learning and culture. The works of Hippocrates, Galen and other famous physicians were translated into Arabic, preserving the medical knowledge built up since antiquity. Avicenna (980–1037), one of the greatest Arab physicians, added to this knowledge and went on to describe the use of healing plants, spinal manipulation and various forms of massage in great detail.

Meanwhile, in Europe, touch became associated with "carnal pleasures" in the eyes of the Catholic Church, and massage was denounced as a highly sinful activity. Its practice was consigned to the realm of folklore, and knowledge was passed down through the female line – the local "wise woman" or midwife – along with knowledge of herbs and other healing remedies. This information was regarded with suspicion and could lead to persecution as a witch.

The Renaissance saw a revival of interest in classical medicine, and massage gradually became more respected by mainstream society. Ambroise Paré, a 16th-century physician to the French court, used massage in his practice. European journeys of exploration also revealed how other cultures valued massage. Captain Cook described how massage cured his sciatic pains in Tahiti, and in the 1800s there are records of the Cherokee and Navaho peoples of North America using massage on their warriors.

towards the modern age

However, it was at the end of the 19th century that a Swedish gymnast, Per Henrik Ling (1776–1839), restored to favour therapeutic massage in Europe. Having cured himself of rheumatism, Ling developed a system of massage that was based on physiology, gymnastic movements and massage. Receiving royal patronage for his work, Ling's methods laid the foundation for modern physiotherapy with the establishment in 1894 of the Society of Trained Masseurs. A few years later, St George's Hospital in London opened a massage department, and "Swedish" massage therapy soon became part of mainstream medical practice.

This emphasis continued unchecked until the 1960s, when personal growth centres, notably the Esalen Institute in California, adapted massage therapy into a holistic treatment that could balance mind, body and emotions, rather than simply relieving muscular aches and pains. This holistic approach is now widely used alongside mainstream medicine as a complement to conventional medical treatments.

The power of touch

Touch is a basic human instinct and it has the power to comfort and reassure on many levels. It can relax the body, calm the mind and encourage healing and well-being.

a natural impulse

To touch others or to be touched is one of our most instinctive needs. The sense of touch is the first to develop in the embryo, and babies require and thrive on close physical contact with their mothers and fathers. The caring, loving touch of another is fundamental to the development of a healthy human being. This need to be touched does not stop as childhood ends, yet as we grow to adulthood many of us become afraid to reach out and touch one another. Mistrustful of our instinctive loving impulse, we have lost touch with ourselves and with the wisdom of the body. One of the most appealing aspects of practising therapeutic touch techniques is that we can begin to re-establish contact with ourselves – and others – in a way that is safe, caring and non-intrusive.

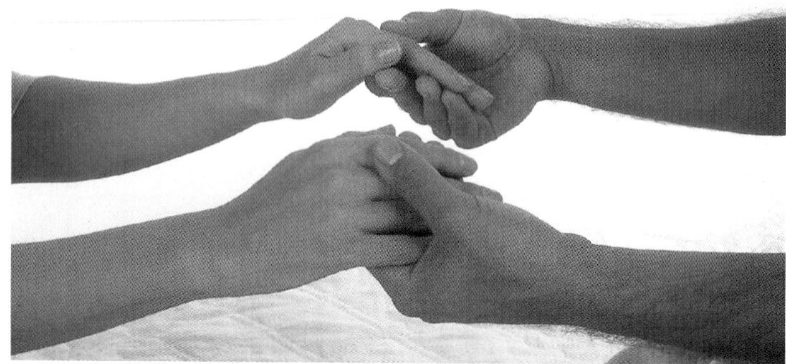

△ **It is a natural reaction to reach out and touch, very often with the intention of soothing and comforting, so it is not surprising that the hands have come to be seen by many as the focus and centre for healing energies.**

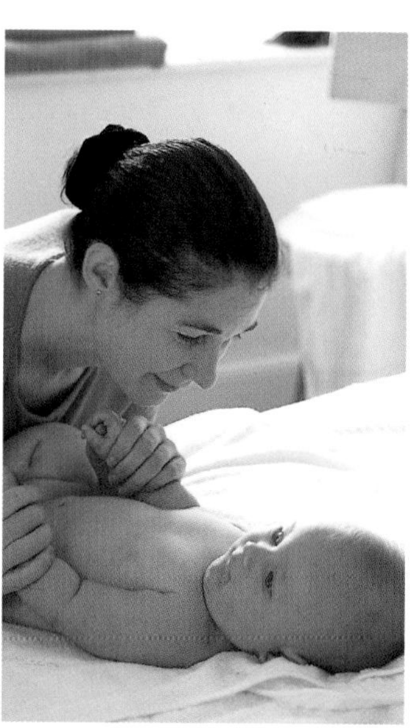

benefits of touch

Awareness of the therapeutic value of touch is growing and many touch therapies are widely used in conventional healthcare to treat pain, ease discomfort and to improve the functional workings of the body. Given the pressures of modern-day living and the increased incidence of stress-related illness, touch therapies also have an important part to play in everyday life. Aching backs and shoulders after a tiring day at work hunched over a computer or spending most of the day on your feet, strained leg muscles after excessive exercise, or circulatory problems from a sedentary lifestyle are some of the occupational hazards of adult life. Through the healing power of touch we can learn to take better care of ourselves. Taking time to channel healing energy or enjoy a soothing foot massage can ease some of the day-to-day tensions of life and put us back in touch with ourselves and our priorities, to feel relaxed and at home in our bodies.

◁ **For a baby, being touched, washed, held, carried, caressed and dressed is a fundamental part of existence, and touch is essential for healthy growth and development, both physical and emotional.**

▷ **Most of us, almost unconsciously, rub tense, aching muscles to bring comfort and relief.**

touch therapy

Working on both physical and psychological levels, massage has the ability to relax and invigorate the person receiving it. While the

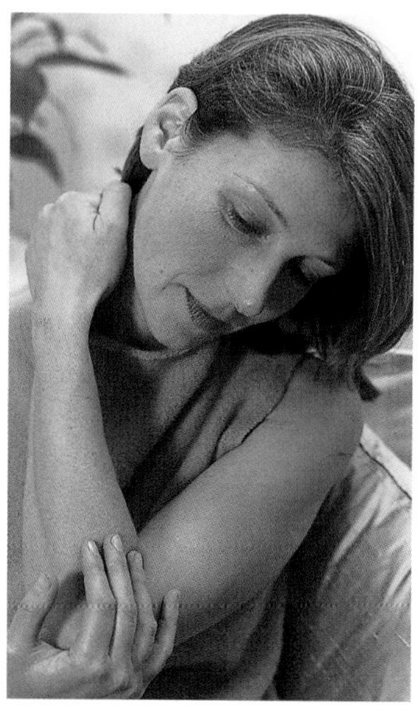

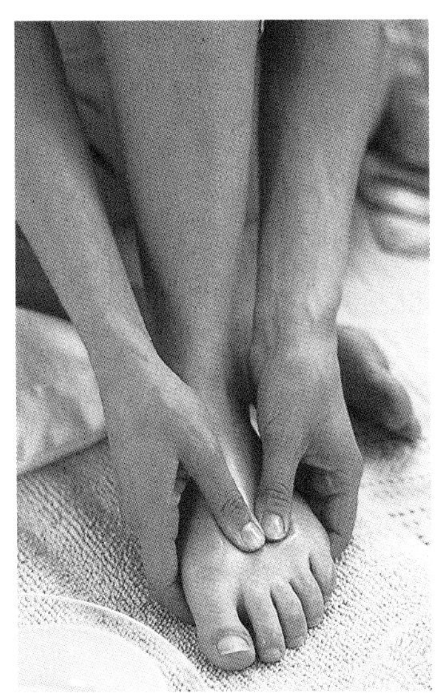

◁ **Our hands are a vital tool in daily body care. Touch can help us identify problem areas, as well as keeping skin healthy and smooth.**

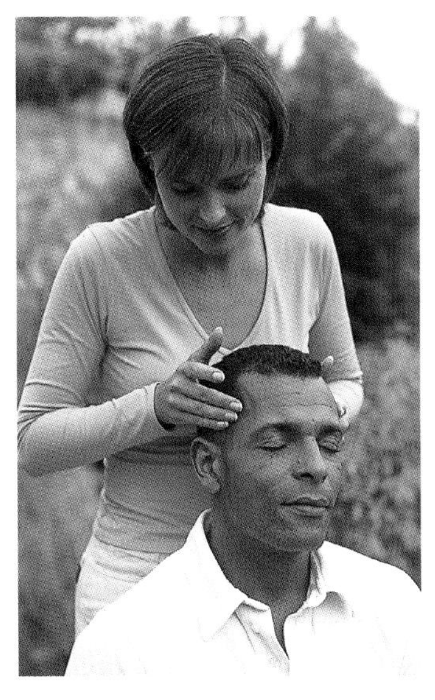

▷ **Massage contributes to our minimum daily touch requirements, now recognized as fundamental to good health and well-being.**

techniques and strokes of massage can ease pain or tension from stiff and aching muscles, boost a sluggish circulation, or eliminate toxins, the nurturing touch of the hands on the body soothes away mental stress and restores emotional equilibrium at the same time. As tensions dissolve there is an ensuing integration between the physical body and underlying emotions, which breaks the vicious cycle of tension between mind and body.

soothing hands

Massage allows time for the replenishment of innate resources of vital energy. This is particularly relevant in a modern world when stress is known to be the root cause of many serious physical and mental conditions. Stress is a natural factor of life, and moderate levels of stress can be beneficial for certain activities. However, if stress is not discharged appropriately, or is suffered for a prolonged period of time, it robs the body of health and energy. Stress can also lower the natural defences of the body's immune system and its ability to fight disease. When a person is constantly exposed to the adverse effects of stress, anxiety, depression, lethargy, insomnia, and panic attacks can result. Increasingly, both the medical profession and the public recognize the benefits of massage as a successful treatment of symptoms arising from stress.

emotional health

Massage provides a safe and neutral situation in which to receive loving touch and stimulation of the skin senses, which are so important for emotional health and self-esteem. Touch is fundamental to the development of a healthy human being, and touch deprivation in the early stages of life is known to inhibit the emotional and physical growth of a child. Since touch is so bound up with the emotions, it can also lead to feelings of vulnerability, so massage needs to be practised in a safe environment, with great care and sensitivity. A loving touch can heal, share empathy, and comfort, and massage should combine skilful techniques with loving touch, so that as the hands stroke the body, they unlock not only the physical tensions trapped in muscles, but also acknowledge, with complete acceptance, the essence of the person within. While massage itself is active, the underlying quality of the touch is one of stillness and calm, a sense of being totally present with that person. For all these reasons, massage is a highly beneficial therapy, because it helps the person receiving it to feel safe enough to relax completely and unwind from the deepest parts of the mind.

▽ **Throughout life, touch has the power to comfort, reassure and relax.**

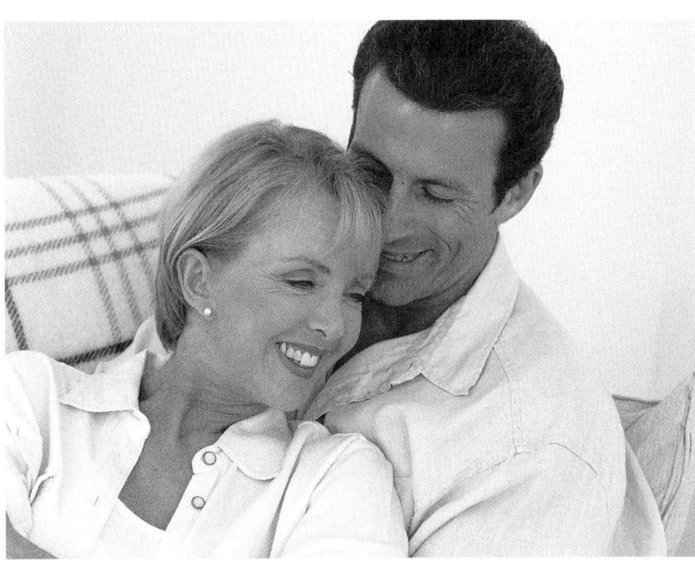

How massage works

On a physiological level, massage affects all the body systems, resulting in improved general functioning, as well as relieving specific conditions. It can also assist with self-esteem, release emotional blocks, increase mental clarity, and help you to connect with your "inner light". Having a massage is simultaneously relaxing and refreshing. It is about taking time out to restore harmony and well-being so that you feel ready to take on the world again.

body systems

The skin is the body's largest sensory organ. When it is touched, thousands of tiny nerve receptors on its surface send messages to the brain via the central nervous system. The brain interprets these messages and returns them to the muscles. Stroking can trigger the release of endorphins (the body's natural painkillers) and send messages of calm and relaxation. More vigorous massage works on the body's underlying muscles, easing tension and stiffness.

▽ **A soothing self massage of tired legs and feet can relieve muscle tension, improve circulation and calm and relax the whole body.**

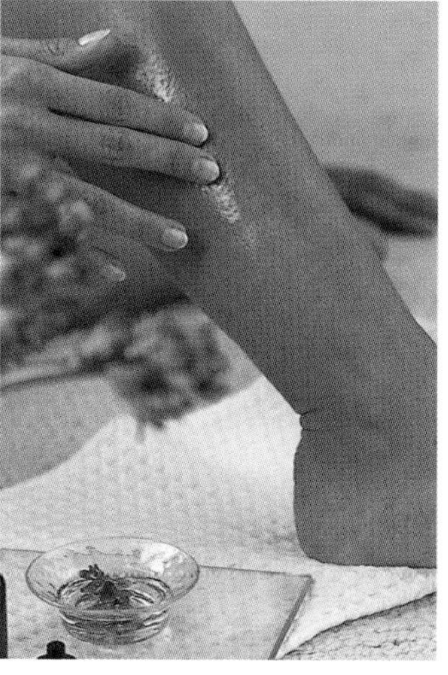

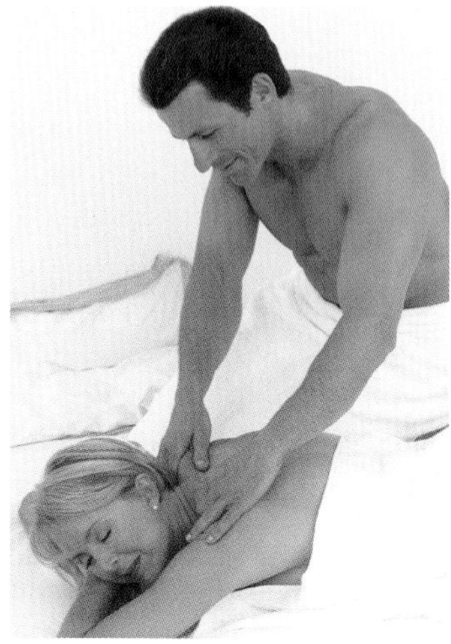

physical benefits

A sound circulatory system is vital for the healthy functioning of the whole body. Massage causes breathing to deepen and the blood vessels and capillaries to dilate, which boosts the circulation and helps oxygenate the blood. Improved circulation also means that vital nutrients are carried around the body more effectively, while temporarily reducing blood pressure and pulse rate and so relaxing and calming the body and mind. Massage stimulates the functioning of the skin's sebaceous and sweat glands that work together to moisturize, clean and cool it. Massage also has an exfoliating action, helping to eliminate dead skin cells and thus resulting in a fresher appearance to the skin. Boosting the circulation improves the supply of necessary nutrients needed for healthy hair, nails and skin, and can also help relieve a range of problems including headaches and digestive disorders.

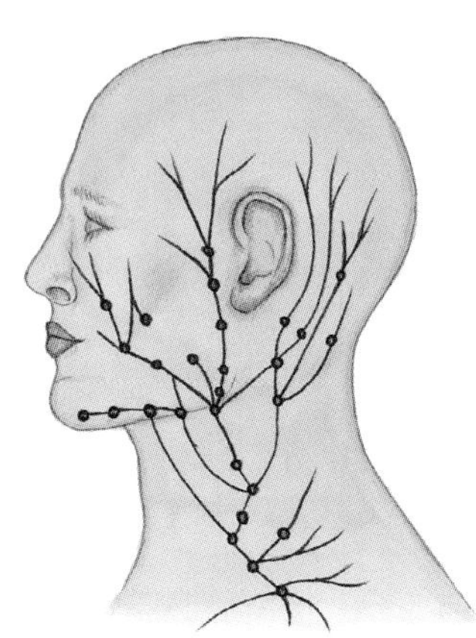

△ **Lymph nodes and ducts in the face and neck help eliminate toxins. Massage stimulates the effectiveness of this cleansing action.**

◁ **Regular massage is a good immunity booster. Research has shown that it can have a protective effect on the body for up to a week after a single treatment.**

Massage also has a direct benefit on the body's muscular structure. By relaxing and stretching muscles that have become contracted and shortened with tension, massage helps the body to regain its flexibility as the elasticity and mobility of the body tissues is restored. These actions can help to ease painful muscles and improve posture by helping to bring the body's musculature back into a more balanced position. It can also help to restore muscles that have become weak and flaccid through underuse. The physical action of massage also works directly on the lymphatic system, helping the body eliminate lactic acid and other chemical wastes that contribute to pain and discomfort in the joints and muscles. Many lymphatic nodes are situated in the neck, back of the head, face and jaw.

As a massage treatment progresses and the body relaxes more deeply, there is a gradual switching over in body functioning towards the parasympathetic nervous system. This system operates outside of our conscious control and is related to the hidden work of general maintenance and repair, and essential functions such as digestion and elimination. We are often in

▽ Blood is transported around the body by a complex network of arteries (shown in red) and veins (shown in blue). Massage increases peripheral circulation and assists blood flow through the system.

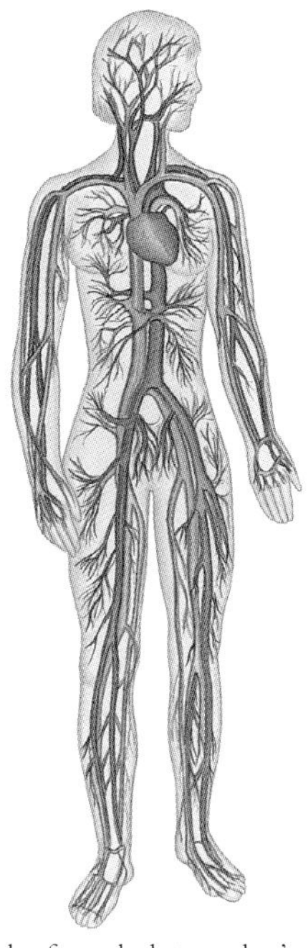

▽ Movement in the body is produced by the action of muscles. It is these skeletal muscles that register discomfort, or ache when we get tired or put them under strain. Massage works directly on these key muscle groups.

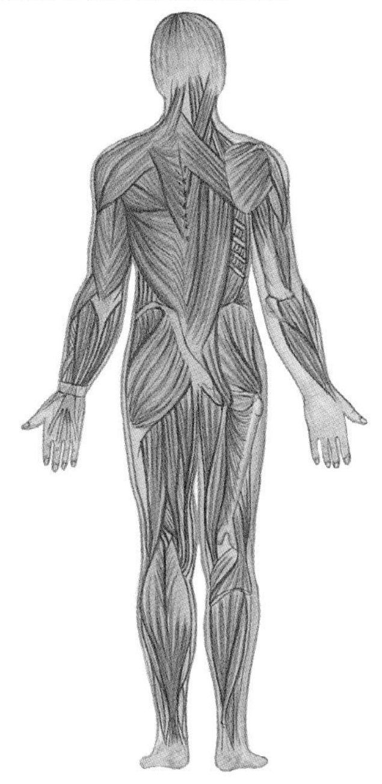

▽ Messages are transmitted between the brain and receptors and nerves through the body's "wiring system", which runs via the spinal cord. These include messages of relaxation from massage action.

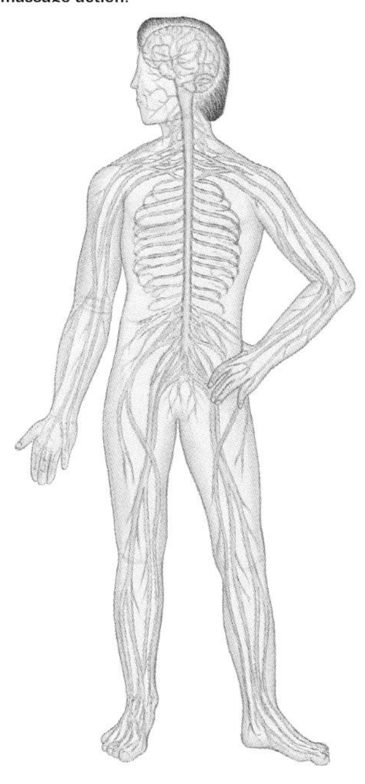

so much of a rush that we don't give our bodies enough time for this important work. Massage is a good way of giving the body a "pit stop", where it can attend to its inner workings.

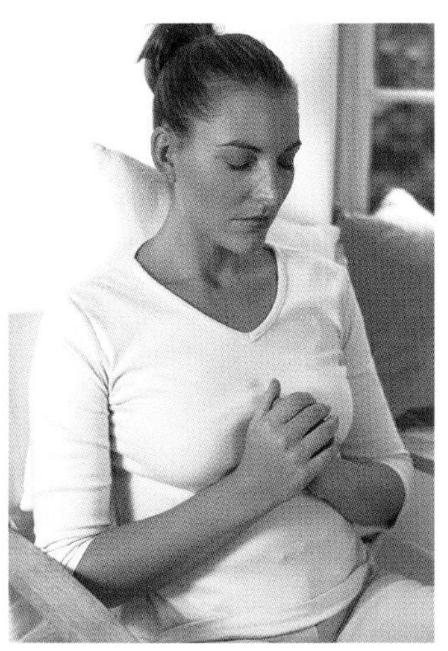

◁ Glowing hair and skin, relaxed muscle tone and an upright, balanced posture are some of the visible benefits of massage.

mind and emotions

An extensive body of research supports the therapeutic claims of massage, with growing evidence that it can contribute to the relief of conditions such as stress, depression and anxiety. Head massage in particular has a significant impact on a mental level. The physical release of muscular tension and the increased blood supply to the head results in improved mental functioning and a greater sense of clarity. There is a reduction in mental exhaustion, feelings of irritability or being overwhelmed and a corresponding increase in alertness, mental agility, concentration and insightfulness.

Massage is also valued for its "feel-good" factor. As the body releases tension, a weight is lifted, leading to an increased sense of lightness and happiness. These emotional shifts correspond to the hormonal changes that occur in the body during a massage treatment. Research indicates that the level of stress hormones such as cortisol falls during massage, while the level of feel-good bonding hormones, such as oxytocin, significantly increases. Stress hormones have a weakening effect on the immune system.

nourishing the soul

Massage can also work on the energetic balance of the body through the chakra system, which centres around its spiritual dimension. By aligning body and soul through massage, a deep sense of peace, calm and balance can be achieved. The sense of lightness that people often feel after a treatment can also bring an increased awareness of their spiritual identity or inner light. After a massage, people often feel more at one with themselves. Some people report an improved perspective on life, the return of their sense of humour, or say that they are simply more relaxed and comfortable within their own bodies.

Energy work

There is more to the body than meets the eye. As you approach another person, they may be able to sense your presence before you touch them. That is because you have entered their "energy field" or aura, the invisible vibrations that radiate from our bodies. The stronger and healthier we are, the bigger and more expansive our aura; when we are tired or sick, this field is smaller and closer to the body. The chakra system is part of this energy field and some understanding of it is useful in massage. Although you may not be able to see it, you will be affecting the way it functions through your touch.

health and the chakras

The chakras represent energy points in the body. The word *chakra* means "wheel" in Sanskrit, indicating that the chakras are like spinning vortexes, receiving energy from the universe and transforming it to be utilized by the body. In energy-based medicine, the first signs of ill health are believed to show up as blockages or disturbances in the chakras. If these imbalances are not sorted out then the issue will eventually show up as a physical problem. Keeping the chakras working effectively is important for good health.

the chakra system

There are seven major chakras, each having its own characteristics and correspondences. They are found at points that run up the body from the base of the spine to the top of the head, and can be located on the front and back of the body. Each chakra is associated with different organs and systems of the body and with a different colour, although there are some variations according to which chakra system you are using. It is a dynamic and ever-changing interaction of energies.

▽ **Spiritual awareness is part of Eastern culture, and in India it is commonplace to see the "third eye" marked by wearing a bindi.**

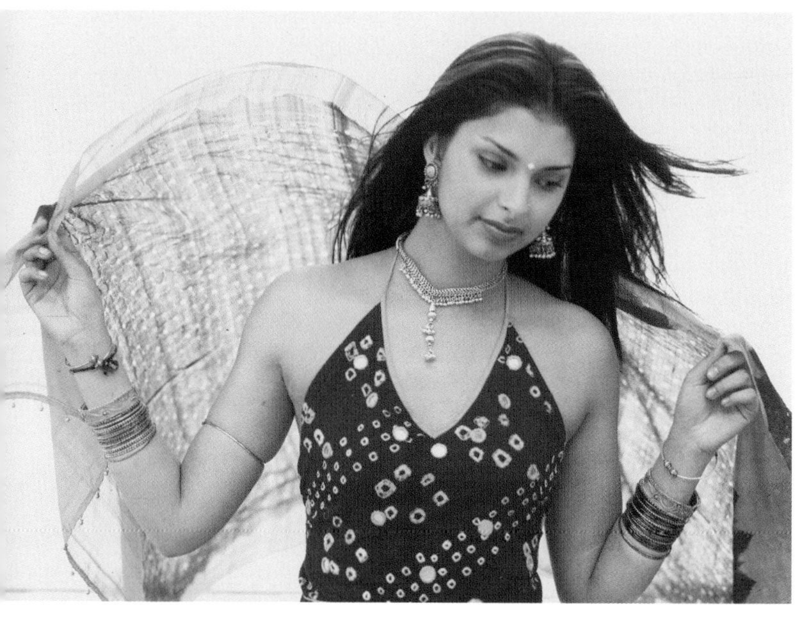

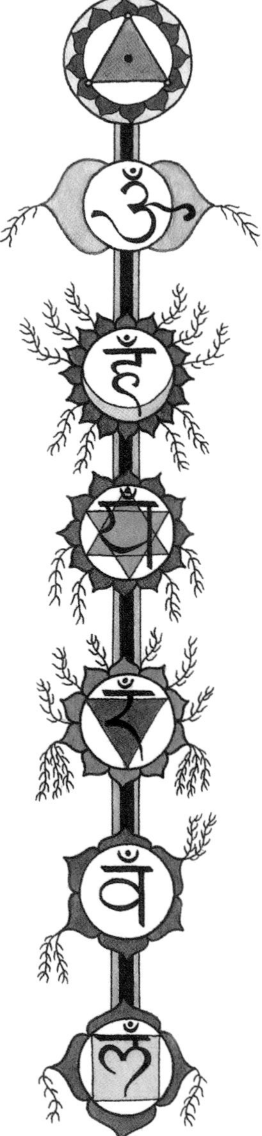

△ **The seven major chakras are energy centres for accessing and distributing *chi* or *prana* or life force around the body through the system of meridian channels.**

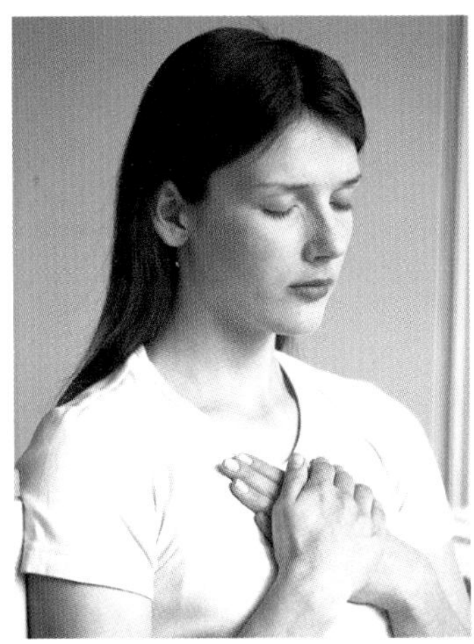

△ **Resting your hands over your heart centre and breathing into the hold will help you feel your own heart energy through which love and healing forces flow.**

the seven chakras

The base chakra, at the base of the spine, is related to the testicles or ovaries in some systems, and in others to the adrenal glands.

The sacral chakra is located in the lower abdomen and is associated with emotions and sensuality.

The solar plexus chakra, found at the front of the body between the bottom of the ribcage and the navel, is related to personal energy and power. It is associated with the adrenal glands and the pancreas.

Roughly halfway up the spine, the heart chakra corresponds to unconditional love, compassion and friendship. It relates to the thymus, heart, lungs, bronchial tubes, upper back and the arms. Physical release points are in the shoulders, the intercostal muscles of the ribs, the upper arms, under the chin and at the base of the skull.

The throat chakra is located at the base of the neck where it connects to the shoulders. It is concerned with all forms of communication and self-expression. It relates to the thyroid, ears, nose and throat, the neck and teeth. Physical release points are in the neck, shoulders, fingers and toes.

The "third eye" chakra is located in the middle of the forehead or the brow. Its energy release points are in the eyes, temples, forehead and at the base of the skull. It is concerned with the development and deepening of intuition and soul knowledge. It regulates the energies of the pituitary and nervous systems, as well as the brain, head, eyes and face.

The crown chakra is located at the top of the head. Its energy release points are in the head, hands and feet. It is concerned with higher consciousness and spirituality.

working with the chakras

As you massage, you can become aware of these energy centres, especially when working near the areas of the body where they reside. At the end of a treatment, when your partner is still, you could experiment by using "holds" over one or two chakras. To do this, place one hand gently over the other and let them rest lightly over a chakra spot for a few moments. Follow your intuition when choosing each spot. For instance, if you sense your partner needs comfort and reassurance, then you may feel drawn to the heart chakra in the middle of the upper back. Or if your partner has communication issues, then a gentle holding on the throat chakra at the back of the neck may be helpful. As you "hold" imagine healing energy flowing from your heart chakra down your arms and out of your hands into your partner, and intend that it goes where it is most needed.

When you have finished, take your hands away slowly and carefully. See if you can feel your partner's energy field and notice the point at which your hands finally leave it. It is likely that after a treatment their energy field will have expanded, as the chakras have become more balanced and their energies are flowing more efficiently.

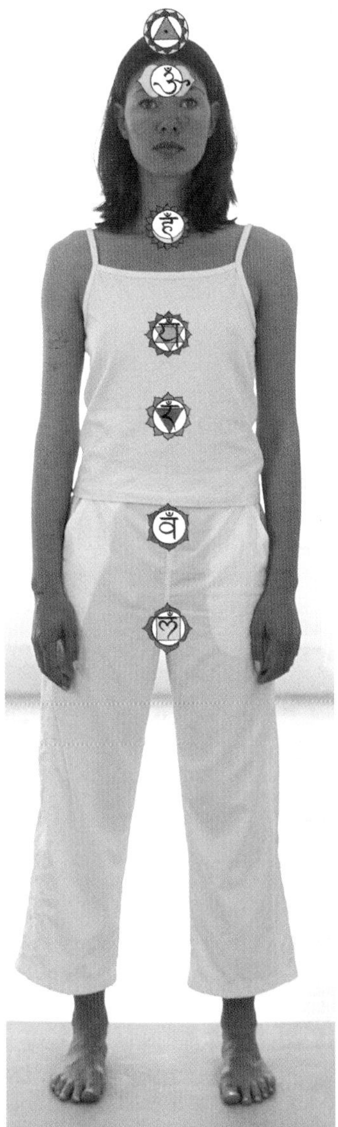

△ **The chakras are located in key areas and these energy centres nourish, and have correspondences with, the physical and emotional dimensions of the whole person.**

Massage systems

There are various approaches to the art of healing through touch, massage, and bodywork. Some systems focus directly on the physiology of the body, and others on the release of emotional tension. Others work more subtly on energy levels within the body. These days, many touch therapies combine ancient and modern techniques drawn from both the East and the West. What they all have in common is the aim to bring harmony and well-being to the recipients by releasing tension and congestion, thereby allowing the restoration of natural vitality.

soft tissue massage

This system makes use of a variety of techniques to stroke and manipulate the skin and the superficial muscles and tissues in order to alleviate pain and tension. The strokes themselves help to boost the circulatory system and increase the exchange of tissue fluids. Variations such as Swedish massage, sports massage, physiotherapy, and lymphatic massage are particularly beneficial for these purposes, as they work directly with the anatomy and physiology of the body to restore vitality and a state of relaxation.

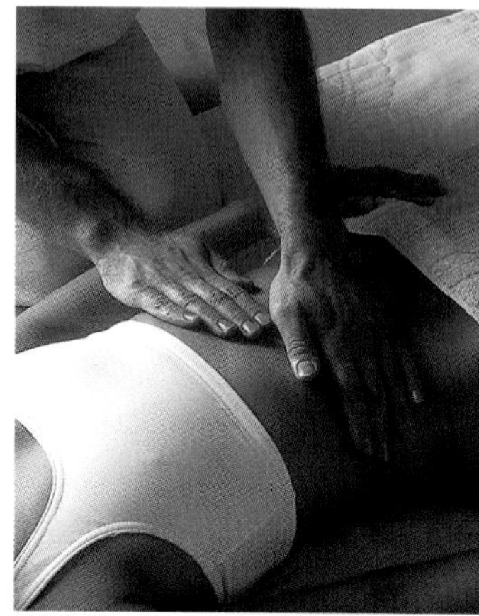

◁ Soft tissue massage uses a variety of techniques to stroke and manipulate the skin and the superficial muscles and tissues to alleviate pain and tension, and restore vitality.

Holistic massage also works with the body's soft tissue, but is generally more concerned with psychological relaxation. Soporific strokes predominate, lulling the mind, calming the nervous system, and restoring a sense of equilibrium, thereby producing an inner release of tension. A nourishing touch and the delivery of massage in an atmosphere of loving care is seen as the main medium of transformation. A holistic session can also combine the strokes of therapeutic and remedial massage, but its main emphasis always remains on relaxing the body and mind.

deep tissue massage

The aim of deep tissue massage is to restore structural alignment and balance within the body by releasing chronic tensions, formed by deep muscular tension, which inhibit postural ease and movement. It works mainly on the body's connective tissue, or fascia, which wraps, binds, supports, and separates all the internal structures, including the skeletal muscles, bones, tendons, ligaments, and organs. This muscular "armour" in the body may be the result of injury, habitual bad posture, or the repression of emotions.

Connective tissue is present throughout the entire internal structure of the body, and is best recognized by its shiny white fibres, which are formed mainly from a type of protein called collagen. When the body is free of trauma (injury) and tension, the fascia is generally elastic, but if the system is sluggish or inactive, or muscular armour has formed in the body, the fascia can become rigid and immobile. Since connective tissue envelops and connects every internal structure, tension in one area can have a detrimental effect on the whole system.

Deep tissue massage strokes manipulate the fascia by the action of friction and stretching, releasing blocks that impede the flow of energy and life force throughout the whole body. This is a skill that requires a professional training and a thorough

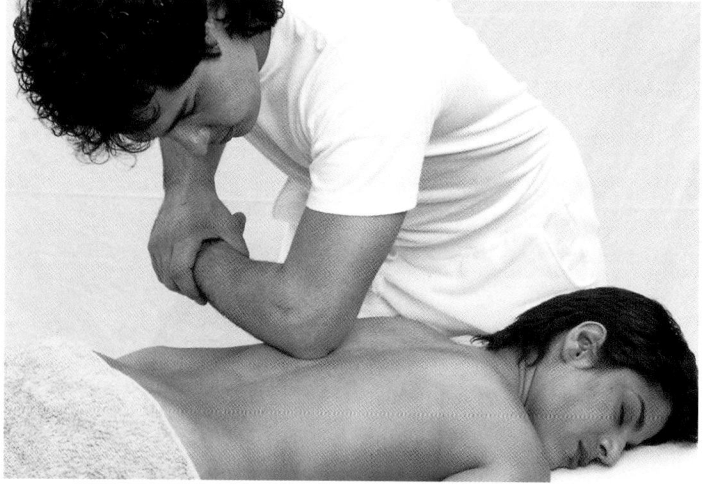

◁ A deep tissue massage may involve applying pressure from the elbow or forearm to sink into the connective tissue before stretching and manipulating it.

▷ **Self-massage can give you a physical and a psychological boost. It is also invaluable for gaining confidence to treat others by practising massage techniques on your own body.**

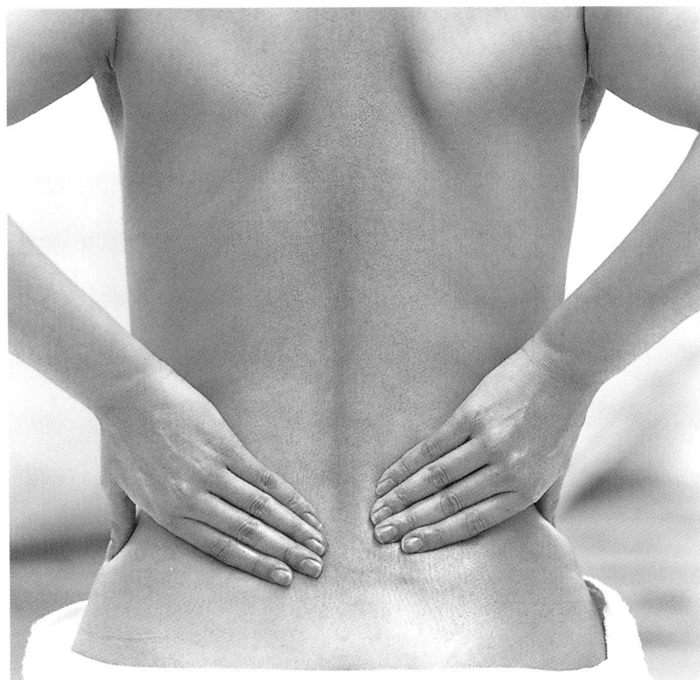

knowledge of anatomy and physiology. While the strokes penetrate the body at a deeper level than in soft tissue massage, the practitioner's hands must work with great sensitivity and patience, and the client must be willing to release tension. Causing undue pain in the attempt to free the body from tension is counter-productive, as the neuro-muscular response of the tissues will be to contract in defence.

Deep tissue massage is usually based over a series of at least 10 sessions, so that the whole structure of the body can be balanced and realigned. In the process of breaking down chronic tensions, breathing becomes deeper and the body regains its vitality and feeling. Emotions and memories that have been repressed within the body by the muscular armour may be released. It is important, therefore, for a deep tissue bodyworker to be aware of the psychosomatic link between the emotions and physical tension, and to understand that behind the most defended areas of the body there is a great deal of vulnerability.

A deep tissue practitioner may use the thumbs, fingers, knuckles, and forearms to stretch and manipulate the fascia. Pressure is applied slowly, and in conjunction with the client's awareness and breathing. The tissue is then stretched and moved in specific directions, depending on its location in the body. By ungluing and freeing the fibres, the tissue becomes warm and revitalized, and returns to its natural fluidity. When the whole body is treated systematically in a series of sessions it is able to regain its vitality, structural alignment, and ease of movement.

▽ **Rolfing can appear to be quite rough, as the connective tissue is manipulated using deep tissue massage techniques.**

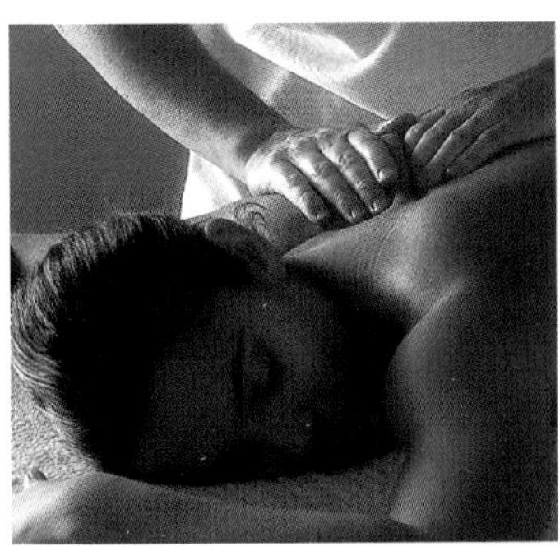

There are a number of schools of deep tissue bodywork. The most established of these is rolfing, also known as structural integration, which was founded in the United States by Ida Rolf. Rolf pioneered many new techniques in her work with connective tissue, and it is her profound understanding of its role in the body's structural balance that has laid the foundations for the ensuing development of connective tissue massage.

head massage

For centuries, head massage has played an essential part in Ayurvedic medicine, widely practised throughout India and some parts of Asia. In India it is still a regular aspect of daily life, and head massage is frequently practised on street corners. However, this ancient art is also highly practical and relevant to the Western world.

Head massage combines energy-based pressure-point techniques with more traditional massage strokes such as rubbing and stroking, thus working on the body's energy system as well as its physical structure. In addition to focusing on the head, it also targets the upper back, shoulders, and neck area – significant places in the body where we store tension.

▽ **Head massage is particularly helpful for relieving tension commonly found in the upper back, shoulders and neck areas.**

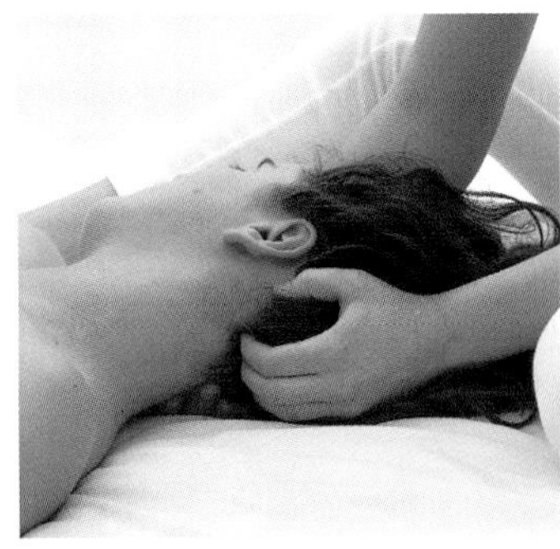

foot massage

Like head massage, foot massage has become increasingly popular in recent years because it is simple, fast and effective, as it focuses on a relatively small area of the body.

The feet are highly sensitive and very responsive to touch: they contain more than 14,000 nerve endings between them. Foot massage uses a combination of the energy-based pressure-point techniques of acupressure and reflexology and more traditional massage strokes aimed at relaxing and soothing as well as improving circulation. A foot massage can be carried out as a quick-fix soother, using an appropriate aromatherapy blend, after a busy day's shopping. Combined with the principles of reflexology it can also be used to treat a range of problems and disorders.

reflexology

A reflexologist believes that energy is channelled through the body along specific paths, or meridians. When a person is healthy, energy moves freely along these channels. However, if the energy is impeded or blocked through tension, congestion, imbalance, or sluggishness within the system, then all those organs and internal structures that lie in the energy path have the potential to succumb to disease.

▽ **A qualified reflexologist will be able to detect or locate a disorder in a corresponding body part because of tenderness or the accumulation of granular deposits at certain points of the foot.**

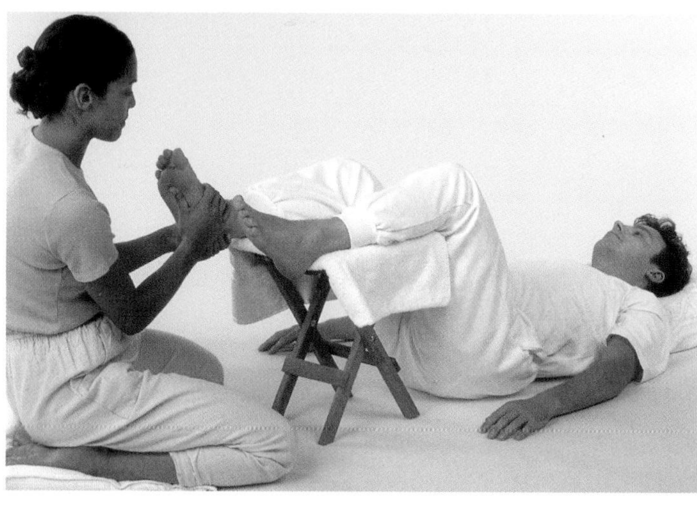

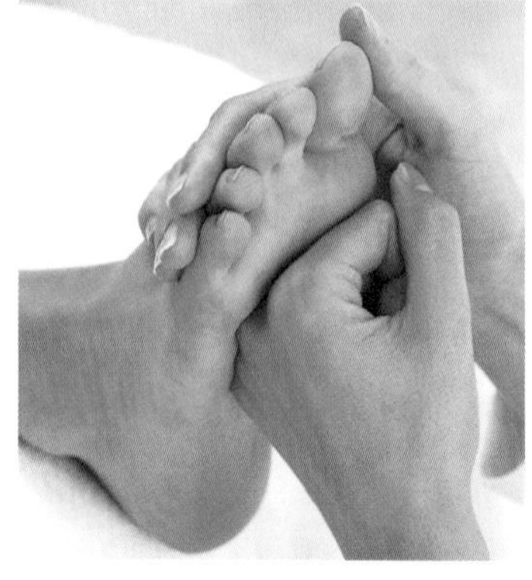

△ **Foot massage is easy to learn and quick to apply. A soft-tissue massage using a relaxing oil blend and soothing, flowing strokes can be highly therapeutic.**

Reflexologists maintain that an individual's health can be restored when pressure is applied to certain points on the body, generally the feet and sometimes the hands. This helps to unblock the energy channel, thereby having a revitalizing effect on all the organs, glands, and other structures that lie within its zone.

Reflexologists divide the body into 10 vertical zones, 5 on each side of the medial line that runs from the top of the head to the tips of the fingers and toes. Although the pressure-point therapy can be applied on the hands, the treatment is usually more effective when used on the feet.

The technique involves applying pressure to the reflex points on the sole or palm, sides, and top of each foot or hand in turn, for up to three seconds – using the top or side of the thumb or finger to apply pressure – before walking, or inching, the digit to its next position. The foot or hand must be securely held and supported, and leverage applied by the fingers or thumb opposing the movement.

While no scientific explanation, as yet, can be given to explain exactly how reflexology works, it is widely accepted as a successful treatment for a number of ailments. When applied skilfully the techniques can help to relax and invigorate the entire physiology of the body, stimulating the nervous system and the blood circulation, and boosting the elimination of toxins, in addition to clearing congestion within the organs. Reflexology is now firmly established as a complementary healing art.

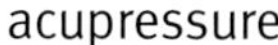

acupressure

An ancient Chinese therapy, acupressure is based on very similar principles to acupuncture. In common with acupuncture and reflexology, it is based on the belief that the body's energy flows through channels called meridians.

Acupressure uses the same points as acupuncture, but instead of using needles, it uses the fingers to apply gentle but firm pressure on the key points. This pressure stimulates the flow of energy and helps to release blockages, thus alleviating many common complaints and disorders and restoring harmony and balance to the body, mind and spirit.

▽ The bladder meridian is the largest in the body and runs down each side fo the spine to the back of the pelvis. In acupressure, a steady thumb pressure applied on the sacral points can relieve sciatica and lower-back pain.

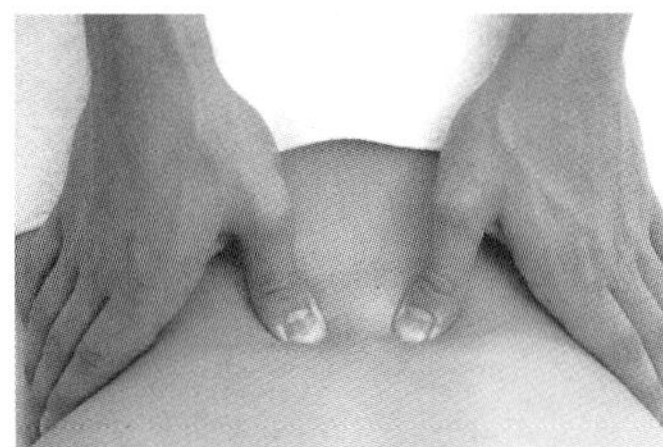

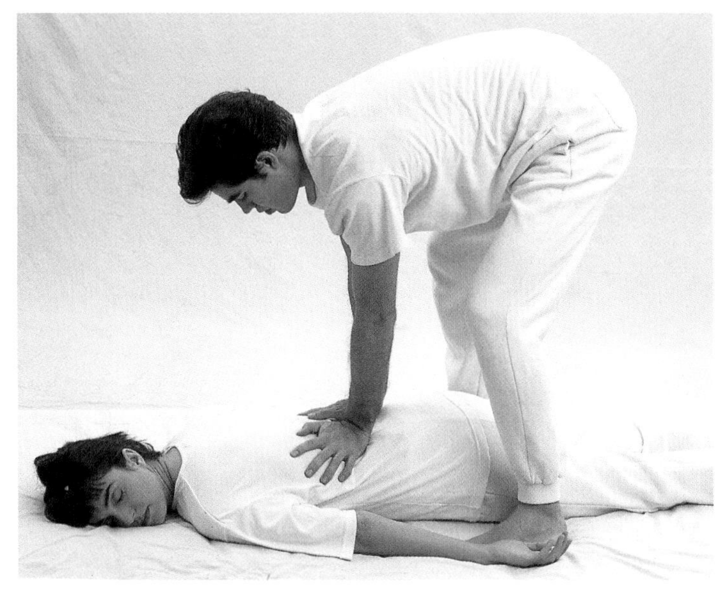

▷ The shiatsu therapist also uses the palms and heels of the hands to press firmly but gently. Here the focus is on the bladder meridian points.

shiatsu

A relatively modern Japanese body therapy, shiatsu derives its principles from the ancient wisdom of Chinese medicine. It operates on the belief that health is restored when a balance is reached between the energetic forces of yin and yang within the body, mind, and spirit. Yin is feminine and passive, yang is masculine and active. Shiatsu helps to bring a harmony between the yin and yang energies of the body and its internal organs. In shiatsu there are 14 energy meridians, and pressure is applied to key points along those pathways where the energy, or *ki* (*chi*), is blocked or over-stimulated. The word "shiatsu" translates literally as "finger pressure", although the practitioner can use the hands, elbows, knees, and feet to apply pressure on specific meridian points to stimulate or massage them. Shiatsu can also incorporate the passive movements of Western osteopathy to stretch and manipulate the joints and ease tension from the major segments of the body, thereby helping to clear congestion in the energy pathways. The aim of shiatsu is to restore a balance in the flow of *ki* as it interconnects the vital organs.

Shiatsu works on our *ki* or life force, which maintains and nurtures our physical body and so also affects our mind and spirit. The flow of *ki* can be disturbed by external trauma such as injury or internal trauma such as anxiety or stress.

The shiatsu practitioner assesses the client's health through observation, or by taking a case history. Steady weight is then applied to the key points of the relevant meridian for up to 10 seconds before slowly releasing the pressure. A whole body session can be given as a maintenance treatment or to detect an imbalance between the organs.

Ancient and modern techniques drawn from traditions of the East and the West can be combined to provide truly holistic massage therapy for body, mind and spirit.

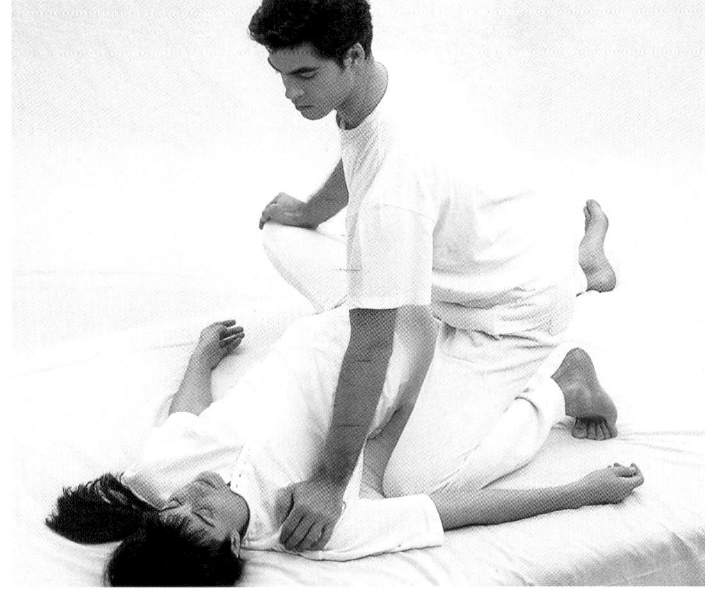

▷ Passive stretch movements increase the effects of shiatsu treatment by relaxing joints and unblocking congested energy meridians.

Body awareness and visualization

Massage is an ongoing process of learning about the human body in all its holistic aspects, and the best place to explore the relationship between mind, body and spirit is within your own body.

If you are giving massage on a regular basis it is important that your body is strong and flexible. Exercise regularly to relax and strengthen your muscles and, in particular, to provide support for your spine and back. Visualizations will help you contact your energy resources and cleanse and relax your body, mind, and spirit.

exercises for strength, flexibility and energy

The following exercises will help you to learn how to breathe deeply and synchronize your breathing with your movements, so that your strokes become fluid and you remain energized. The more you learn about your own body, the better able you will be to pass on that knowledge through your massage to help others.

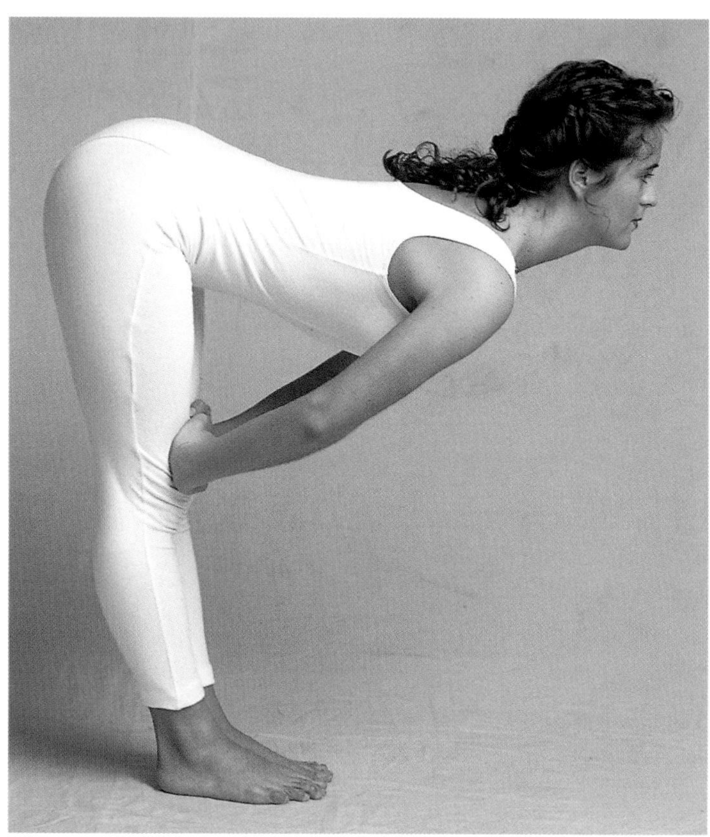

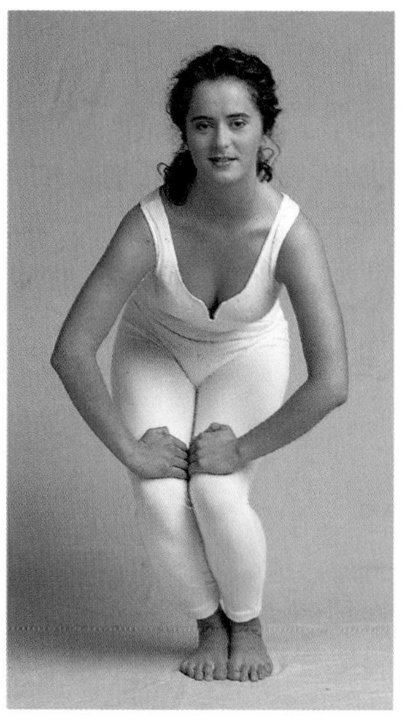

creating a stable foundation

Your legs help you to maintain a balanced and stable posture as you massage. They provide a firm but flexible foundation to support your body weight and to connect you to the ground, so that you can release tension away from your spine and back as you work. This exercise helps you gently to warm and loosen the ankle and knee joints, areas that are vital to structural support.

◁ **1** Rest your hands on your knees without straining your shoulders. Place your feet together and, bending your knees, rotate them in circles, first in one direction and then in the other. Begin with small circular movements and gradually make larger ones as your joints and muscles warm up.

△ **2** Straighten the knees slowly and gently press your abdomen down in the direction of the floor to create a stretch in the hamstrings at the back of your legs. Alternate this step with the knee circles carried out in step 1, repeating them two more times.

warming up

You will probably not have time to do all these exercises before every massage session, but it is a good idea to combine at least one or two of the sequences as a warm-up and to focus your mind.

breath and movement

The next exercise is a series of continuous flowing movements adapted from the t'ai chi form, a Chinese martial art. It helps to create stability and strength in the legs, while making pushing movements with the arms and hands. The complete motion is made in conjunction with your cycle of inhaling and exhaling. This makes the exercise particularly appropriate when learning how to apply long effleurage strokes with a graceful posture and synchronized breathing.

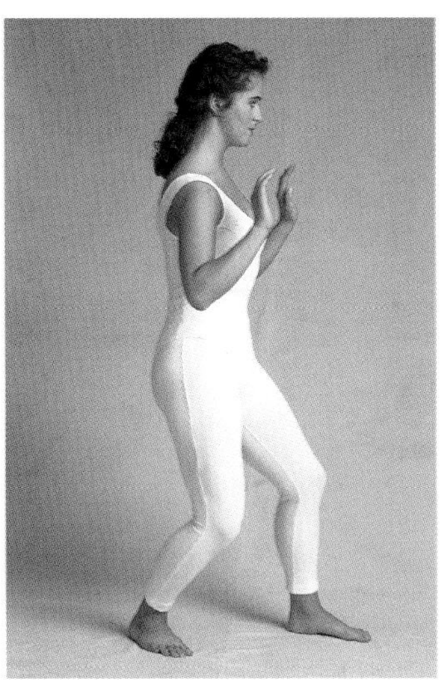

△ **1** Begin with the basic stance of good posture, keeping both feet parallel and the knees slightly flexed. Step forwards with the front foot and turn the back foot out at an angle of 45 degrees. As you breathe in, bend your elbows and draw both hands to chest level, palms facing outwards.

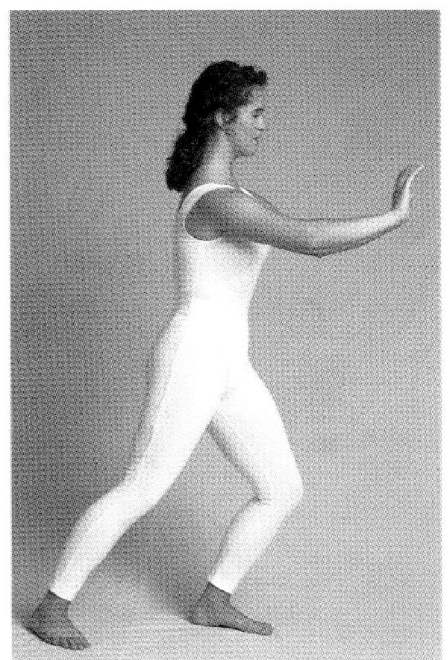

△ **2** Keeping both feet flat on the floor and the spine erect, transfer your weight to the front foot and push your hands away from your body while you exhale. Your torso should be facing in the direction of your front foot.

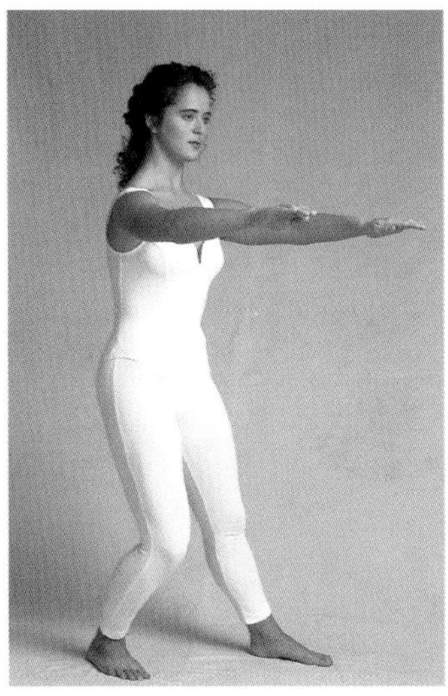

△ **3** As you inhale, move your weight to the back foot, allowing your body and arms to swing around to face the same direction. Draw your hands back to chest level. Continue breathing in as you turn towards the front foot to repeat the full movement again. Repeat 10 times before changing the position of your legs and repeating the full flowing cycle from the other side.

swinging the torso

Limbering up the spine and torso prevents strain and tension from gathering in the back while giving massage. It keeps the body supple, enabling it to turn easily while performing some of the longer strokes. The key to the following exercise is to transfer weight from one foot to the other as you swing around, leaving the other foot feeling "empty" and weightless. Flex both knees so your height never changes during the exercise, and your head rests comfortably on top of your spine. This gentle spinal twist will relax your muscles and nerves and stimulate your breathing.

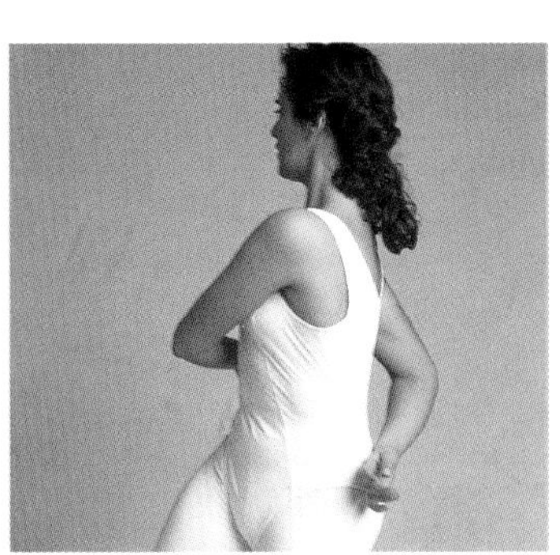

▷ **1** Begin the exercise with your feet parallel, and more than the width of your hips apart. Transfer your weight on to one foot, leaving the other weightless. Swing your torso and arms around to face the "empty" foot, letting your arms flop against the sides of your body.

◁ **2** Swing your torso back to the other side as you transfer your weight across to the other foot. As you turn, relax the gaze of your eyes so they take in a moving picture of your surroundings without fixing on any point.

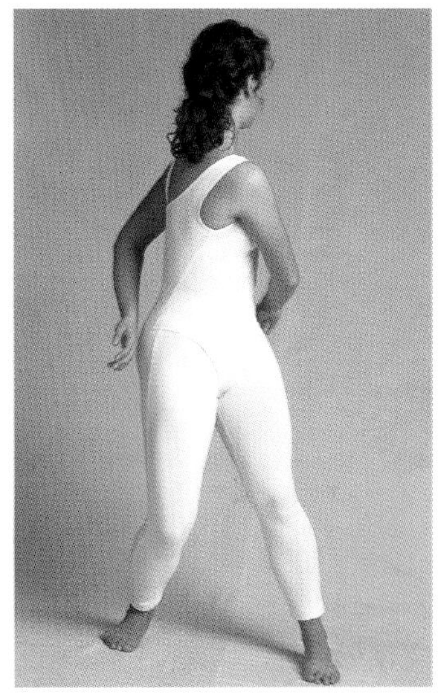

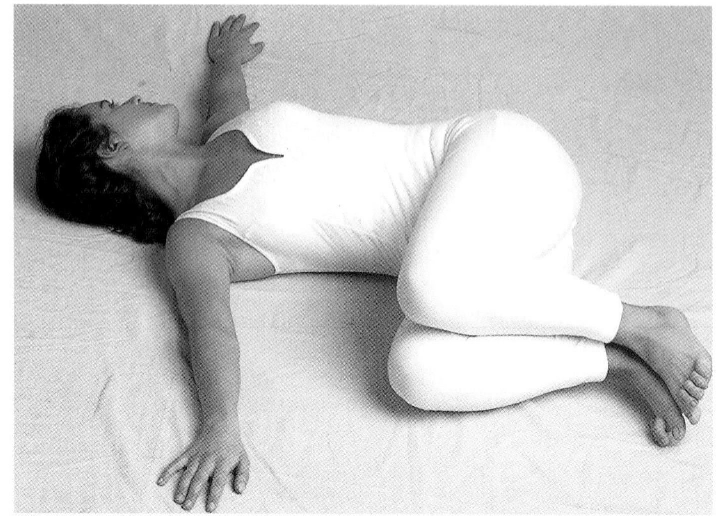

strengthening abdominal muscles

The abdominal muscles flex and support the spine, and it is important to strengthen them in order to safeguard your back while giving massage. A firm but relaxed abdomen will allow tension to sink away from the upper back and shoulders, while stabilizing the lumbar region. The belly is also the source of power and vital energy. These exercises will bring it strength and relaxation, helping you to gain stamina. Perform them slowly and carefully to avoid strain, and gradually build up to 10 complete movements for each exercise.

▷ **1** Lie on your back with your knees bent towards your chest and your feet flexed. Begin to make circles in one direction with your knees, making certain you keep them together. Gradually enlarge the circles, keeping the middle and base of your back in contact with the floor at all times, as this will activate the abdominal muscles. Remain lying down on your back and spread your arms to the sides of your body, palms facing downwards. Bend your knees towards your chest and flex your feet. Breathe in.

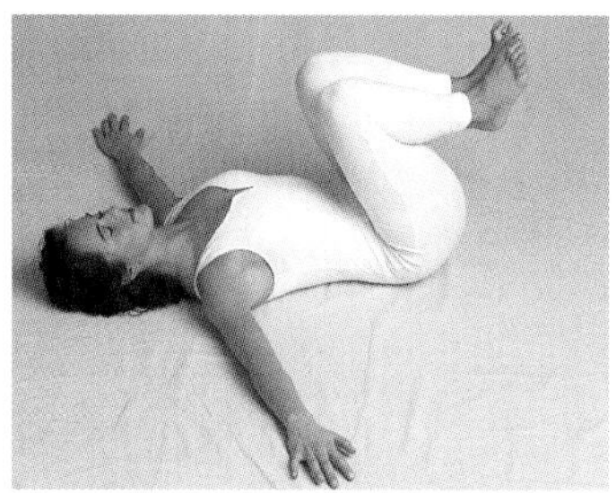

△ **2** Breathe out as you take your knees to one side of the body as far as they will comfortably go, keeping them close together. At the same time, roll your head in the opposite direction. As you inhale, return both head and knees to their original position. Repeat the exercise, moving your head and knees to the other side of the body.

visualizations for healing energy

Visualization is a powerful tool frequently used in healing work. It allows an intuitive use of the imagination to bring about subtle and beneficial changes in the body and mind. Within massage and body awareness work, imagery combined with "good intention" can be used in relaxation exercises as a means of directing the movement of energy within the body, or to "see" and heal its internal structure and physiology.

tuning in to light and energy

When massage is performed with a relaxed posture and breathing, the experience can be equally as nourishing and invigorating for both people involved. If you believe, however, that you are using up all of your own energy while giving a massage, then the experience can sometimes leave you feeling tired or drained. This visualization exercise helps you to replenish your vital resources by opening you up to the idea of a constant stream of energy, or light, that passes through you to your partner. You can practise this during the massage, with or without a partner; it is an excellent way to start or finish a session.

▷ Stand with your feet apart and with your arms slightly out in front of your body, palms facing downwards. As you breathe in, imagine a white light descending through the crown of your head and filling your body with vital energy. Breathe out and visualize the light flowing out of your arms and through your hands to the person beneath them, or towards the ground. As you continue to inhale and exhale, repeat this visualization several times.

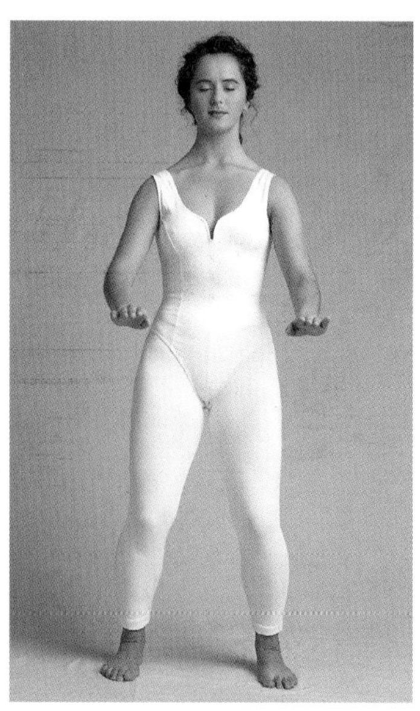

bone breathing

During massage, your hands are mainly in touch with the body's skin, soft tissues, and superficial muscles. However, it is also beneficial to gain a sense of the skeletal structure, which is vital to the body's support and locomotion. Try this exercise to provide a mental image of the bones, and to encourage a sense of relaxation into the core of the physical body.

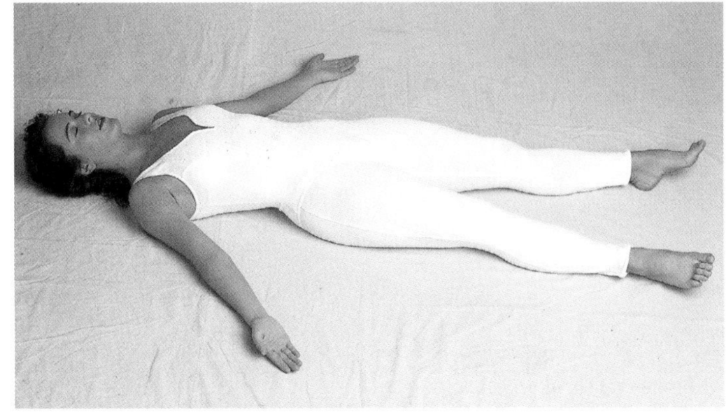

△ Lie on your back. As your breathing deepens, focus your attention on your right leg and consciously relax the muscles from the foot up to the hip. Then try to visualize the bones as they link together from the toes, through to the ankle and knee joint and up to the hip socket. Now imagine that the bones are hollow, so that as you breathe in, a white light is drawn in through the toes and is pulled up through the bones to the top of the leg. As you breathe out, the light returns via the same pathway and out of the body.

Repeat this visualization several times with the right leg before repeating the exercise with the left leg. Finally, breathe in deeply and draw the white light up the right leg and into the belly. Hold your breath for a few moments and breathe out, before sending the light down through the left leg. Reverse the imagery so that you draw the light from the left to the right side of the body. The same visualization can now be applied to the arms and chest.

opening the heart centre

Just as it is essential to connect through breath and awareness to your abdomen during massage – in order to work from your source of power and vital energy – it is also important to allow your heart and feeling centre to open and expand. This allows the essence of life to flow to your hands, enlivening them with a nourishing and healing quality of touch. In this visualization, you imagine that your heart is like the bud of a flower. As you focus your breath towards your heart, allow the flower to open its petals until it fills the whole of your chest.

◁ To help you connect with the heart centre, sit and close your eyes while breathing, holding your hands just in front of your heart.

Aromatherapy and massage

When essential oils are used for aromatherapy massage, different oils are combined to increase their therapeutic effect. As you become more practised in the art of blending you will begin to develop a nose for compatibility, in much the same way as a perfumer blends scents, and you will be able to judge the best blend for your requirement by its aroma. Once you have mixed your oils, store and use them immediately, as they are perishable.

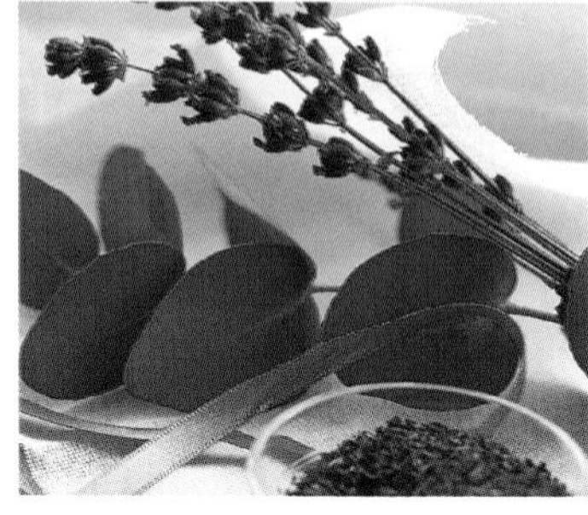

◁ Lavender is one of the most useful essential oils, and it combines well with peppermint and eucalyptus for a relaxing, yet stimulating, blend.

useful conversion guide

1ml	=	20 drops of essential oil
5ml	=	1 teaspoon
30ml	=	2 tablespoons
600ml	=	1 pint

blending essential oils

Blending oils for massage enables you to alleviate various physical and emotional symptoms in a single treatment, and while the combination of therapeutic properties is of prime importance, the value of fragrance should also be taken into account – nobody enjoys taking unpleasant medicine, so don't underestimate the beneficial effects of a pleasing and sweet-smelling odour when mixing your oils.

The ratio of essential oil to carrier oil may vary, but as a general rule, 5 drops of essential oil in 10ml (2 tsp) carrier oil is enough for a body massage. This gives a standard 2.5 per cent dilution, the recommended dilution for most purposes. However, if you are using oils for purely emotional problems, half the number of drops can be equally effective, while physical symptoms often respond better to a slightly higher percentage of essential oil. If your massage partner has a lot of body hair you will need to use more carrier oil, but keep the amount of essential oil the same. If you are using bottles or jars bought from the chemist they will usually have their capacity marked on them. To work out how many drops of essential oil you will need in a container, simply divide its capacity by two. For example, if you have a 30ml (1fl oz) bottle of carrier oil you will need to add 15 drops of essential oil, or for a 50g (2oz) jar, 25 drops of oil.

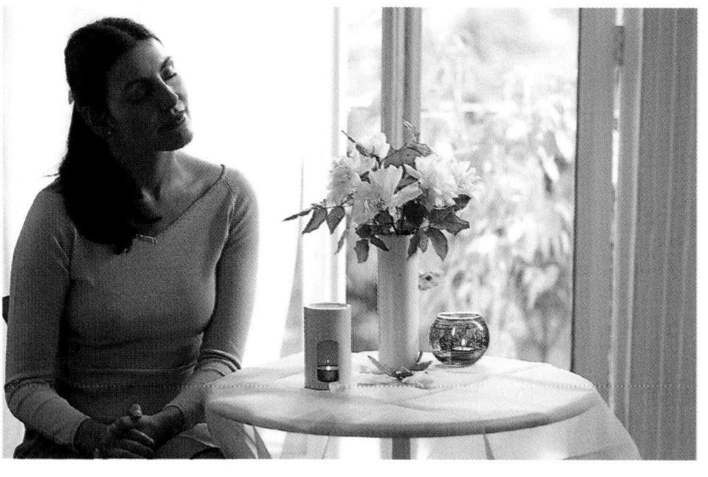

synergy

When essential oils are blended, a chemical reaction occurs and the oils combine as a new compound. For example, when lavender is added to bergamot the sedative qualities of bergamot are increased; but if lemon is added to bergamot, then its uplifting, refreshing aspect is enhanced. This process is known as synergy. Using this principle, oils can be blended so that they treat a person's emotional and physical needs at the same time. The blend can also be modified from treatment to treatment, depending on the time of day or the person's mood (for example, changing the balance of the blend, or substituting a different oil to the basic blend, can raise someone's spirits if they are low).

top, middle, and base notes

Essential oils are categorized by what are known as top, middle, and base "notes", which is how perfumers categorize scents, using different combinations of notes to create a new perfume. A good blend combines an oil from each category, and each oil is classified according to its dominant characteristic. It is not always

◁ You will develop a nose for top, middle and base scents, but generally fresh, herbaceous oils such as lemon, eucalyptus, or tea tree are good top notes. Floral oils and some herb oils make up the majority of the middle notes, while woody, resinous oils are base notes.

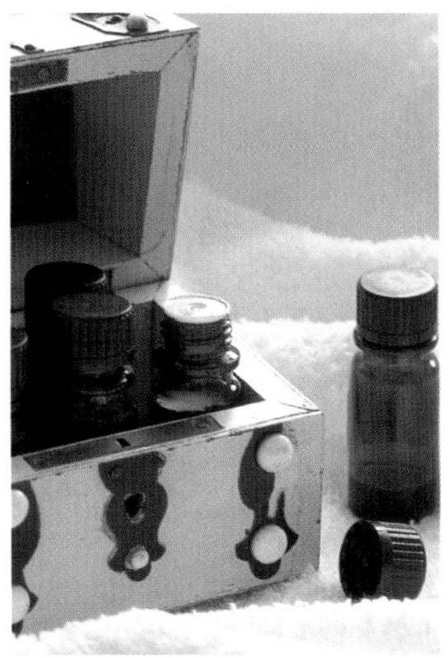

◁ Essential oils should be stored away from direct light and heat. Specially made boxes are ideal and must be kept out of reach of children.

▷ A soothing blend of essential oils and an appropriate carrier oil can make all the difference to a massage to relieve a headache.

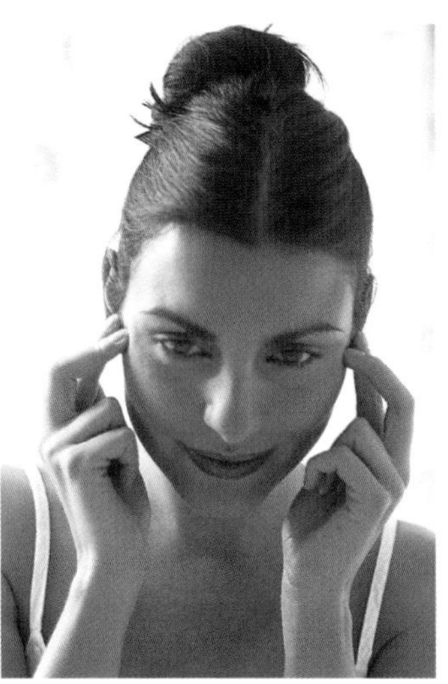

simple to classify oils by note. For example, rose and jasmine are heady fragrances, and are floral oils but are usually considered to be base notes. Because they evaporate quickly, most blends should contain a higher number of top-note oil drops to middle-note and base-note oil drops. For example, a well-balanced blend would be made up from three drops of orange (top note), two drops each of clary sage and geranium (both middle notes), and two drops of cedarwood (base note).

buying and storing essential oils

Make sure the oils you buy are pure, undiluted essential oils. In general, price is an excellent guide, and it is wise to compare various suppliers' prices so that you can recognize an expensive oil and a very cheap one. Be aware that essential oils are easily adulterated, and that there is no such thing as cheap rose oil, for example; cheap rose oil is probably a similar-smelling product to which geranium or palmarosa oil has been added. If you buy from a reputable source you will also avoid buying oils from a second or third distillation. These contain only a few active ingredients as the majority are removed during the first processing.

It is useful to know the Latin, or scientific name of each oil because most reputable suppliers put this name on the label of the bottle. If you are in any doubt about where to buy oils, seek the advice of a qualified practitioner, who will recommend a reputable retail supplier.

Essential oils last for a relatively long time if a few simple precautions are taken. They should be bought and then stored in dark-coloured glass bottles with a stopper that dispenses them a drop at a time. Keep the lid firmly closed to prevent evaporation, and store them in a cool place out of direct sunlight. Citrus oils tend to go off more quickly than other oils, so it is a good idea to buy them in small quantities as you need them. It is easy to tell if an oil has deteriorated because it will become cloudy and give off a distinctly unpleasant odour.

carrier oils

Massage is a wonderful way to use essential oils, suitably diluted and blended with an appropriate carrier oil. Suitable carrier oils for massage include sweet almond oil (probably the most versatile and useful), grapeseed, safflower, soy (a bit thicker and stickier), coconut and even sunflower. For very dry skin, a small amount of jojoba, avocado or wheatgerm (except in cases of wheat allergy) may be added.

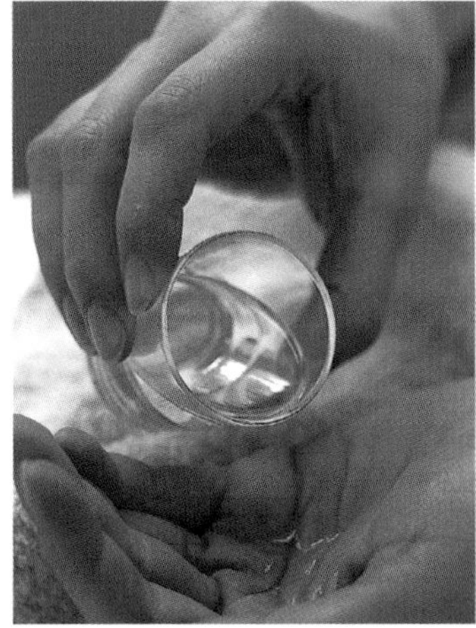

▷ Vegetable carrier oils are ideal for massage. Essential oils readily dissolve in the carrier oil, and the blend allows the hands to move over the skin without dragging or slipping.

cautions

- Never take essential oils internally, unless professionally prescribed.
- Always use essential oils diluted.
- Do not use the same essential oils for more than one or two weeks at any one time.
- In pregnancy, some oils can be dangerous. Do not use without professional advice.
- For problem or sensitive skin, dilute the oils further, and if any irritation occurs, stop using them.
- Some oils, such as bergamot, make the skin more sensitive to sunlight, so use with caution in sunny weather.
- Anyone with a specific complaint such as epilepsy or asthma must be treated with extra care. If in any doubt, seek professional advice.

More information on essential and carrier oils is provided in the appendix at the end of the book.

Cautions and contraindications

Although the massages in this book are well-established, safe techniques for working on the body, as with any therapy, it is important to be aware that there are certain situations where you should be particularly careful or where a treatment may be contraindicated. If you are in any doubt, always ask a doctor or professional therapist for advice before giving any treatment.

At the beginning of the session make sure you have time to ask your partner how they are feeling, and find out if they have any medical conditions and/or are taking any medication. You should also check for any recent injuries, fractures or surgery. If your partner is feeling unwell, it is best to postpone the treatment, as it could aggravate their condition. This might include anything from a cold or a temperature to a serious skin condition or an acute infectious disease.

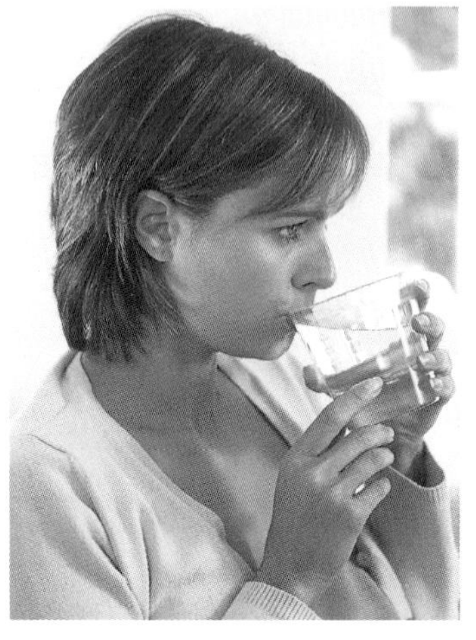

△ **Drinking a glass of water is a good way to begin and end a massage treatment, as it is cleansing and grounding for the system and will aid the elimination of toxins from the body.**

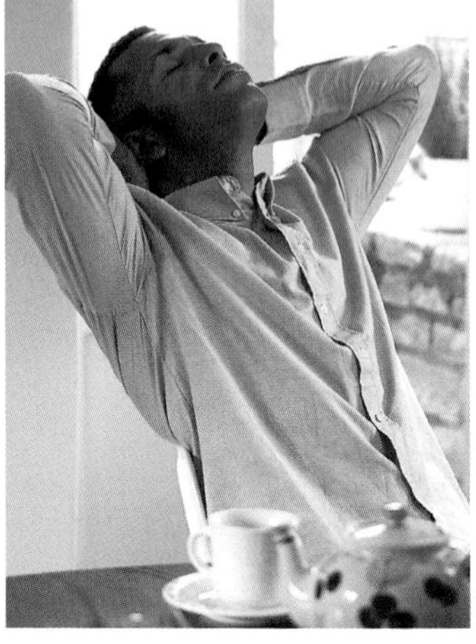

△ **If your partner is particularly tense, and their muscles are sore and tender, always make sure you massage with caution in order not to aggravate their discomfort.**

▽ **Make sure you take enough time to talk through the massage with your partner to establish a rapport and sort out any concerns he or she may have about the treatment.**

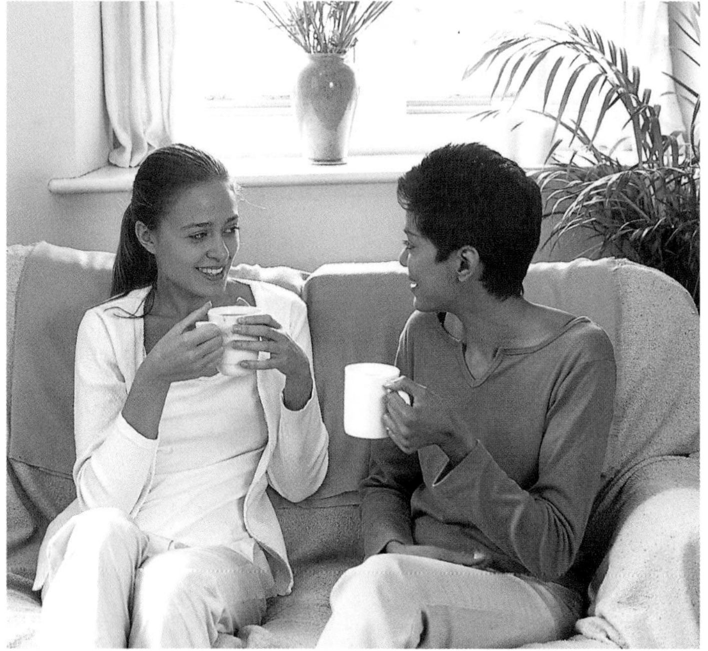

skin conditions

Be aware of any cuts, bruises, open sores, blistering, redness or swelling. These areas will be painful when touched and could become infected, so are best avoided. Any contagious skin conditions, such as ringworm, impetigo, scabies or herpes (cold sores), should also be avoided to prevent the risk of you picking up the infection.

Large areas of bruising on the skin may indicate internal injuries, so massage could be extremely dangerous.

Ringworm is a fungal infection. It begins as small red papules that spread to form red, itchy, shiny circles under the skin over the body. Impetigo is a highly contagious bacterial skin condition, usually found around the mouth, nose and ears, in which raised, fluid-filled sores seep and leave honey coloured crusts on the skin. Scabies is

▷ **For babies, gentle body and foot massage can be soothing and nurturing. However, as babies' skulls are so delicate, due to the unfused fontanelles, massaging the head is not advisable.**

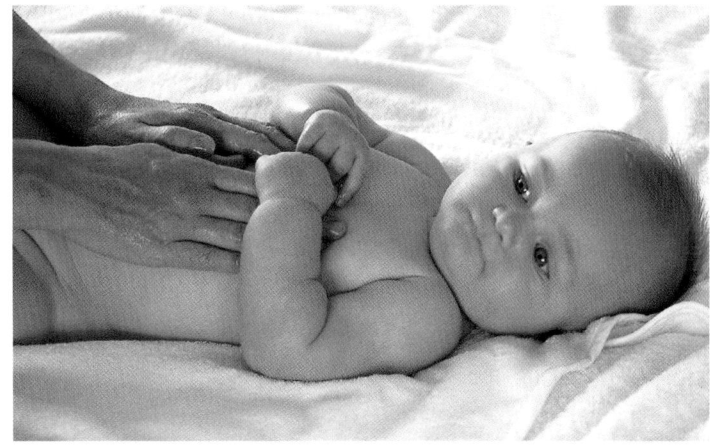

identified by small reddish marks around the wrist and between the fingers, and is very itchy. Herpes is a viral infection that erupts in sores around the mouth and nose, particularly after exposure to the sun or during times of stress.

Eczema and psoriasis may look unsightly, but they are not contagious, and unless the skin is broken, they are not contraindicated for massage. However, it is best to check with your partner that they find it comfortable to be touched in these areas.

Scalp conditions to be aware of include head lice (nits), ringworm and folliculitis. The latter is a bacterial infection with swelling and pain around the hair follicles.

the skeleton

Conditions relating to the bones and the skeleton, which include brittle bones, osteoporosis and spondylitis, are clearly contraindicated for massage because of the high risk of injury to your partner. Bone diseases, congenital problems and habitual poor posture can cause spinal weakness. In such cases it is advisable to massage only after you have sought medical advice.

You should also be aware of any head, neck or shoulder injuries, such as whiplash. Massage could make these conditions worse, so check with a doctor.

circulatory problems

With high blood pressure there could be a risk of clotting, so always seek medical advice. When this is related to high stress levels, massage can be effective in reducing stress triggers, but do seek medical advice first. Low blood pressure increases the likelihood of feeling faint so make sure your partner gets up slowly after the massage. Recent haemorrhages, a history of thrombosis and embolisms are other blood disorders that can cause problems. Anyone with any of these conditions should not be massaged in the absence of medical supervision. Although massage can be helpful in boosting circulation, varicose veins should be treated with great care and no pressure should be applied to affected areas.

epilepsy

This condition requires medical advice before carrying out any treatment. Epilepsy is normally controlled and stabilized by medication, but it is thought that stimulating massage, particularly to the head, can trigger an attack.

cancer

Massage is contraindicated with cancer, but it is increasingly recognized as having a supportive role in palliative care. Always seek medical advice first. It is not advisable to massage immediately after chemotherapy or radiation treatment.

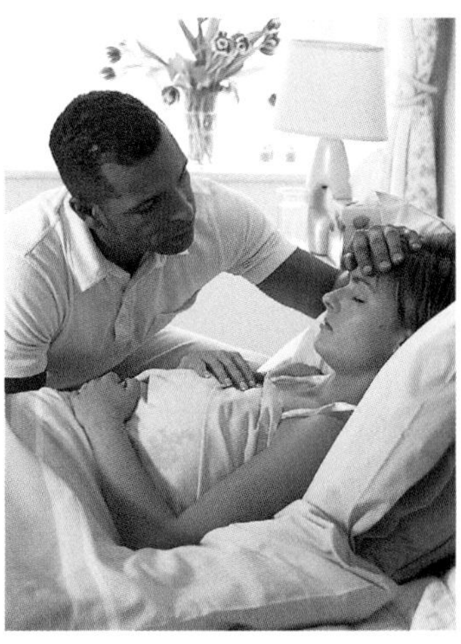

pregnancy

Massage can be helpful during pregnancy but remember that you are treating two people, not one, so be particularly sensitive. Avoid the abdomen, and use a lighter pressure than normal, and this is particularly crucial during the first trimester.

Head massage is an ideal treatment during pregnancy, as it is possible to remain sitting rather than lying down, which can be awkward and uncomfortable.

children and the elderly

The rule of working lightly also applies to children, the frail and the elderly. Adjust your pressure to the energy of the person you are massaging. Even when treating robust-looking older children, it is advisable to work lightly until you are both familiar with massage. If it is done too strongly it can stimulate a rise of energy that is too much for your partner's young body and could cause them to faint.

emotional response

People can have emotional reactions to massage such as feeling tearful or upset. This is because the effect of massage can be to release pent up feelings. In these situations, be sensitive in your response and check if your partner would like you to continue or to pause for a while before carrying on with the massage.

◁ **During illness it is not advisable to massage deeply, although a tender loving touch can be comforting and healing – to give and to receive.**

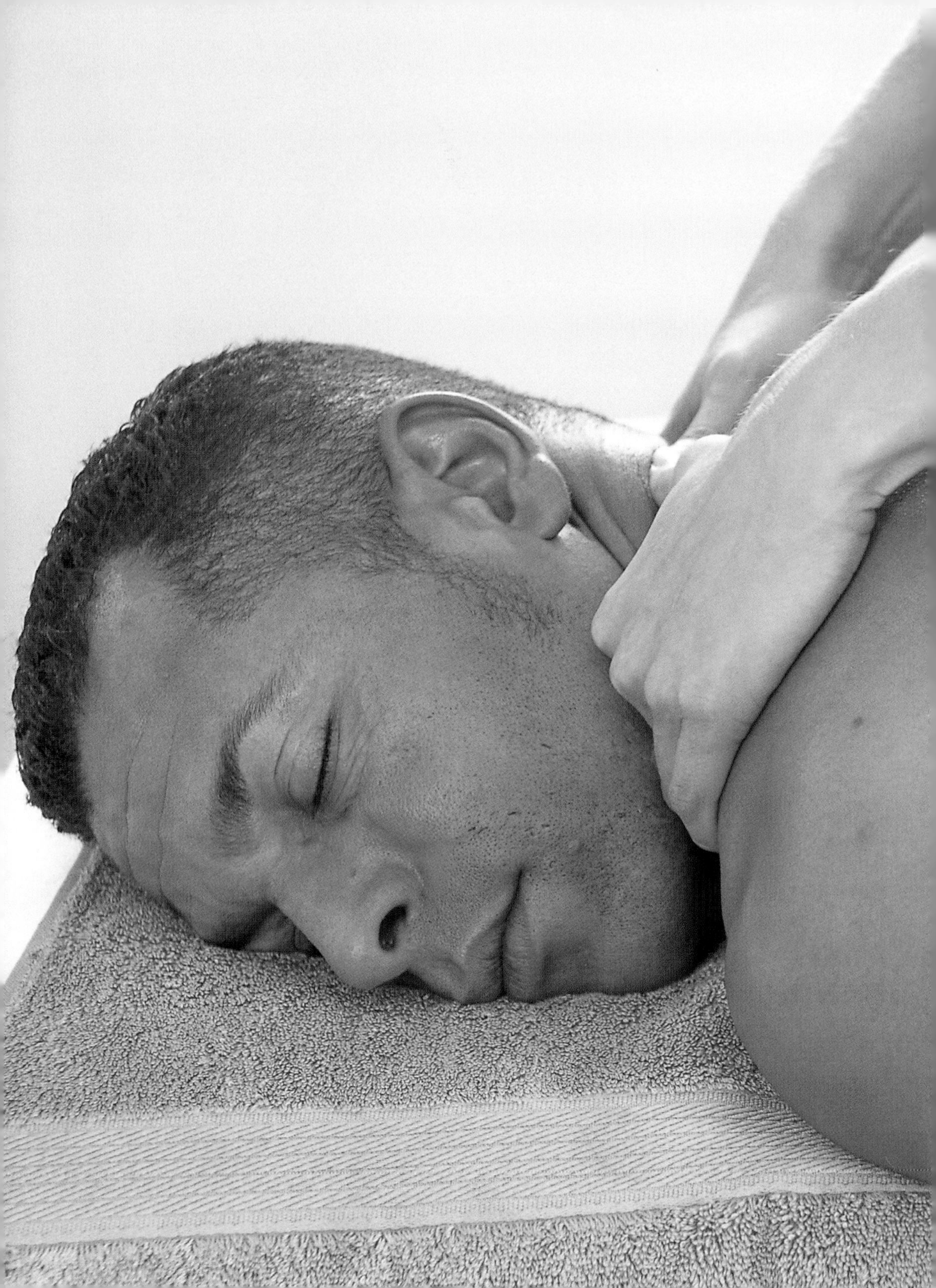

Part Two
Head Massage

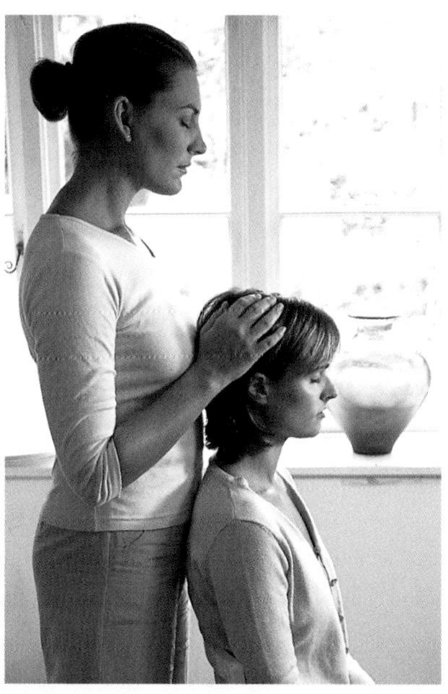

Introduction

Unlike many other healing traditions, Indian head massage is as widely practised today as it was thousands of years ago. It has its roots in Ayurveda, one of the oldest healthcare systems in the world. Dating back more than 4000 years, Ayurveda is grounded in the philosophical and spiritual traditions of India. It offers comprehensive and practical guidelines for how to achieve health and wellbeing, and covers many different aspects of daily life.

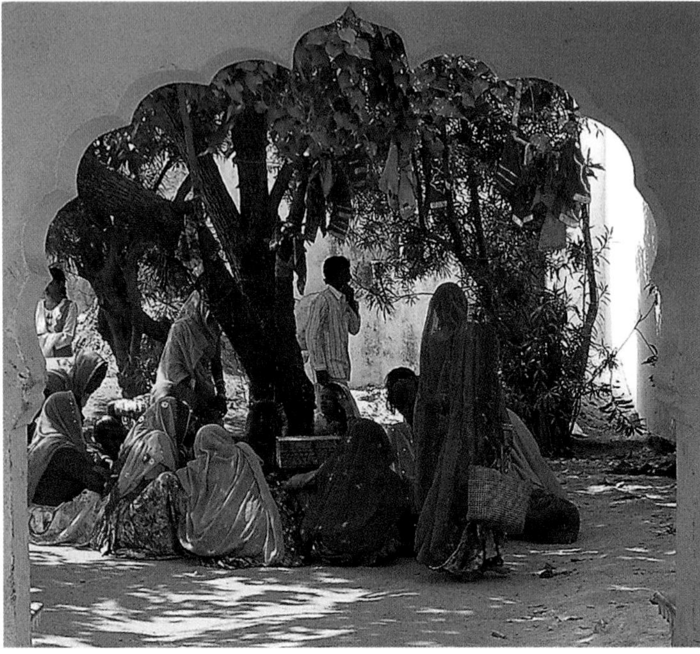

the science of longevity

Ayurveda is known as the "science of longevity". It is based upon the holistic principle that illness or disease is created when we are out of balance. It describes three energy forces (known as the *doshas*), namely *vata*, *pitta* and *kapha*, each having its own characteristics and purpose. All physical, emotional and mental functions are controlled by the *doshas*. When they are balanced and working in harmony, we feel vibrant and enjoy good health.

▽ **Indian women have been admired throughout history for their long, lustrous, thick black hair that is traditionally nourished, maintained and groomed with oils and by head massage.**

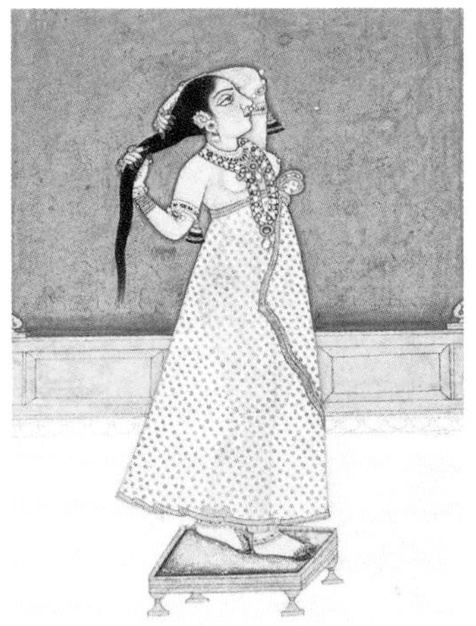

The Ayurvedic healthcare regime is comprehensive. It covers diet and exercise, yoga and meditation, detox and herbal remedies, as well as regular massage treatments using essential oils. A weekly head massage is highly recommended as a way of restoring and maintaining balance in the body's systems. Specific oils and herbs are used with head massage to help to stabilize the *doshas*. For instance, a *vata*-type imbalance may manifest as dry skin and hair, in which case sesame oil, with its strengthening and nourishing properties, would be recommended.

touch culture

The healing power of touch to restore and maintain wellbeing is deeply embedded in the culture of India, and head massage has to been seen within this context. Massage plays an important part in many major life events, such as marriage and pregnancy, or

△ **An Indian wedding is about to begin. The ritual of preparing the bride and groom for the ceremony will have included head massage.**

in looking after babies and children. It is customary to give massage to both the bride and groom before they get married. This involves ritual and the use of specially blended herbs and oils designed to strengthen, beautify and bless the couple in preparation for marriage.

The practice of baby massage is also widespread. Even at the poorest level of society, where people live on the streets, and deprivation and hunger are rife, mothers can be seen oiling and massaging their babies every day, regardless of the traffic, dogs, pedestrians and street sellers all around them. In India, massage is not seen as a luxury, but as one of life's essentials. Daily massage continues until the child is about three years old, when it is reduced to twice a week. From the age of six, children then take part in a weekly massage ritual with other members of the family, even learning to exchange massage with one another.

male and female traditions

Historically the practice of Indian head massage is carried through both the female and male line, each having a different emphasis. The female line is primarily concerned with grooming, bonding and nurturing. Every week, head massage is carried out in the family home, where mothers nourish and condition their children's hair with oils and scalp rubs. For daughters and women, the weekly ritual is elaborate and time-consuming, involving lengthy preparations. That is because in India a woman's hair carries great status, so taking care of it is extremely important. There are many different traditions and ways of doing this. In the villages, it is usually a communal outdoor activity. Women of all ages get together once a week and sit in the sunshine to indulge in head massage and brush and groom each other's hair. The heat of the sun allows the oils to penetrate into the hair shaft, nourishing and conditioning it. The ritual is very much a social activity that gives the women involved a chance to talk and relax with one another.

Men also enjoy a tradition of head massage, which is practised by barbers. Treatments take place in shops, in the home, and also on many street corners. It is a more vigorous style of massage than for women, designed to energize and stimulate. Sometimes manipulation is also involved. As with the women's tradition, different kinds of oils are used at different times of the year and to treat a range of different conditions. Because of its cooling properties, coconut oil is often used in the summer, for example, while mustard oil may be preferred in the winter because it is warming. Being a head masseur is a fully recognized profession, and there is even a special caste attributed to it, in which the skills and expertise are handed down from father to son through each generation.

Experiencing an Indian head massage usually leaves the recipient feeling relaxed and unburdened. Some people even report a deep feeling of peace, such as may be experienced after meditation. Perhaps this is because the practice has its roots in India, where spirituality is so much an integral part of everyday life.

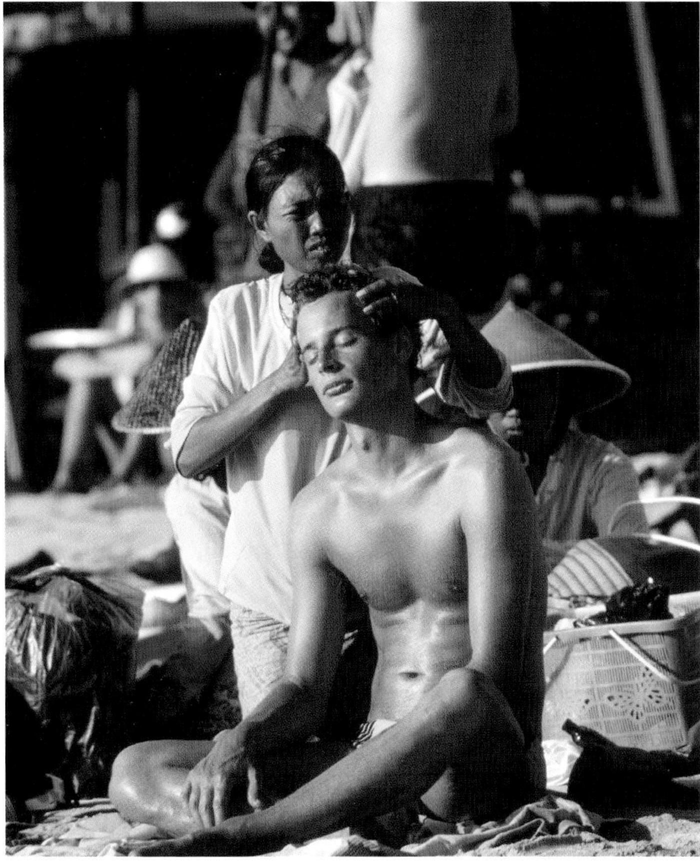

△ In India head massage is traditionally practised on the streets by male masseurs. In areas frequented by tourists, however, women have taken up this public work.

▽ *Shirodhara*, the sensual ritual of running warmed sesame oil on to the middle of the forehead, is a relaxing and therapeutic part of traditional Ayurvedic practice.

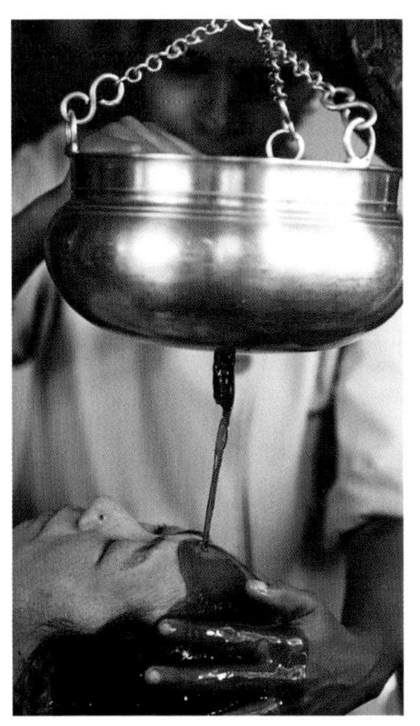

Combining the traditions

Traditional Indian head massage is somewhat different from the style of head massage that is generally practised in the West today. There are a number of reasons for this, although both styles of massage are equally effective and appropriate to the culture in which they are enjoyed.

head massage in India

Traditional Indian head massage is carried out in the context of a culture where social etiquette dictates that the masseur and recipient should be the same sex as one another. In India, a woman's hair is one of her most valuable beauty assets, and a great deal of time is devoted to cultivating the long, lustrous well-oiled locks that are so highly prized. The pace of life is unhurried, and it is quite possible to spend several hours a week enjoying massage and beautifying rituals as a regular social activity. Personal grooming is carried out either in the home or the community, an excuse for friends, family and neighbours to gather together to exchange stories and catch up with one another. Even when life is fast, the therapeutic value of massage is so much a part of everyday life that people still seem to find enough time to enjoy its simple and sensual pleasures.

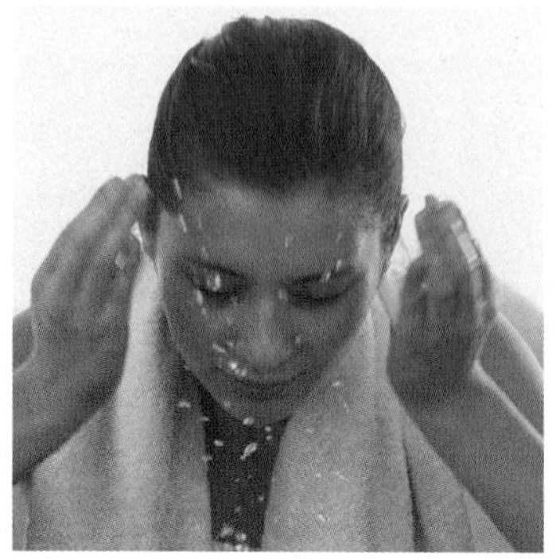

△ The trend in the West towards a faster lifestyle has meant that there is less time available for lengthy grooming procedures.

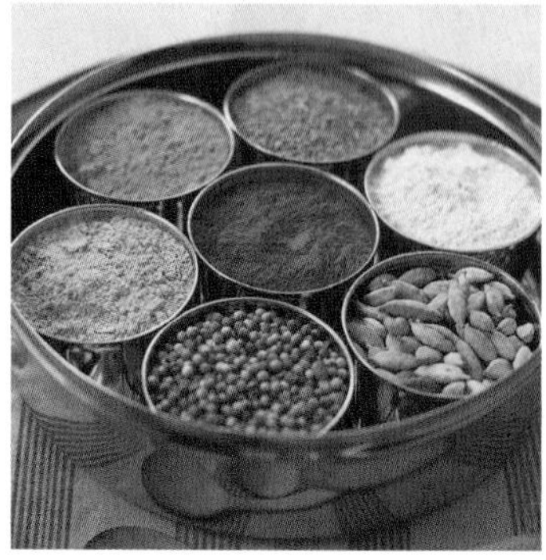

△ Traditional Indian head massage uses Ayurvedic oils from spices and plants, such as mustard, sesame, cinnamon, and cardamom.

▽ Massage is part of the everyday culture in Indian society, and its benefits are increasingly appreciated by tourists.

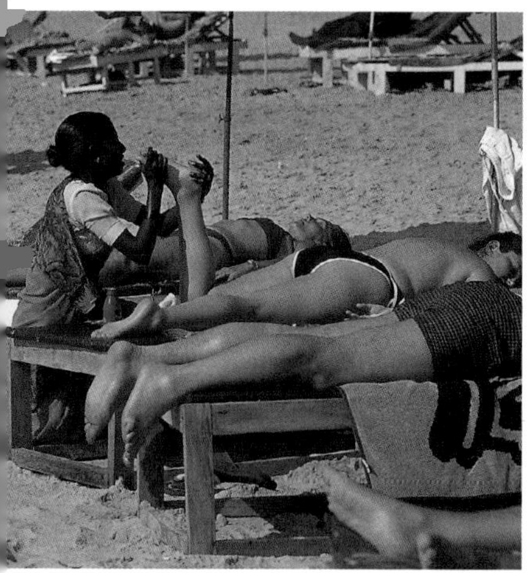

the Western tradition

It is not so long ago in the West that practices such as hair-washing or bathing would also have taken up a large chunk of time each week. Today, however, the pace of life demands that grooming practices be as fast and practical as possible. In the Western world, the last fifty years or so has seen the accelerated development of a lifestyle based on speed, quantity and production. Showers, hairdryers and special beauty products, such as shampoos and conditioners "in-one", are designed to cater for our overriding need for speed and convenience, and a more perfunctory "wash-and-go" attitude towards personal maintenance has taken over.

redefining our values

This emphasis on speed and convenience means our primal need for touch is largely unmet, and there is a danger that living life in the fast lane is at the expense of a real quality of life. Stress-related conditions are on the increase, and despite our material abundance many people experience a sense of emptiness. This has caused many Westerners to look for ways to discover their inner values and a more fulfilling lifestyle. The growing wave of interest in holistic

▽ The daily practice of yoga is part of the holistic Ayurvedic system of health, of which head massage is an integral component.

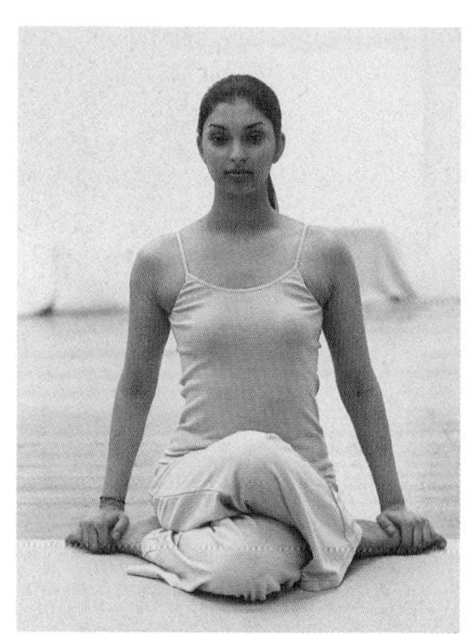

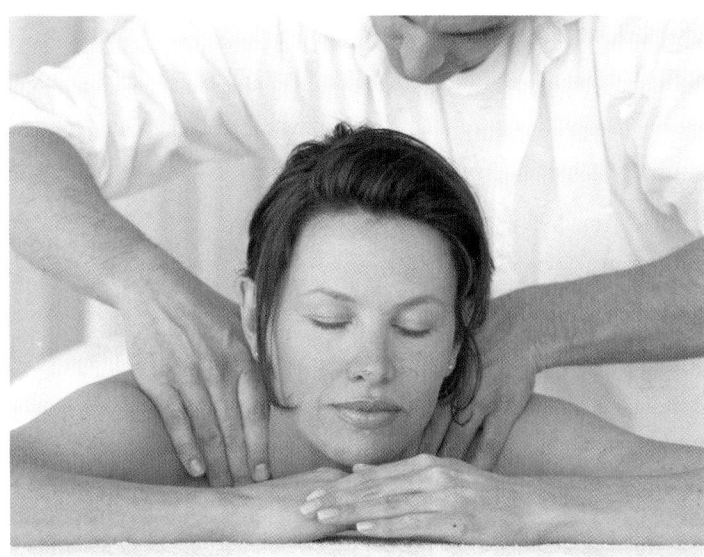

◁ As life continues to speed up, the need to slow down increases, and massage is increasingly being offered as a relaxation treatment in the Western beauty industry.

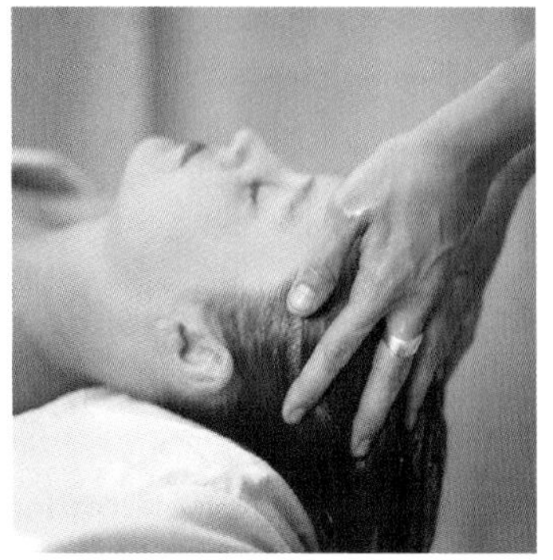

△ A head massage with oils is one of the most luxurious and relaxing treatments available for unwinding at the end of a day.

therapies, which take into account the emotional, mental and spiritual aspects of a person as well as the physical body, is part of this trend, with Indian head massage being just one of these.

a treatment for the modern world

Indian head massage is now finding and filling a niche in Western society. Gradually it has moved from being an "alternative" or "fringe" therapy to something that is becoming more widely recognized; many hairdressing salons now offer head massage as a service to their clients, for instance. However, the type of head massage being practised has been adapted to suit the constraints and demands of our culture.

Our work and lifestyle patterns have been changing, with the emphasis shifting away from physical activity to a more sedentary lifestyle. Every day we are confronted with huge amounts of information, which has to be processed, and we tend to live very active mental lives. Typically we suffer from mental overload, and because of our lack of physical activity, the resulting tension can get stuck in the body and emerge as discomfort.

Despite its name, the Western head massage routine includes more of the body than just the head. It also embraces the upper back, shoulders and neck, the main areas where we store tension in the body. While in India it is customary to use treatment oils on the hair and scalp, here head massage is done dry for the most part, although it is also possible to use oils for a special treatment every now and again. One of the great advantages of head massage (both Eastern and Western varieties) is that it is done clothes-on. This, together with its "dry" aspect, makes it highly versatile. Head massage can be carried out in a variety of settings, both at home and in the workplace. Consequently, many massage practitioners are able to run a mobile service, travelling to people's homes or places of work to deliver head massage treatments for stress relief. It is important that the spiritual origins of head massage should not be forgotten, for it does much more than simply relieve physical tension. It also calms the spirit and helps to rebalance the body's own vital energies.

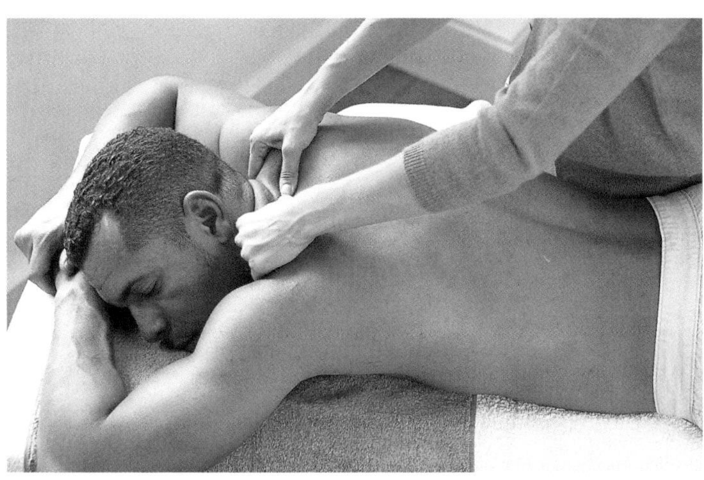

▷ Massage is becoming increasingly mainstream and is recognized for its effective role in helping to get rid of stress and maintain balance.

Head Massage Techniques

It is not difficult to learn how to practise Indian head massage. By mastering a few basic strokes and techniques you will soon be on the way to becoming a proficient masseur. However, although the strokes are important, they are not the only elements of a good massage. How you give the massage is equally important. Your ultimate aim is to give a treatment in which all the strokes and techniques blend together, each flowing seamlessly from one to the next. To achieve this level of mastery takes practice.

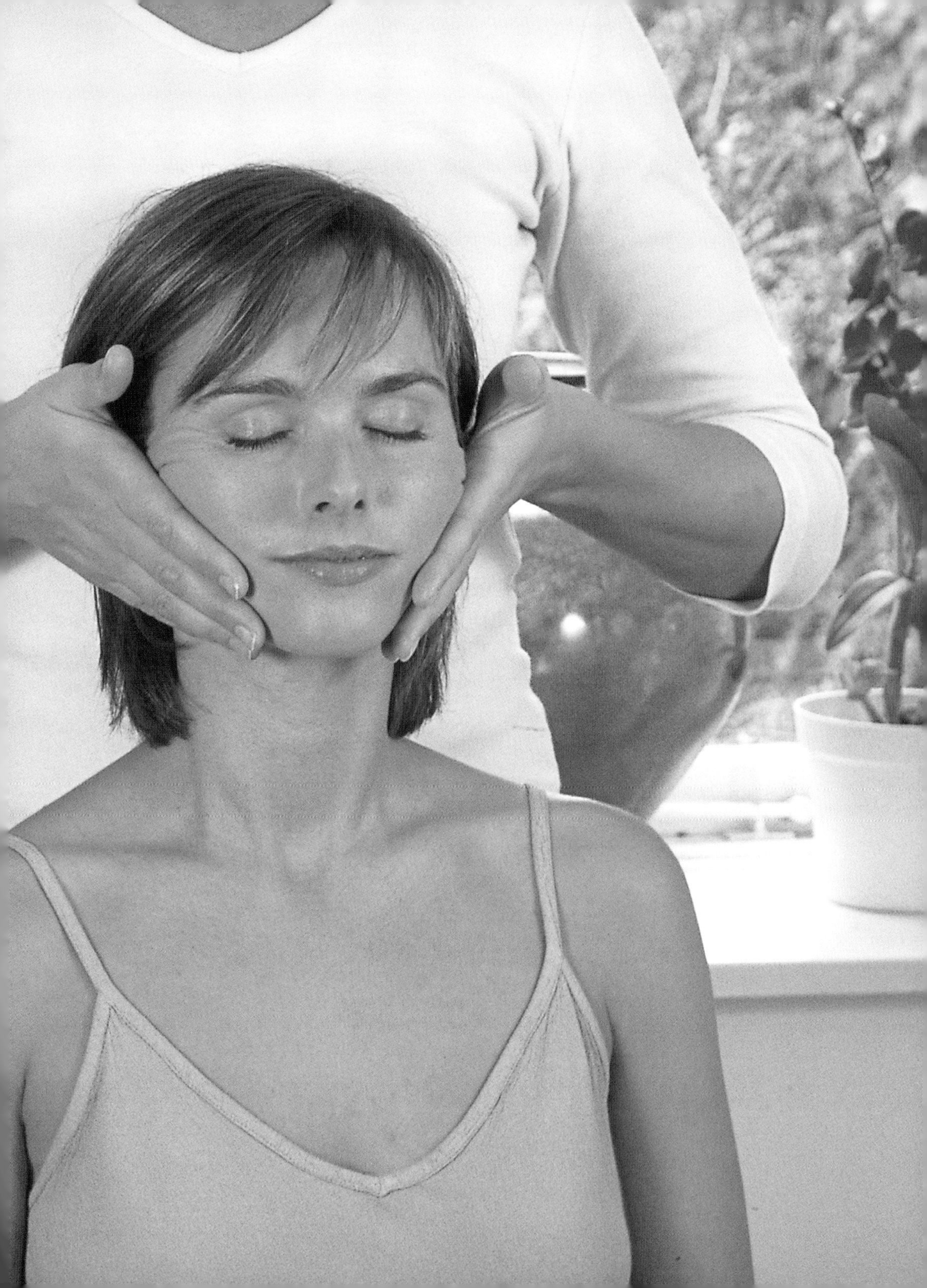

Head massage basic strokes

Giving a head massage can be likened to playing music, with the basic strokes as the notes that are used to create the overall effect. Like musical notes, the strokes vary enormously, each one having its own particular quality and being used for different reasons to create different effects. The speed and depth with which you apply the strokes also affects how they come across.

stroking

One of the most basic and familiar massage strokes is stroking. It can be done with the hands, fingers or forearms over the head and body. Stroking has a calming and soothing effect on the nervous system, sending messages of relaxation to the brain via the skin's sensory nerve endings. Sometimes it connects to body memories of nurture and is a comforting, reassuring and affirming action. Strokes such as smoothing, ruffling, sliding or gliding are derived from stroking.

Stroking helps prepare the body for deeper massage work. It is also good after deep or vigorous actions such as pressure or kneading. This makes stroking a useful linking stroke to use in between different movements. It is also useful for travelling from one part of the body to another when working over different areas. This maintains contact with the body and keeps a sense of continuity. If you take your hands off the body or move away too quickly this disrupts the energetic flow and can feel strange for your partner.

friction strokes

Applied with the fingers and heel or sides of the hand, friction strokes use a rubbing or chopping motion. They are used on the head, shoulders and upper back and are vigorous and warming, stimulating the circulation and bringing heat and energy to the area being worked on. These strokes are useful for loosening muscle fibres and connective tissue that have become compacted with tension over a long time. Friction strokes feel exciting and energizing to receive, but some people also experience them as relaxing when done repeatedly.

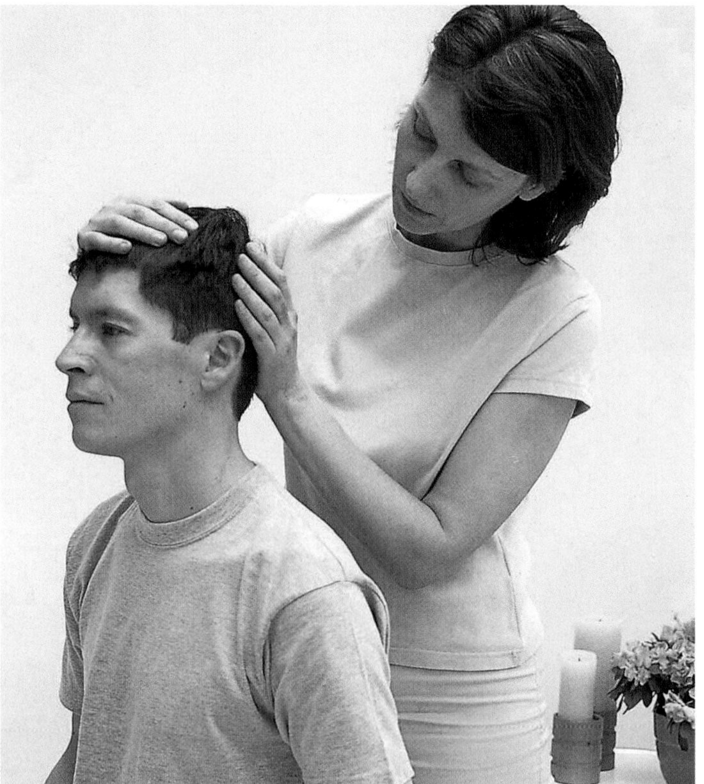

◁ **For whole hand stroking, use the flat of your hand with your fingers pointing forwards and bring it slowly down over the back of the head. Let one hand follow the other in one flowing movement, and always support the head.**

▽ **Stroke over the upper body, shoulders or arms, working in a smooth and repetitive circular, zigzag, or back-and-forth action.**

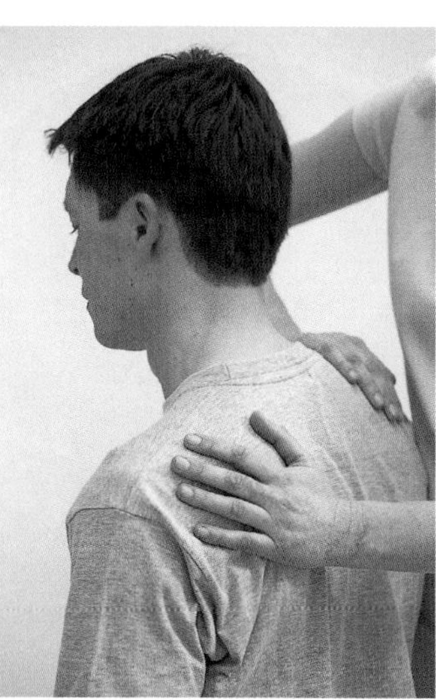

▷ **Circular friction strokes with your thumbs will loosen tightness at the base of the neck and the tops of the shoulders. Begin in a small area, then make the circles wider as you work.**

pressure strokes

Pressure strokes work in a number of ways. Sometimes the whole hand or forearm may be used to apply pressure, such as when pushing or pressing down on the shoulders or chest. These strokes work on releasing the body's deeper muscle layers. At other times, the fingers or thumbs are used to work on the body's energy system by applying pressure at specific release, or acupressure, points along the meridians (energy channels). When pressure is applied at such a point it helps to clear the energy channels so that the body's vital energies can flow freely. This helps to restore a sense of balance and equilibrium to the person.

Pressure points can be tender so your pressure needs to be firm but not cause undue pain. Gradually exert pressure on the points using your thumbs or fingers and hold it there for a few seconds before slowly releasing and moving on.

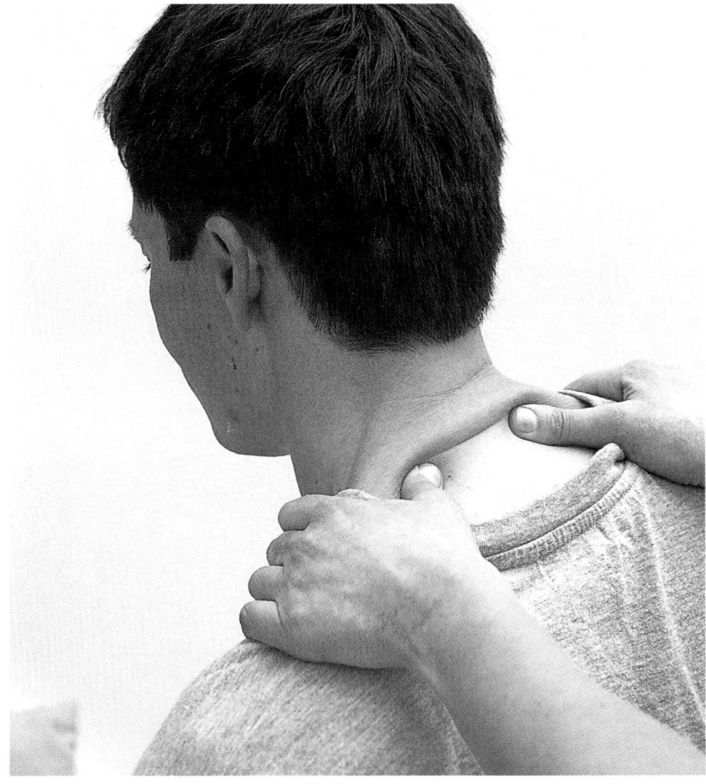

▽ **Use firm pressure for friction strokes on the upper body, keeping your fingers straight but not rigid. Working rhythmically, you can build up momentum and massage at a fast pace.**

▽ **When doing friction strokes on the head, remember to support it with your other hand. Allow your own body to adjust and go with the momentum of the movement.**

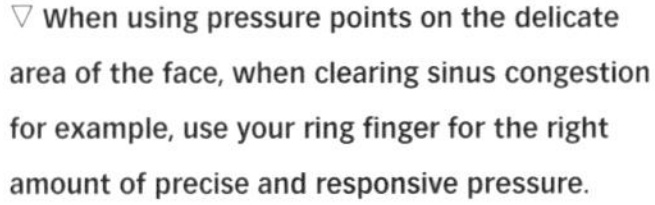

▽ **When using pressure points on the delicate area of the face, when clearing sinus congestion for example, use your ring finger for the right amount of precise and responsive pressure.**

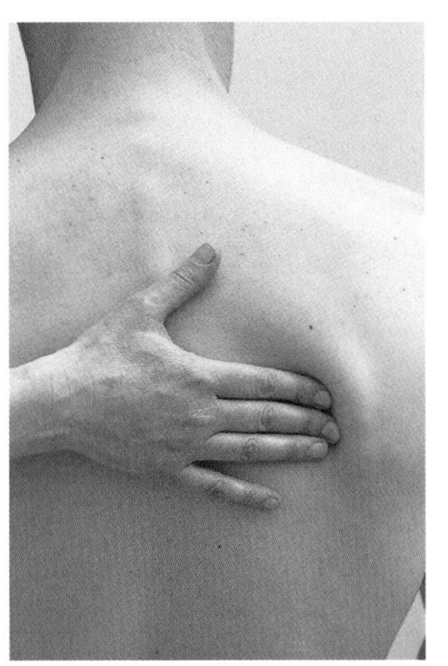

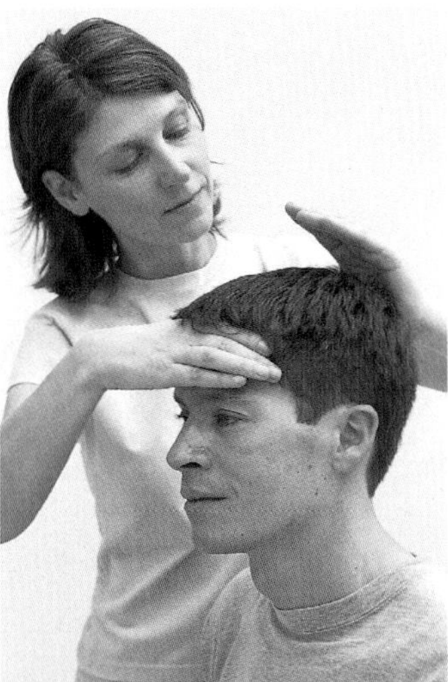

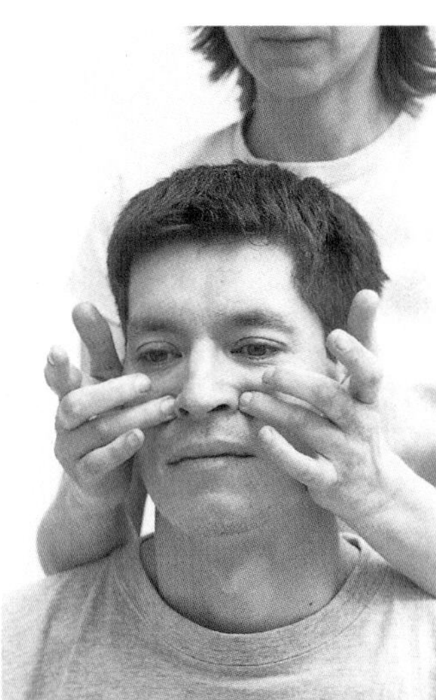

▷ **When you do tapotement all over the scalp, as one hand rises let the fingertips of the other hand gently fall on the scalp.**

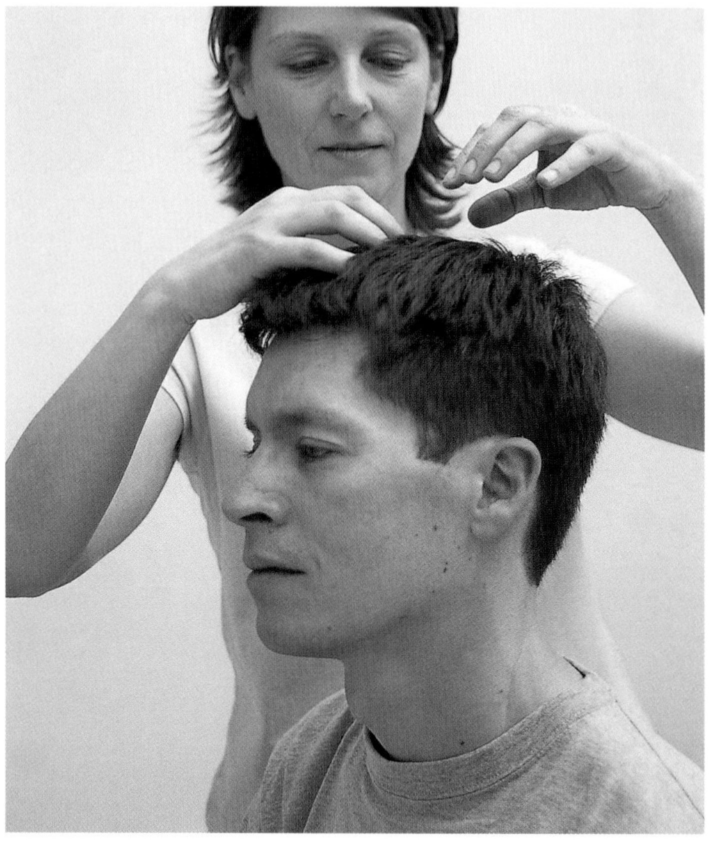

tapotement

Also known as "percussion strokes" or "hacking", tapotement is a kind of tapping action. It is applied with the sides or tips of the fingers, and you can think of it as being a bit like playing a drum. One hand goes up as the other goes down. Tapotement is used on the head, the upper back and shoulders. This stroke works on the nervous and circulatory system. It has a stimulating effect and is light and refreshing to receive.

pulling and lifting

There is a range of strokes used in head massage that involve pulling, lifting, stretching and tugging. Most of these are done on the head itself, although some, such as lifting the shoulders, are also done on the body. They are done using the fingers and thumbs. These strokes work on the principle of tension followed by release, which leads to greater relaxation or increased mobility. As these strokes work in a lateral direction, that is away from the body, they also serve to direct and draw unwanted energies released by the massage, away from your partner's energy field.

▽ **When doing tapotement remember to keep your fingers soft as they land. Keeping your fingers spaced out a little will help with this.**

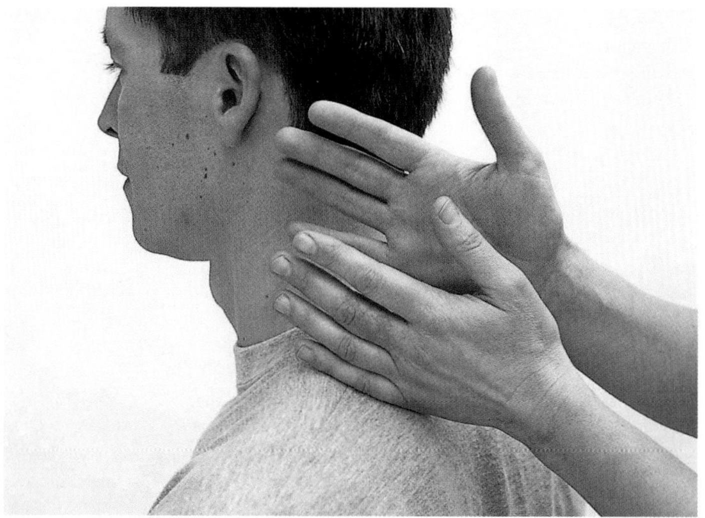

▽ **For a lifting action, gently pull your fingers to the very tips of your partner's hair. Let long hair fall through your fingers as you pull through.**

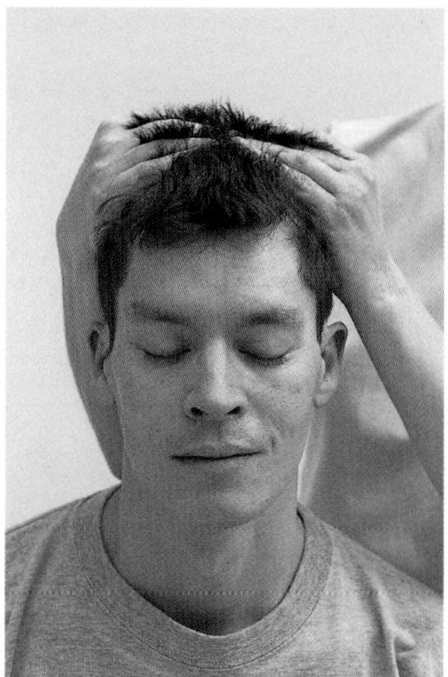

▷ When using a holding stroke, gradually let your hands descend on your partner and let them rest there in a relaxed and focused way for seven seconds or so.

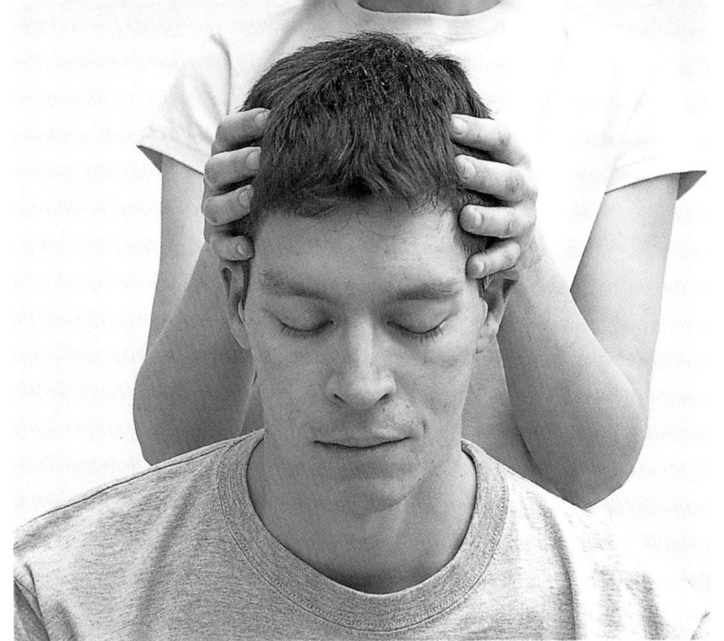

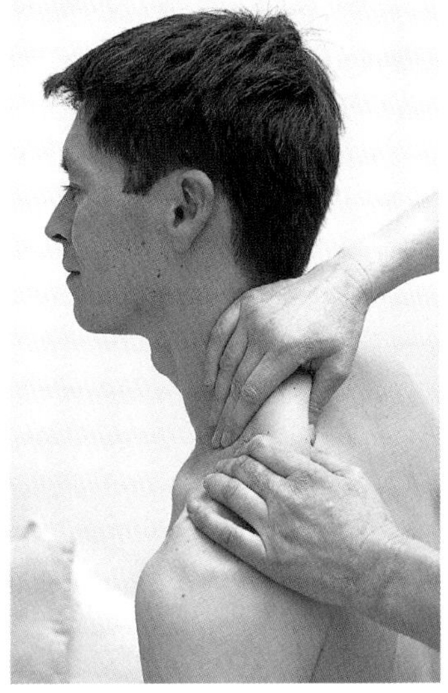

△ Knead the shoulders in a rolling action, not unlike working dough. Check the comfort level with your partner. If the shoulders are tight, reduce the pressure.

▽ When kneading in a small area such as under the chin, use a rolling action, working your fingers and thumbs together as you massage.

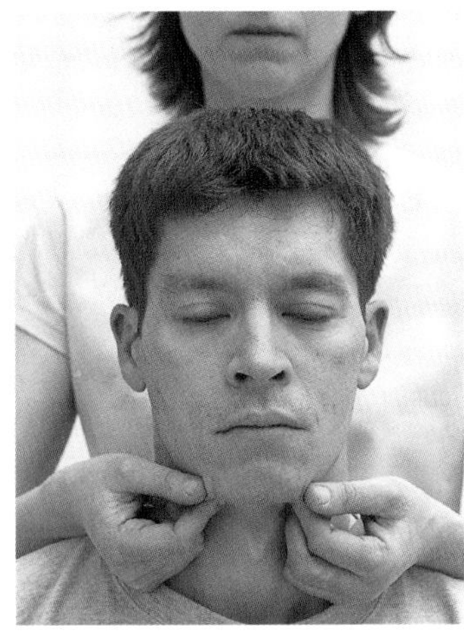

kneading and squeezing

The bread and butter of massage strokes are kneading and squeezing. In head massage these strokes may also be referred to as circling, rolling or pinching. Using the whole hands or thumbs and fingers, these strokes involve picking up the flesh away from the body and manipulating it in various ways. Kneading and squeezing strokes are appropriate for the more fleshy parts of the body such as the shoulders, the base and back of the neck, the chin and the outer edge of the ears.

holding

Although head massage is about movement, it is also about stillness. Holding involves keeping your hands still on your partner's head or shoulders, with a relaxed yet aware presence. It is often used to create a boundary around the session by marking its beginning and end. At the beginning, holding establishes initial contact with your partner and creates an energetic link between the two of you. It establishes communication through your hands, using massage as the language. At the end of the session it is a signal that the circle of energy between you and your partner is now complete and that you are about to move away. Holding can ground the treatment by holding the energy, and give healing, love, and energy to your partner.

key principles

There are a number of principles to keep in mind. The first is to stand at a comfortable distance from your partner when you work, not too close and not too far away. This is so that you can get a good leverage and your partner can feel your reassuring presence.

Second, stay as relaxed as you can and do not hold yourself tense or rigid. You need to be like a dancer, having your feet on the floor yet allowing your movements to be free and flowing.

Third, tune into and be sensitive to your partner's changing energies and moods through the different phases of the massage.

It may take a little practice and trust before you feel confident enough to be able to pick up and respond to the subtle nuances. If your partner is ticklish, omit stroking and light touches and instead use the flat of your hand, a firmer touch and work at a lower speed. Try and enjoy yourself, as how you are feeling will be communicated to your partner through your hands.

Using oils in head massage

There are many benefits of using oil in head massage, the most obvious being the conditioning effect on the hair and scalp itself. The effects of stress, chemical hair treatments, central heating and poor nutrition can all be seen in the health of our hair and scalp. Similarly, frequent hair washing and the use of hairdryers and heated hair-styling devices strip the hair of its natural oils, making it dry and brittle. Using oils can help restore the hair to its optimum condition, penetrating deep into the hair shaft to strengthen the hair. Unlike most ready-made products they do not contain any harsh detergents or chemicals and can be custom-blended to suit your specific needs. There is a wide array of suitable oils for use in head massage. These fall into two broad categories: carrier oils and essential oils.

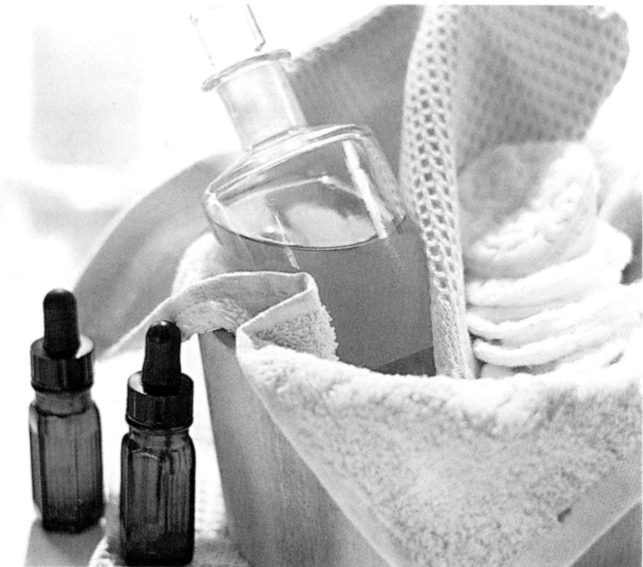

△ **Using oils as part of your regular beauty routine can be of lasting benefit in helping you to keep looking and feeling good.**

carrier oils

Traditionally, carrier oils are used in their own right in head massage, but they can also be used as a base to mix with essential oils. Sweet almond is one of the most versatile carrier oils. It is easily absorbed and is a warming, light oil. It can help reduce muscular pain and stiffness.

In Ayurveda, sesame oil is very popular for massaging the head and body. It helps to strengthen, condition and moisturize the skin and hair. It is a balancing oil and can help to reduce swelling, pain and stiffness.

Deep yellow mustard oil is thick and heavy. Its strong characteristic odour makes it unsuitable for blending with essential oils, so only use it by itself. Mustard oil has a stimulating effect on the circulatory system, helping to increase body heat and warm up the muscles and joints. Its properties help to ease general aches and pains, tension and swellings. It is a good oil to use in the cold winter months or when the body is chilled. Another thick and warming oil that can ease muscular pain and stiffness is olive oil. Use the best quality virgin, extra virgin or cold-pressed oils as these contain high levels of unsaturated fatty acids that are nourishing for dry skin and hair.

Light coconut oil is used extensively in southern India. It is easy to use and blends well with essential oils. It has softening and moisturizing qualities that makes it ideal for dry, brittle or chemically-treated hair. You can also leave it on the hair to give a high gloss sheen or "wet look".

Finally, luxurious jojoba oil is rich in protein, minerals and vitamin E. It is ideal for use on all skin and hair types and mixes well with essential oils. Because it is expensive, jojoba is usually used in a mix with another carrier oil.

▽ **Used regularly in traditional Indian head massage, light coconut oil, sweet almond oil and sesame oil have therapeutic properties.**

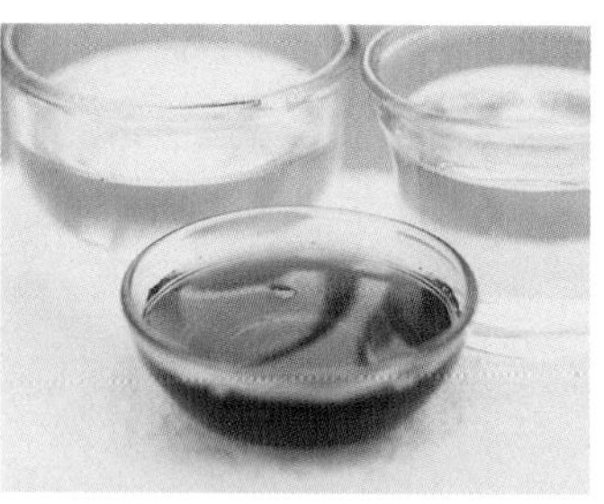

▽ **Olive oil has been used in skin treatments for centuries in the Mediterranean region for its nourishing properties and versatility.**

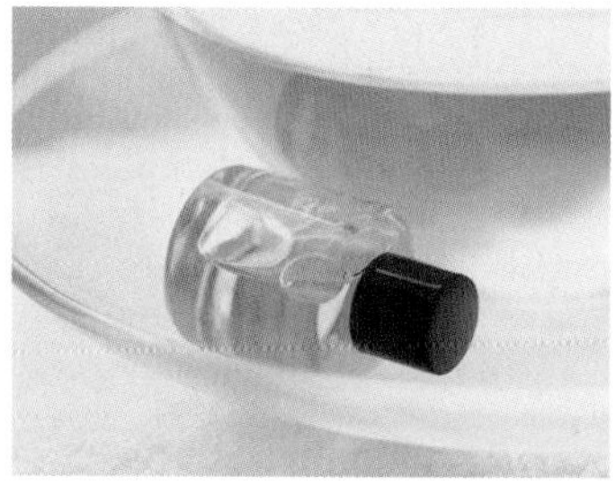

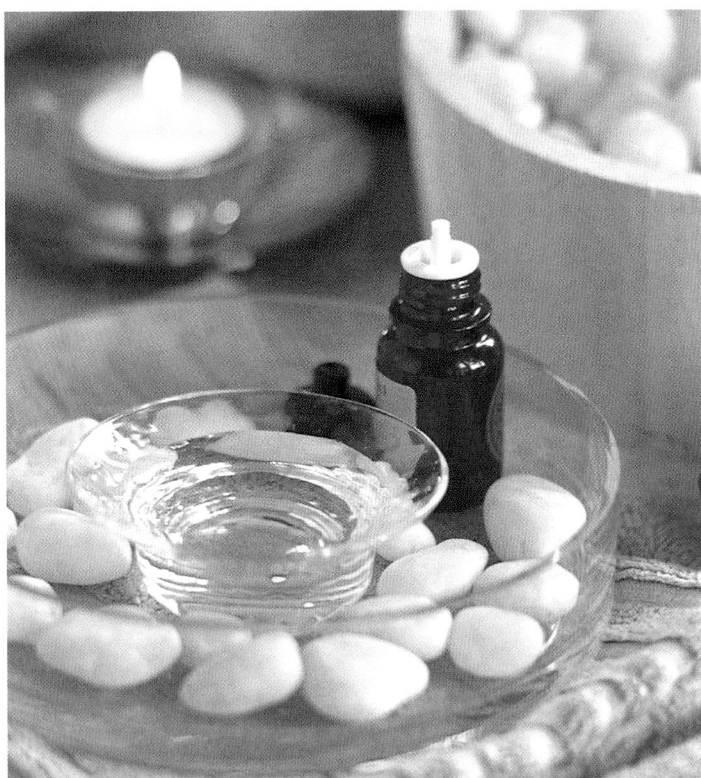

▷ **A relaxing bath fragranced with essential oils will round off a head massage. Alternatively, it will help you to fully unwind at the end of a long and tiring day.**

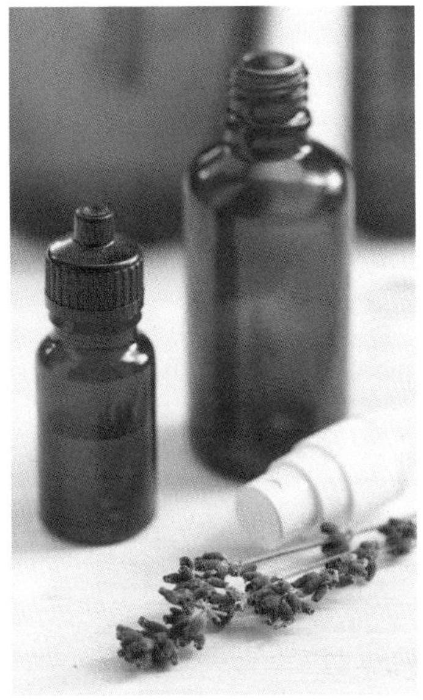

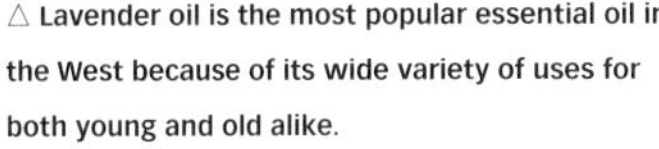

△ **Lavender oil is the most popular essential oil in the West because of its wide variety of uses for both young and old alike.**

essential oils

You can choose an essential oil, or a blend of several oils, on the same basis as for any aromatherapy treatment – each oil has distinctive properties, as well as contributing to the pleasure of the experience. However, certain oils are particularly useful in head massage, and the following are all recommended. Remember that essential oils should never be used undiluted.

lavender One of the most universal of all the essential oils, lavender's relaxing and balancing properties make it useful for stress, insomnia, anxiety and depression. It is useful for treating dandruff, hair loss and lice and blends well with geranium and rosemary.

rosemary The refreshing and stimulating properties of rosemary oil have a head-clearing effect, so it is useful for periods of mental work. Rosemary is also a good treatment for greasy hair and skin, dandruff and hair loss, as well as restoring the shine to dark hair. It blends well with lavender.

sandalwood This oil's woody, haunting aroma quiets the mind and relaxes the nervous system, making it useful for stress-related conditions. Its softening and soothing action is good for dry skin and scalp conditions, while its aphrodisiac properties lend itself to sensual massage. Sandalwood blends well with bergamot, cedarwood, jasmine, palmarosa, vetiver or ylang ylang.

frankincense This has calming and relaxing properties for body, mind and soul. Because it deepens and slows down breathing, frankincense is good for respiratory conditions such as asthma, blocked sinuses, coughs or colds. Its moisturizing properties make it especially nourishing for older skin. Frankincense has a tradition of use in sacred ceremony and is helpful for inner journeys or a process of change.

geranium A light floral fragrance with a refreshing and balancing action, it is used to normalize very dry or very greasy skin and hair conditions by bringing them back into balance. Emotionally it is calming, restoring, uplifting and useful for anxiety or depression. It is an oil to use if you are uncertain which to choose. It blends well with lavender, sandalwood, rose, bergamot, marjoram, lemon or orange.

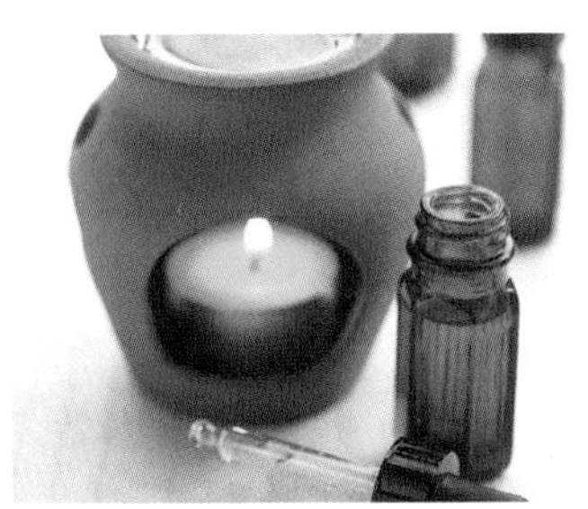

◁ **Using essential oils in a burner will enhance the ambience of the space you work in and help transport you to another dimension.**

Working with oils

Oils are messy to work with so you need to make sure your partner is not wearing anything that could be spoiled – an old t-shirt is ideal. Keep a couple of towels specifically for this purpose, and drape one around your partner's shoulders. Have a good supply of tissues to hand and gather together all your oils, plus a suitable spoon and mixing bowl. Put the equipment on absorbent paper to soak up any accidental spills. You will also need a shower cap or silver foil to wrap your partner's hair up in when you've finished. If your partner has long hair, it is best to apply oil in sections over the head, in which case you will also need a comb, tinting brush and hair clips.

using essential oils

The head is a sensitive area, so essential oils should be used sparingly. As a rule, they should be blended with a carrier oil at a ratio of 2 drops to every 10 ml (2 tsp) – weaker than for a body massage. Exceeding the recommended dose could result in toxicity. Sometimes essential oils can cause allergic skin reactions. If you are using an oil for the first time, it is a good idea to do a patch test by dabbing a little of the blended oil on the inside of the wrist or elbow. Wait for 24 hours to see if there is any adverse reaction before using the oil.

Because of their potent effect, do not use essential oils with babies, young children or in pregnancy. When treating older children or the elderly, it is best to halve the dilution to 1 drop essential oil to every 10ml (2 tsp) carrier. If you are in doubt, consult a qualified aromatherapist.

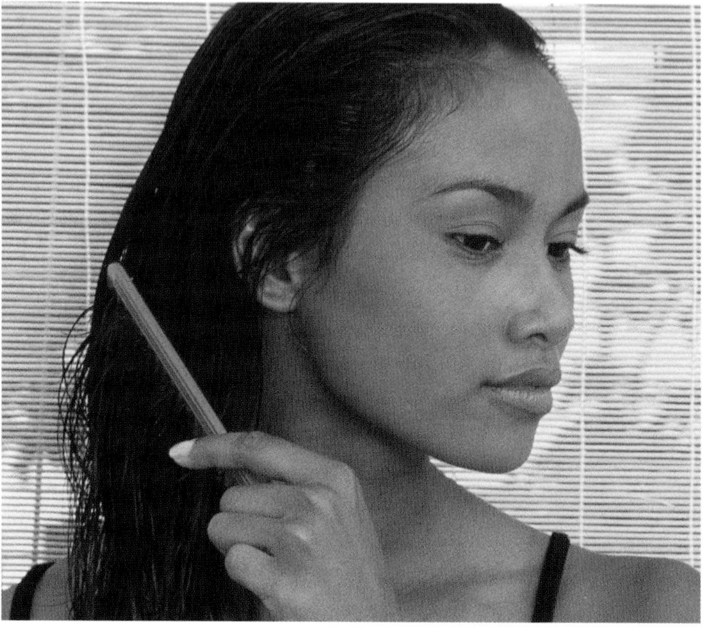

△ Leaving the oils in your hair after an oil massage is a holistic treatment and helps leave your hair and scalp in excellent condition.

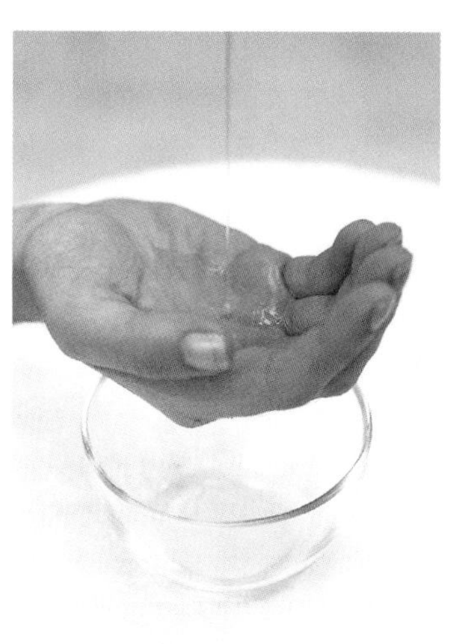

△ Warm the oil up in the palm of your hand or on a radiator before applying it, as heated oil is more easily absorbed and feels nicer.

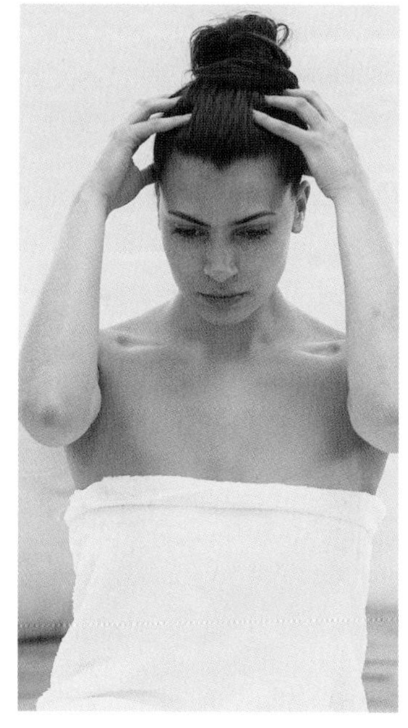

▷ Applying nourishing oils to your hair as part of your weekly beauty routine can be combined with a relaxing head massage.

oils for the hair and scalp

Choose from the following recipes to give your hair and scalp a nourishing conditioning treatment.

normal hair
carrier oils: almond, coconut, jojoba
essential oils: rosemary, lavender, geranium

dandruff
carrier oils: jojoba, olive, coconut, sweet almond
essential oils: rosemary, lavender, eucalyptus, geranium

greasy hair
carrier oils: sweet almond, sesame, jojoba
essential oils: rosemary, lavender, sandalwood, lemon

thinning hair
carrier oils: sesame, olive
essential oils: rosemary, lavender, geranium

dry or chemically-treated hair
carrier oils: sesame, coconut, jojoba, almond
essential oils: lavender, rosemary, geranium, sandalwood

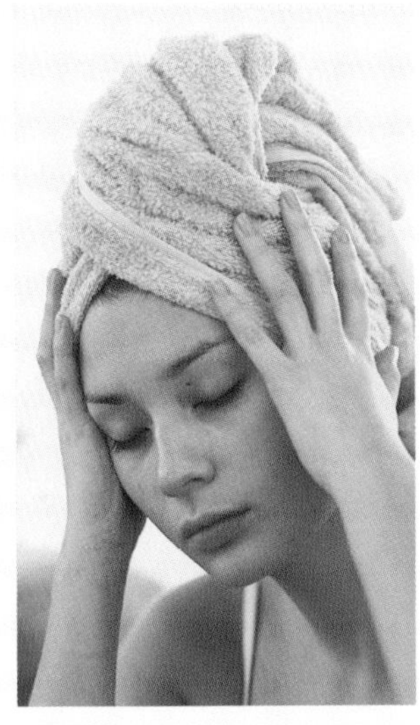

hair and scalp treatments

Mixing up your own blends of oils for your treatments is both very satisfying and beneficial. It is empowering, and you can also ensure that the ingredients you are putting on your hair and scalp are fresh and potent (all the oils have a limited shelf life) and are of a high quality. Because you are choosing the raw ingredients, you can guarantee that the blend you make is appropriate and of nutritional benefit to your body. Choose a carrier oil and an essential oil or two from the category on the left that best describes your hair. As a rough guide, 10ml (2 tsp) carrier oil should be sufficient for short hair, 15ml (1 tbsp) for medium length hair, and 30ml (2 tbsp) for long hair. The amount of oil you will need will also depend on the texture and thickness of the hair.

Measure the carrier oil into the mixing bowl. You may use more than one carrier oil if you wish, but mix them well together. Next add your chosen essential oil(s). Try not to make up more than you think you'll need, as it is best to work with a fresh mix each time. If you do have any left over, you could rub it into areas of rough skin, such as the elbows or heels. To get the most from the treatment, leave the oils on the hair for as long as possible, from a minimum of 30 minutes to up to 12 hours.

treating head lice

Head lice (nits) are a common problem among school-age children, and they can be difficult to eradicate. Using essential oils is becoming a popular treatment, as it offers a natural rather than a chemical approach to the problem. When treating lice it is essential that the whole family is treated to prevent the risk of cross-infection, and that all bedding, clothes, combs and brushes are washed to remove the eggs.

The quantity given below is sufficient for one complete treatment for one person. It comprises three separate applications, so you will have to store the remainder of the mixture in a sealed dark glass jar or bottle. It will keep for up to 12 months.

Use 30ml (2 tbsp) coconut or almond oil (or a combination of the two if you prefer). Add 5 drops lavender, 5 drops geranium and 5 drops eucalyptus oil. Apply the mix all over the head and hair, massaging it in well. Cover the head and leave the oils in for a minimum of 4 hours, although overnight is better. To remove the oil, massage the shampoo well into the hair before applying water. Wash and rinse as normal. Comb through the hair with a lice comb. Repeat the whole process after 24 hours and again after 8 days. This will give you the opportunity to treat any lice that have hatched since the first treatment and to ensure the head is clear.

▽ **Oil treatments can be therapeutic, and the treatment of head lice with oil blends is very effective, toxic-free and pleasant.**

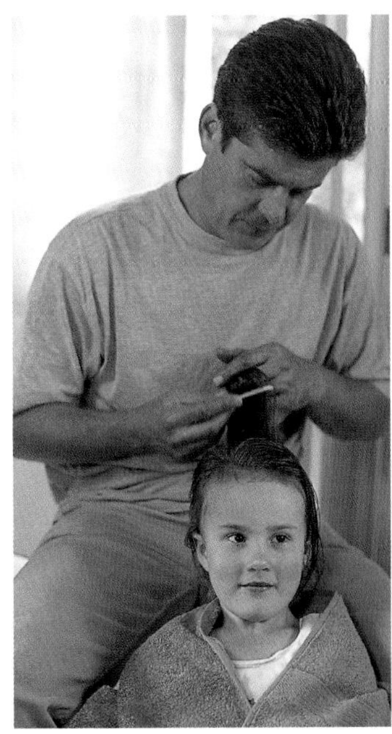

How to apply oils

The tradition of anointing the head with oil dates back to antiquity. There are many references to the practice throughout the Bible, while it has always played an important part in Ayurvedic medicine. In India, the practice of putting oil on the head begins at birth when a piece of soft cloth soaked in oil is placed over the fontanelle (the "soft spot") on a newborn baby's head. There are also complex ritual procedures within Ayurveda for applying oils to the head. Today traditional methods for applying oils have been integrated into a style more suited to a Western approach. Oil can be applied with your partner lying on a couch or sitting upright on a chair. Whichever method you use, warm the oil first. Warm oil not only feels nicer but it is more easily absorbed by the hair and scalp. To warm the oil, place it in a bowl on top of a radiator, or in a pan of hot water. Make sure the oil is not too hot before putting it on your partner's head. Take some time to discuss with your partner which oils and aromas they prefer, let them sniff the bottles and together work out a mix that will suit their state of mind and preferences.

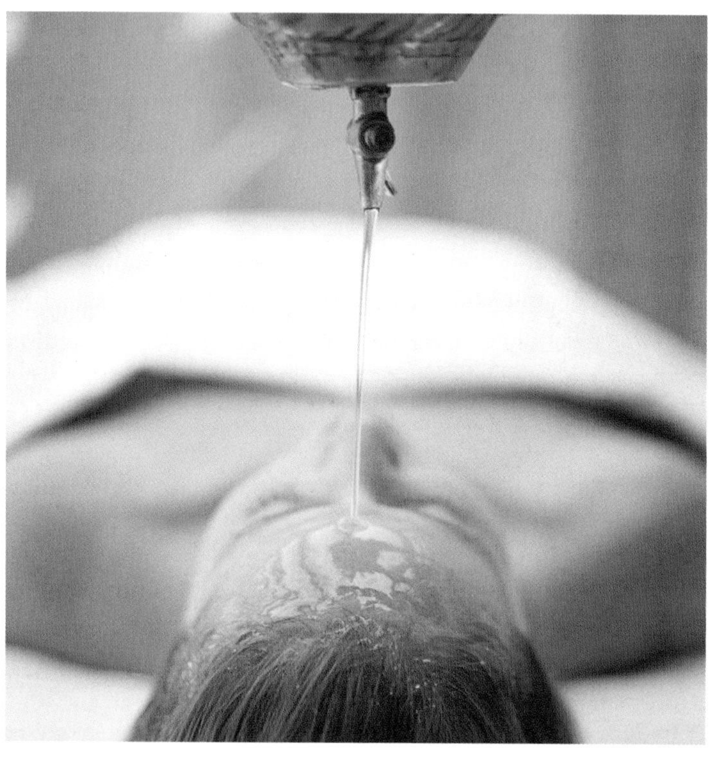

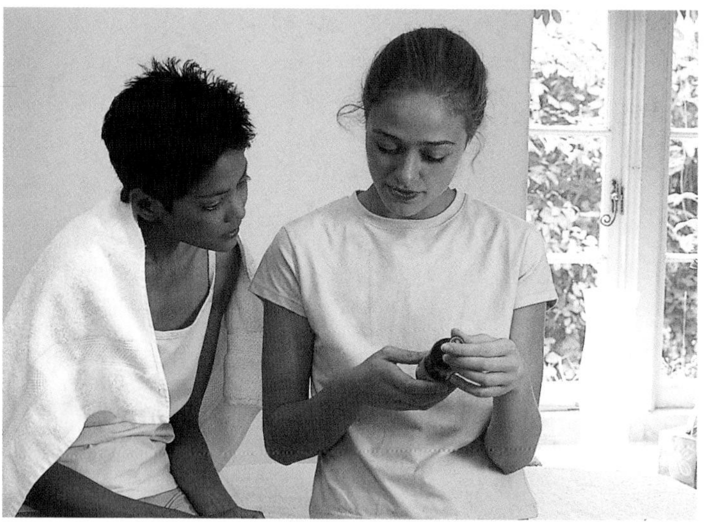

△ In Ayurvedic medicine the calming treatment of slowly and steadily pouring warmed oil over the forehead soothes and uplifts the spirit.

◁ Choosing which oils to use is part of the session and it is a good idea to discuss any preferences with your partner before starting.

lying-down method

Cover the surface of a couch or bed with suitable towels and have your partner lie down with their head near the edge. It's also a good idea to put a towel on the floor immediately below your partner's head.

Pour a little of the warmed oil directly on to the crown of your partner's head – it is a wonderful feeling as the oil seeps across the scalp. If you prefer, you may find it easier to pour some oil into the palm of your hand

▷ **Make sure you have assembled everything and that it is to hand before you begin working with oils, as they can be messy.**

and put it on top of your partner's head like that. Work the oil into the scalp, applying more oil should you need to.

Pour more oil into your palm and massage up from the sides of the head towards the top. Put some more oil in your hand and apply it to the front of their head and work it upwards towards the middle. Then apply oil to the back of the head. Make sure that you have covered the whole head with oil. You can use this method with your partner sitting in a chair, too. You are then ready to proceed with the head massage routines described in the following section. The strokes are the same; the only difference is the presence of the oil.

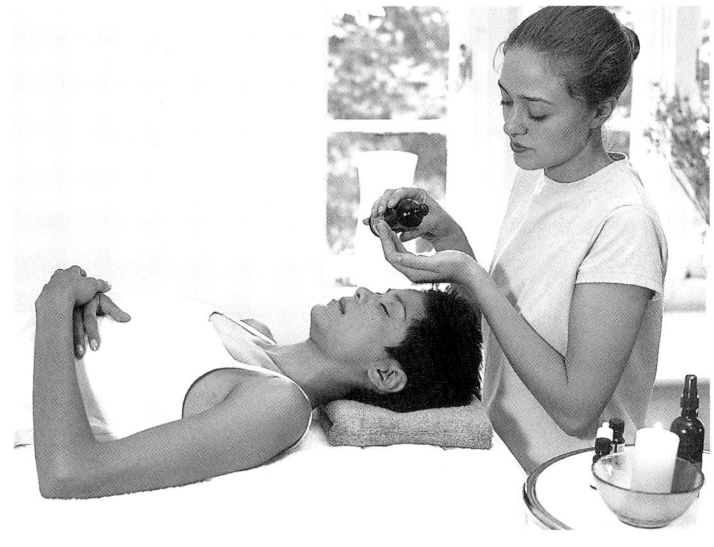

▽ **Use your hands to apply a little oil into the hair at a time, working it well into the hair and scalp for a nourishing treatment.**

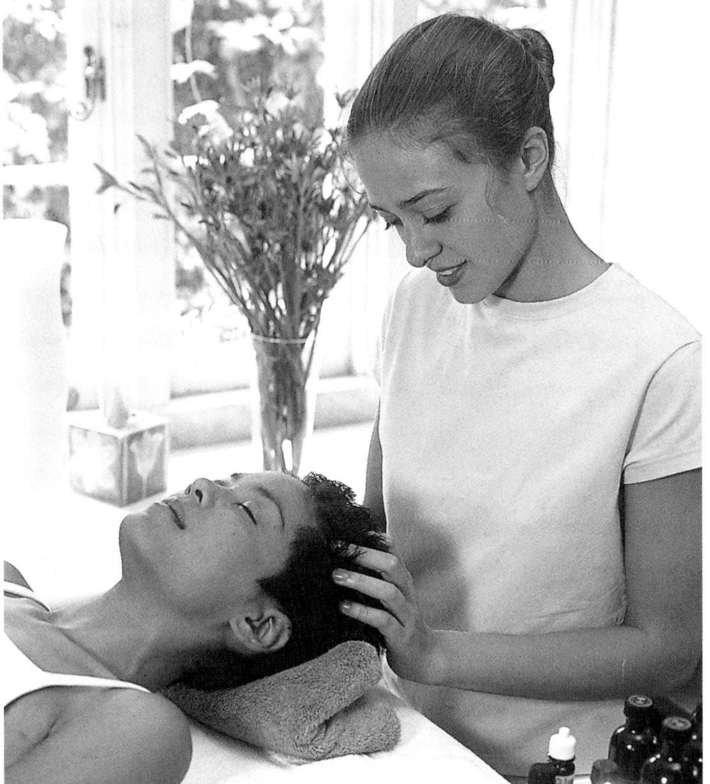

sectioning method

This method applies the oil in sections and works well for longer hair. You will need hair clips and a comb.

Divide the head into eight or so sections, clipping the hair out of the way. Starting at the front of the head, take down a section and comb the oil through, beginning at the roots and working down to the hair ends. Working with one section at a time, continue until the whole head is covered, then proceed with your head massage sequence.

▽ **The sectioning method ensures that the oil is evenly applied all over the head and hair.**

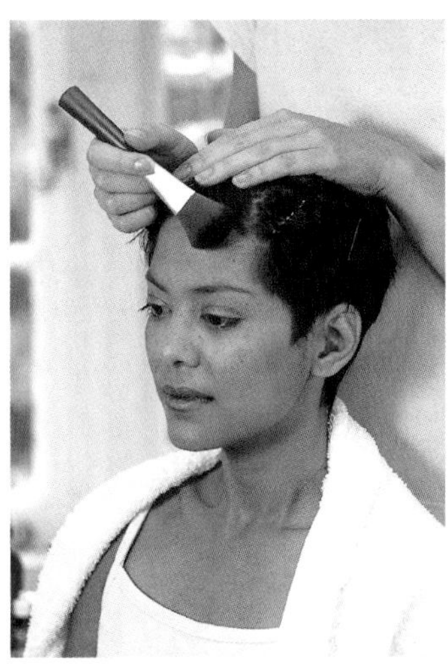

leaving and removing oils

To get the most out of an oil treatment the oils are best left on the head for some time. This maximizes their beneficial effects, giving them a chance to sink into the hair shaft and nourish it at a deep level. They will also be absorbed through the skin and enter the bloodstream where they will work their benefits through the whole body. Oils can be left on the hair from anything from 20 minutes to 24 hours. When it is time to remove them, there are a few guidelines for leaving your hair grease-free.

leaving oils on the hair

Once you have put the oils on, you will need to cover up your head. This will trap body heat and help the oils sink further into the hair and scalp. It may also feel more comfortable, particularly if you have long hair. You can do this by wearing a shower cap or by covering the head with silver foil, and bending it round at the corners to form a cap. You can then wrap a towel round your head to keep warm.

If you are keeping the oils on for an evening, then the treatment can be made part of a general pampering session combining self- or partner massage and other "feel-good" treats, such as a relaxing aromatherapy bath. Alternatively, leaving the oils in overnight will provide your hair and scalp with a deep conditioning treatment.

▽ **Leaving oils on your hair gives them a chance to sink in and deeply condition while you relax and take some quality time out.**

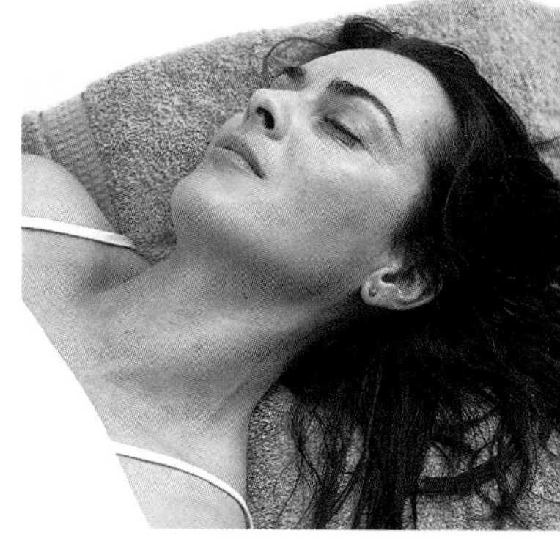

△ **For a really deep conditioning treatment, oils can be left on overnight and can continue working while you recharge with a restful sleep.**

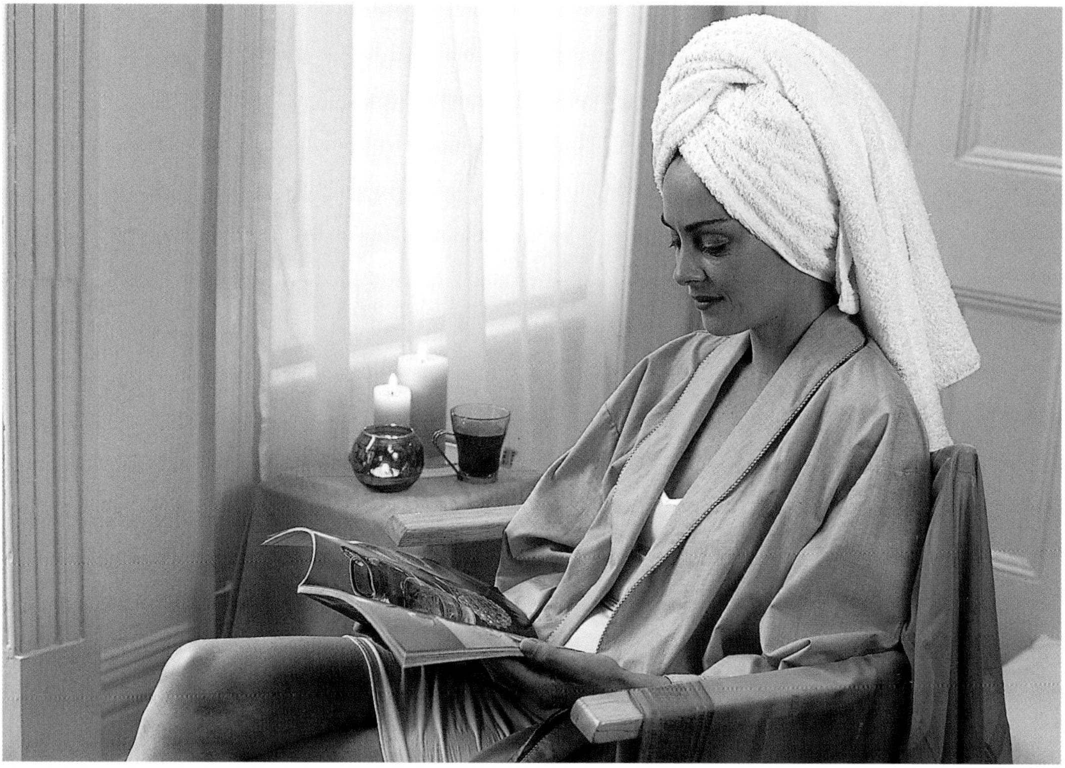

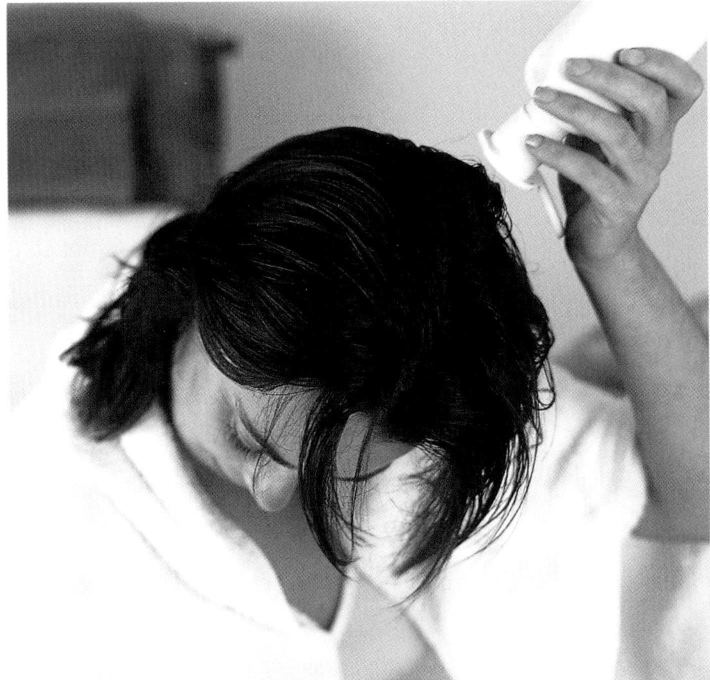

◁ **When removing oils, always apply liberal quantities of shampoo directly onto the hair itself and work it repeatedly into the hair shafts and scalp before rinsing.**

If you plan to leave the oils on overnight, then you may find it more comfortable to have the hair loose and use old towels or sheets to protect the bedding.

removing oils

When it comes to removing the oil from your hair, it is vital to use lots of shampoo at the start.

Do not wet your hair, but put the shampoo on first. If you put water on your hair it will interfere with the break down of the oil molecules and will make the oil harder to remove – it's the same principle as using oil paint and then trying to clean your brush with water. On the other hand, shampoo without water emulsifies with the oil, making it easier to rinse out later. You will probably need to use a lot of shampoo, but don't be alarmed at the amount you are using as it will take a lot to get the oil out of the hair. It is unlikely at this stage that you'll notice any lather. Once you have thoroughly shampooed your whole head, begin the whole process again as if you were starting from scratch.

Still without water, shampoo over your whole head and hair, working it well into the hair fibres. If you have long hair, take a handful and rub it between your hands as if you were scrubbing. At this point, it is likely that you will begin to see some lather. This is a good sign and indicates that you are well on the way to being able to wash out the oil successfully. Work your way round the whole head, rubbing your hair between your hands. When this is all worked in, shampoo again for a third time, working it in as before. When this stage is finished you are ready for rinsing.

Using warm water (once again the temperature will help break down any residual oil), thoroughly rinse out the shampoo. For a final time, shampoo your hair again. Your hair should be a mass of lather and soapsuds by now, so you should only need to use a little shampoo for this final wash. Rinse out as usual. Your hair is now ready for your usual drying and styling.

aftercare

To maintain the good you've just done to your hair, follow some of the advice suggested in the section on hair care. Particularly, try to leave your hair to dry naturally if you have the time. If you only have a little time to spare, and need to use a hairdryer, remove any excess water from the hair by towel-drying it first. This reduces the drying effects of a hairdryer.

▽ **Your hair should be free of oil and full of foamy suds by the end of the oil-removing session. It should be in tip top condition.**

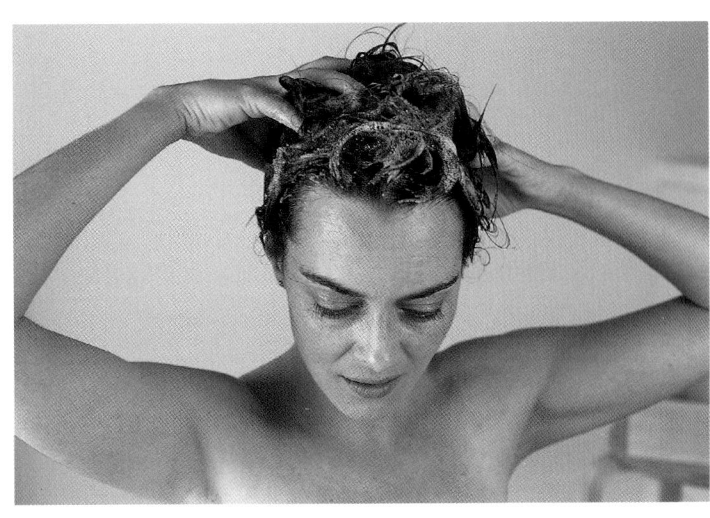

Getting started

One of the beauties of Indian head massage is that it can be performed almost anywhere and doesn't need a lot of equipment. The essentials are a suitable chair, a pair of hands, a willing heart and knowledge of what to do. To get the most out of it, a few preliminaries will help put you and your partner in the right frame of mind. These include getting all your equipment together, scene setting, and preparing yourself and your partner for a treatment.

seating

The best chair is one without any arms and a relatively low back to give you easy access to your partner. Cushions or pillows can be used to soften or raise seating or to provide comfort or support. However, you can always adjust the massage according to the situation. For instance, if you can't get to your partner's arms easily then just stroke them gently. If your partner is too tired to sit up, they could sit astride the seat and lean over the back of the chair, supported by cushions. The most important thing is for them to be comfortable.

▽ Make sure that you prepare a relaxing space and have everything to hand before you begin so that your massage will go smoothly. A low backed chair without arms is ideal.

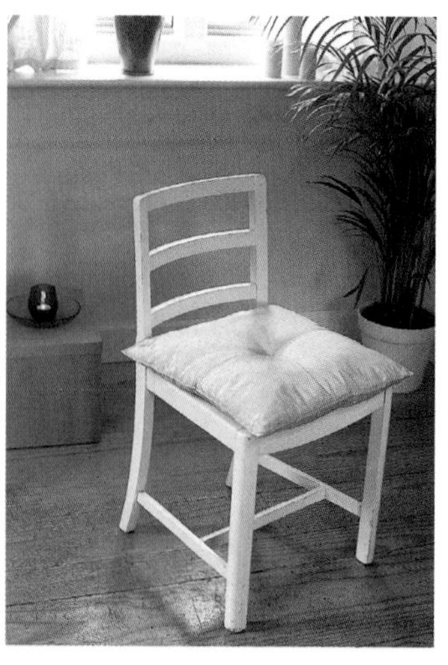

preparation

Clean and tidy the room to create a harmonious space that is easy to work in. Make sure that it is warm, and eliminate as many potential distractions as you can. Unplug the phone, turn off any mobiles, and put a "do not disturb" sign on the door.

Next think about mood setting. Sound, lighting and fragrance can all be used to help create a particular ambience and turn the room into a healing space. Candles give a soft and subdued light, while certain types of music can help you relax. Burning incense or vaporizing essential oils will fragrance the air, as well as helping to clear impurities. If you want to use music and/or scent, choose something that both you and your partner will enjoy.

Make sure that you are wearing loose comfortable clothes, and take a few moments to make the following preparations. You also need to take a few

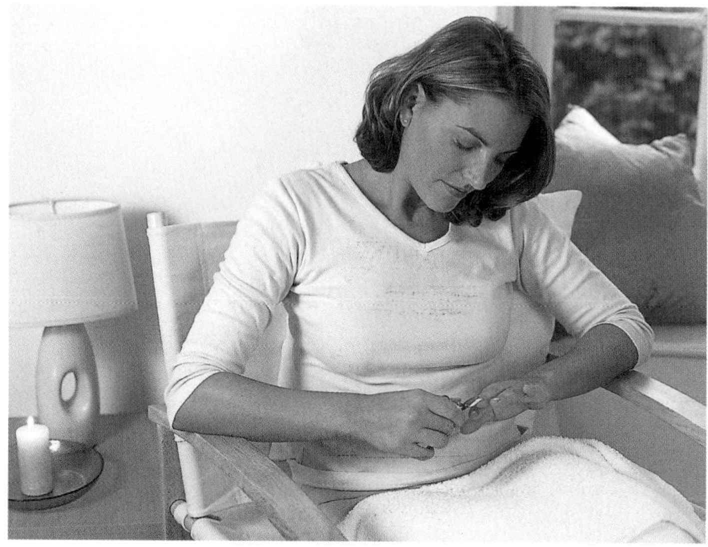

△ Remove your watch, and any rings or bracelets, and wash your hands. File your nails so that they are short and smooth to the touch.

▽ Make sure your hair is tied back or clipped up so that it does not fall over your face as you massage, as this is distracting.

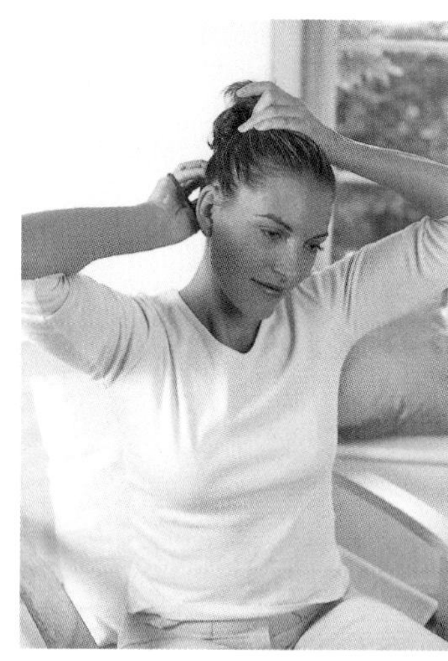

▷ Spend some talking with your partner so you can check for contraindications as well as tune in to each other and establish a smooth rapport before beginning the session.

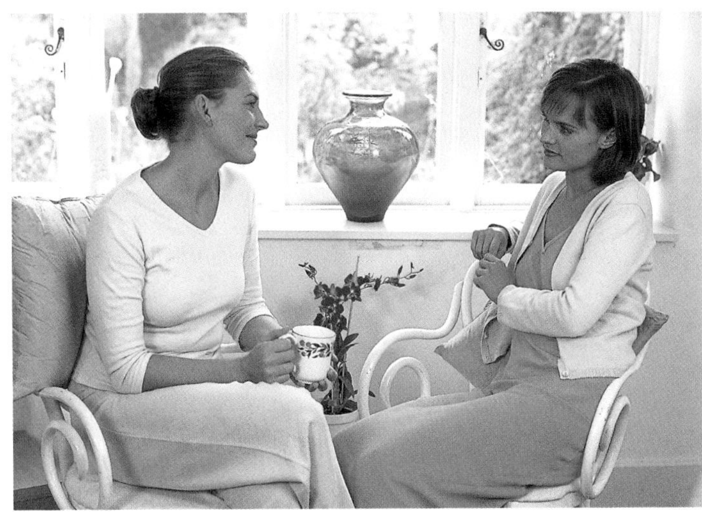

equipment

If you are using any oils, set them out with a little bowl for mixing. You will also need a pack of tissues for wiping your hands and a blanket to cover your partner if they get cold. Also have plenty of drinking water available for yourself and your partner.

moments to make sure you are "grounded". To do this, sit in a comfortable chair and relax. Now close your eyes and take a deep, slow breath into your belly. As you breathe out, imagine channels of energy travelling down through your body, legs and feet and into the ground. Think of your feet having extensions that stretch deep down into the earth like the roots of a tree. As you breathe in, imagine the energy coming up again through the roots and into your body, replenishing you with new energy. As you breathe in and out, see this continuous movement of energy. Once you are grounded, you are ready to warm up.

▽ Take some time to breathe deeply, relax your own mind and body and tune in and calm yourself, otherwise known as grounding.

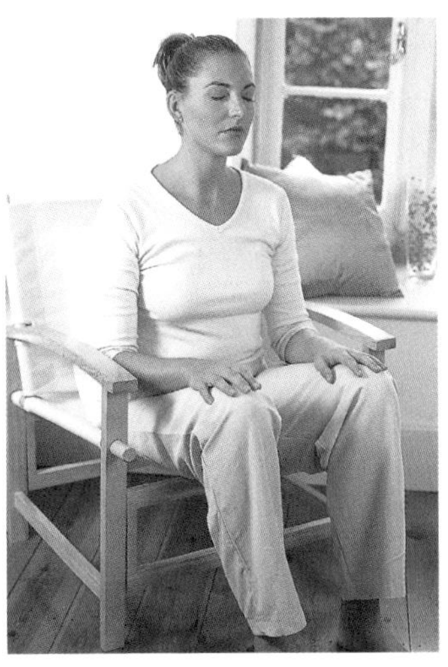

warming up

Giving yourself a shake-out will warm up your body and help you let go of tension. Stand in a clear space and have a chair to lean on, if necessary. Pick up one leg and shake it out so that it wobbles. Circle your foot at the ankle in both directions. Repeat on the other side. Next move to your arms and repeat. Circle your hands at the wrists in both directions and shake them out.

making contact and tuning in

Sit with your partner and spend a few moments checking in together, making sure there are no contraindications. Review any areas of tension and find out where they would like you to prioritize. Have them remove any jewellery and loosen their hair, if necessary. It is best if they are wearing a loose t-shirt or vest top. Make sure they are sitting comfortably, with both feet placed squarely on the ground. You might like to put a pillow under their feet for comfort. Ensure there is enough space for you to work around them freely. Ask your partner if they will let you know if there is anything they don't like or is uncomfortable during the massage, and give them permission to relax their body and mind and switch off during the treatment. You are now ready to tune in to your partner.

Stand behind your partner and place your hands on top of their head. Close your eyes and let go of your thoughts, tuning in to your partner's breathing and energy field. If you have a spiritual belief, you might offer it up as a type of prayer. Then very gently move your partner's head, first forwards and then backwards, and then to the right and left. Finally, let your hands slide lightly down from the head, over the neck to a point level with the bottom of the shoulder blades. You are now tuned in and ready to begin.

▽ The beginning of a massage always begins with a non-verbal tuning-in as your hands touch the head and your energies merge.

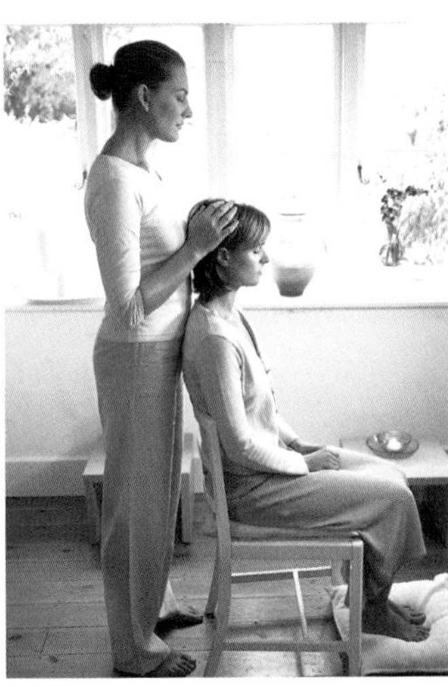

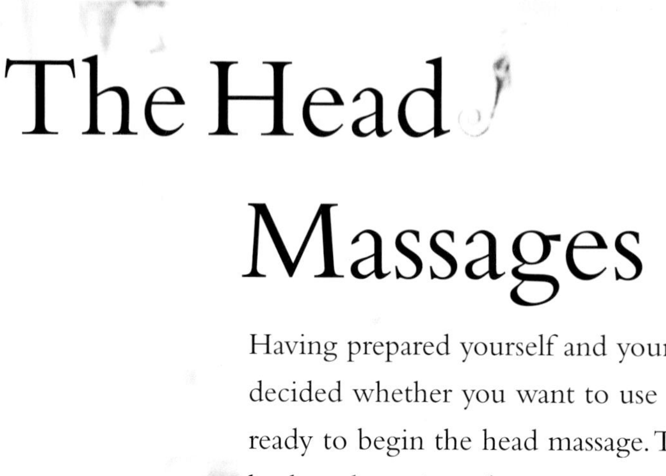

The Head Massages

Having prepared yourself and your partner, and decided whether you want to use oils, you are ready to begin the head massage. This section is broken down into short sequences focusing on a specific area of the body or using a certain technique, so that you can build up your routine in easy stages. Quick-fix and self-massage sequences are also included. As your confidence increases and you become more adept, you will develop your own style of working, uniquely suited to your circumstances.

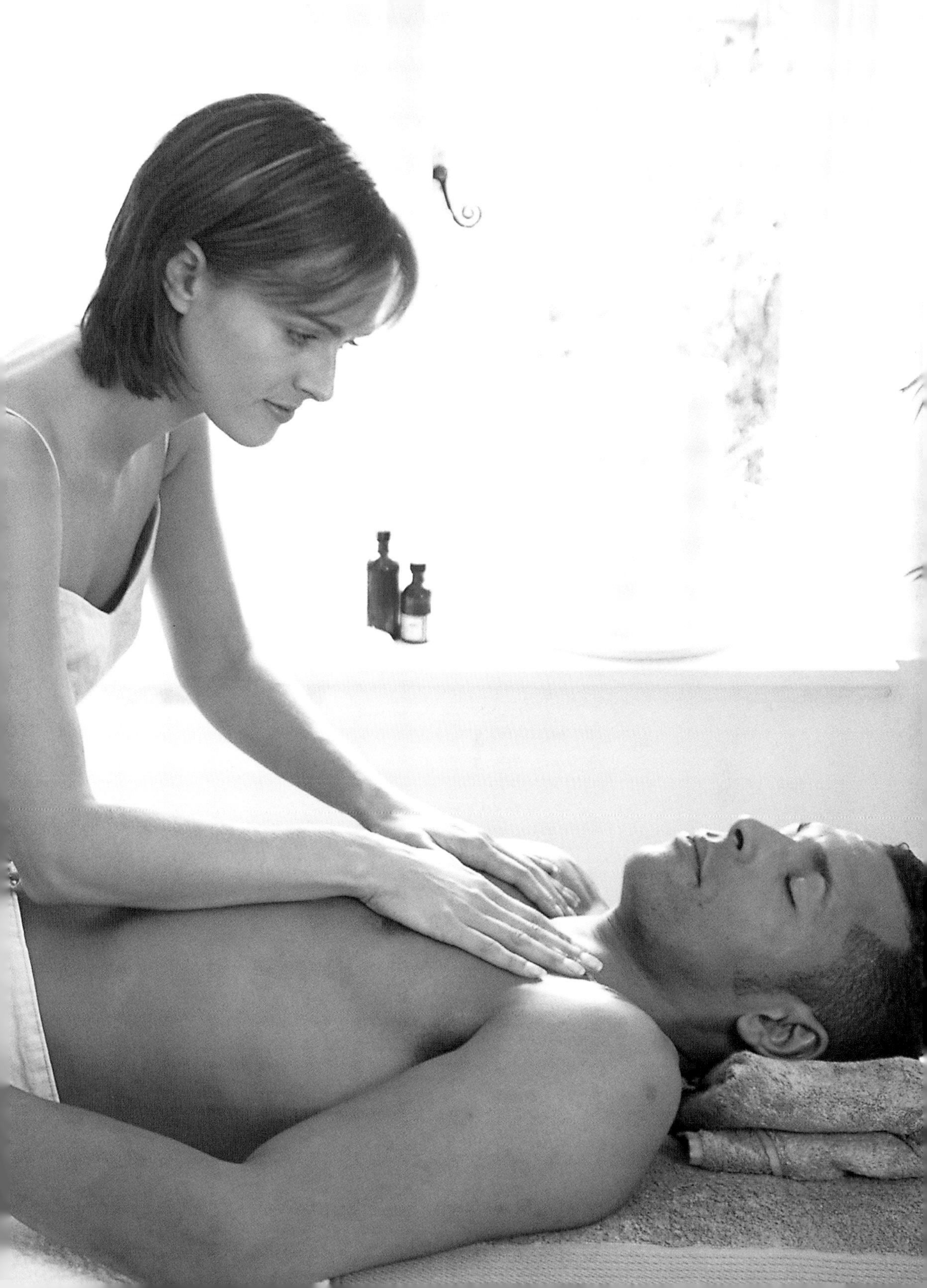

Head massage with a partner

Once you have made all the necessary preparations and have spent a few moments tuning in with your partner, you are ready to begin giving a head massage treatment. The following pages give detailed instructions for a sequence of movements using the basic strokes. To help you, this sequence is divided into sections, each relating to the area of the body being worked on. It begins with the upper back.

the upper back

The strokes outlined here help to relax and release tension in the upper back. Many aches and pains, including tension headaches, begin in this area, particularly in the trapezius (the large muscles over the back of the neck and shoulders). Never work directly on the spine.

▽ **1** Place your thumbs in the ridge that runs up either side of the spine at a point roughly parallel to the bottom of the scapulae (shoulder blades). Spread your other fingers on the back to support your thumbs. To increase your leverage and to prevent back strain, you may need to take a step backwards or bend your knees as you do this stroke.

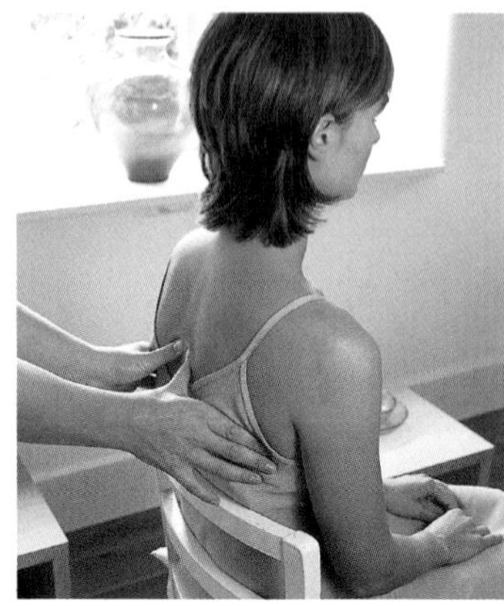

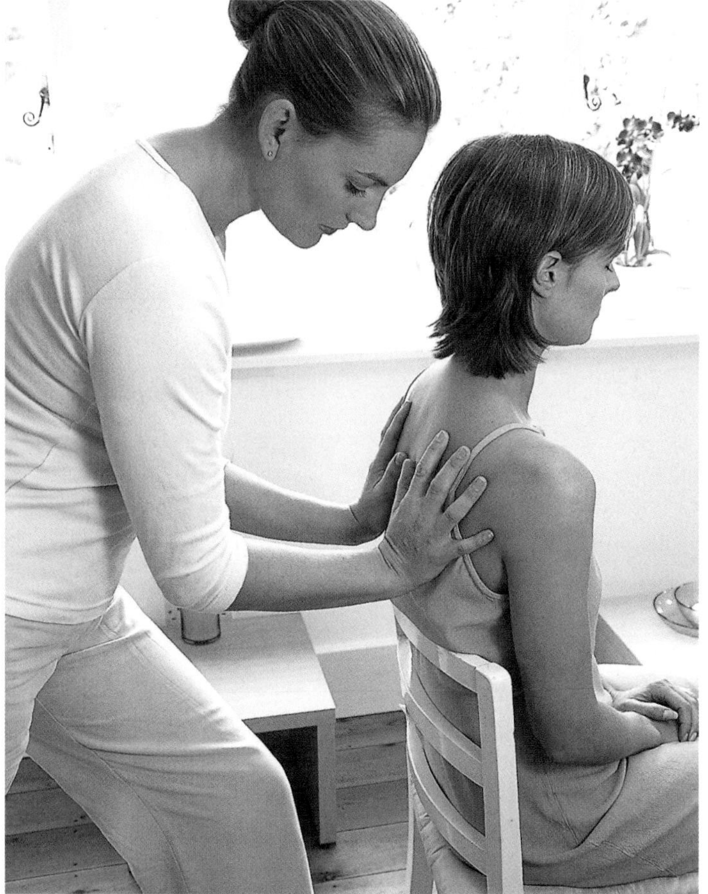

△ **2** In an upward movement, slide and push your thumbs up on either side of the spine. Continue up the back and neck to the top of the spine at the base of the skull. Go back to the starting position and repeat three times, increasing the pressure with each movement. This stroke helps release tension in the muscular attachments that run up the back.

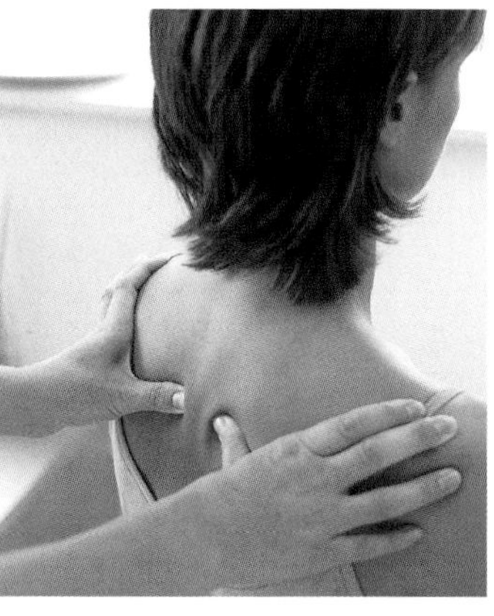

△ **3** Find the muscles that run up either side of the spine, about 2cm (¾in) out. You can feel their line with your fingers, like a rope or a cord down the side of the spine. Using your thumbs or the small bony part on the outside edge of the wrist, make small circular strokes on the belly of the muscle. Work from the middle of the back up to the shoulders.

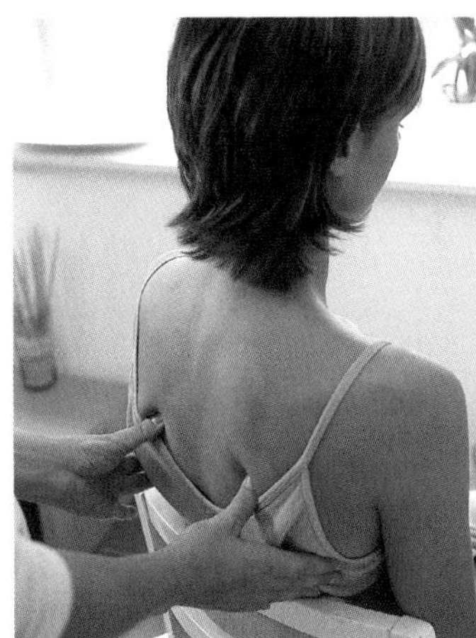

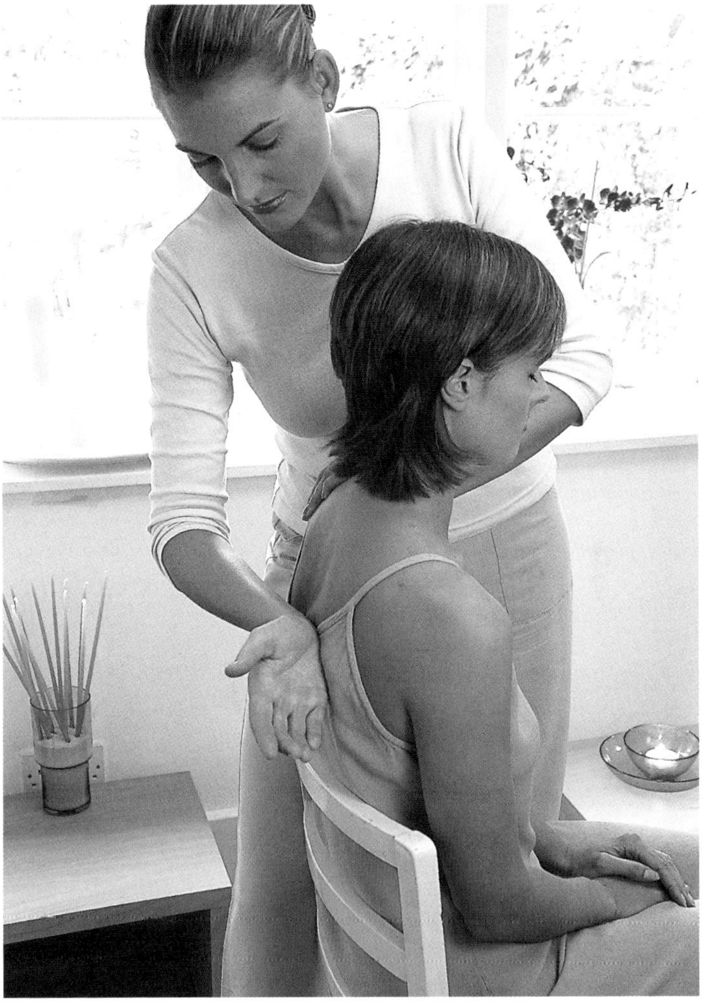

△ **4** Place both your thumbs at the bottom outside edge of your partner's scapulae. Push and slide your thumbs in an upward direction, moving along the edge of the scapulae all the way round to the top of the shoulders. Sweep round to your starting point and repeat three times. This helps release the trapezius attachments around the scapulae.

▽ **5** Move to the left side of your partner and place your left hand gently on their shoulder. Position the fingertips of the first two fingers of your right hand at the base of your partner's right scapula. Using a fast jabbing motion move your fingertips back and forth in a friction movement against or underneath the outer edge of the scapula. Work upwards to the outside edge where the arm attaches and repeat two more times. The most vigorous of the strokes described here, this action releases tension in the muscle attachments and layers.

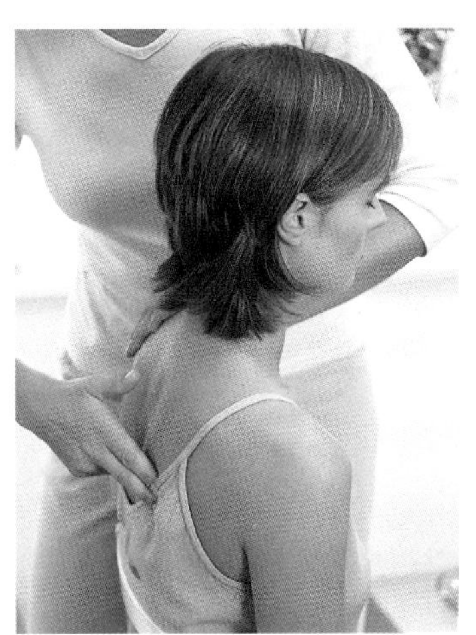

△ **6** Follow the same path around the edge of the scapula, this time using the side of your hand and wrist. Place the side of your hand and the small bony ridge of your wrist at the base of the scapula. Using a circular movement, as if drawing little circles, follow around the edge of the scapula as you progress in an upward direction. This stroke helps to flatten and smooth out the muscles. Repeat three times.

▷ **7** From the top of the scapula stroke the whole shoulder joint in a wide generous movement, using the whole of your hand. Make the circles increasingly wide to take in more and more of the upper back. This is a calming action after the vigorous strokes earlier on. Once you have finished, move round to stand at the other side of your partner and repeat steps 5–7 on the other side.

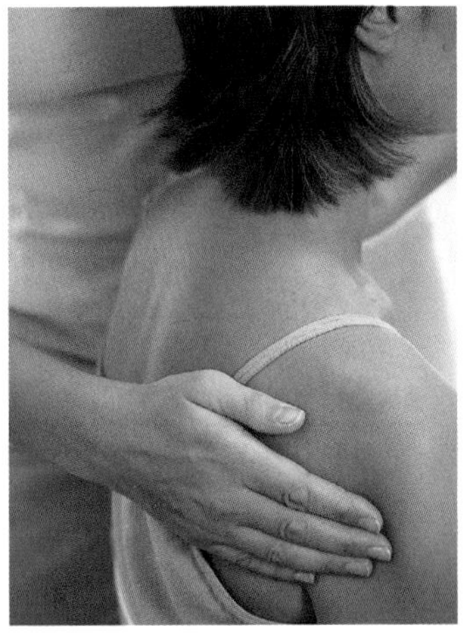

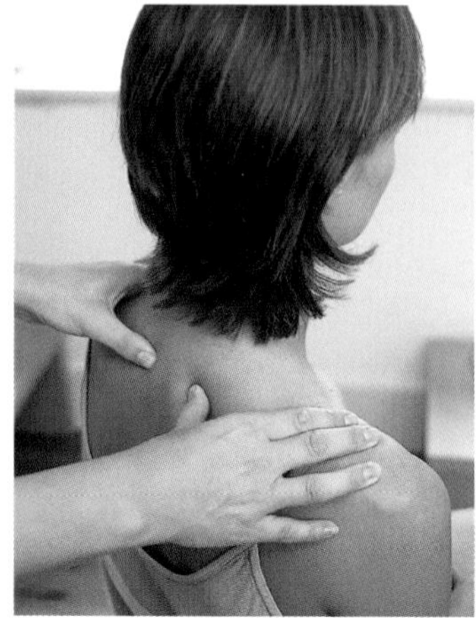

shoulders and arms

After the upper back, the next part of the massage sequence is to work on the shoulders and arms. When you get to this part of the massage, most people are usually very grateful, as the arm and shoulder area is generally very tight and achy. Our arms perform countless tasks that we take for granted – pushing, pulling, lifting and carrying all manner of things, big and small. Shoulder tension is also connected with emotional burdens and responsibilities from "carrying the world on our shoulders".

When massaging the shoulders, it is best to proceed cautiously as the muscles can have a tendency to contract even further, particularly in response to deeper massage. If you feel this happening then change immediately to lighter, more sweeping strokes.

▽ **1** Rest your hands lightly on your partner's shoulders, and as they breathe out, use your body weight to gently push down on their shoulders. Notice with your hands when you feel the resistance and release. Next use both hands to make a wide sweeping movement, brushing across the tops of the shoulders away from the body. Do this a few times. It is a gentle stroke that warms up the area and prepares the body for deeper massage.

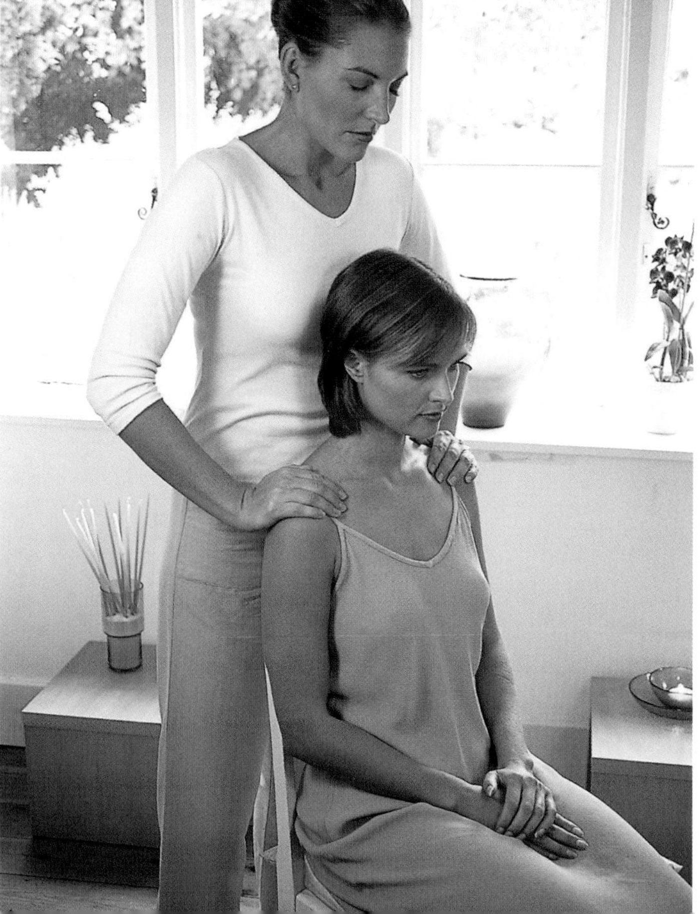

△ **2** Rest your thumbs at the base of your partner's neck. Using the pads of your thumbs, make circular, pressing stokes over the whole of the trapezius muscle that runs along the base of the neck, top of the back and across the shoulders. This warms up the muscles and makes them more pliable for kneading. How hard you press will depend on the feedback you receive from your partner.

▽ **3** Pick up a roll of flesh from the trapezius muscles with the thumb and fingers of one hand and slide it across to feed the other hand in a smooth rhythmical way. Repeat the movement with the other hand. This kneading action is similar to kneading bread dough. Keep this up for a few minutes and establish a regular rhythm, adjusting the speed and pressure according to your partner's needs. This is a very popular stroke for a key area of tension. Work for a few minutes on each shoulder without overworking the muscles.

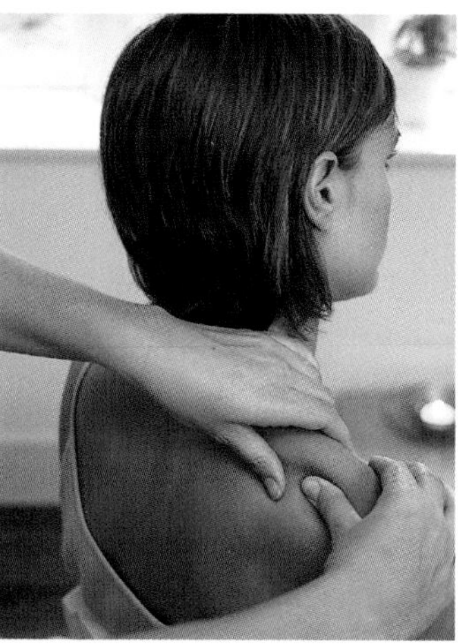

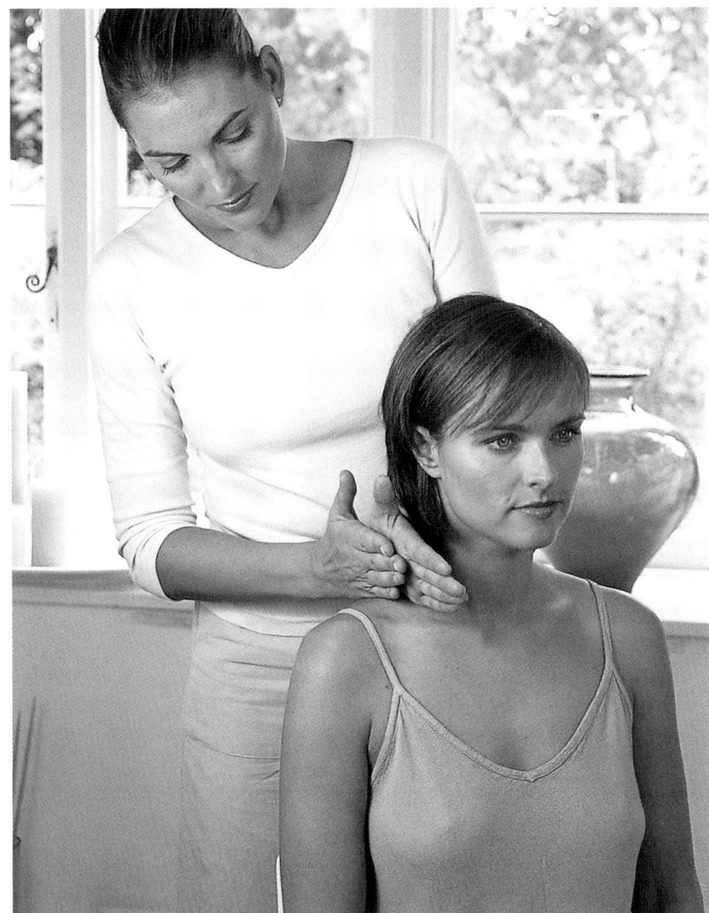

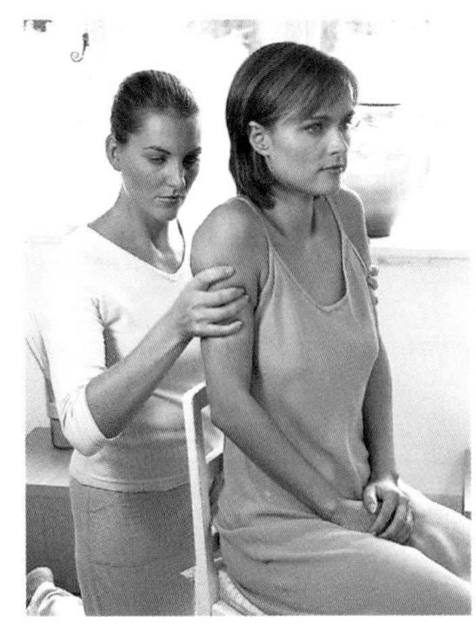

△ **6** Slide your hands down to the tops of your partner's arms and hold there for a moment in preparation for the shoulder shrug. Ask your partner to take a deep breath in and as they do so lift their arms slightly so that their shoulders are raised near their ears. As they breathe out, let go of their arms. The shoulders may drop down abruptly. Repeat once.

▽ **7** Place the heel of each hand at the top of your partner's arms. Roll down the arms, turning your wrists in a circular action. Use firm pressure as you go and continue down to the elbow joint. In a continuous movement, roll around to the back of the arm and move back up. Roll over the tops of the shoulders and continue down the arms again until you have completed the whole cycle three times.

△ **4** Place both hands together as if in prayer position and put them side-on near the base of your partner's neck. Slowly rub your hands together, applying a little pressure as you move across the surface of your partner's shoulder in a sawing action. Build up speed as you get into the rhythm of it. Travel across the top of one shoulder and saw down a little into the upper back area, working on the muscles either side of the spine. Then in a continuous movement, jump your hands over the spine and continue working on the opposite side of the upper back, travelling up and across to the other shoulder. Repeat three times.

▷ **5** Lift and drop your hands alternately. As each one descends, let the sides of your fingers hit down lightly on the skin for this hacking stroke. Your fingers should be soft as they knock together on impact. Move across the shoulders and upper back, building up momentum. Work over the area three times. Slow down gradually to bring to a close.

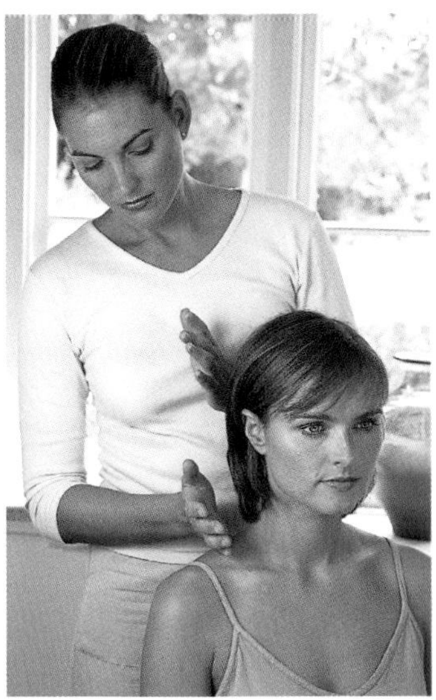

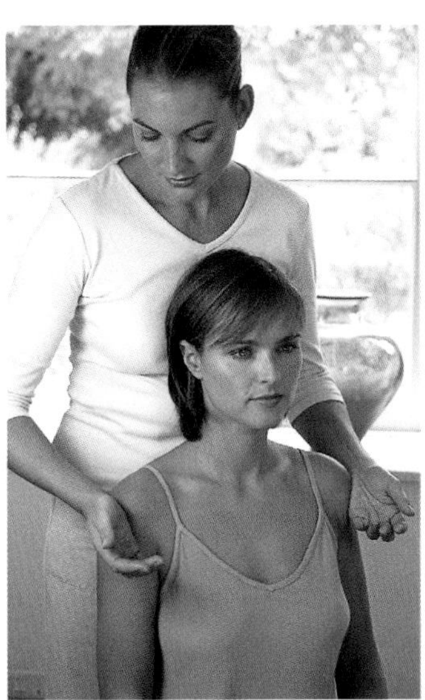

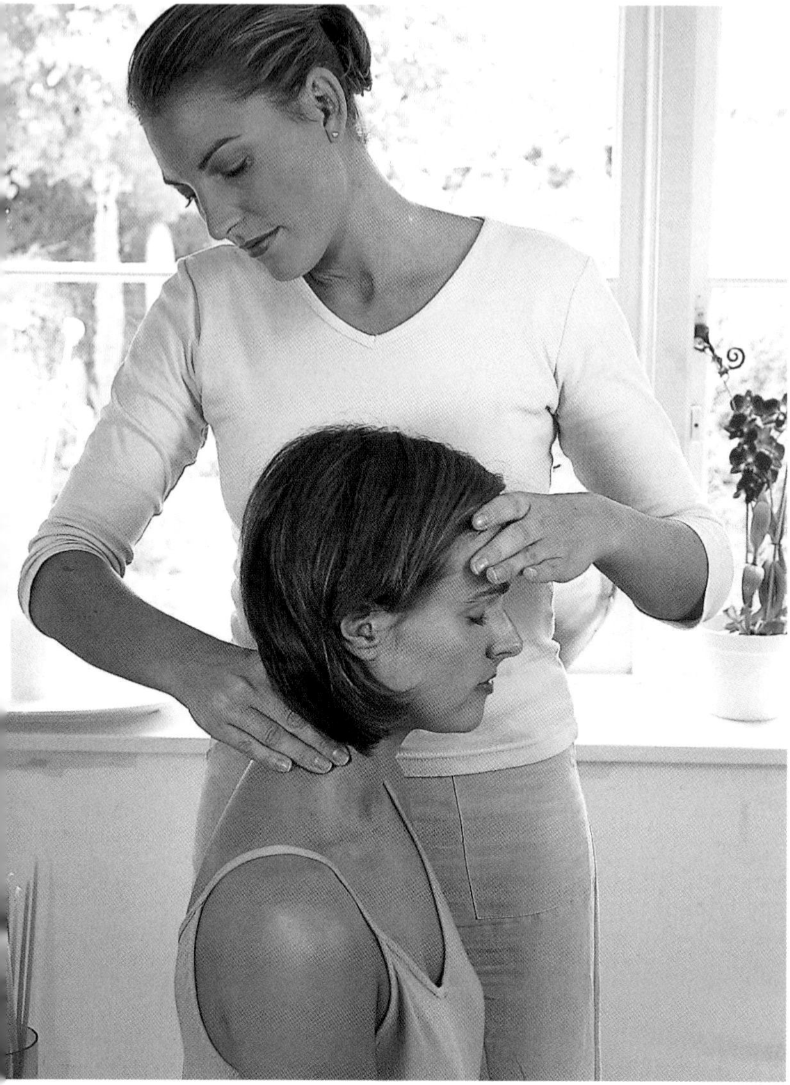

the neck

The head, neck and back are held in dynamic relationship. When all three are working as they should, we tend to feel good in every respect. The neck has a particularly important part to play. It should be long, stretching up and away from the shoulders, supporting the head with a wide range of movement. Poor posture and stress cause tension in the neck, the muscles to become imbalanced and the head to be thrown forward. Due to the uneven strain, some neck muscles can be in a permanent state of contraction, with tension knots particularly at the base and top of the neck. This imbalance puts a tremendous strain on the upper back and shoulder muscles because they are part of the same muscle group. Over time this can build up and become chronic, making the neck more prone to injury. Tight neck muscles are one of the main causes of tension headaches.

Massaging the neck helps to ease out tension and stiffness, giving greater comfort and increased mobility. It can also help to relieve headaches. When working on the neck you need to support your partner's head with one hand. Swap hands as often as you need to, but keep the movement flowing. Make sure you work at a level that is comfortable for your partner.

◁ **1** Stand to the left of your partner. To support your partner's head, place the thumb and the middle finger of your left hand on either side of their forehead, using a firm but soft grip. Place your right hand at the base of the neck and with a wide span, grasp and pull back the neck's flesh and muscles. Sweep your hand up a little and repeat the movement in the middle and at the top of the neck. Repeat the whole sequence three times. This warms up the neck and loosens the muscles.

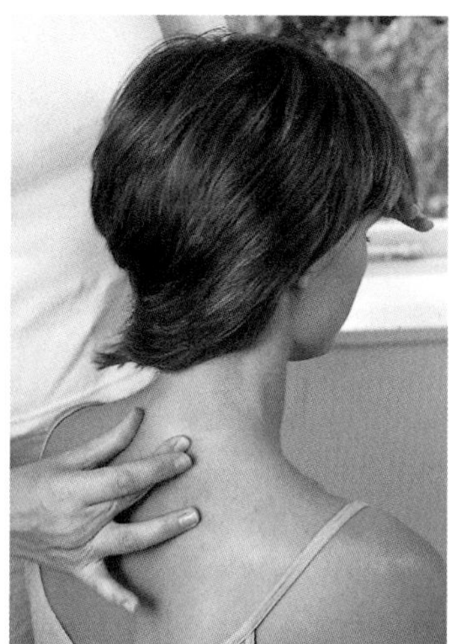

△ **2** Continuing to support your partner's head with your left hand, use your right thumb to slide up the muscles, massaging in a circling action. Continue to the top of the neck where the skull attaches. Bring your thumb down and repeat. Follow with some circular strokes (petrissage) around the back and sides of the neck, using your fingers and thumbs together in a circling upward movement. Do not go as far round to the front as the windpipe or cause your partner any discomfort.

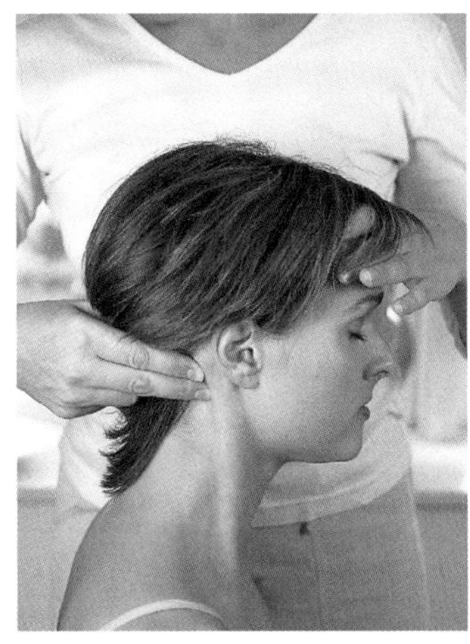

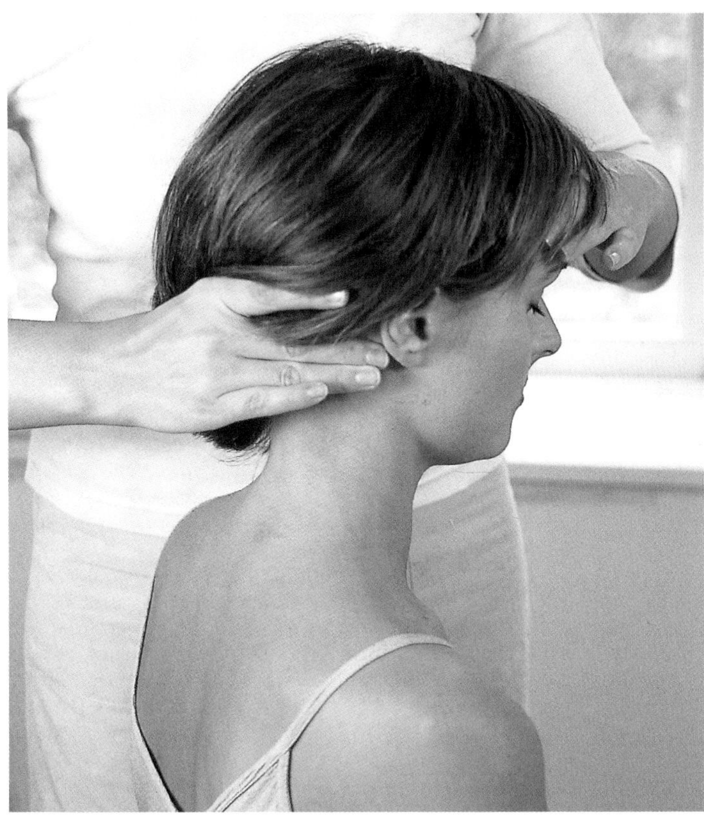

△▽ **3** Starting at the bony ridge behind the back of the ear, make small circular strokes across the base of the skull to the middle of the neck, using the first two fingers of your right hand. Continue the stroke down the middle of the neck along the ridge by the side of the spine. Repeat three times. Work very sensitively, as this area is often tender. Gently increase the pressure as the neck muscles release. Swap hands, move to your partner's right side and repeat steps 2–3.

△ **4** Stand on your partner's left and, supporting their head (step 1), stretch out your right hand to reach either side of the base of their skull with your thumb and middle finger. Press and slide your outstretched fingers along the base of the skull to the middle and then move down the neck on either side of the spine. Repeat three times. This stroke works on the lymphatic system and helps flush out toxins released earlier. The hand position is good when using your thumb to work on pressure strokes to the neck.

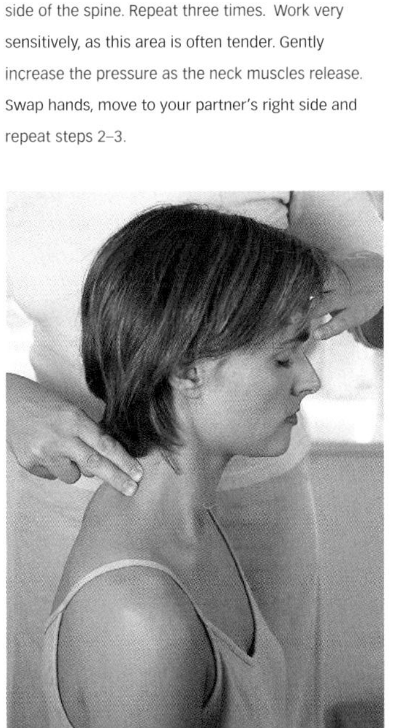

pressure strokes for the neck

As you perform this massage routine, you will be stimulating acupressure points that can have a therapeutic influence on specific body organs and systems and help relieve symptoms of ill health. It can also release endorphins, serving to unblock stuck energies and restore balance to the body as a whole. When massaging over these points, be sensitive to the amount of pressure you apply. Exerting pressure on the various points around the neck can help stiffness and pain, headaches, eyestrain and imbalances in the eyes, ears and throat. Massage here will also have a positive effect on relieving stress, exhaustion and irritability. In the case of pregnancy avoid pressure strokes to the neck and shoulders.

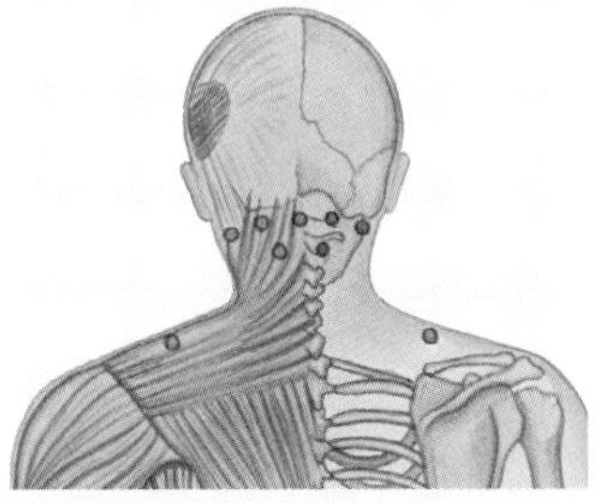

the face

Facial expressions and "character" lines can tell us a lot about someone. Our facial muscles are highly versatile and work hard in transmitting – or concealing – information about ourselves. From a young age, we learn how to "pull ourselves together" or to put on a "brave face" to avoid showing certain emotions. This results in tension being stored in the facial muscles and is compounded by the stress of ordinary living. Typically, worry lines develop across the forehead, the jaw is clenched tight and the eyes can assume a hard, staring look, even appearing to stand out of their sockets.

Because of the very high number of nerve receptors on the facial skin's surface, face massage is a mainline to relaxation. It not only helps the muscles let go of tension, but also sends relaxing signals to the brain, which are then transmitted to the rest of the body.

Facial expressions can be part of our protective armour, and people can look much more youthful and open after a massage because defensiveness has been dropped, and the face restored to a state of natural relaxation.

△ **1** Stand behind your partner and softly draw your hands down over their face to cup the bottom of the face at the jaw. Then slowly draw your fingers and palms up over the face, trailing them across the cheeks and up to the tops of the ears. Extend this stroke to sweep over the eye sockets and take in the forehead. Repeat this upward movement a few times.

▽ **2** Return your hands to cup the bottom of the face, and place the thumb and index finger of both hands in the middle of the chin. With your thumbs on top and the index fingers underneath, gently pick up the fold of flesh along the chin and roll it between your fingers. Work along and just under the edge of the jaw line towards the ears. Repeat three times.

location of the lymph nodes

Part of the body's immune system, the lymphatic system plays a key part in eliminating toxins. The lymph nodes make and store white blood cells and process wastes and bacteria before passing fluids back into the circulatory system. Fluids are delivered to the nodes via ducts located throughout the body. The ducts depend on suction and muscle pumping to work effectively, and they have one way valves. Without bodily movement to trigger its mechanisms, its functioning can become sluggish and impaired. An increase in pollution and toxins, compounded by today's sedentary lifestyles, can often result in the lymphatic system becoming overloaded.

Massage action can stimulate the effective functioning of the lymph. Face massage works directly on the lymph nodes located in the face and neck and can directly support and benefit detoxing.

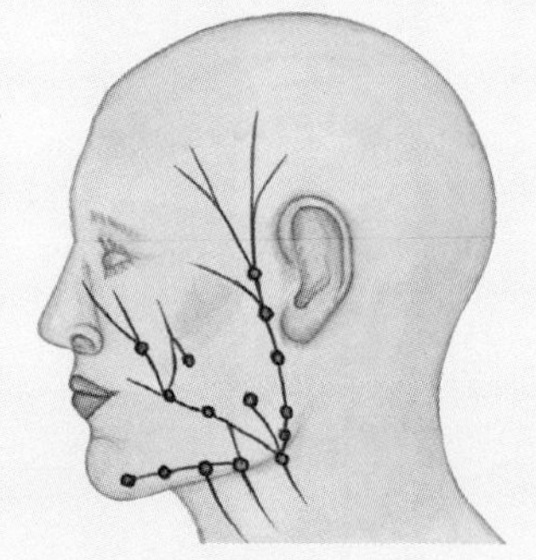

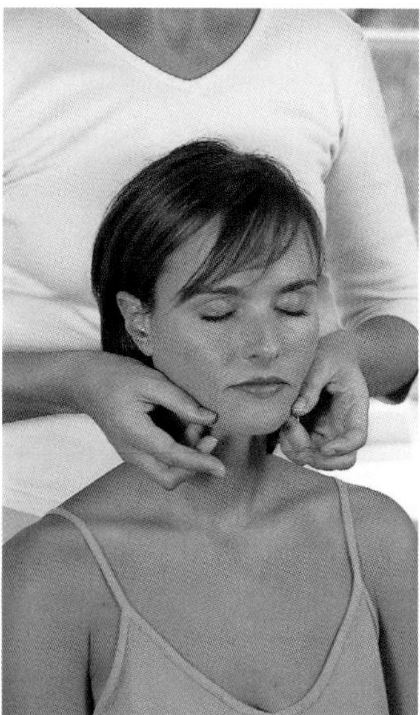

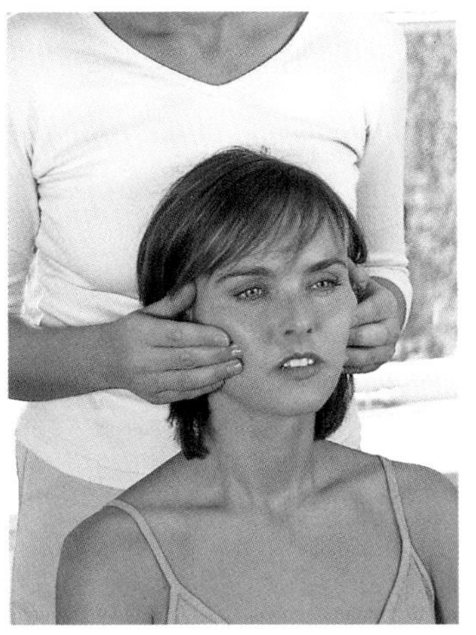

△ **3** At the jaw socket by the ears, make circular strokes with your fingertips, paying particular attention to the hinge area. If your partner is holding their jaw tight, you may be able to feel it release and drop as you work. You could also ask them to drop their mouth open, which will help release jaw tension.

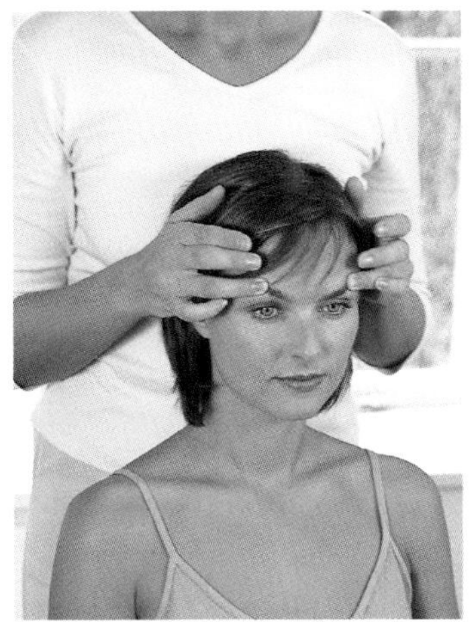

△ **4** Use your ring fingers to gently press at three evenly spaced points along the eyebrow. Begin at the inner edge and finish at the outer. Repeat the stroke directly above these points in the middle of the forehead and then at top of the forehead. Repeat the sequence two times. Finish by stroking the forehead.

the ears

In Chinese medicine, the ears are seen as a microcosm of the whole body, rather like the feet in reflexology. The earlobe corresponds to the head and the face areas, the outside edge to the spine, and the middle to the body's inner organs. In such a small surface area, the ear is highly concentrated in acupressure points. Massage to the ears can stimulate the brain, improve the movement of lymph, help circulation and alleviate pain and stiffness generally from the muscles and joints.

The ears are full of nerve endings and their massage can feel wonderfully pleasant, intimate and stimulating for the recipient. When massaging use your fingers and thumbs to work along the outside edge, and only use your index or ring finger to trace inside the hollows of the ear because it is so sensitive here. Work both ears simultaneously, and use your fingers to twiddle along the outer edge or gently pull down on the ear lobes. A calming way to end a massage is to cover your partner's ears with the palms of your hands for a few moments.

▽ The ear has a high concentration of pressure points, and according to Chinese medicine can be seen as a microcosm of the entire body.

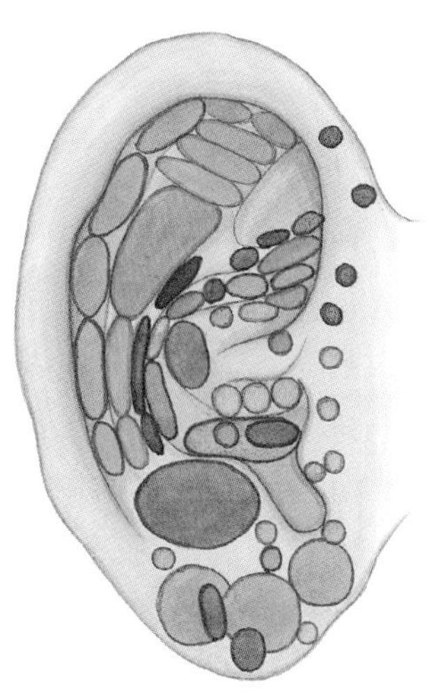

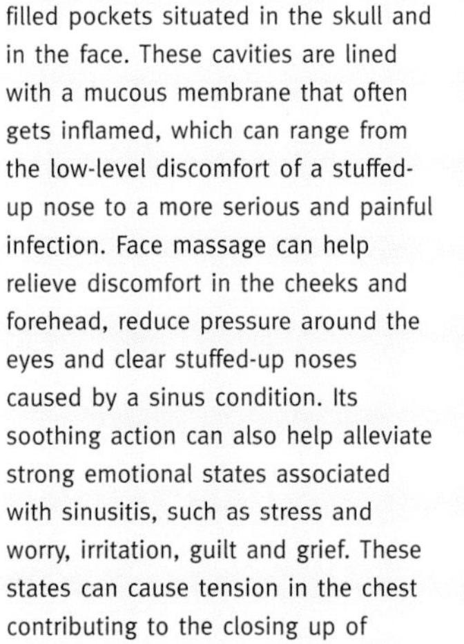

location of the sinuses

Structurally the sinuses are four air-filled pockets situated in the skull and in the face. These cavities are lined with a mucous membrane that often gets inflamed, which can range from the low-level discomfort of a stuffed-up nose to a more serious and painful infection. Face massage can help relieve discomfort in the cheeks and forehead, reduce pressure around the eyes and clear stuffed-up noses caused by a sinus condition. Its soothing action can also help alleviate strong emotional states associated with sinusitis, such as stress and worry, irritation, guilt and grief. These states can cause tension in the chest contributing to the closing up of the sinus passages.

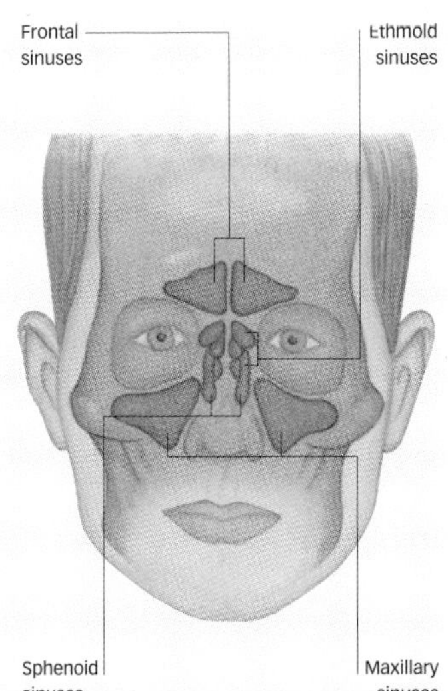

the head

The final part of the massage sequence is spent working on the head, which contains many pressure points that relate to other parts of the body. People are often surprised by how much tension is stored in the musculature of the head. This may be related to tension held in the back muscles travelling up the spine and into the head, or it may be caused by mental overload. Massaging the head is a very effective antidote to stress, as it loosens tension in the scalp and benefits the whole body.

Keep your hands moving as you use the several different strokes, keeping a sense of rhythm and flow as one stroke moves into the next. As you start each different stroke, begin slowly, building up the pace before slowing it down again as you draw to a close and move to the next movement.

▽ **1** Stand to the left of your partner and support their forehead. Put the right hand at the front of their face before the ear by the hairline. Using three or four fingers, rub the scalp briskly back and forth in a vigorous sawing movement. This is known as the "windscreen wiper" stroke. Work from the front of the head down to the hairline at the back, moving across the whole of the left side of the head. Do this three times, then repeat on the other side of the head.

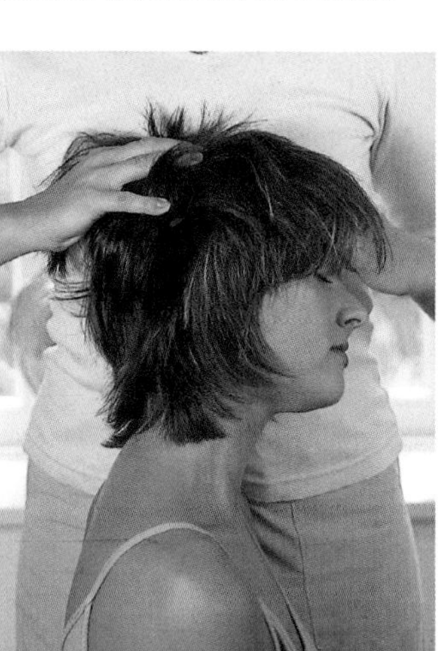

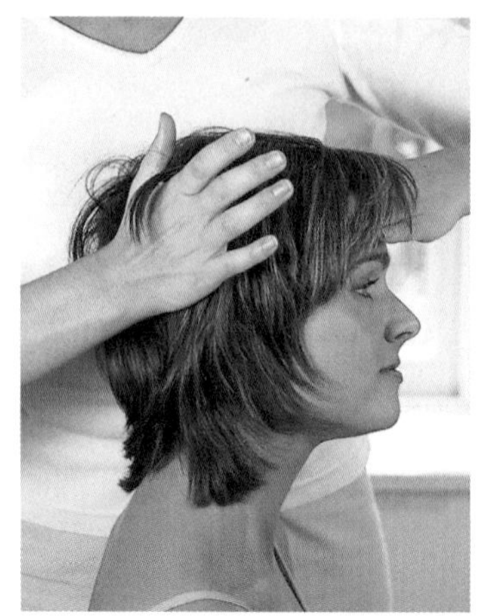

△ **2** Without stopping, use the heel of your right hand to rub briskly over the whole head as if you were buffing it up. Use firmer pressure at the base of the skull, repositioning yourself, if necessary, to get the heel of your hand under the occiput. Repeat three times. These strokes will increase circulation to the brain, improving efficiency.

▽ **3** Standing behind your partner, slide both hands round to the side of the head. Spread your fingers wide and, with slow deliberate movements, make small circles on your partner's head, applying pressure with your fingertips. You should feel their scalp moving slightly. Using this "shampooing" action, work across the whole head. Repeat three times. This stroke releases the deeper layers of muscle that cover the head.

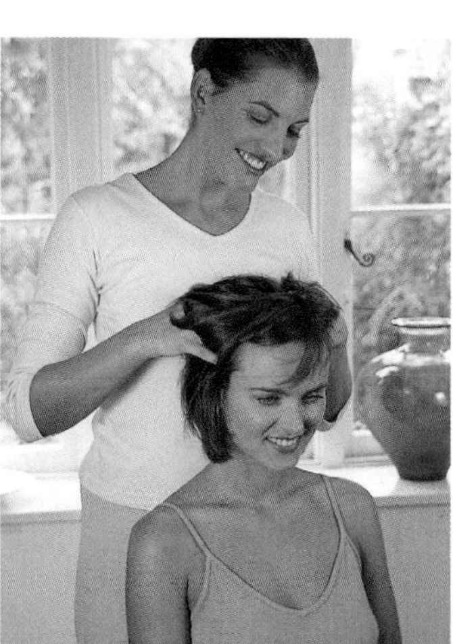

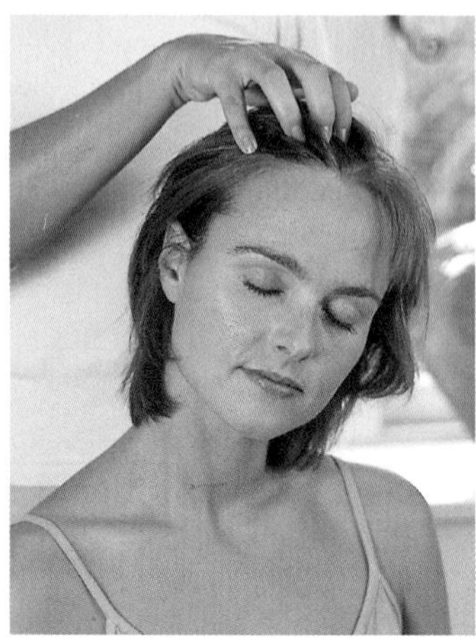

△ **4** Placing one hand at the top of your partner's forehead at the hairline, pull your fingers backwards through the hair in a strong raking movement. Let your other hand follow suit, building up a circular flow so that your partner doesn't have a sense of where one stroke begins and the other ends. Work over the whole head three times. Repeat this action with a slower, gentle ruffling movement through the hair, moving over the whole head three times.

▽ **5** Starting at the front hairline, use the whole of your hand to lightly stroke over your partner's head. Let one hand follow the other in a continuous movement and work down to the base of the skull. Work over the whole head a number of times. This stroking action is calming and soothing to the nervous system.

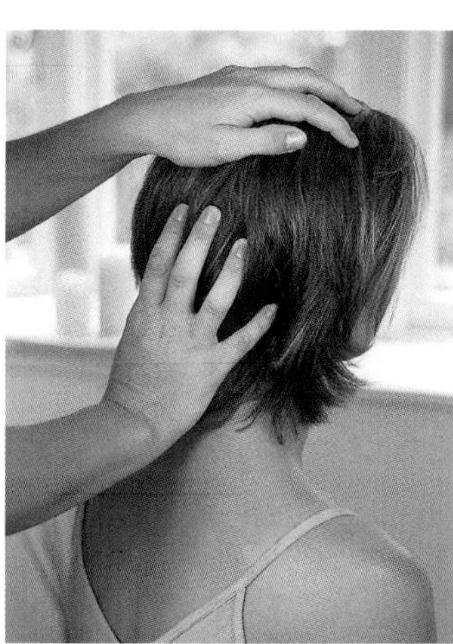

closing the sequence

The feeling of the ending is what will stay with your partner after the massage has finished, so make sure you don't end it too abruptly or insensitively. To round off your treatment, slow your actions down and take your time. Gentle stroking or holding are ideal strokes to use, as the hands gradually trail off the body. Make sure your partner doesn't get up too quickly at the end, but give them a glass of water and leave them to sit for a while.

▷ **1** To close, trail your hands over the top of the head and down the back using a brushing action as if sweeping off cobwebs. Use one hand after the other or both hands together, gradually coming to a stop. Begin slowly and lightly. For a calming, reassuring end, finish in this way, and for an invigorating effect increase to faster, firmer dynamic pressure.

▽ **2** Make sure that your partner is fully alert before getting up, as massage works deeply, and it may take them a while to come round.

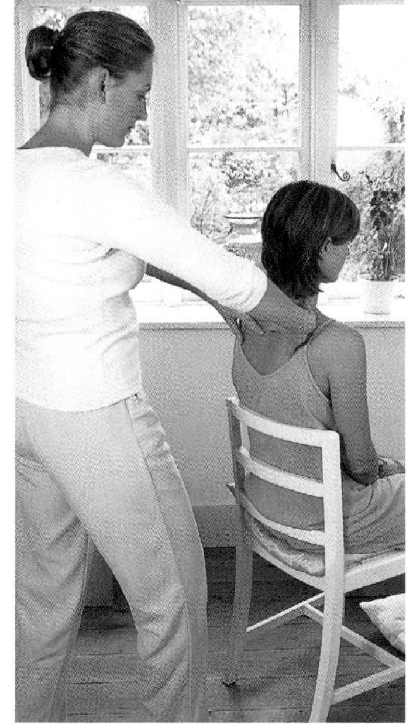

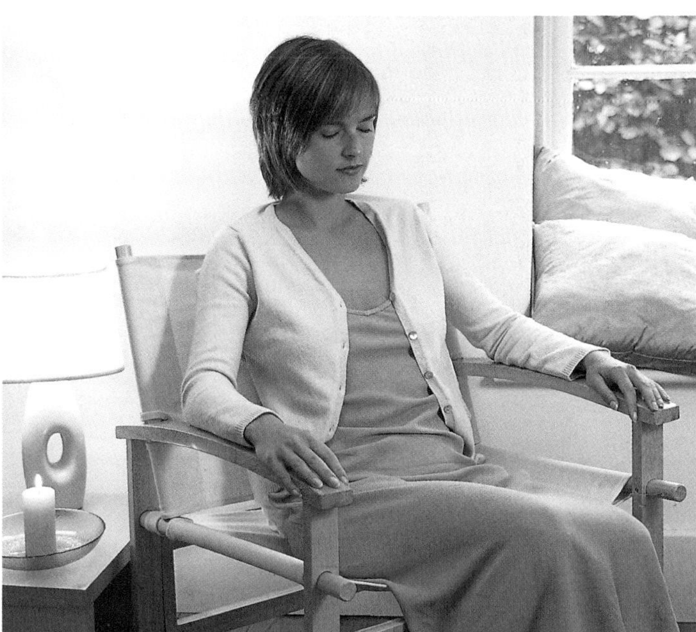

pressure points on the head

The head contains some key pressure points. Massage strokes that work well on these acupressure points include friction strokes, as in steps 1–3, and tapotement or percussion and pressure strokes, as in the basic strokes section. If you wish to apply direct pressure on the points themselves, use the pads of your fingers and gradually increase and decrease the pressure as you come off the points. Hold the pressure for a few seconds only before moving to the next points. Only press as far as feels comfortable for your partner.

Massage on the top of the head relates to improvement in memory and increased mental clarity. It also helps to calm the spirit and clear psychological conflicts. The points at the base of the skull relate to headaches, migraines and stiff necks. The two points on the face are connected with tension in the shoulders and neck, and clearing the lungs and chest of wheezing and coughing.

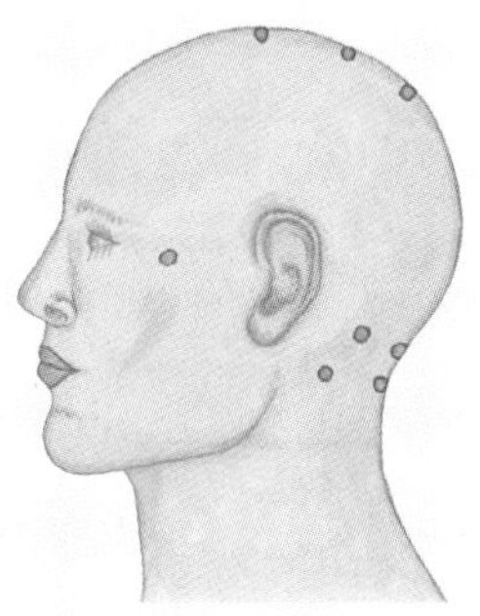

△ **The location of the pressure points on the face, head and base of the skull.**

Head massage lying down

Sometimes you may prefer to give head massage with your partner lying down. This is ideal for when your partner has a headache, is very tired or has a backache from sitting all day. The advantage of lying down is that the neck and shoulder muscles no longer have to support the weight of the head and so have more chance to relax. The routine is similar to the sitting-up sequence except your partner is lying down.

preparation

The same preparation guidelines apply as with the standard sitting-up head massage routine, with one or two additional points to bear in mind. Before you begin, make sure that both you and your partner are comfortable. If your partner feels any discomfort, give their body some more support with cushions or towels beneath the knees or neck. If your partner wears contact lenses, they may want to remove them. Working from a kneeling or sitting position can be tiring, so have a cushion to sit or kneel on. Being uncomfortable during the massage is not only unpleasant for you but will also be communicated to your partner. Have a small bottle of lavender oil to hand in preparation for the face sequence.

▽ Before you begin the massage make sure your partner is comfortable, and then ask them to lie still for a few moments with their hands resting gently on their stomach.

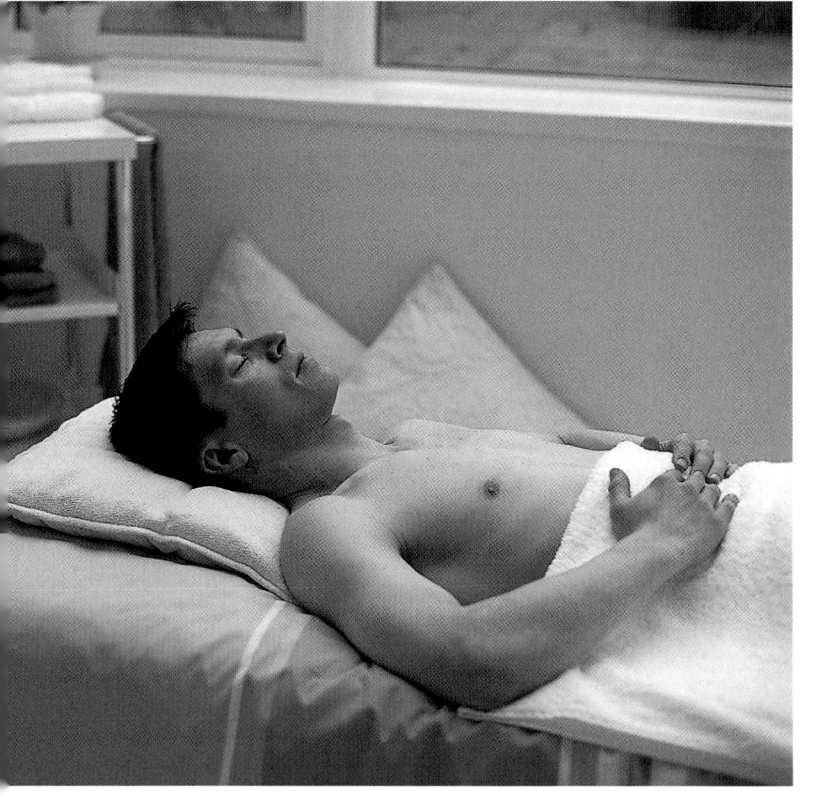

head, neck and shoulders

If you are short of time, you can concentrate on massaging the head, neck and shoulders without having to work on the face.

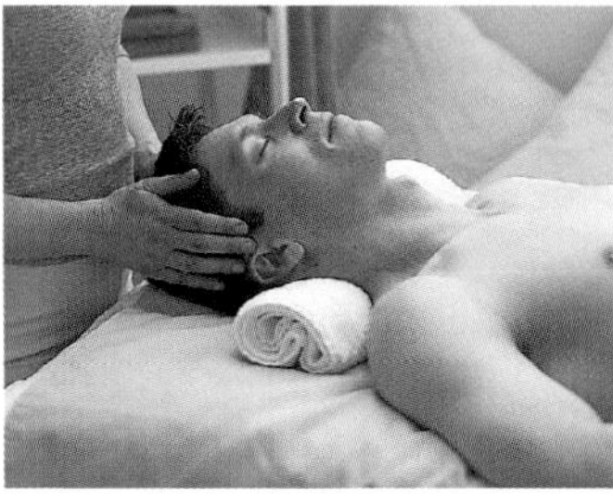

△ **1** Begin by gently placing your hands either side of your partner's head and hold it in this cradled position. Stay still for a few moments and attune your breathing with your partner's.

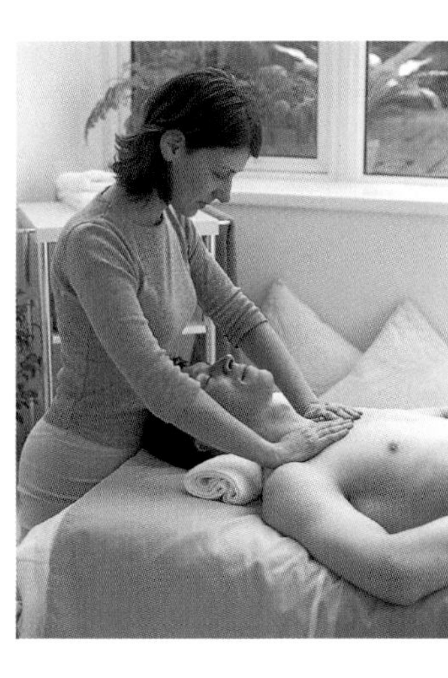

△ **2** Keeping contact with your hands, slide them down to the front of your partner's upper chest to just below the collarbone. The heels of your hands should be resting on the shoulders, with your hands forming a 'V' shape. Ask your partner to take a deep breath in; on the out-breath, press down with your hands, holding the pressure for as long as they breathe out. Repeat.

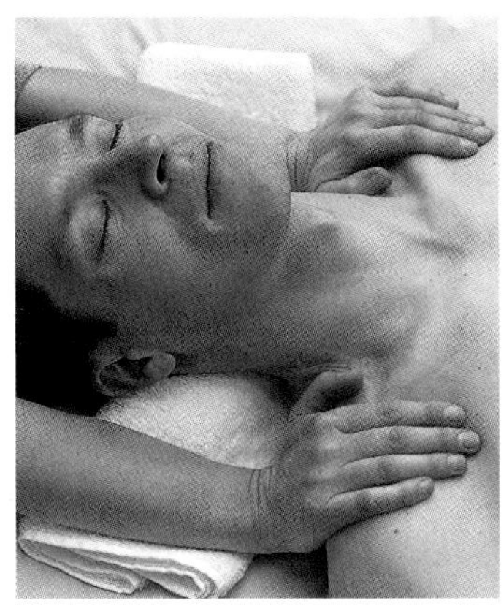

△ **3** Slowly draw your hands up to rest over the top of the shoulders. Listen to your partner's breathing, and as they breathe out push down on the shoulders in the direction of the feet. Repeat twice more.

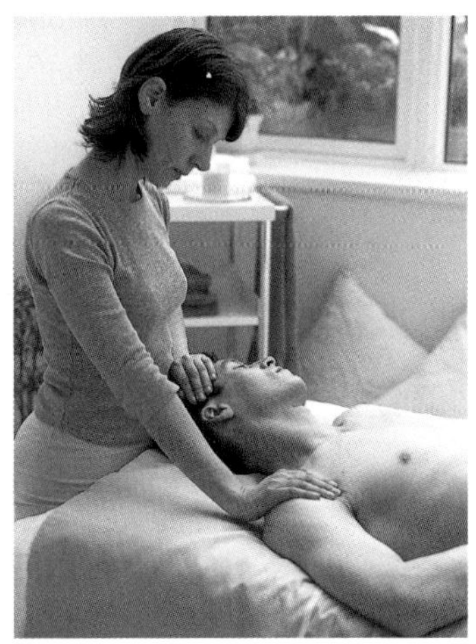

△ **4** Slide both your hands up to the sides of your partner's head and gently turn their head to one side. Keep one hand in position so it is cradling the head. Slide your other hand down the side of your partner's neck to the top of the shoulder. As your partner breathes out, push the shoulder down into the direction of the couch or floor. Repeat twice more.

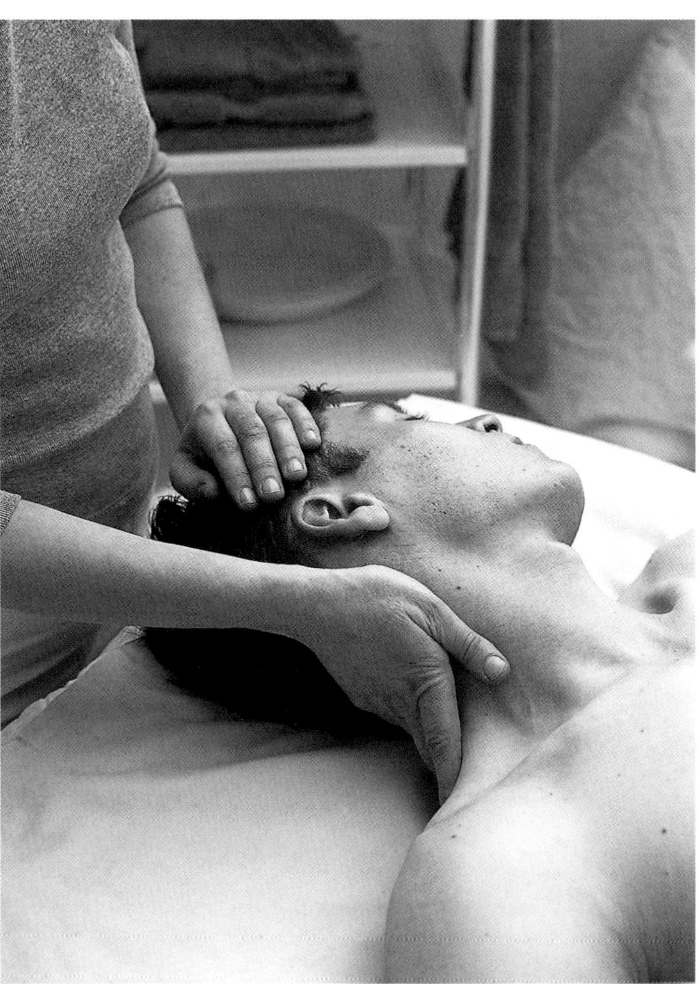

△ **5** Place the palm of your hand at the base of the neck. Using the pads of your fingers, make circular strokes all the way up the side of the neck, being careful to avoid the windpipe area at the front. Then continue circling along the base of the skull, working from the middle towards the ear. Repeat twice. Then slide your hand to the side of your partner's head and turn the head back to a central position before repeating steps 4–5 on the other side.

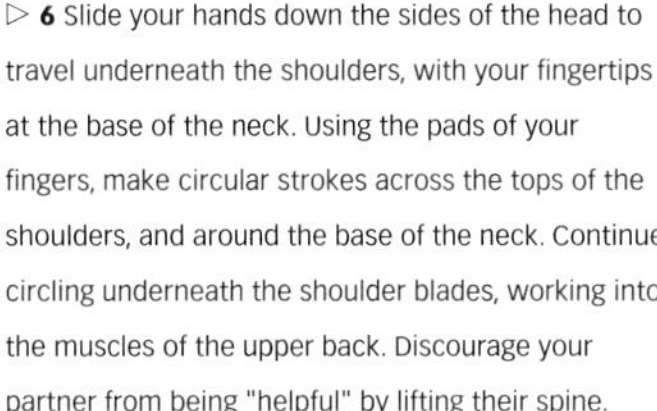

▷ **6** Slide your hands down the sides of the head to travel underneath the shoulders, with your fingertips at the base of the neck. Using the pads of your fingers, make circular strokes across the tops of the shoulders, and around the base of the neck. Continue circling underneath the shoulder blades, working into the muscles of the upper back. Discourage your partner from being "helpful" by lifting their spine.

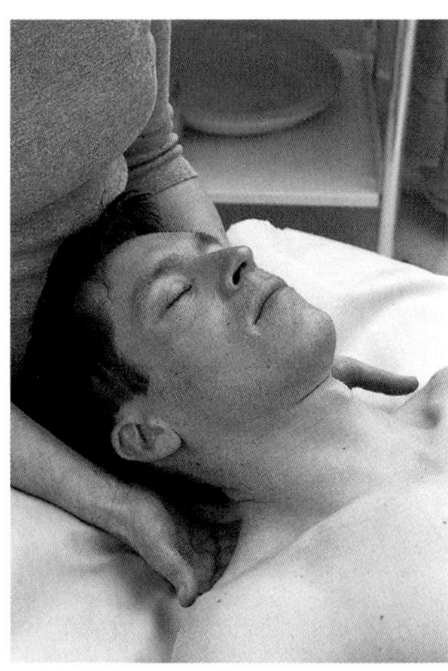

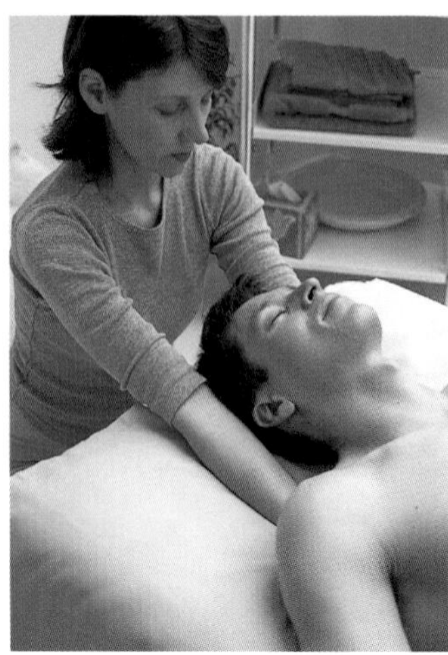

△ **7** Keep your hands underneath the back, palms facing up. Place your middle finger in the ridge that runs either side of the spine – it may be possible to reach as far down as the bottom of the shoulder blades. Ask your partner to take a deep breath in; on the out breath, slowly pull your hands up either side of the spine towards you. Continue the movement through to the top of the neck. Remove your hands and repeat twice more. This is a wonderful stretching stroke for the upper back and neck.

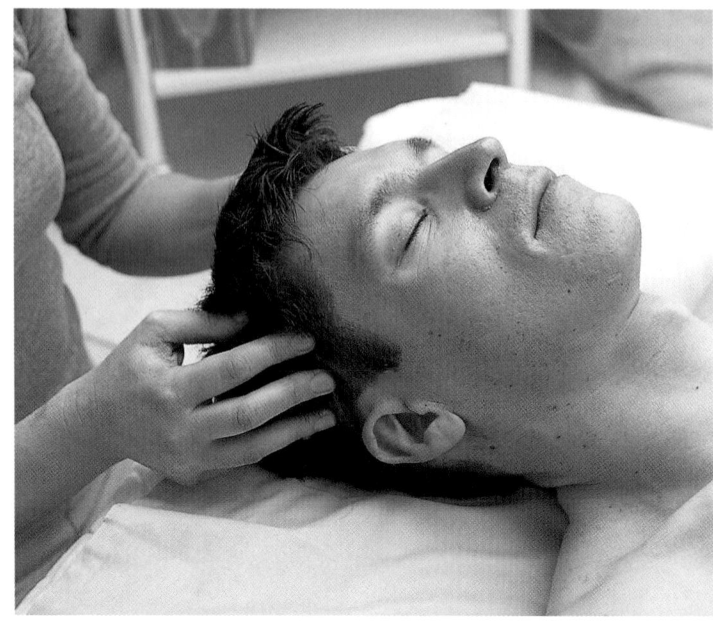

△ **9** Slide your hands to the back of the head. Starting at the back of the ears, use your fingertips to make circular strokes over your partner's scalp. You can either do this with both hands at once, or you may prefer to use one hand to work and the other to support the head. Pay particular attention to the area around the base of the skull, as a lot of tension accumulates here. As the tension loosens, try to feel the scalp moving underneath your fingertips. Work over the scalp three times.

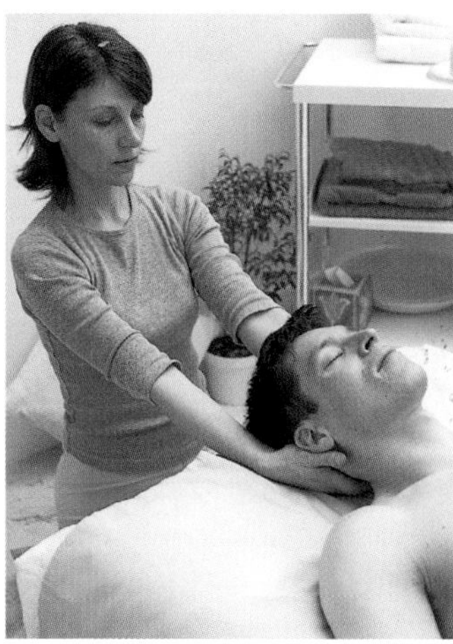

△ **8** Place both hands, one resting on top of the other, to cup underneath the neck. Slowly pull your hands up the length of the neck, gently lifting and stretching it towards you. Hold for a few seconds. Continue moving up and under the head, pulling your hands apart as you go until they come off the body at the top of the head. Repeat twice more.

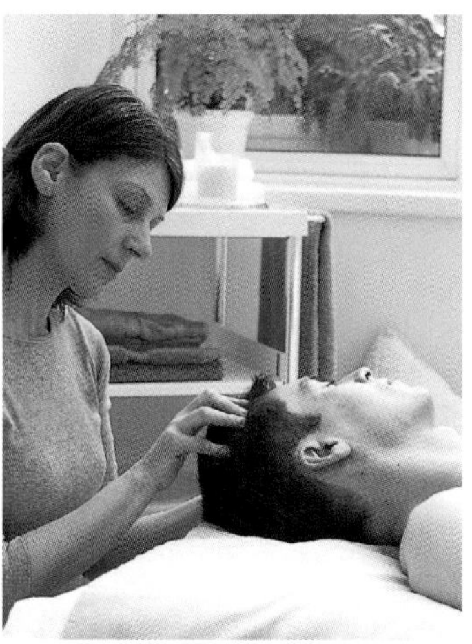

△ **10** Position your right hand at the side of the head to support it and place the left at the base of the skull. Using the pads of your fingers, rub across the surface of the scalp in a zigzagging "windscreen wiper" movement. Work your way around the ears, increasing the depth of your massage to release tension. Cover the whole head three times.

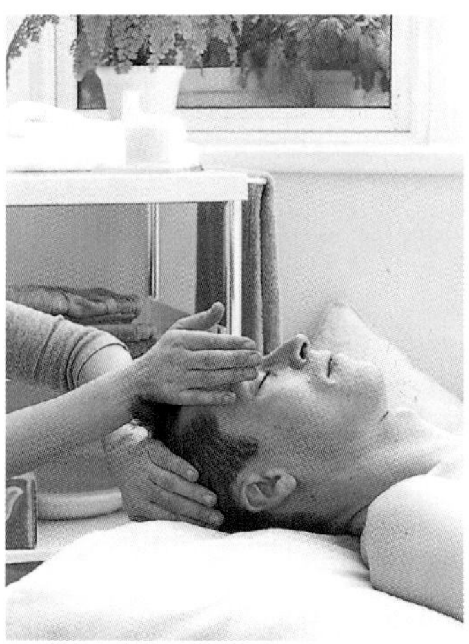

△ **11** To finish on the head, stroke or comb through your partner's hair, using either your whole hand or just your fingers. Begin at the hairline and bring your hand down over the hair towards the back of the head. Let one hand lead and the other follow so it feels like a continuous movement. Cover the whole head three times, using lighter pressure to close.

working on the face

Ideally the full head massage sequence continues on the face, but you can perform this routine as a short facial sequence if you wish. When you have finished on the head, rub a drop of lavender oil between your palms to clear any residual smell from the scalp sweat glands and to provide a pleasant and calming aroma. The face contains many nerve endings that are very receptive to massage, accelerating the relaxation process.

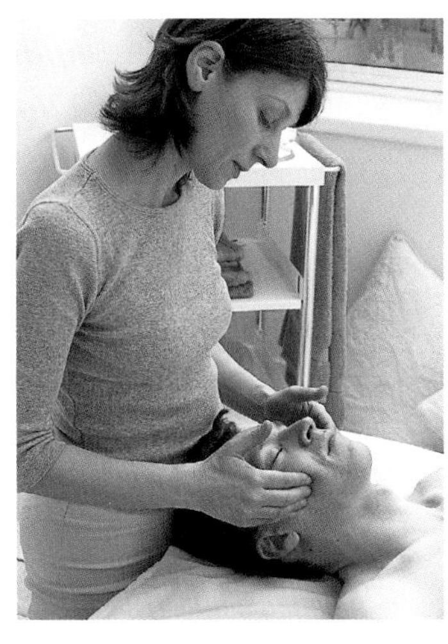

△ **2** This stroke involves circling movements over different areas of the face. Make sure that you cover each section three times and that you move smoothly from one area to the next. Using your fingertips, make small circular movements over the chin and above the upper lip. Continue with this circling action over the face, working well into the cheek and jaw area, which are both high tension spots, and using only feather-light pressure around the eye area.

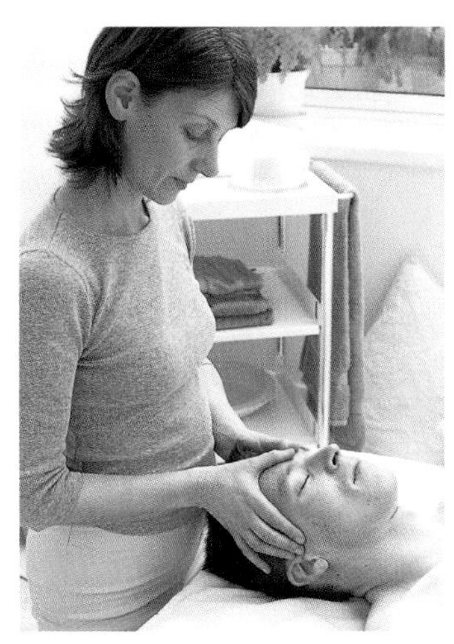

△ **4** Move your hands to the brow and let your thumbs meet together in the middle by the hairline. Using medium pressure, glide your thumbs in a straight line along the forehead and out towards the temples. Return your thumbs to the middle and work below the area just covered. Continue smoothing out the brow until the whole area is covered. Repeat twice more. This gentle but firm ironing out with the thumbs help to ease out worries and concerns registered in the lines of tension in the forehead.

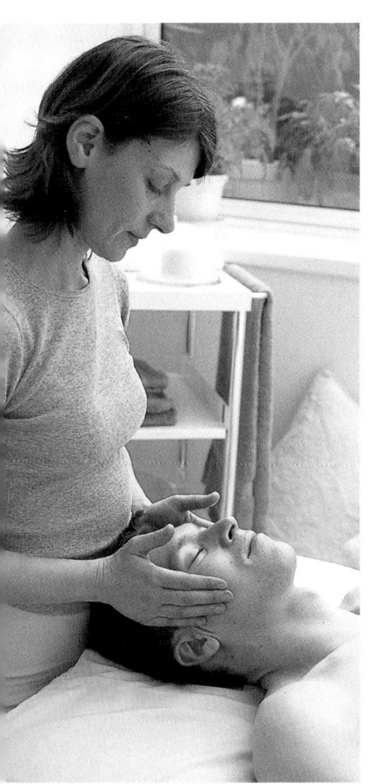

△ **1** Gently place both your hands on your partner's face, with your palms on either side of their chin. Lightly slide your hands up from the chin, stroking across the cheeks and up to the forehead. Repeat slowly several times, avoiding the delicate area around the eyes, and making your strokes a little firmer each time.

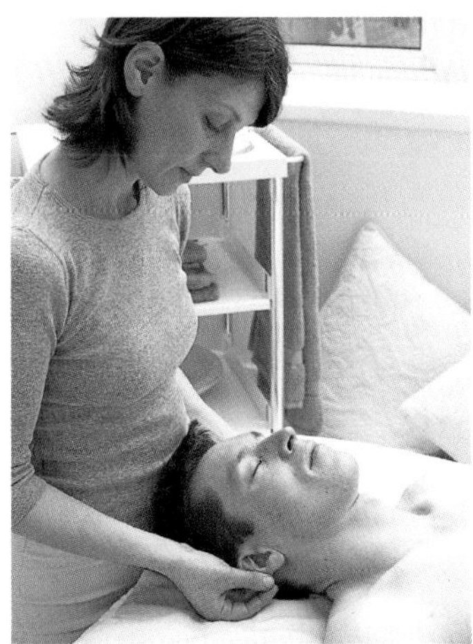

△ **3** Slide your fingers to your partner's ears. Starting at the top, use your thumbs and forefingers to lightly pinch or squeeze the ears' outer edges, working your way down to the base of the ear. End by pulling on each earlobe for a couple of seconds. Repeat three times and then cup your hands over the ears and hold for a few moments.

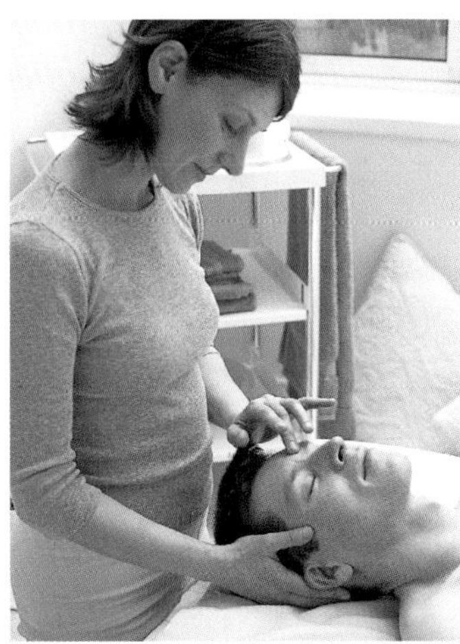

△ **5** To finish, place one finger in the "third eye" area, just above where the eyebrows would meet. Using light pressure, make small, slow circles over the surface of the skin, gradually increasing their size to take in more of the brow area. Make the circles smaller until your finger comes to a final resting place or stillness in the middle of the "third eye".

Self-massage

There are times when we could just do with a massage but there is no one around to oblige. Rather than give up, we can take a tip from other cultures, particularly those of the East, who have a longstanding tradition of self-massage. What we find is that head massage can be adapted into a self-treatment routine to suit ourselves in a wide variety of situations, as and when the need arises.

the shoulders and neck

You can follow the whole self-massage sequence, or if you have less time you can just work from the relevant section. It begins with the shoulders and neck. Make sure you are sitting comfortably with enough support for your spine, particularly if you feel tired. Many people find sitting cross-legged against a wall works well. Use cushions to give your back extra support if necessary.

▽ Prepare a nurturing space for yourself in which to self-massage, as this helps to create a healing atmosphere and to slow you down.

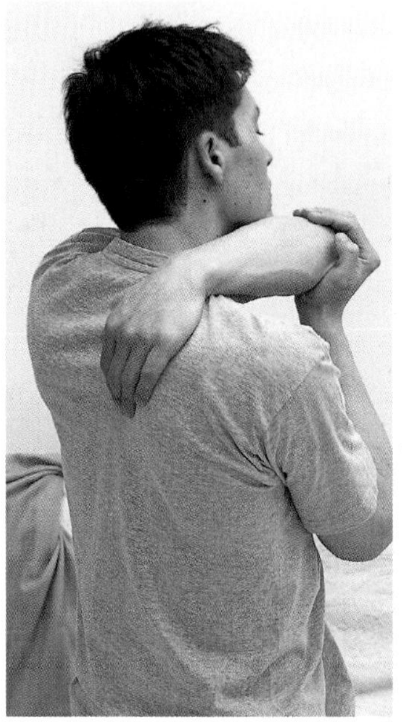

◁ **1** Take a deep breath in and out from your belly and place one hand on the opposite shoulder. This is your working hand. Lift your other hand and cup it over the elbow of your working hand for support and to provide leverage. Use your supporting hand to push the elbow up so that the working hand finishes as far down the upper back as is comfortable. Using the pads of your fingers make circular strokes, working your way upwards over the muscles that lie in between the shoulder blade and the spine. You can also massage around the line of the shoulder blade up to the top. Repeat twice more. Swap hands and repeat on the other side.

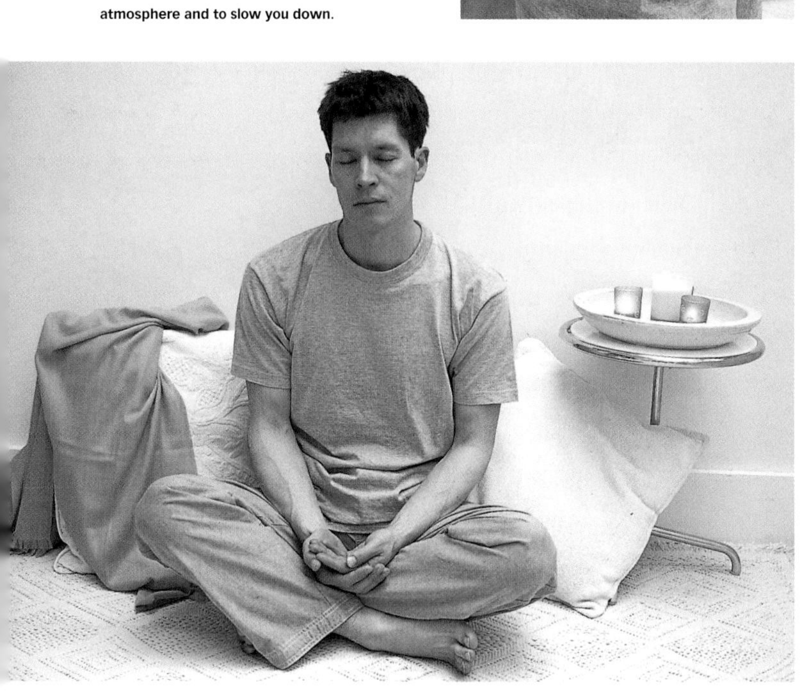

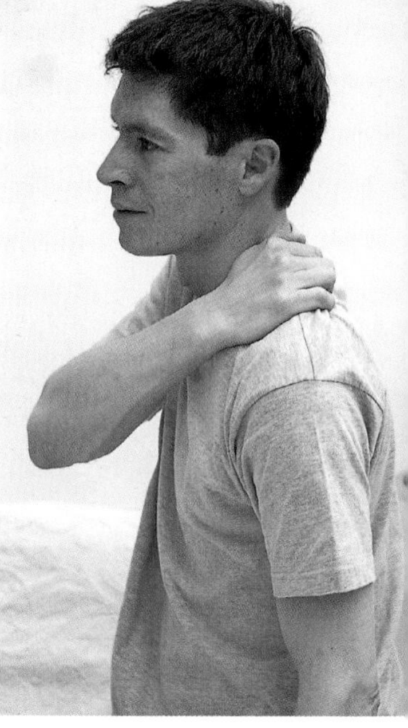

△ **2** Place your working hand near the base of your neck on the opposite shoulder. Using your whole hand, gently squeeze the muscle that starts here. Work your way along the top of the shoulder in this way, continuing down the upper arm to the elbow. Increase the intensity of pressure as you go if it is comfortable. Hold and release. Repeat three times. Swap hands and repeat on the other side.

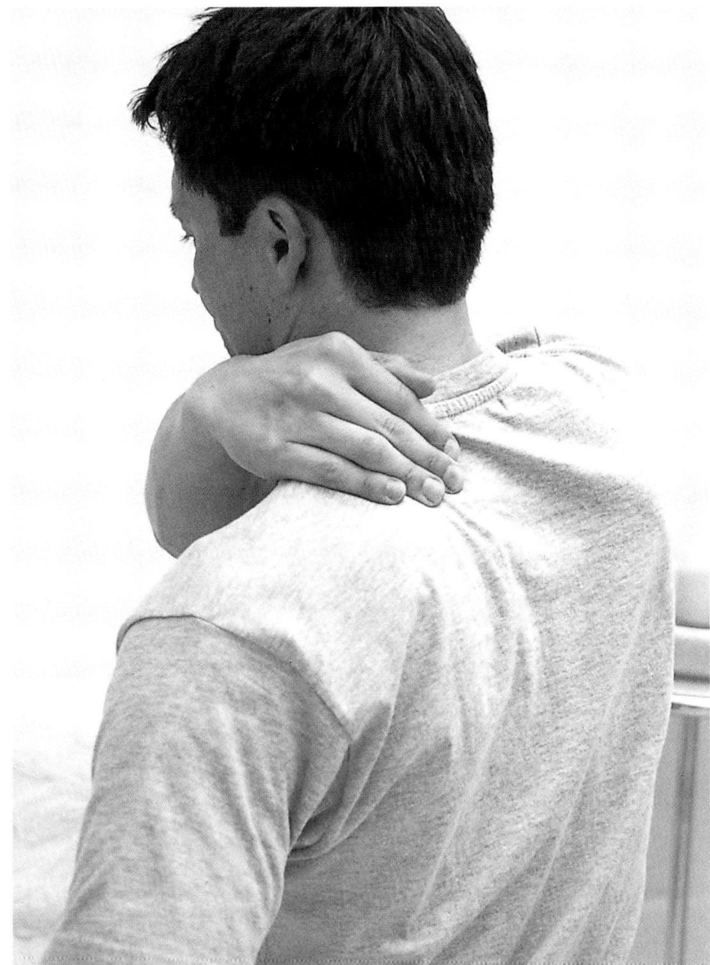

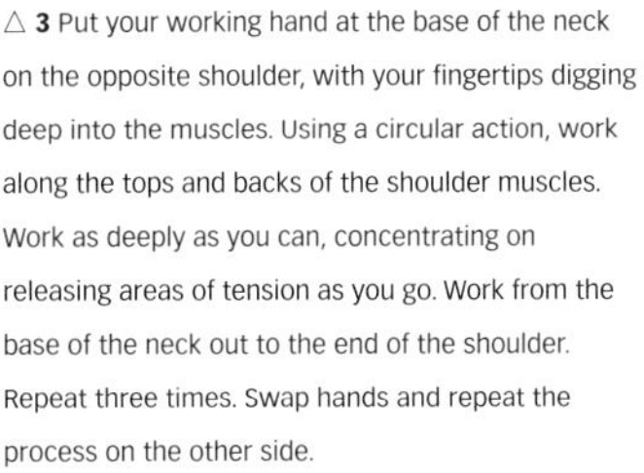

△ **3** Put your working hand at the base of the neck on the opposite shoulder, with your fingertips digging deep into the muscles. Using a circular action, work along the tops and backs of the shoulder muscles. Work as deeply as you can, concentrating on releasing areas of tension as you go. Work from the base of the neck out to the end of the shoulder. Repeat three times. Swap hands and repeat the process on the other side.

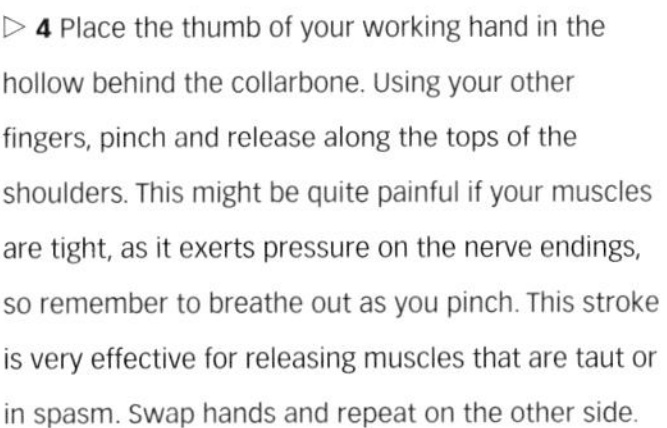

▷ **4** Place the thumb of your working hand in the hollow behind the collarbone. Using your other fingers, pinch and release along the tops of the shoulders. This might be quite painful if your muscles are tight, as it exerts pressure on the nerve endings, so remember to breathe out as you pinch. This stroke is very effective for releasing muscles that are taut or in spasm. Swap hands and repeat on the other side.

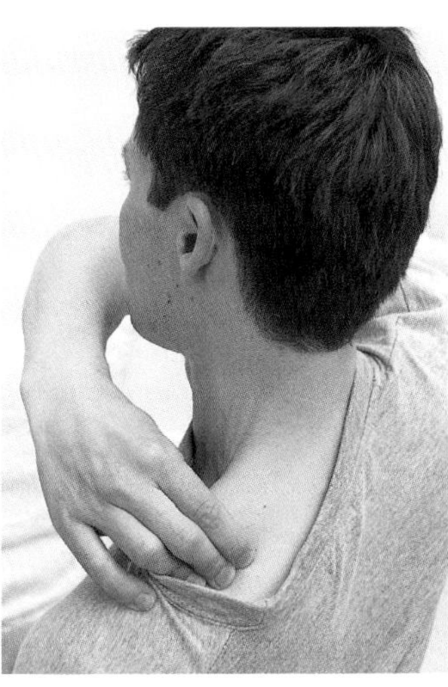

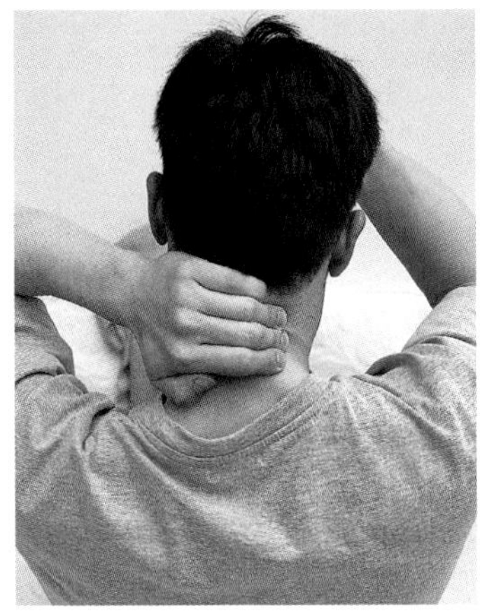

△ **5** Place one hand on your head and your working hand at the back of the neck. Tilt your head forwards a little. Starting at the top of the neck, use circular finger strokes to roll down the sides of the neck. Then use your whole hand to squeeze and pull down the back of the neck. Repeat three times and swap sides.

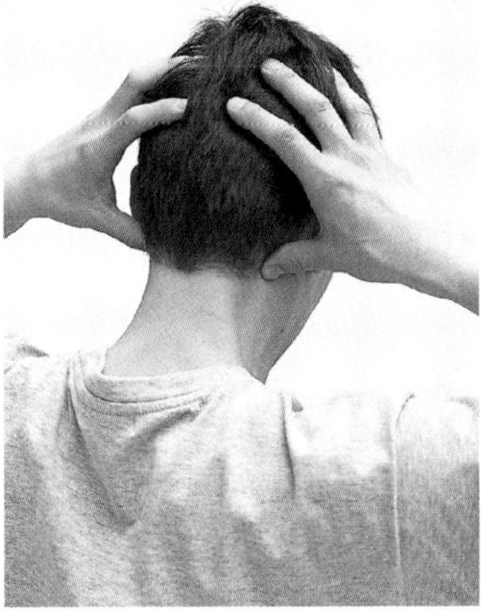

△ **6** Using both hands, clasp the back of your head and place your thumbs at the bony point just behind the ears. Work from here along the ridge of the skull, using thumb pressure and circular strokes from the middle outwards to the end to release tight muscle attachments. Repeat twice more.

the head

For the head part of the self-massage sequence, make sure you are sitting comfortably and adjust your position if necessary. Some people like to kneel or have their legs stretched out in front rather than sit cross-legged, which can be tiring. You can also do this sequence sitting down, with your elbows supported on a table.

▽ **1** Place your hands on your head and use the pads of your fingers to make circular strokes across your scalp. Work with medium pressure so that you feel the surface of the scalp move against the hard surface of the skull. You should feel this movement increase as you work. Cover the whole surface of the head three times, making sure that you work right down to the hairline.

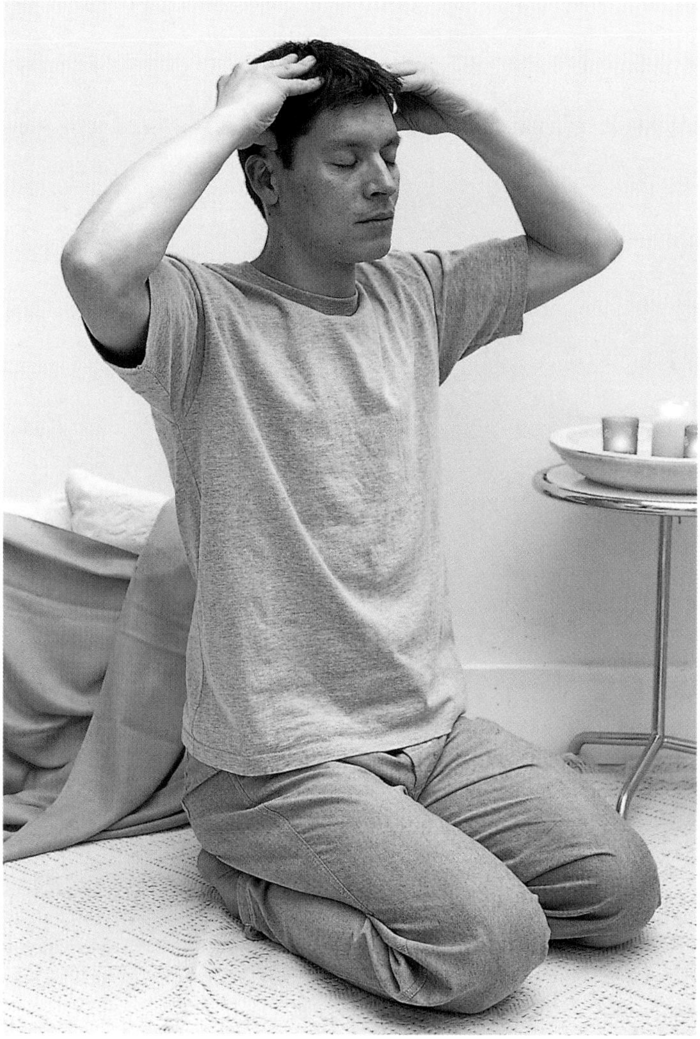

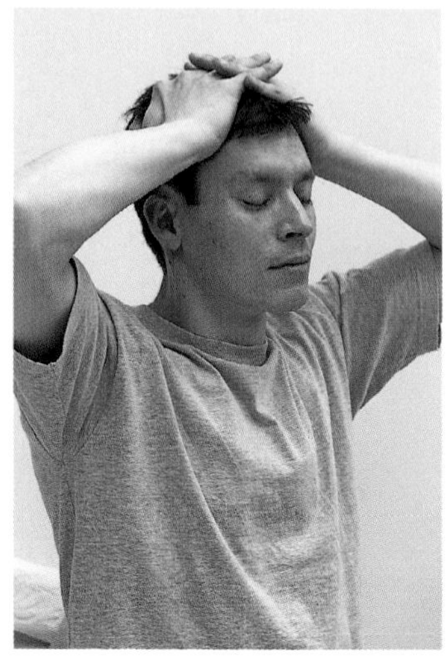

△ **2** With your hands on top of your head, interlock your fingers, press your palms into the sides of your head and lift them upwards. You should feel the scalp lift underneath your hands. Move to another part of the head and repeat, working in sections until the whole scalp is covered. If your hair is long enough, you can extend this lifting stroke by grabbing a fistful of hair with each hand and tugging it from side to side, keeping your knuckles close to the scalp.

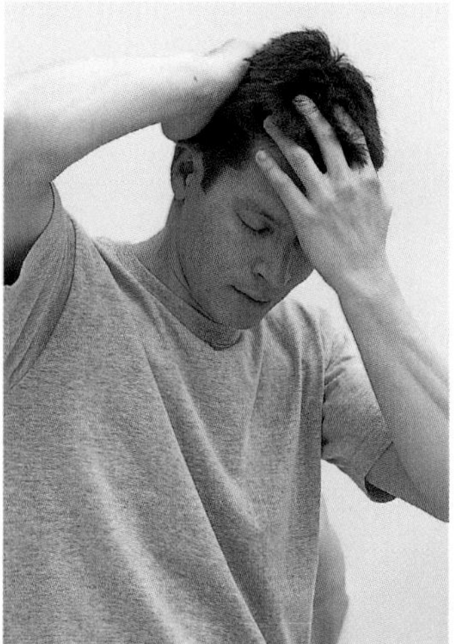

△ **3** Using both hands, use your fingers to rake through your hair and over your scalp. For a calming effect begin at the front of the head and work backwards to the nape of the neck. For an energising effect, begin at the nape of the neck and work forwards to the front. Repeat three times.

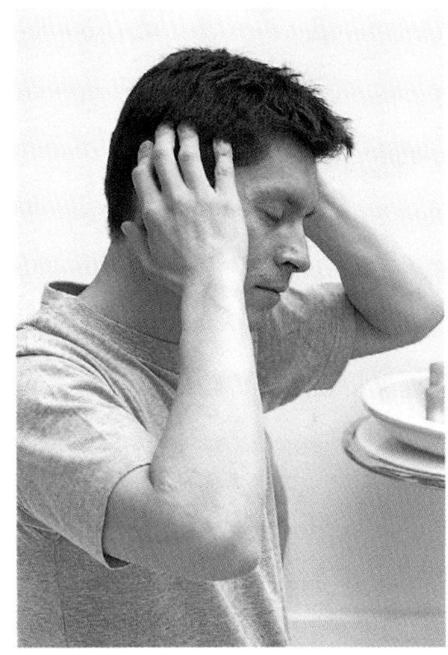

△ **4** Support your head with one hand on the side and put the other hand at the front of the ear by the hairline. Using the pads of your fingers, rub vigorously backwards and forwards in a friction stroke, applying medium pressure. Pay particular attention to releasing the muscle band that runs around and across the top of the ear. Massage the whole head using this stroke three times, working in a fast rhythmical way and changing hands when necessary.

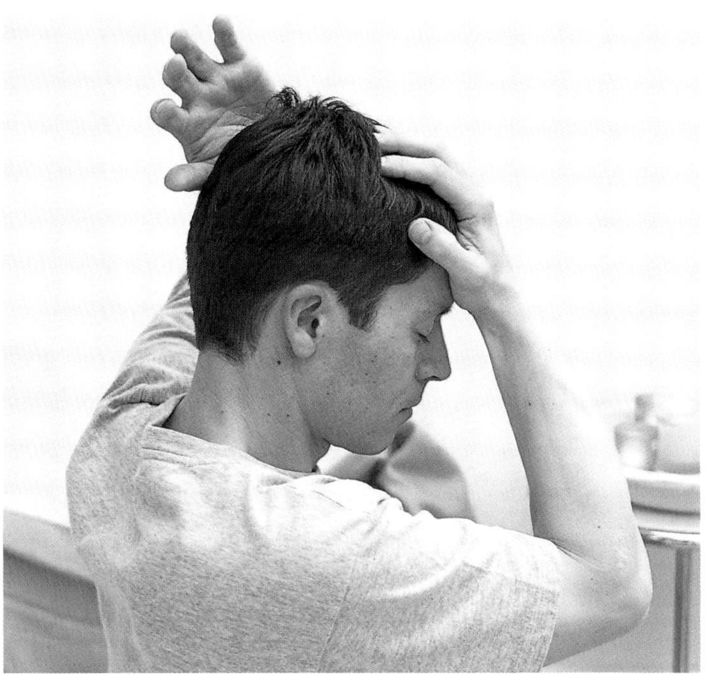

△ **6** Use one hand to support your head at the front. Put your other hand at the base of the skull in the middle and use the heel of your hand in a zigzagging motion to rub up and over the back of the head until one side is completely covered. Change hands and repeat on the other side.

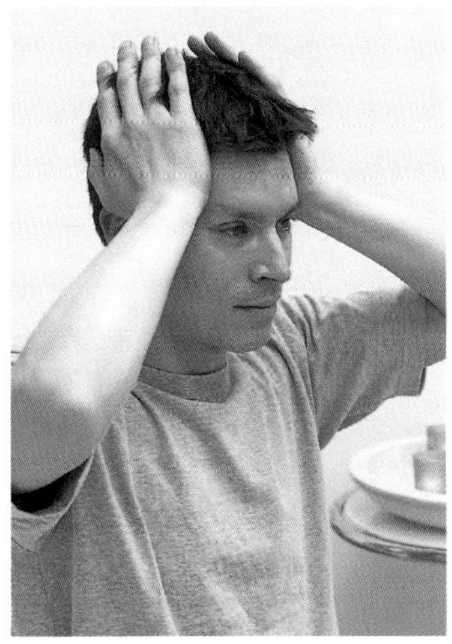

△ **5** Place the heels of both hands on your temples. Press in slightly and make circular actions with your hands. Keep your movements slow and work in a clockwise and then an anti-clockwise direction. Adjust pressure so that it is comfortable to receive. Repeat five times in each direction.

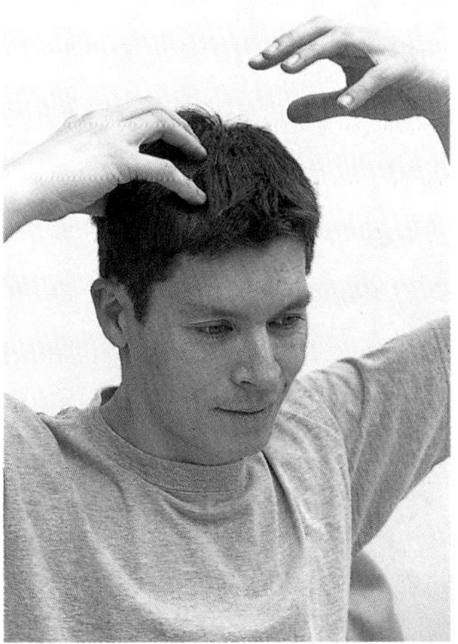

△ **7** Place the tips of your fingers on top of your head and begin to tap lightly all over the surface of the head, building up a smooth rhythm as you work. Keep your fingers soft so that your touch is light and your fingers spring off the surface of the head. Work over the whole head three times.

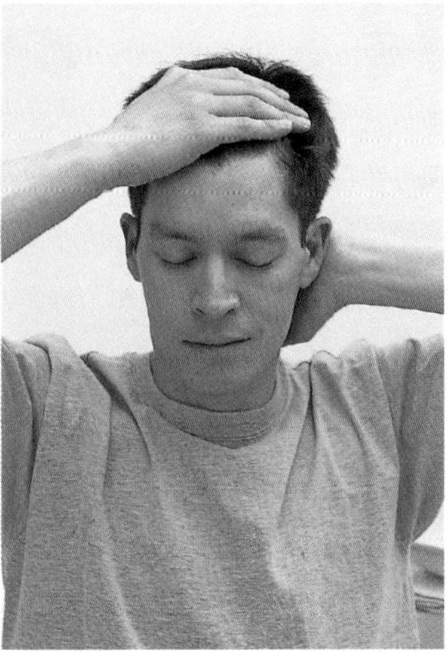

△ **8** Make long stroking movements working from the front of the head to the nape of the neck. As one hand comes off the head, let the other come down so that one stroke flows seamlessly into another. Cover the whole head a few times, gradually slowing down until you finally come to a stop.

the face

Most of us are unaware of how much tension we store in our faces, particularly around the jaw area. The tightness it registers leaves us looking tired and strained. Using self-massage on your face is soothing and relaxing, especially at the end of a long and stressful day, and will help restore a fresher look to your face. This sequence can be done as a facial massage in its own right. Again make sure you are sitting comfortably with your back well supported.

▽ **1** Place your thumbs just under your chin with the pads of your fingers resting on top. Now, pressing your thumb and fingers together, pinch your way along the whole of the lower jaw line. As you get to the outer edge of the jaw, you can increase the pressure as a lot of tension is usually held here. Work along the whole area three times. There are a lot of lymph nodes along the jaw line and this action stimulates their function to eliminate toxins from the body. Extend this stroke by making circular strokes with your fingers over the chin and lower jaw area.

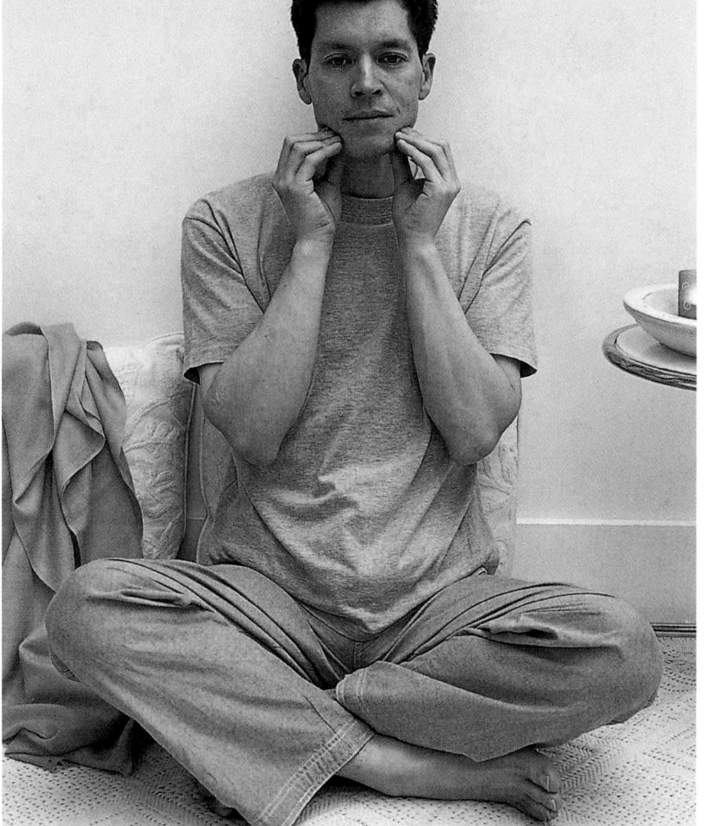

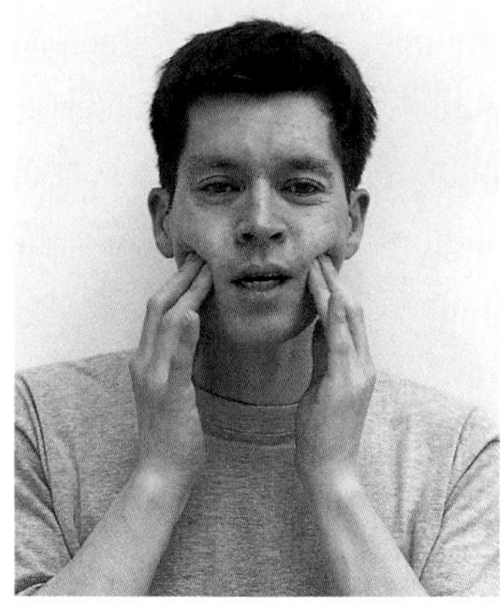

△ **2** Using the pads of your fingers, make circular strokes across the whole of your face. Begin at the bottom by the jaw line and work upwards using light pressure. To avoid stretching the skin, only use the pressure on the upward movements and be especially careful with the delicate area around the eyes. Cover the surface of your face three times. Around the jaw area and cheeks you can make your circling action slower and deeper, working deeply into the jaw socket itself to release tension.

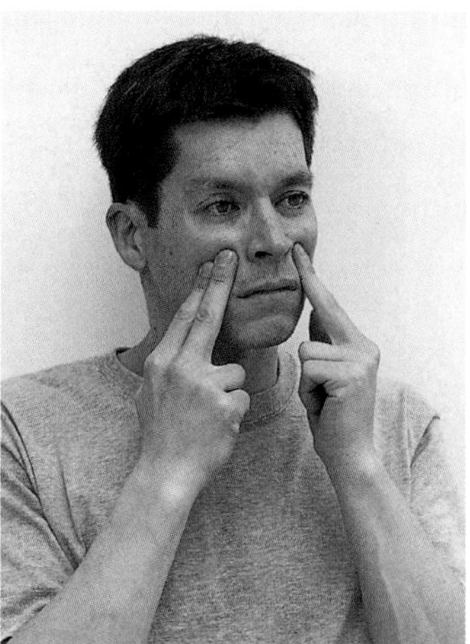

△ **3** Place your first two fingers on the underside of your cheeks, near the hollow at the base of your nose. Press in gently against the bone, hold and release. Move along the cheekbone with this action until you get to the hinge by the jawbone, then work your way back to the middle of the face. Repeat this movement three times. Any tender spots can indicate areas of sinus congestion, which may be helped by this particular massage action.

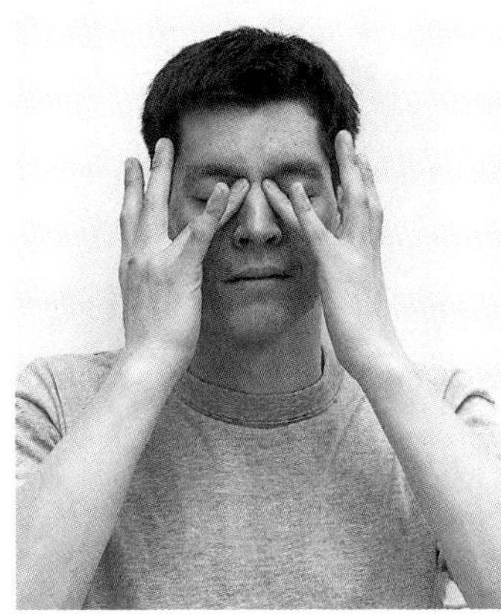

△ **4** Close your eyes and put the pads of your ring fingers at the inner edge of your eyebrows by the bridge of the nose. Gently but firmly press inwards and upwards, hold for a few seconds and then release. Repeat a few more times if the area feels tender, which indicates congestion. Continue with this pressure stroke, working out along the lower edge of the eyebrow and back underneath the eye, tracing the bony rim of the eye. Complete three full circles in this way.

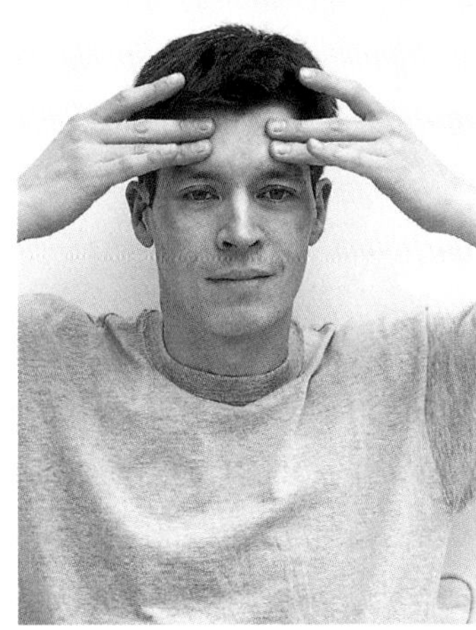

△ **5** Place your middle fingers on your forehead so that they face tip to tip in the middle of your lower brow. Slowly draw your fingers apart across the brow towards the hairline. Move your fingers a little higher up the forehead and repeat. Continue to work up the brow in sections, smoothing out lines of worry and tension as you go. Cover the whole area three times. To draw to a close, use your fingers to trace increasingly light circles around the "third eye" area.

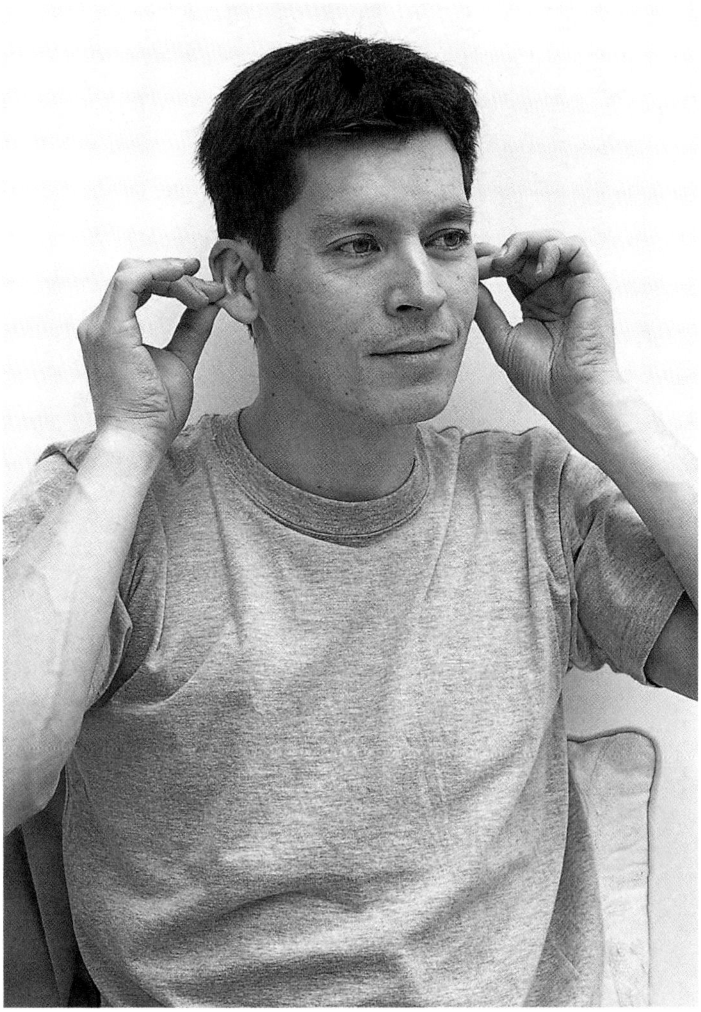

△ **6** With thumb and fingertips at the bottom of both earlobes, gently squeeze and roll along the outer edge of the ears, working up to the top. At the top, continue squeezing and rolling down the inner edge of the ears, back to where you began. Repeat this movement twice, then gently pull down on the earlobes to release them. Next place your palms over your ears and rub over the area, exerting a comfortable pressure. Do this a number of times. You can rub quite briskly till your ears are quite warm for a stimulating effect. This ear massage action will have an energizing result and will help relieve pain being experienced elsewhere in the body, as the ears contain correspondences to the whole system. The stimulating effect will activate the body's energy channels (meridians). To finish the massage sequence, gently place your palms against your ears for a few moments and slowly release.

Oil massage with a partner

Sometimes you and your massage partner may decide to opt for using oils when giving a head massage. Sharing an oil massage can be an enriching experience, depending on the need at the time and the oils used. It will add another dimension to the routines described elsewhere in the book. Oils also make it easier to extend a treatment to take in a general back and upper-body massage.

With a wide range of oils to choose from, you can make up your own concoctions to suit the particular situation – to enhance moods, relieve physical conditions or to facilitate emotional and physical healing. Take some time to assess your partner's particular need, and together choose the oils that seem most appropriate.

You can use a carrier oil on its own or you can add essential oils to the base oil for a broader effect. Several useful oil blends are suggested below. If you need more information on oils generally, see the previous chapter.

a sensual experience

A massage that involves any kind of oil feels very different from one without, as the increased lubrication is smoother and feels more sensual. The addition of aromas to the oils can make the massage even more luxurious, shifting the emphasis from mainly therapeutic to something more special.

Using oils also enables you to extend a head massage to include an upper-body massage and so share a more relaxing and intimate experience with your partner. You can follow all the steps in the lying-down routine, but the oils will give the massage a very different character.

Warm your hands before applying oil, and use wide stroking movements to spread the oil evenly over the surface of your partner's skin. Apply more oil to the skin

▽ **As you apply nourishing oil to your massage partner's body allow your hands to mould over the contours in a smooth gliding way, with long stroking movements.**

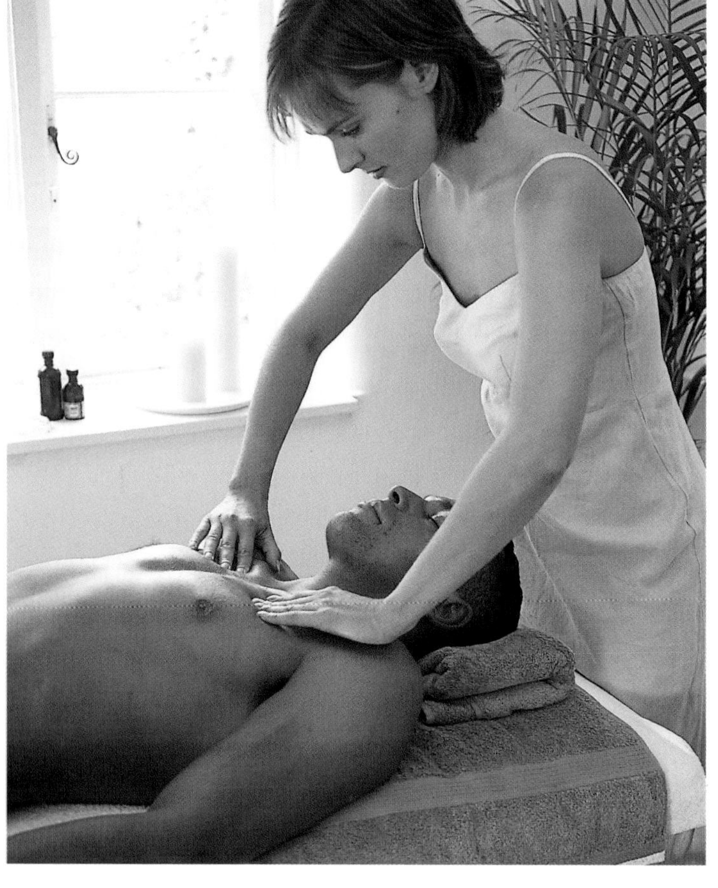

essential oil blends

Outlined here are a range of useful essential oil combinations that are appropriate for a range of needs and conditions. Use 2 drops essential oil for every 10ml (2 tsp) carrier oil. Sweet almond is one of the best multi-purpose carrier oils you can use.

general aches and pains: lavender and rosemary

stress: sandalwood, lavender and geranium

mild depression: geranium and lavender

pampering and nourishment: sandalwood or geranium, mixed with coconut base oil because of its softening qualities

spiritual transformation: include frankincense, as this helps to break links with the past and facilitates moving forwards.

as you need to, but remember to always keep your other hand on your partner's body in order to keep the flow and a sense of continuity. Stroking, holding, circling and smoothing strokes can all be used effectively anywhere on the body when you are using oils.

Allow the nature of the oil as a medium to guide how you work. The oil on your hands will enable them to glide smoothly over your partner's skin. It will also make it easier for them to mould over the shape of the body and to follow its natural undulations. The strokes you use will be more gliding, stroking, smoothing and caressing in nature. You should also let yourself work at a slower pace than you normally would and take pleasure in the sensual nature of the oil itself.

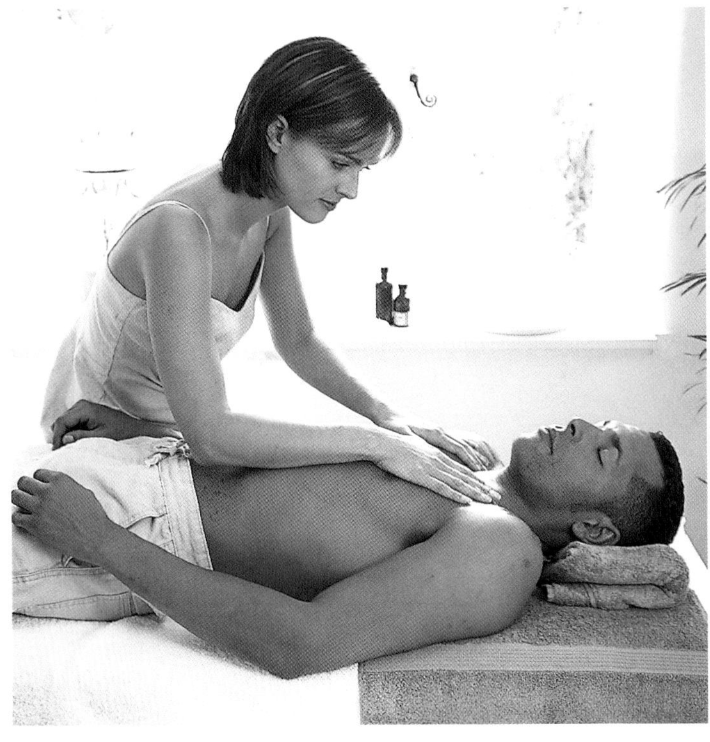

▽ **Allow your hands to glide over the shoulders and back of the neck, easing out tension. Avoid working on the spine itself.**

△ **Using oils in a massage slows you down and if done regularly can be part of quality time with your partner as you connect on other levels.**

▽ **When done with oils, a tension-releasing shoulder massage can become a luxurious experience that is a pleasure to give and receive.**

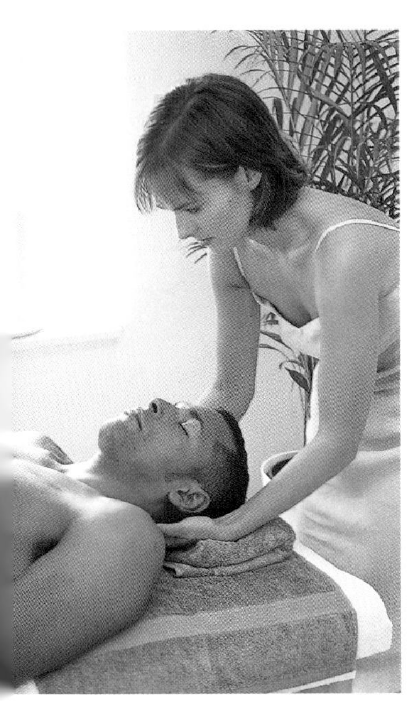

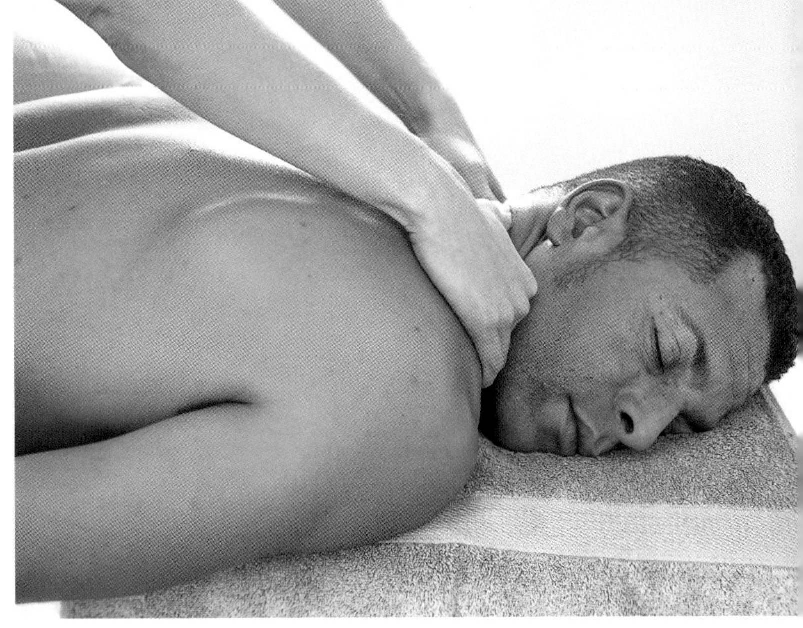

Self-massage with oil

You may not think so at first, but giving yourself a head massage with oil can be as nourishing as receiving it from someone else. It is definitely worth trying, for it is very rewarding and is something that can easily be incorporated into your normal pampering and body-care routine. As oils have such a therapeutic effect, it would also be an ideal opportunity to extend the massage to other parts of the body, rubbing and smoothing oil on other areas, such as your arms, legs and feet as well as your face and neck. Always work up towards the heart when massaging other body parts.

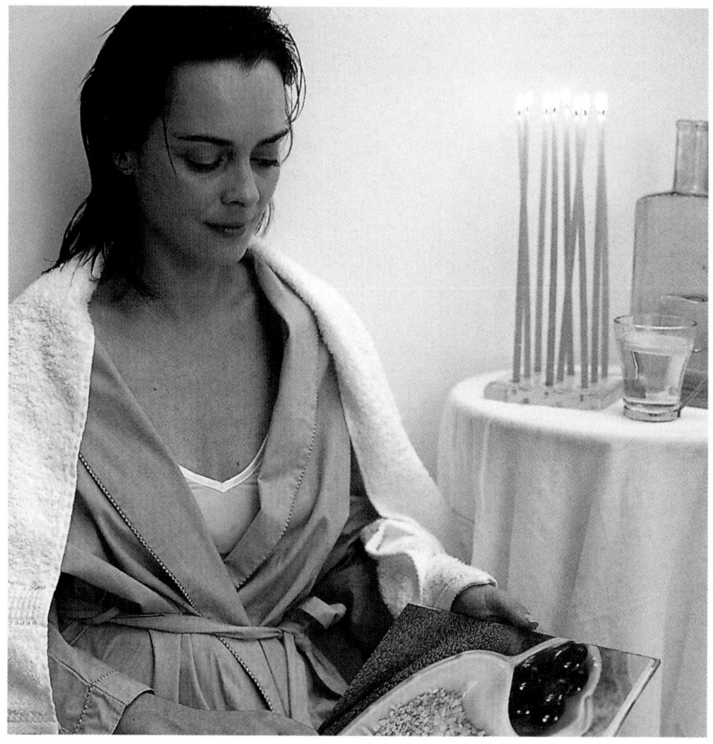

getting started

Preparing the space for yourself is as important as if you were preparing it for someone else. In Western culture we are not used to self-massage and reactions such as futility, doubt and dissatisfaction are common to begin with. Giving positive attention to creating the right atmosphere sends a strong message to your subconscious mind that you are worth it. This is a good opportunity to play self-healing or affirmation tapes, while relaxing background music will give you something to focus on if you feel bored. Wear something loose and comfortable and that won't matter if it gets marked. Prepare everything else you may need for your pampering session. This will include a few towels to wrap yourself or your hair in, plenty of tissues, some water or herb tea and maybe some reading material and beauty preparations. You also need to have all the oils ready to hand plus a suitable mixing bowl and comb.

▽ Make sure that you have everything ready before you apply oils to your hands, as working with oils can be messy.

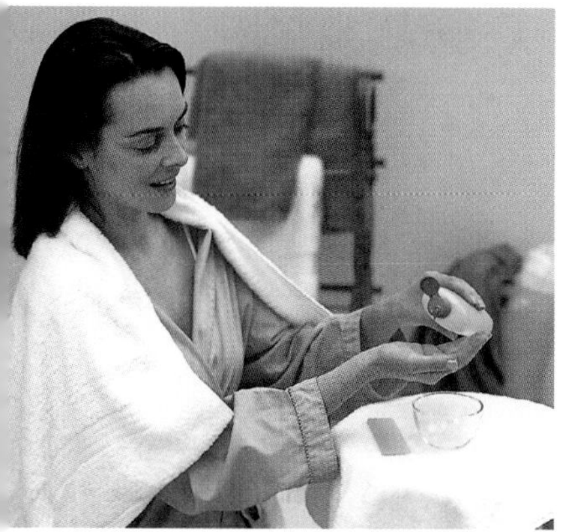

Warm up a little oil in the palm of your hand and apply it to the top of your head. Loosely ruffle your hair and work it in. Then apply some oil to the sides of your head and work this in. If you have long hair, you may need to lift it up and work outwards from the roots to the tips. Apply more oil, working from the front to the back of the head.

△ Allowing time for the oils to sink in provides an opportunity to spend some quality time on yourself for self-nourishment and to rebalance. Use it to do something you really enjoy.

Using the pads of your fingers, go on to make circular strokes across your scalp with medium pressure. Work methodically from the front to the back, covering the whole head. You should feel your scalp move underneath your fingers. When you have finished, cover your head and leave the oils to sink into your hair and scalp to do their work. This can be anything from 20 minutes to 24 hours. Using a warm towel around your head accelerates the penetration of the oils into the hair and scalp. Wrap it around your head "turban style" and use the time to catch up with yourself and relax.

▷ **For a truly nourishing experience, use oils to help you massage away tensions and knots and to help create a greater sense of ease within your own body.**

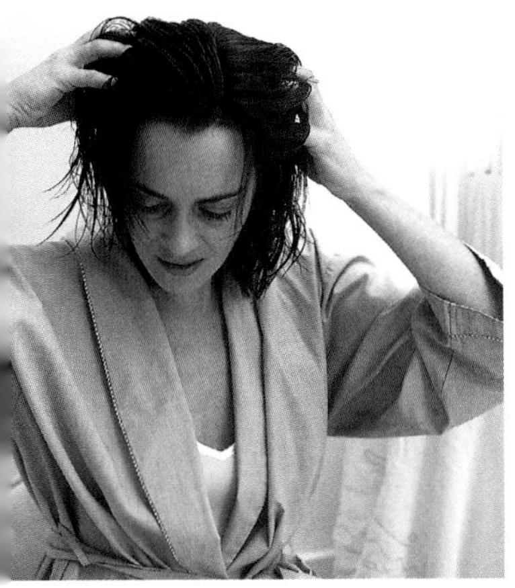

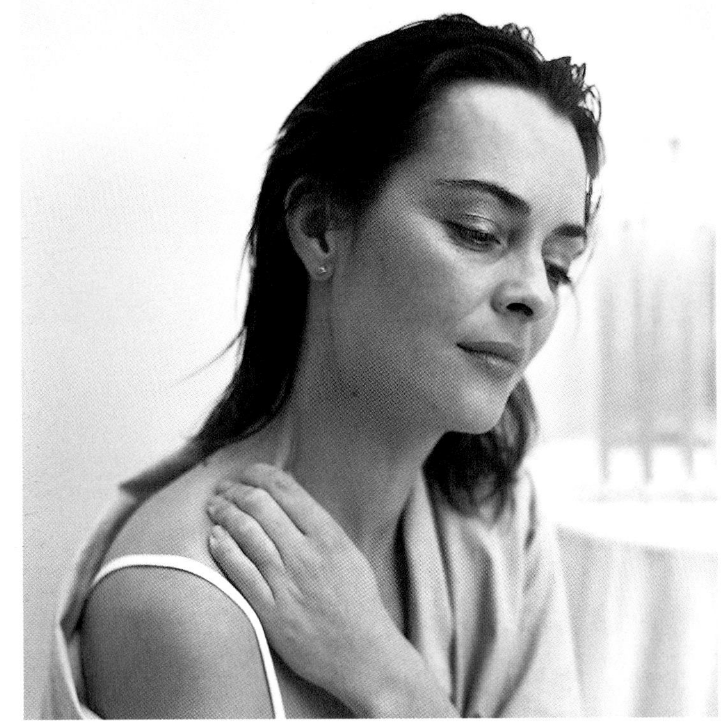

△ **Release tension in the head and discharge mental stress and worries by working them out through massage with oils. Then you can wash them all away.**

To continue working with oil you can follow the basic self-massage sequence outlined earlier in the book. However, because of its slippery nature there will be more "give" with oil, and you will have less of a grip than with dry massage, so the experience will feel very different. With oils your strokes are likely to be smooth, gliding over the skin in a continuous movement.

After you have finished with your hair, you may want to use up any remaining oil on your face and neck. Place your hands on your face and gently smooth the oil into the skin with small circular strokes, being particularly careful around the eyes. Move to your neck and glide your hands up and out to the sides. You can leave the oil to soak in or wipe it off with a tissue.

Remember that when giving self-massage you are both the giver and the receiver. As the giver you are your own therapist, so be sympathetic and understanding to how you feel inside. As you massage you could inwardly thank the different parts of your body for serving you so well each day. You may also notice how your thoughts stray away or become negative, worrying or busy. When this happens, bring your attention back to the self-massage. As the receiver, you have the opportunity for self-empowerment and healing. If it hurts, you can instantly lighten the depth of your touch. Alternatively you can apply pressure for much longer than is conventional if it feels good to you. You also know exactly where it hurts and can find the precise location of any knotty and painful spots.

As you massage, make sure that your strokes give you pleasure, adjusting the pace so that it is faster, slower, deeper, or more loving. Be responsive to your own needs and be flexible in your approach. A basic guideline is to recognize that the body has a wisdom of its own and that if something feels good, it is likely to be doing you good.

▽ **Relieve tension in your face with an oil facial that will leave you feeling good and your skin soft, smooth and glowing.**

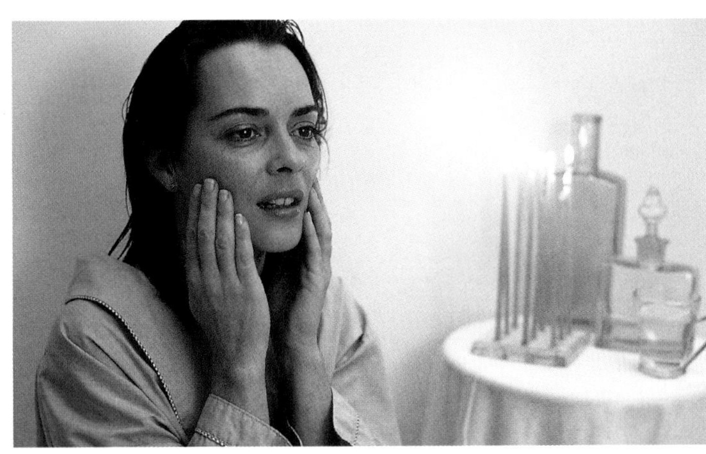

Five-minute fixes

When you don't have enough time for a complete self-massage sequence, there are some quick-fix routines that can be done at home or at work. They will give you an energy boost, keep your body loose and help improve posture. The first five-minute routine is based on shiatsu-style massage and works on energy channels; the second sequence focuses on neck care and includes a sequence of movements that can be done at any time during the day.

energy channels booster

The following massage routine is energizing and invigorating. It works by activating the energy channels (meridians) that run throughout the body through the use of tapping and pummelling movements. It "wakes up" the whole body and is therefore ideal for first thing in the morning or if you need recharging in the middle of the day. The energizing, pummelling action of your knuckles also has a stimulating effect on some of the muscles, increasing peripheral circulation and loosening tension through its vibrations.

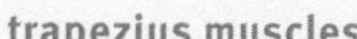

trapezius muscles

Under stress these muscles tighten and can pull the muscles around the neck and on the attachments to the skull, resulting in headaches, stiffness, and impaired breathing. Stretching helps reduce and prevent this build-up of tension.

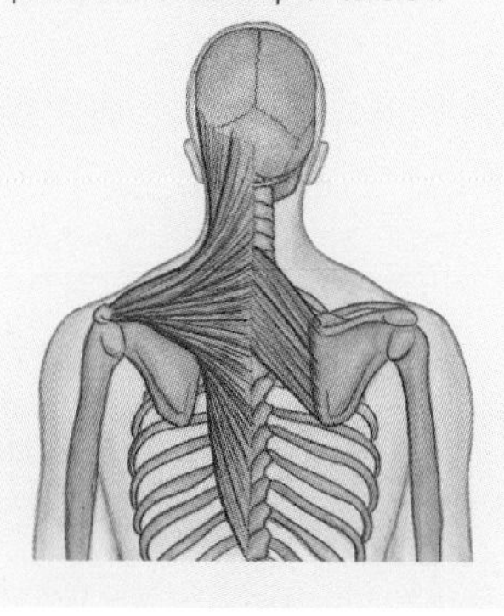

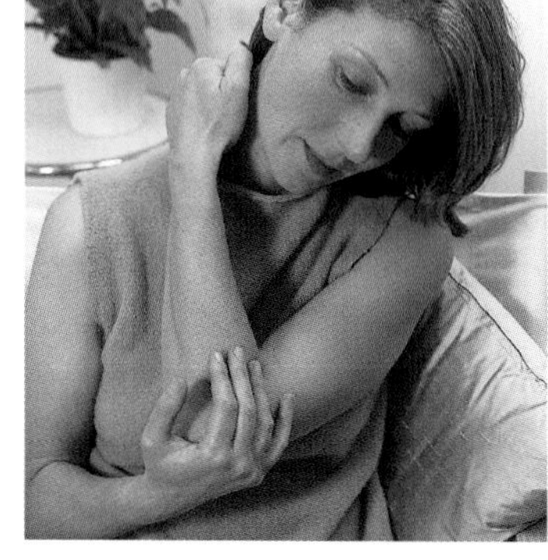

△ **1** Sit with your shoes off. Spread out your toes and plant your feet firmly on the ground. Cup your left elbow in the palm of your right hand and use your left knuckles to tap the right side of the body. Tap down the side of the neck and continue over the top of the shoulder and down into the upper back. Work as far down the back as you can, using your hand on your elbow for leverage. Repeat on the other side.

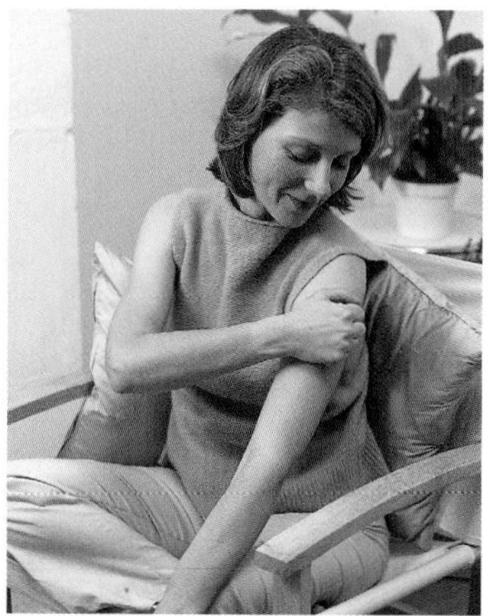

△ **2** Continue tapping down the outside of your arm to your hand. Then tap up on the inside all the way up to the armpit, over the shoulder joint and then back down the outside of the arm once more. Repeat three times, then swap hands and do the other arm.

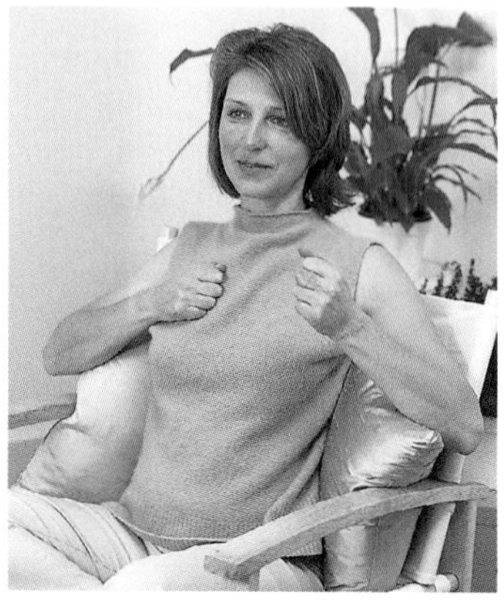

△ **3** Now use the same tapping stroke on your chest. Sit back in the chair and, keeping your wrists soft, tap across the upper chest. Work from the middle of your chest outwards towards the shoulder. This is a very invigorating and sometimes quite amusing movement. Repeat three times.

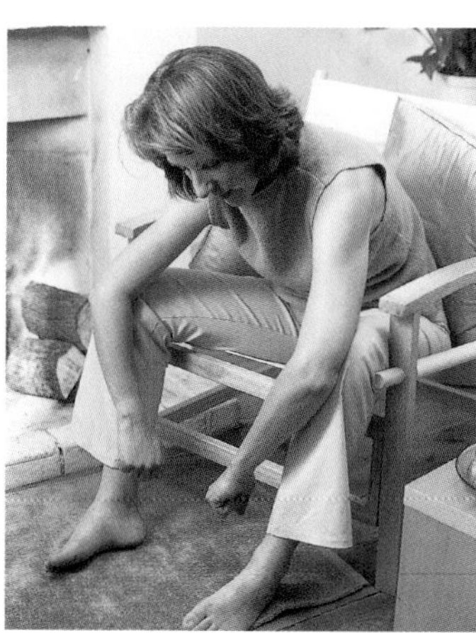

△ **4** Place your feet slightly apart on the ground, and pummel down the outside of both legs at the same time. Repeat this action three times. Finish by pummelling up the inside of both legs. Repeat three times. Slowly sit up and take a deep breath to finish.

essential neck care

Weaknesses, tension and imbalances in the neck are helped and can even be corrected by exercise. These gentle movements will loosen up and strengthen the neck, giving greater freedom of movement and reducing the risk of strain or injury. They only take a few minutes and are effective for stretching out the muscles and connective tissue and energizing the body. They can also help improve posture. It is important to keep breathing during exercises to encourage the flow of oxygen to the muscles and assist the releasing process.

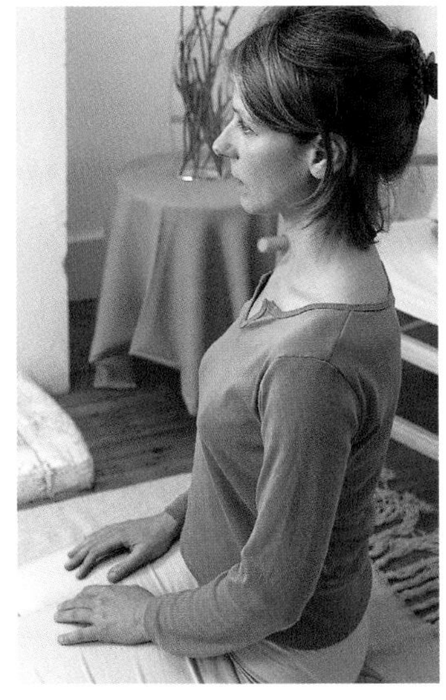

To improve your posture, kneel on the floor, take a deep breath in, and on the out breath drop your shoulders. Imagine your head is attached to a cord tied to the ceiling. Every time you breathe out imagine the cord pulling your head up, and your spine lengthening and straightening.

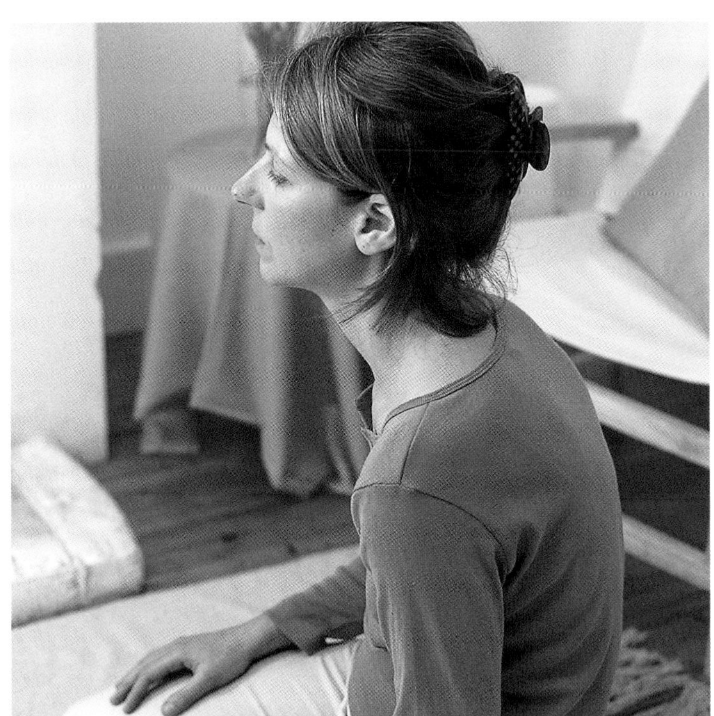

▽ A poor posture profile, such as a curved back, slumped shoulders and a head that juts forwards is commonplace. Stretching, exercises and massage help reverse the trend and prevent this posture becoming a long term hump that is set and irreversible in later years.

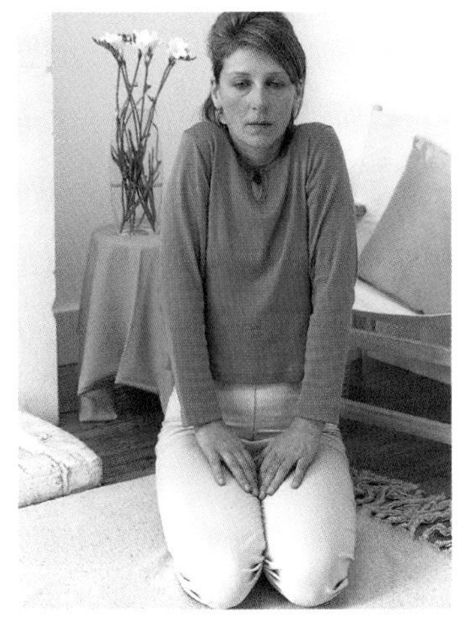

△ **1** Take a deep breath in and slowly begin to lift your shoulders up and back as far as they will comfortably go. On the out breath, slowly release, beginning the upward movement again on the next in breath. As your shoulder blades come down, imagine them meeting together in the middle of your back. Shoulder shrugs help to release tension in the large muscles of the upper back that pull on the neck.

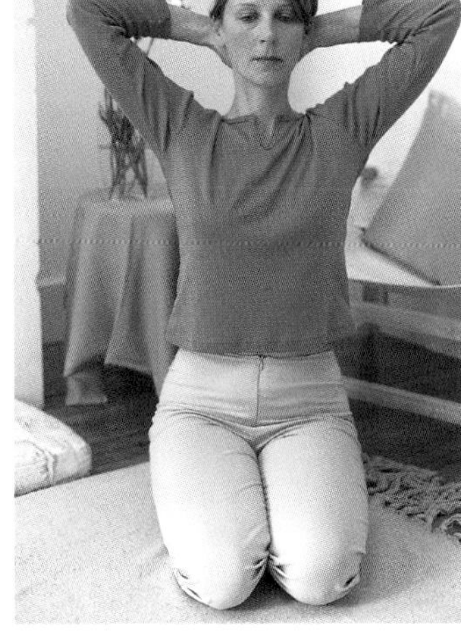

△ **2** Centre your head and tuck your chin in. Tuck your hands behind your head, push your head against them and hold for 3–5 seconds. Repeat 10–20 times. Then place one hand on the side of your head. Tuck your chin in, push your head against your hand and hold for 3–5 seconds. Repeat 10–20 times. Swap hands and repeat on the other side. These movements help to strengthen the neck muscles.

End of the day de-stresser

Being able to relax and leave work behind is essential if we are to make the most of our time off. Yet with the day's work over, many people find that switching off is not so simple and have trouble letting go of stress and tension. Head massage is a fantastic tool for de-stressing after a long day, whether you've been out at work or involved in childcare at home. Many people find it much more effective than other quick-fix solutions, such as drinking alcohol, as its benefits are longer lasting and it has no harmful side effects. An end of the day de-stress routine can be done with a partner or by yourself – even if you feel too tired to bother, it's usually well worth the effort.

partner shoulder massage

Massage with your partner gives both of you the opportunity to relax and to re-connect after being in different worlds all day. It can form part of winding down and spending quality time together, and after just a few minutes of massaging the shoulders the cares and tensions of the day will start to fade as your muscles begin to unwind.

▽ **1** Briskly rub the palm of your hand over your partner's shoulders and upper back, and use fingers and thumbs to massage knots and tensions away.

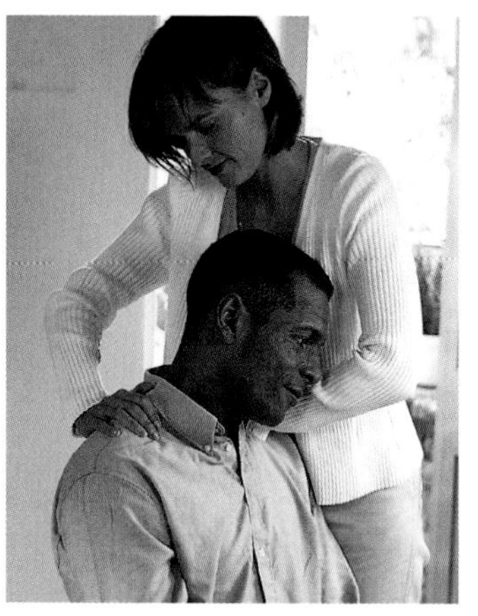

after work de-stresser

After you have been sitting at work all day, the following sequence is specifically designed to target the areas of stress in the body. It is done lying down to give your muscles and spine a chance to decompress. Make sure that you have a firm, comfortable surface to lie on, plus cushions for support and a blanket for keeping warm. Turn the lights down low and make sure the phone is off the hook.

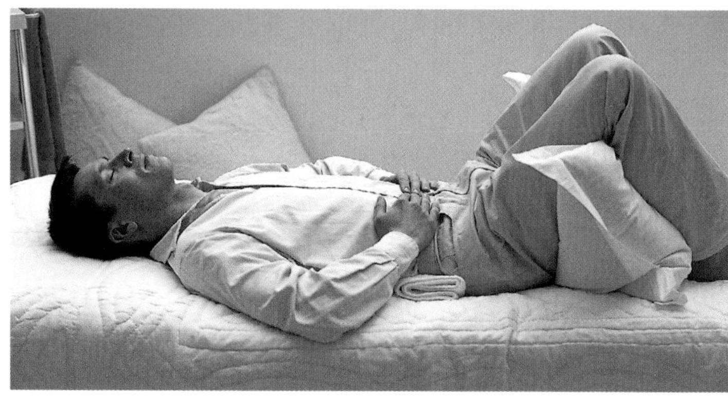

△ **1** Begin by lying flat on your back. Bending your knees is helpful, as it gives the lower back extra support and helps the spine to lengthen and straighten. You could also place a large cushion underneath your knees as a bolster. Place your hands on your belly, close your eyes and take a few deep breaths in and out of your belly. As you breathe in, you should feel your hands lift up slightly and as you breathe out feel your belly contract and your hands come back in. Do this a few times.

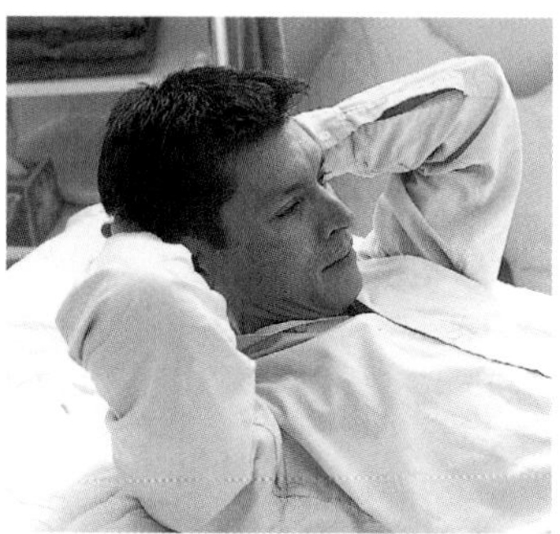

△ **2** Clasp your hands together behind your head. As you breathe slowly out, lift your head up with them. The hands should lead with the head following. Do this slowly, imagining each vertebra lifting one at a time as you rise. When the neck is comfortably stretched, hold for a few moments and release slowly and smoothly, vertebra by vertebra. Repeat twice.

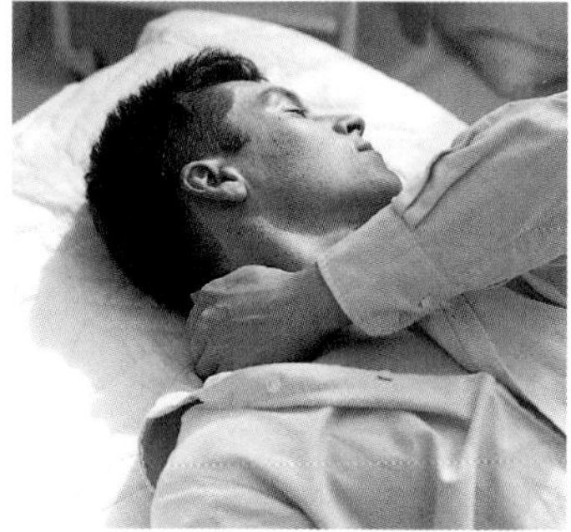

△ **3** Turn your head to the left and place your left hand on the right side of your neck. Using the fleshy pad of your hand (by the base of the thumb), make small circles, working down the neck and continuing across the top of the shoulders. Increase the size of the circles as you go. Repeat three times and then do the same on the other side.

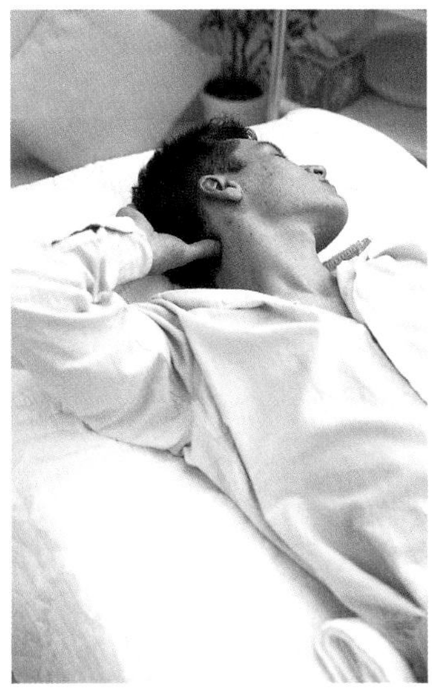

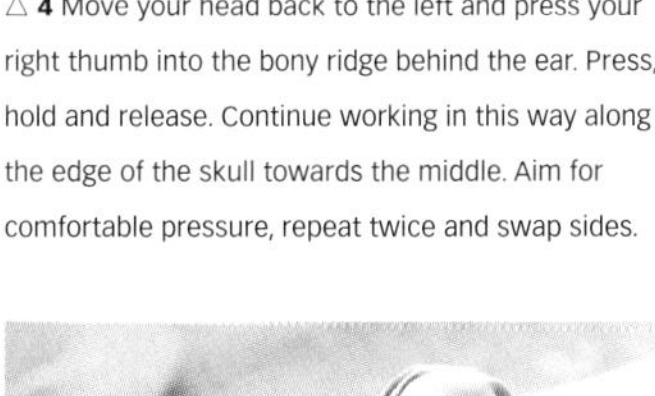

△ **4** Move your head back to the left and press your right thumb into the bony ridge behind the ear. Press, hold and release. Continue working in this way along the edge of the skull towards the middle. Aim for comfortable pressure, repeat twice and swap sides.

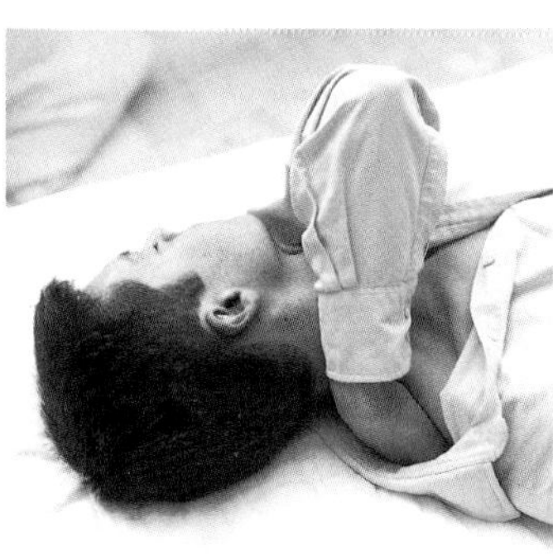

△ **5** With your head on the left, hook your left hand over your right shoulder, resting the heel on top of the shoulder with the fingers pointing down the back. Dig your fingers into the muscle, grab some flesh and drag it up until your fingers slide over your shoulder. Continue finding tight spots along both shoulders. Repeat three times on both sides.

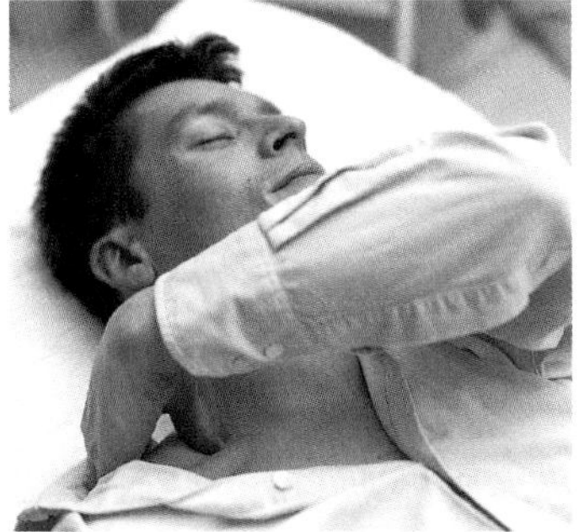

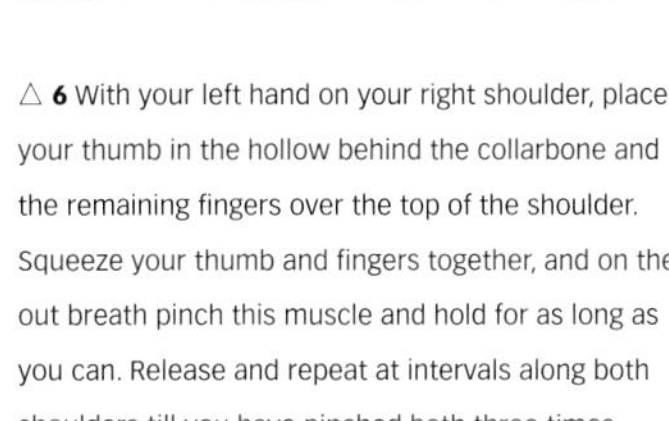

△ **6** With your left hand on your right shoulder, place your thumb in the hollow behind the collarbone and the remaining fingers over the top of the shoulder. Squeeze your thumb and fingers together, and on the out breath pinch this muscle and hold for as long as you can. Release and repeat at intervals along both shoulders till you have pinched both three times.

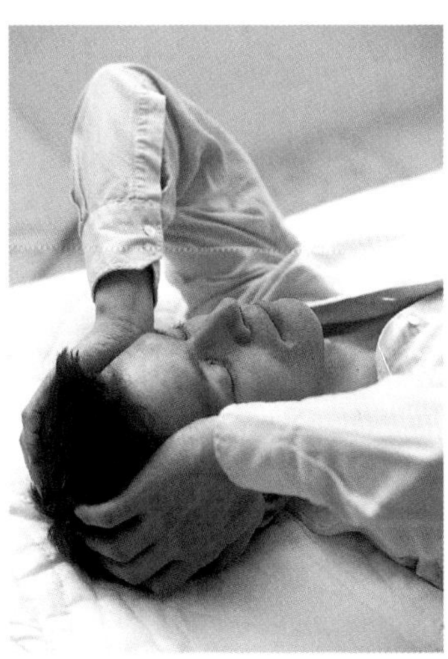

△ **7** Place the heels of your hands on your temples and, using medium to firm pressure, press while simultaneously making circles. Make at least six big slow circles and work into areas of tension. If you wish, you can extend this circling action to include the whole head and scalp, using the heel of your hands or your fingers.

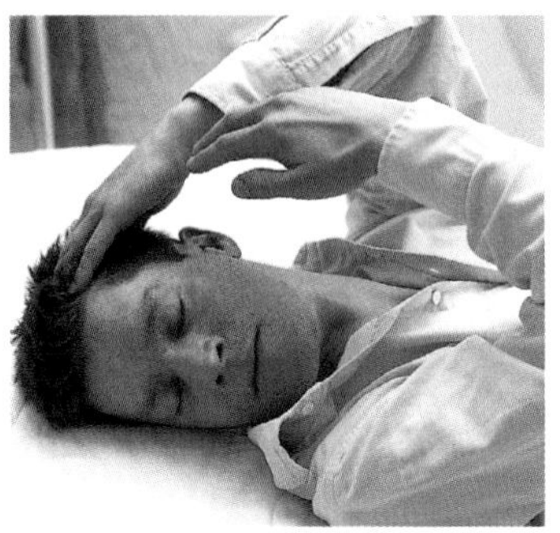

△ **8** Run your fingers across your scalp as if you were combing and lifting your hair away from your head. Flick your fingers away as they come off the ends of the hair. You can either do this stroke softly and slowly for a relaxing effect, or firmer and faster for an energizing clearing effect. Work over the whole of your head three times.

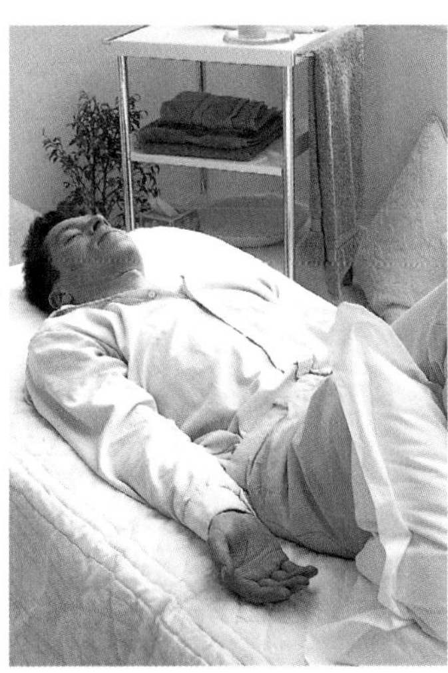

△ **9** To finish, take a deep breath in and out from your belly as in the beginning. Rest for a few moments, covering yourself with a blanket, if you wish. Imagine stale energy and stress leaving your body as you breathe out, and fresh energy revitalizing your body and mind as you breathe in. When you are ready, roll on to one side and get up slowly.

Relieving tension from driving

Driving is an integral part of a modern sedentary lifestyle. We use our cars to make short journeys around town, as well as for longer trips, and we spend a lot of time behind the steering wheel. For most of us, our cars are indispensable, yet driving can also create stress and tension in the body. To minimize this, we can cultivate some good driving habits. These include improving and adjusting our driving posture, taking breaks during long journeys and using some stretching and self-massage treatments to ease out tense muscles.

improving posture

How you sit at the wheel is a key to body tension. Bad habits include craning your neck to peer over the driving wheel or overextending your back by leaning too far backwards. The body's muscles then become tired and stressed, leading to aches and pains. If the back's lumbar region is not supported, it can have a tendency to sag and slump. This pulls on the muscles and puts a strain on the rest of the spine.

▽ **Driving in poor conditions, a hurry or heavy traffic can all contribute to poor posture and can have the effect of making it worse.**

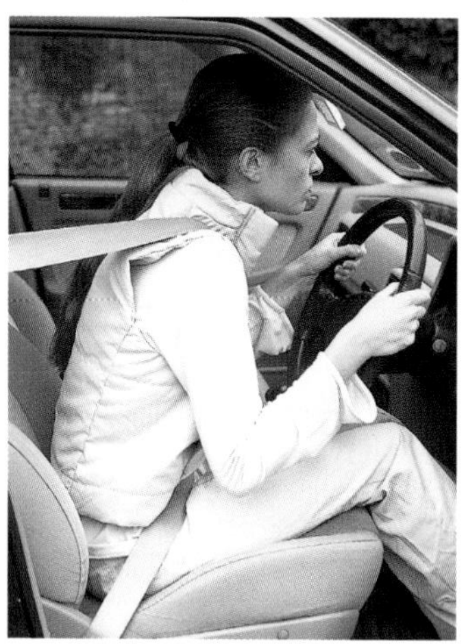

Good posture supports the body's musculature and helps keep its energies flowing. Make sure that you sit up straight and that your seat supports you. You can use cushions to adjust your position, or buy the special back supports now available. Have enough headroom between your head and the roof of the car, otherwise you may slouch to fit yourself into the available space. Adjust all the mirrors so you can see them without straining. Hold the middle of the steering wheel, keeping your arms relaxed. Don't twist your feet. They should be in line with your legs and facing forwards.

Sitting for prolonged periods in the same position impairs circulation and causes the body to stiffen up. This can lead to aches and pains in your neck and back, arms and wrists, or legs and ankles. It can also result in eyestrain and headaches, as well as lower levels of mental alertness.

To avoid freezing in the same position, make little postural adjustments as you drive. For instance, you can wriggle yourself further back into your seat, or if you are stuck in traffic, try relaxing your shoulders by lifting and releasing them. As you drive check periodically that your jaw is relaxed, your shoulders stay soft and that you are breathing from your abdomen.

▽ **Sitting in an upright position with a supported back can help make driving safer and minimizes the build-up of tension.**

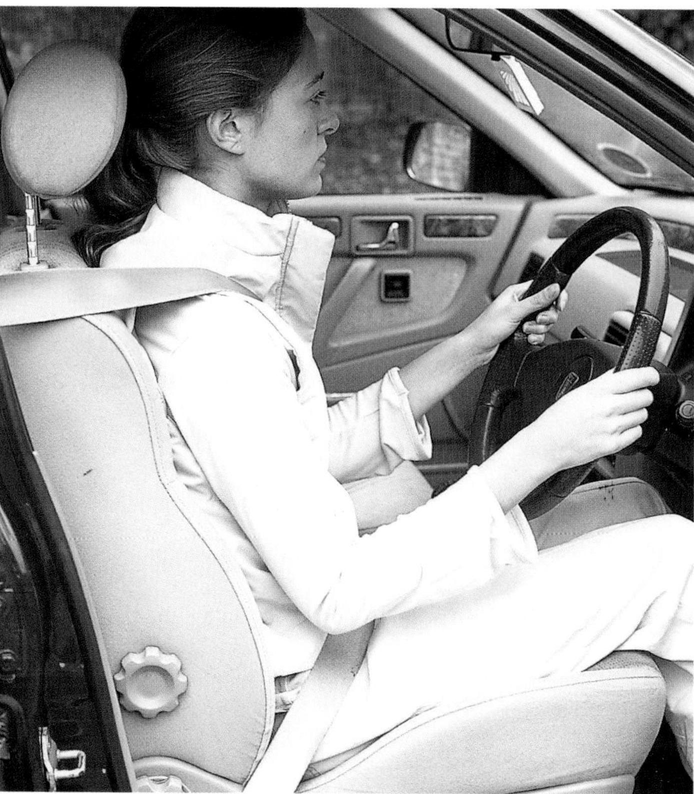

body stretches

On long journeys it is very important to take regular breaks to have some fresh air and a chance to stretch. This will help to release tension, improve circulation and restore concentration, making you a more relaxed and effective driver. Research now shows that taking regular massage and stretch breaks while driving has a beneficial effect on improving driver concentration and on reducing the number of road accidents. It has been shown to be much more effective than coffee breaks.

These stretches and massages are easy to do wherever you take a break from driving. Do each one a number of times. The stretches mobilize the spine, lower back, arms and shoulders.

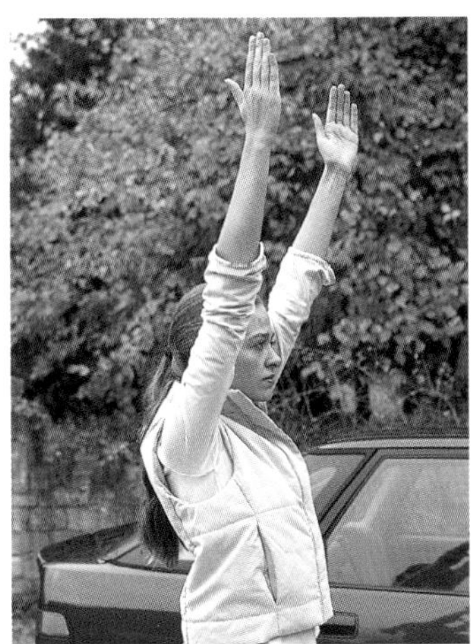

△ **1** Stand with your feet together and facing forwards. Breathe in and stretch your arms up above your head, lengthening up through your spine. On the out breath, bend your knees, tuck your chin in and roll your spine down, vertebra by vertebra, slowly bending forwards as far as is comfortable. Bring your arms down as you do this movement and let them swing gently backwards and forwards. On an in breath, bring your arms forwards and lengthen up through your body to come up to standing.

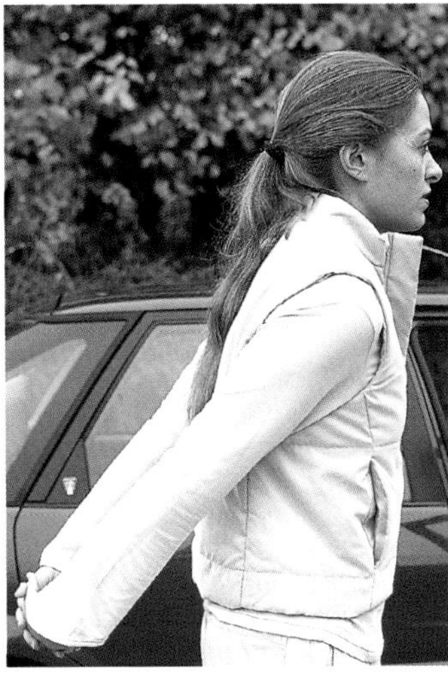

△ **2** Clasp your hands together behind your back. As you breathe out, bring them up slowly as far as possible. Hold and release slowly as you breathe in. Release your arms and let them drop down. Repeat at least three more times. This helps relieve tightness in the shoulders and between the shoulder blades.

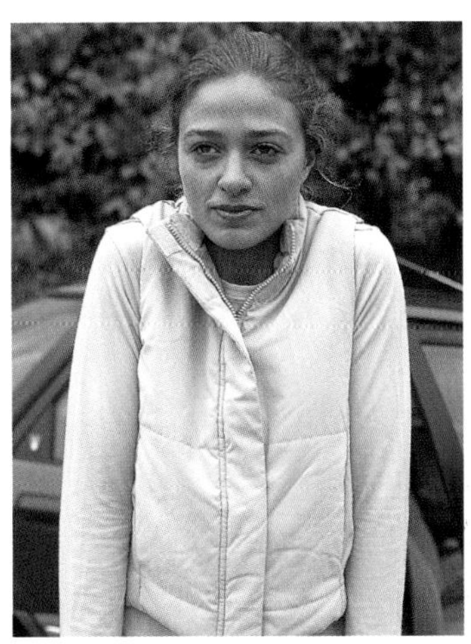

△ **3** Take a deep breath in and slowly begin to lift your shoulders up as far as they will comfortably go. Hold them up tightly as near your ears as possible. As you breathe out, let your shoulders drop abruptly in a release. You can extend this stretch by lifting and rolling your shoulders forwards as slowly as possible. Then change directions so that you roll your shoulders backwards. It can help if you try to imagine your shoulder blades meeting together in the middle of your back as you circle them.

self-massage tension relievers

You can also try this quick-fix self-massage during a driving break or when you get home. It will help to ease out tension in the head, neck, and shoulder areas.

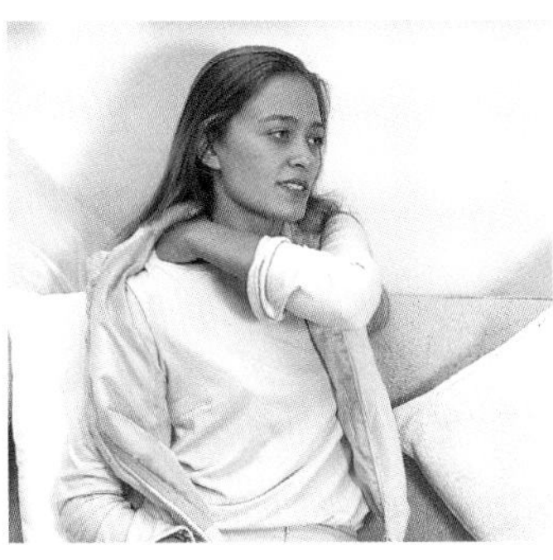

△ **1** Sit with your back well supported and place one hand over the opposite shoulder. Make small circular strokes across the shoulder using your fingertips. Work your way down into the upper back and along the edge of your shoulder blade as far down as you can. As your hand returns up your back, massage the muscles between your shoulder blade and spine.

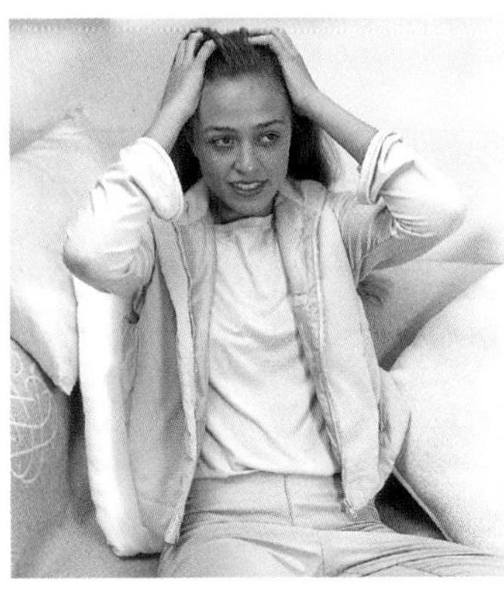

△ **2** Using your fingertips, rub back and forth across the top of your shoulder, following the muscles up into the side of your neck. Continue the movement up to your head, working around the whole head with this rubbing motion.

Sensual massage

Touch is the language of lovers and enjoying massage with your partner adds another dimension to your relationship, becoming part of your intimate exchange and a special way of spending time together. Head massage can be given in such a way that it becomes a sensual experience. Although some of the strokes in a sensual head massage are different from those in the standard routine, the key feature is the sensual quality of your touch and the blending of your energies together. It can be done with or without oils.

mood setting

To set the scene for a romantic and intimate space, think soft and warm. Candles, cushions and an open fire are traditional favourites for creating the right atmosphere; if you don't have an open fire, turn up the heating. Use your creative flair to beautify the space with flowers, fabrics and background music. You could also light some incense or vaporize essential oils in a burner. Many fragrances have sensual, aphrodisiac qualities – some of the most popular include sandalwood, jasmine, ylang ylang, rose and patchouli. Have plenty of towels and warm coverings to hand and a comfortable surface to work on. A duvet, futon, blankets or soft sheepskins make a well-padded surface. Finally, wear something loose and comfortable and appropriate to the romantic occasion.

giving sensual massage

If you are tense it will be difficult for your partner to relax, so make sure you keep your jaw and shoulders soft and breathe from your belly. Focus on giving pleasure to your partner by tuning in to their breathing and being sensitive to their changing responses. Enjoy making your strokes long and lingering or firmer and more stimulating, using your judgement and spontaneity as you work. The massage can be done sitting up or lying down.

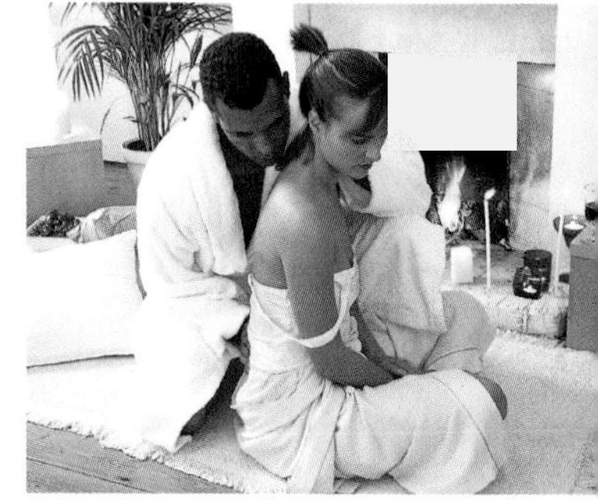

△ **1** This stroke stimulates the release and flow of sexual energy from the sacrum at the base of the spine. Place one hand on your partner's shoulder and the other at the base of the spine. Using your fingertips and very light pressure, make circular strokes in a clockwise direction around the sacrum. Build up a smooth rhythm and make the circles larger till the whole back is circled, each time returning to the sacrum. Gradually decrease their size, finishing at the sacrum.

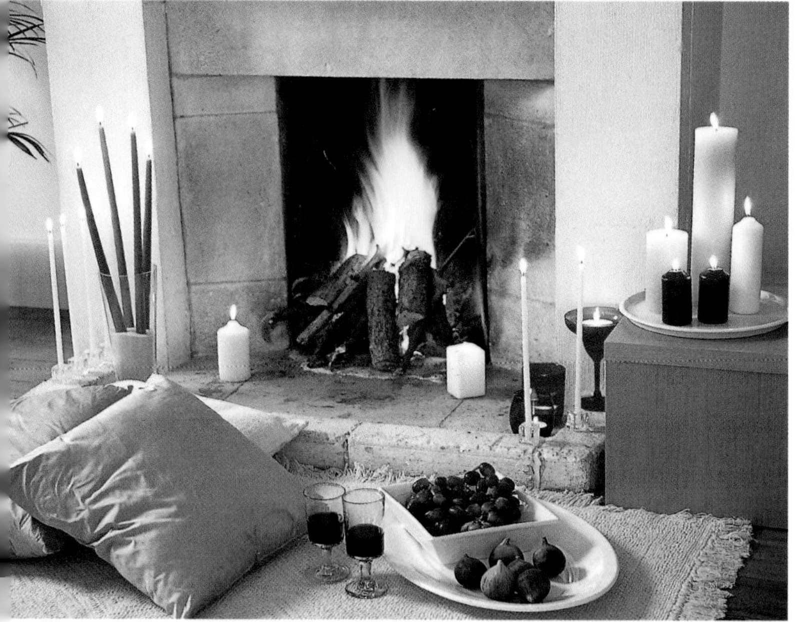

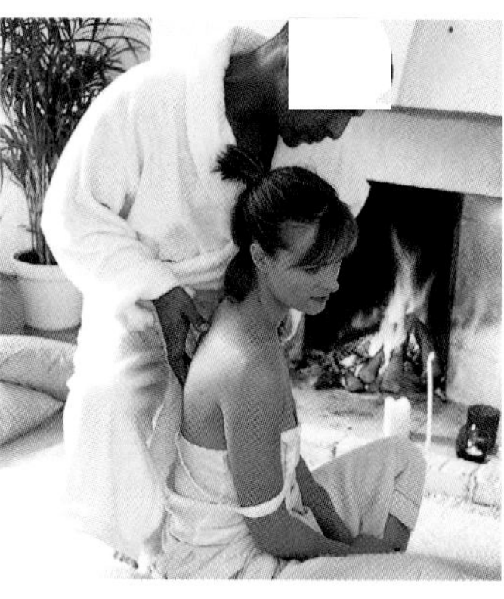

△ **2** With one hand on your partner's head, gently draw the fingers of your working hand up their back to the base of the neck. From here, gently stroke up the back of the neck a couple of times. If you wish you may also blow soft circles of warm air on the back of the neck. Both of these actions stimulate the nerve receptors in the skin and should send shivers of pleasure up your partner's spine.

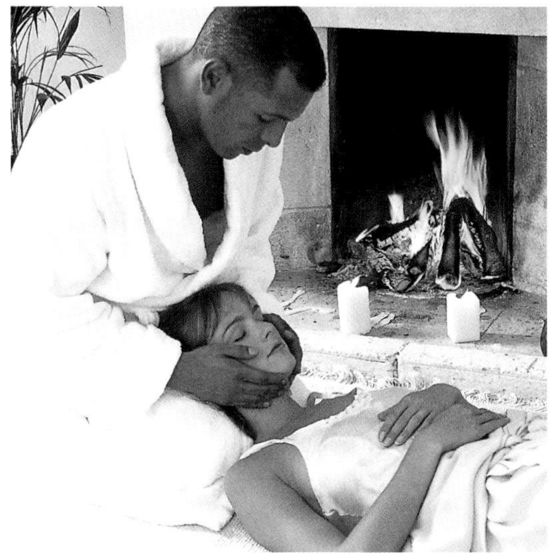

△ **3** For work on the face, your partner may prefer to lie down. Find a comfortable position with their head cradled on your lap or on a cushion. Place your hands at the bottom of their face so that you are cupping their chin. Slowly and gently draw your hands up over the face, up to the forehead and then stroke back down the sides to the chin. Repeat five times. To extend this stroke, use one finger to trace the features of your partner's face, beginning at the lips, and moving up around the nose, cheeks, eye sockets and eyebrows. Trace each feature three times.

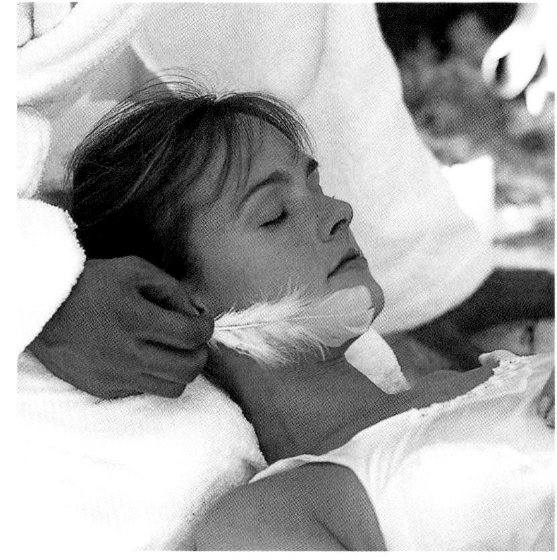

△ **5** Use a feather (or your own hair if it is long enough) for this stroke. Beginning at the chin, slowly trail the feather up the side of the face with slow luxurious strokes. Return to the chin and repeat several times and then switch sides. You can also stroke across the cheekbones and brow, working from the middle out towards the hairline each time. Imagine you are caressing away all cares and tensions as you lovingly stroke. Repeat several times. Should your partner find this ticklish, substitute the feather with some lingering finger-stroking up and across the face.

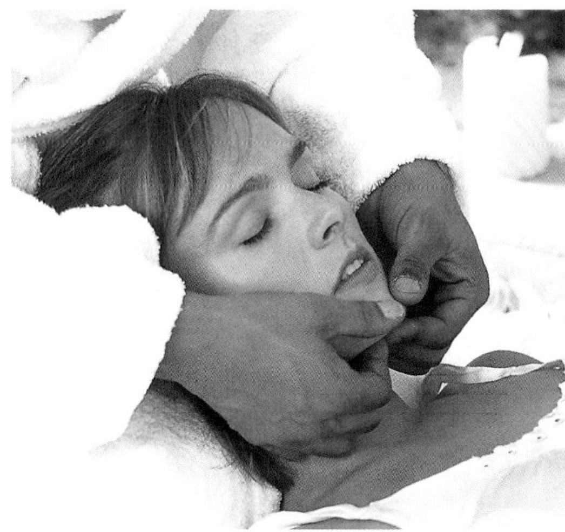

△ **4** Place both thumbs in the middle of your partner's chin, with the index fingers curled underneath. Make small circles with your thumbs on the chin, underneath the mouth and a little out into the lower cheeks, using your fingers underneath for support. As you work, make the circles slightly bigger to include the lower lip. Then gently use your thumbs to pull the lower lip down so that the lips are slightly open. To extend this stroke, continue to make small circular strokes with the pads of your fingers all over the face and forehead. Use a light touch and avoid the eye area.

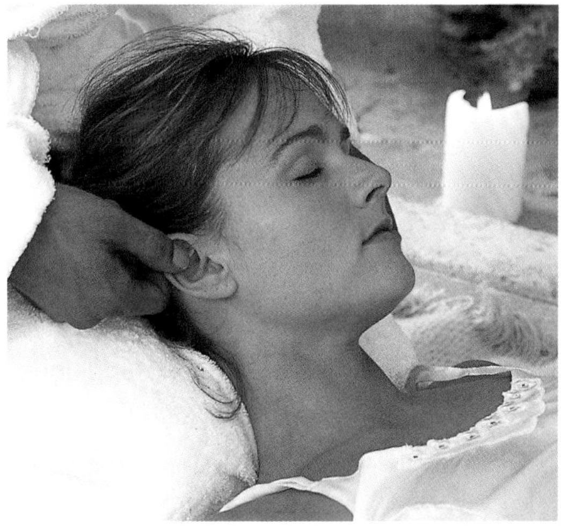

△ **6** Holding your partner's earlobes between your thumb and fingers, gently massage the ears by squeezing and rolling, moving up along each ear's outside edge and then down on the inside edge. Continue working round the ears until you have completed three laps. Then, using your ring finger, trace round each ear's outside and top edge as well as its inside surface. This is a highly delicate area, but done sensitively it can feel very intimate and sensual. Finish by gently pulling down on the earlobes a couple of times.

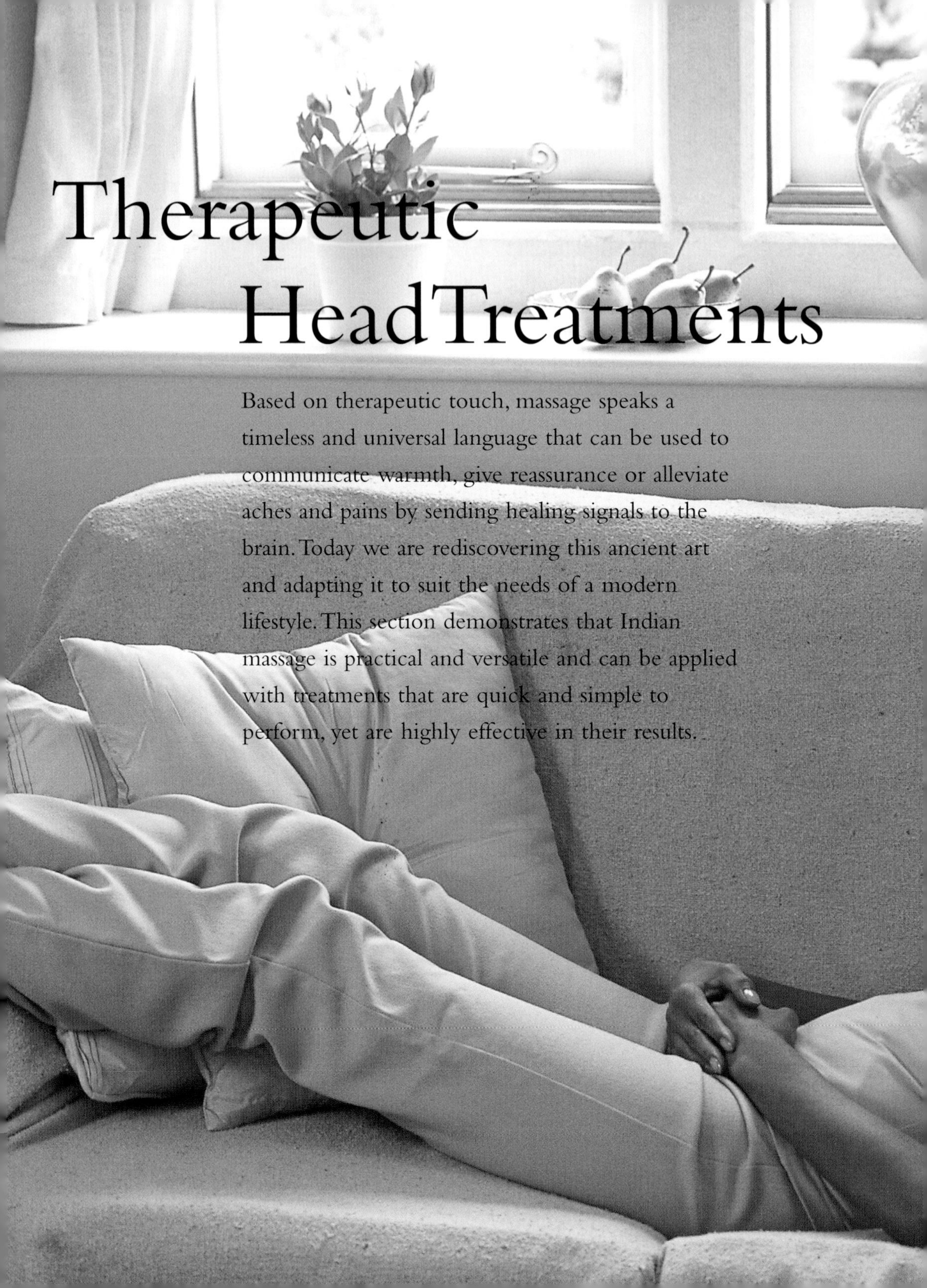

Therapeutic Head Treatments

Based on therapeutic touch, massage speaks a timeless and universal language that can be used to communicate warmth, give reassurance or alleviate aches and pains by sending healing signals to the brain. Today we are rediscovering this ancient art and adapting it to suit the needs of a modern lifestyle. This section demonstrates that Indian massage is practical and versatile and can be applied with treatments that are quick and simple to perform, yet are highly effective in their results.

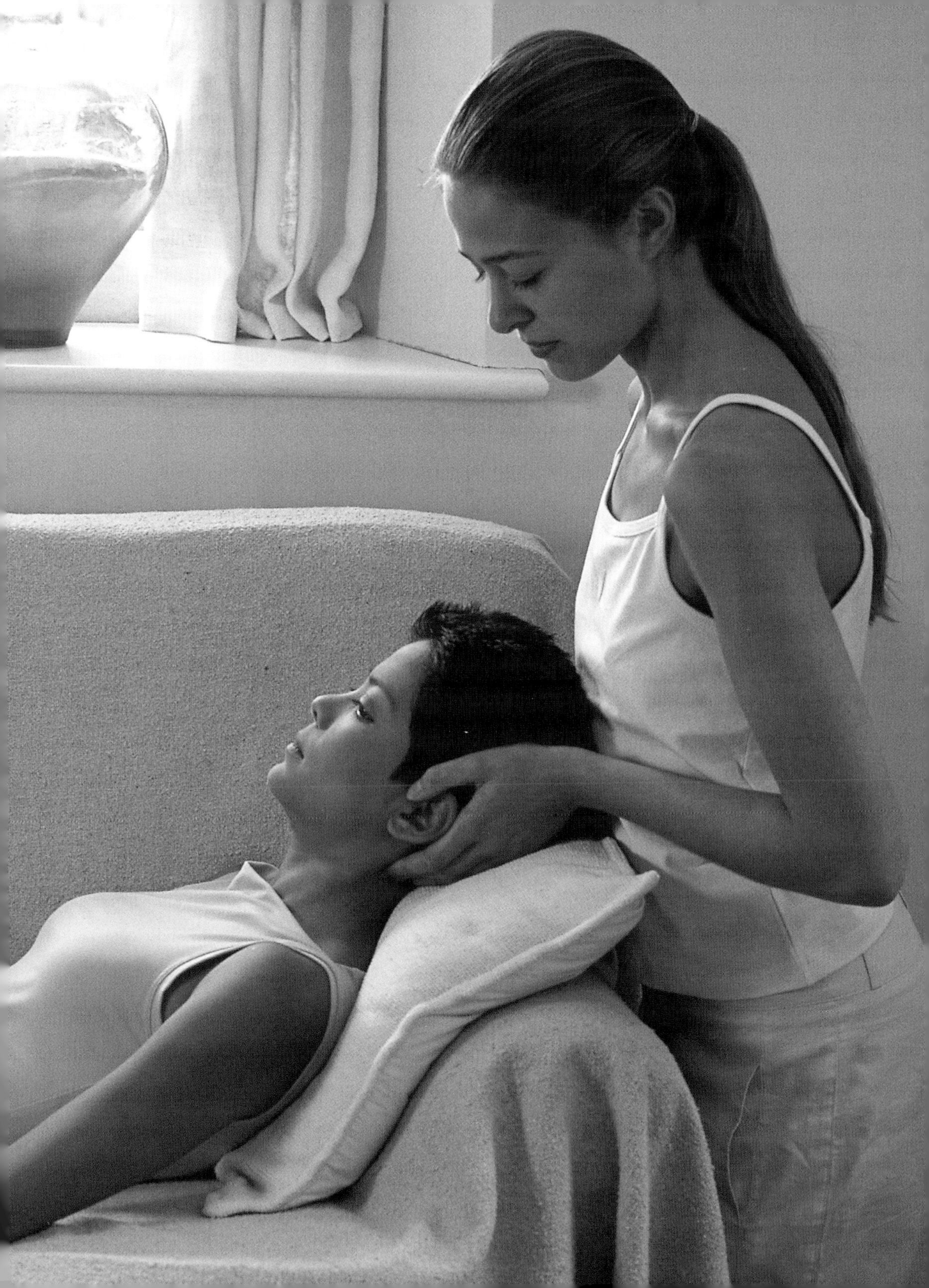

Relieving stress at work

Technological advances have revolutionized our working patterns. Many of these changes are associated with computers and an increase in sedentary jobs, which in turn is leading to a build-up of tension in the body and an increase in emotional stress. This is because our bodies are designed for movement, and our muscular structure functions most effectively when it is used in a whole, active and dynamic way. Increasingly this is not the case. We move in limited ways and hold our bodies in relatively static positions for extended periods of time. This is creating a range of common problems. It is in this context that massage becomes such a valuable tool for relieving stress in the workplace.

work stress

A typical office worker is likely to hold their back, neck, shoulders, arms and eyes in static positions for long periods of time. This causes the muscles to "freeze" into an almost permanent state of tension, in which they no longer work efficiently. The flow of nutrients, oxygen and blood supply is restricted, reducing the efficient circulation of blood to the brain and throughout the body. This leads to tiredness and irritability, as well as poor concentration and difficulties with decision-making. If the muscles are not released through movement or manipulation, they contract and toxins build up in the muscle tissue. This reduces mobility and causes all manner of aches and pains, while specific work-related conditions, such as repetitive strain injury (RSI) and carpal tunnel syndrome, are becoming increasingly common.

On top of the physical stress, many people experience psychological stress at work, which usually makes the physical discomfort worse. Time limits, dealing with frustration or feeling pressurized to perform can all literally become "a pain in the neck" if emotional pressures are not discharged at some point.

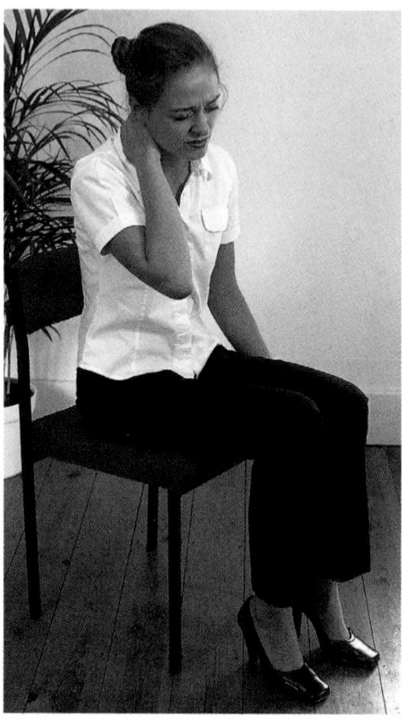

△ **Sitting down working at a desk or computer for long periods of time often causes tension and pain in the neck and shoulders.**

self-help measures

Current thinking says that for every hour that you spend working at a computer screen, you should take a ten-minute break. During this time you should do something active to help discharge physical tension. This could include self-massage, stretch and release exercises or massage with a co-worker. Done regularly, such measures will help discharge tension, particularly from the upper body. They will also help to keep body and mind relaxed and alert during the whole working day.

releasing neck tension

With one hand, grab a handful of flesh from the back of your neck. Squeeze it as hard as feels comfortable and hold the pressure, slowly nodding your head up and down at the same time. Mentally say the word "yes" to yourself as you do this. Keep breathing as you repeat this movement a couple of times. Swap hands, and this time shake your head from side to side, mentally saying "no" inside your head.

neck and shoulder stretch

This stretch helps to release tight neck and shoulder muscles and can be done standing or sitting. Lift one arm and bend it so that your hand is facing palm down on your upper back. Take your other arm and bend it so that your hand reaches up your back with the palm facing outwards. Move both hands towards each other so that the fingers meet and clasp together. If the hands do not reach one another, then rest them as close together as possible. Hold for 15 seconds, maintaining a steady breathing rhythm. Change hands and repeat the stretch on the other side, again holding it for 15 seconds while breathing steadily.

▽ **Taking regular breaks to release taut neck muscles with self-massage contributes greatly to preventing the gradual build-up of chronic tension.**

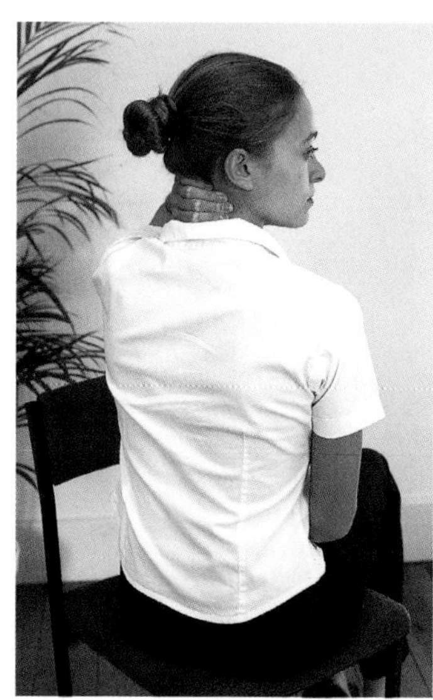

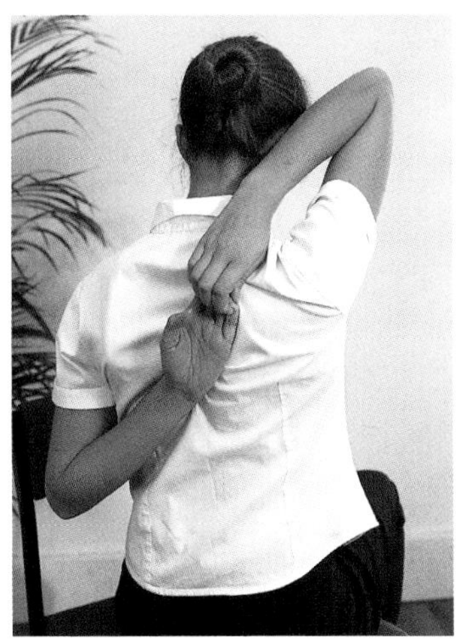

△ **Stretching breaks help release and promote deeper breathing, which oxygenates the body and brain, increasing brain functioning.**

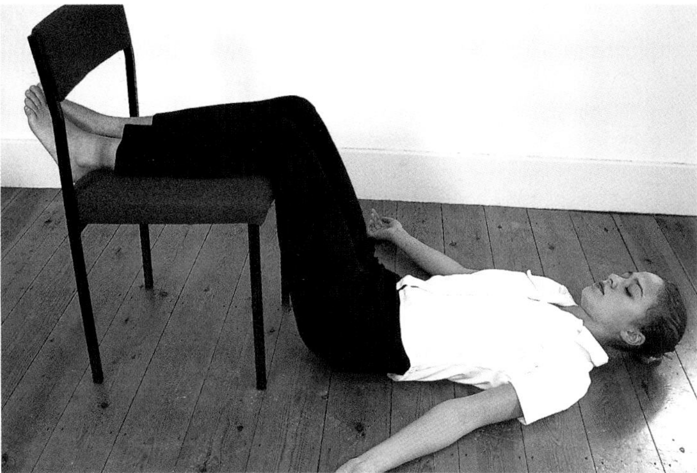

△ **Lying down so that your spine can be supported by the ground gives it a chance to decompress and rehydrate, leaving you feeling refreshed and alert.**

resting the eyes

Our eye muscles get surprisingly tired from focusing for long periods on a fixed plane of vision, such as a computer screen. This simple palming exercise will give your eyes a rest and help to release taut eye muscles. Vigorously rub your hands together so that they become warm and energized, then place them over your eyes, your fingers resting on your forehead. Close your eyes. Hold for a few minutes while your eyes rest in the darkness of your hands. Use the time to tune in to your breathing and focus on letting go of tension as you breathe out.

▽ **It is important to rest your eyes following periods of concentrated work, as this helps to prevent strain and stress, which contribute to headaches and impaired vision.**

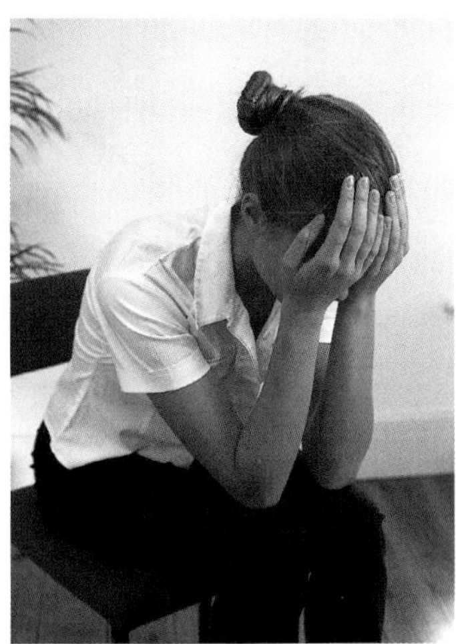

back, neck and shoulder release

The following exercise should help release tension in the upper back, neck and shoulders. It encourages the effective flow of blood back to the head and brain and is ideal after an extended period of deskwork, such as at lunchtime. If you cannot do it at your own desk, you may be able to find another suitable place such as an unused conference or meeting room.

Sit on the floor at right angles to a chair. Then swivel around so that you are facing the chair and put the lower half of your legs up. Your feet and calves should be resting flat on the chair and your knees should be bent at right angles with the floor. Let your arms fall out to the sides with palms facing upwards. Wriggle your back and adjust your position so that your spine is as flat as possible on the floor. It is best if you can close your eyes and rest in this position for at least five minutes.

Gently breathe in and out and use your imagination to visualize the fresh flow of oxygen, blood and nutrients flowing up through your back, shoulders, neck and head to your brain and then down again. This will help to replenish and recharge your upper body and head.

co-worker massage

Massage between work colleagues can create a much happier atmosphere. This is a very quick and easy routine. Sit your partner in front of you and gently rest your forearms on their shoulders. Ask them to take a deep breath in and on the out breath, press down on their shoulders. Then use the whole of your hands to rub briskly over their shoulders and upper back.

▽ **Making co-worker massage part of your work culture makes a noticeable difference in terms of increased creativity and efficiency.**

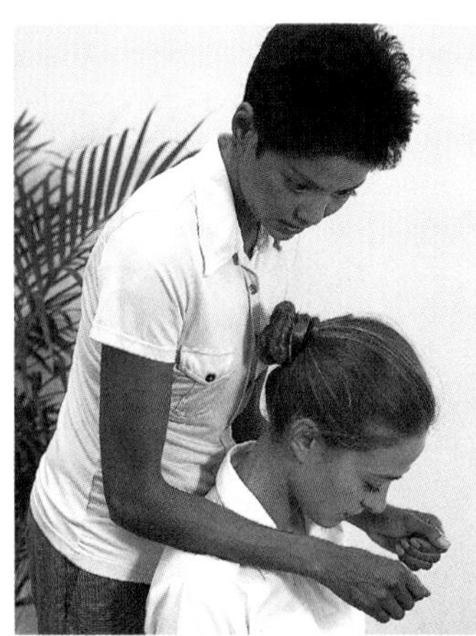

Asthma management

Asthma is a breathing disorder that affects one in seven of the population. It can occur at any age and involves inflammation of the bronchial tubes, excess mucus production and the contraction of muscles in the chest area. This narrowing of the air passages restricts the flow of oxygen and leads to breathing difficulties. These can range from a mild tightening in the chest to restrictions that are so severe that they require urgent hospital treatment. Regular massage to the neck and shoulder area can help reduce both the number and severity of asthma attacks. Massage can also be used to alleviate the symptoms of a mild attack.

a typical asthma profile

Asthma sufferers tend to be highly sensitive and particularly prone to stress and anxiety. Their breathing is rapid, shallow and restricted, with a tendency to breathe through the mouth rather than the nose. They are especially liable to hold tension in the neck, upper back and shoulders. Constriction in these areas inhibits the full expansion of the diaphragm, which in turn restricts lung capacity. Releasing tension in the neck and upper back through massage can help to open up the breathing. It can also help to calm anxiety and help the person to relax.

pressure points on the back

The lung-associated acupressure point, situated on either side of the spine between the scapulae, is associated with relieving the symptoms of asthma and reducing muscle spasms in the shoulders and neck. Massage in between and around the shoulder blades can therefore help relax the muscles and give some relief during an asthma attack.

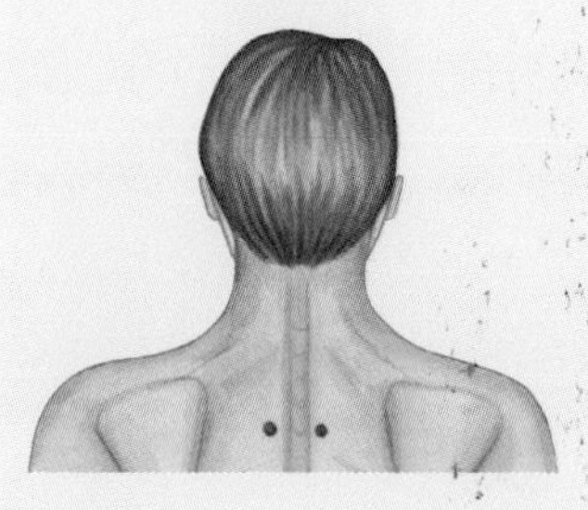

useful essential oils

These are some of the essential oils that help to open up the breathing, relax bronchial spasms and calm anxiety during a mild asthma attack. Use 3–5 drops essential oil added to 10ml (2 tsp) massage oil or lotion, and use as a chest rub. Alternatively, vaporize the oils in a burner.

- eucalyptus or juniper: opens up the airways, encourages expulsion of mucus
- frankincense or marjoram: helps to calm and relax
- rosemary or peppermint: reduces general breathing difficulties

healthy breathing

Research has shown that there are some basic breathing principles that are especially helpful for asthmatics. The first is to develop the habit of breathing through the nose and not the mouth. Breathing through the nose helps to regulate and slow down the breathing. It also means that the air is warmed in the nasal passages before it enters the lungs. Cold air entering the lungs changes the chemical balance and can make the internal environment more susceptible to an asthma attack. Second, it is advised to try to breathe from the abdomen rather than the upper chest. This will help to slow down and deepen the breathing, which helps to stave off an oncoming attack.

causes and effects of asthma

Some types of asthma are triggered by an allergic response to dust, pollen and animal hair, as well as certain foodstuffs, such as dairy products. Other causative factors include stress and exposure to tobacco smoke and high levels of environmental pollution. There can also be cases where a genetic factor may also be involved.

During an asthma attack, the constricted bronchial passages cause wheezing, coughing, and feelings of panic, which serve to exacerbate the symptoms.

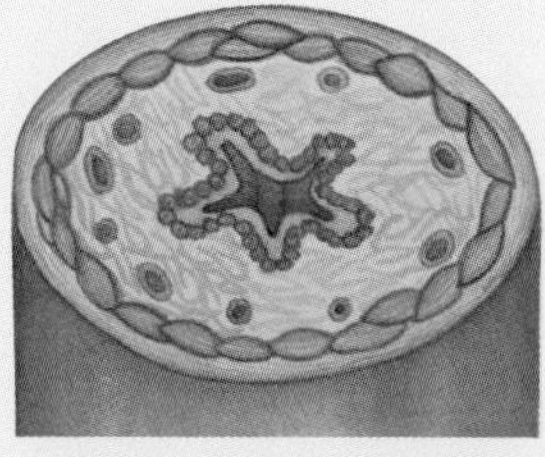

△ **Bronchial passages contract during an asthma attack as the surrounding muscles exert pressure on them, restricting breathing capacity.**

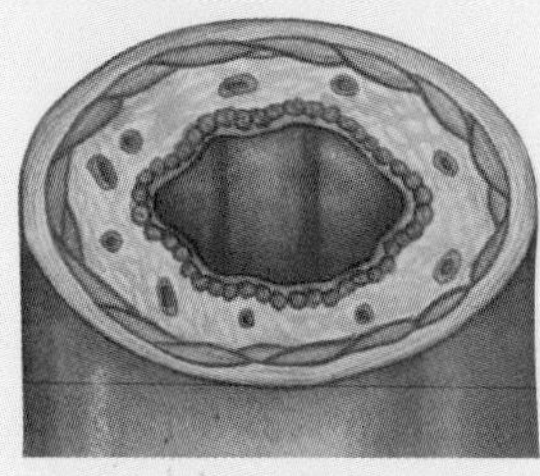

△ **When the attack has subsided and the muscles have relaxed, the airways can expand once more, allowing air to pass through unrestricted.**

massage for asthma

Have your partner sit at a table so they can lean forwards if they want or need to.

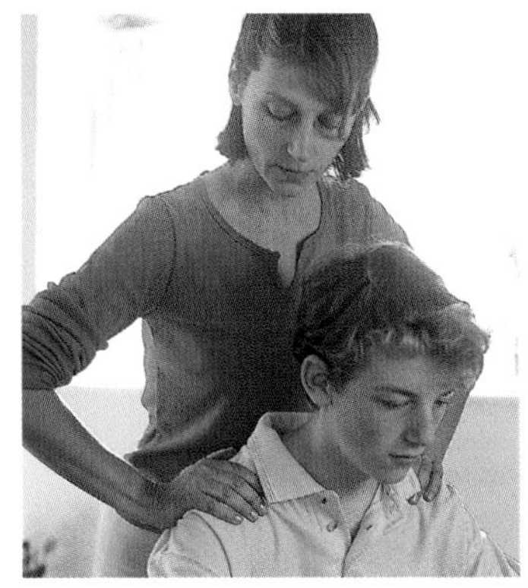

△ **1** Gently place your hands on your partner's shoulders. Ask them to breathe in through their nose and then out for as long as possible. Do it with them. Ask them to take a second deep breath. On the out breath, gently press down on their shoulders, encouraging them to soften.

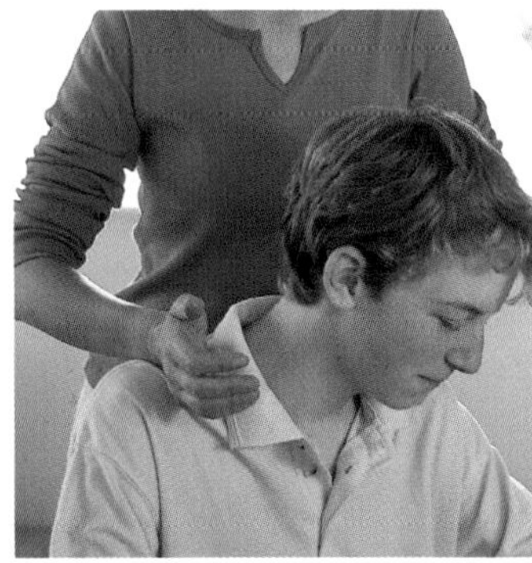

△ **2** Move a little to the left of your partner and anchor your left hand on their left shoulder. Holding your right hand loose and open, use a zigzag rubbing motion with the side of your hand, working along the top of your partner's right shoulder and then down around the shoulder blade into the back. Work the muscles that run between the shoulder blade and the spine itself. Change sides and repeat.

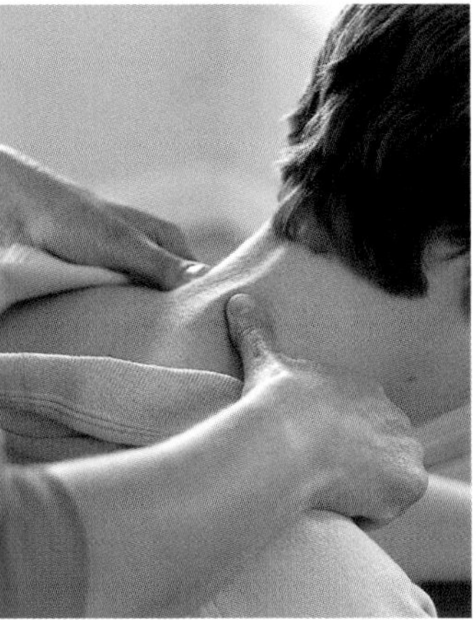

△ **3** Stand behind your partner and hold their shoulders, positioning your thumbs at the base of the neck. With both thumbs working together, make small firm circular strokes across the base of the neck (avoiding the spine), moving a little down into the upper back and a little up into the shoulders.

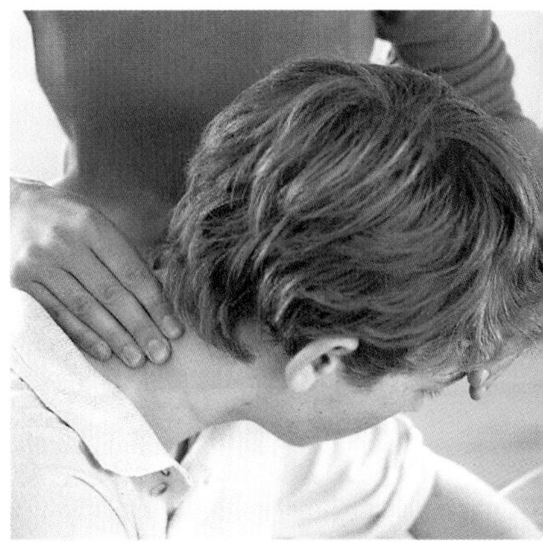

△ **4** Move to the left of your partner. Support their forehead with your left hand. Place your right hand at the base of the neck and, with a wide span, grasp and pull back the neck muscles. Sweep up to the middle and then to the top of the neck, using the same movement. Repeat three times.

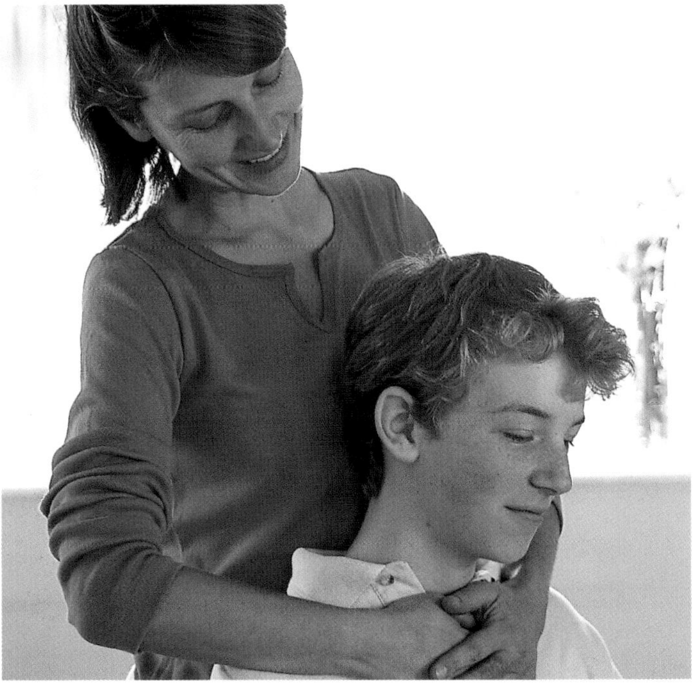

△ **5** To finish the massage, put your hands on the front of your partner's chest just below the collarbone. Using a sweeping stroke, brush outwards and upwards towards the shoulders. Have a sense of your partner's chest opening and expanding as you work. Repeat three times. Come to a rest, putting your hands on your partner's shoulders, and take a deep breath in and out together.

Massage for anxiety

It is more or less impossible to go through life without ever feeling anxious. Any change constitutes some level of stress. Positive life events, such as marriage, the birth of a child or a new job, as well as the more obvious negative ones like divorce, bereavement or redundancy, are fairly common situations, which put us to the test. Sometimes however, anxiety can become a more chronic condition. This happens when we have more stress in our lives than we feel able to cope with and are living in a perpetual state of fear and worry. Massage is an excellent treatment for anxiety. It can reassure and help discharge many unpleasant symptoms.

symptoms of anxiety

Anxiety has a way of pervading the personality so that the symptoms seem to take over. This can show up as someone who is short-tempered, over-reactive, preoccupied and restless, or alternatively as someone who feels overwhelmed, tearful and unable to cope. Anxiety also affects the body. Muscular tension, shallow, rapid breathing, palpitations and aching muscles can all be symptoms of anxiety. Similarly signs of general unease, such as butterflies in the stomach, feeling light-headed or else permanently exhausted are signs that the body is under too much stress.

the benefits of massage

Anxiety is linked with fear and insecurity so the gentle touch of another person can be especially reassuring, helping to alleviate negative symptoms in a safe, supportive environment. A treatment can help the anxious person to relax, leaving them feeling stronger and more able to cope with anxiety-provoking situations. To help with the releasing process, it can help to encourage your partner to sigh as you work, but only do this if you both feel comfortable with it. Other signs that your partner is releasing tension and anxiety during a treatment include reactions like yawning, laughing, shivering or even shuddering. Sometimes they may feel upset and start to cry.

friction strokes

Firm, fast action friction strokes are very effective for cutting through tension. By vibrating the muscle fibres together, they access the deeper muscle layers and nerve bundles and encourage them to relax. It is a little like shaking a bowl of sand, where all the bigger grains and stones are brought to the surface as you shake.

▽ Take time at the beginning of the session to chat with your partner to make sure you have an accurate idea of how they are feeling.

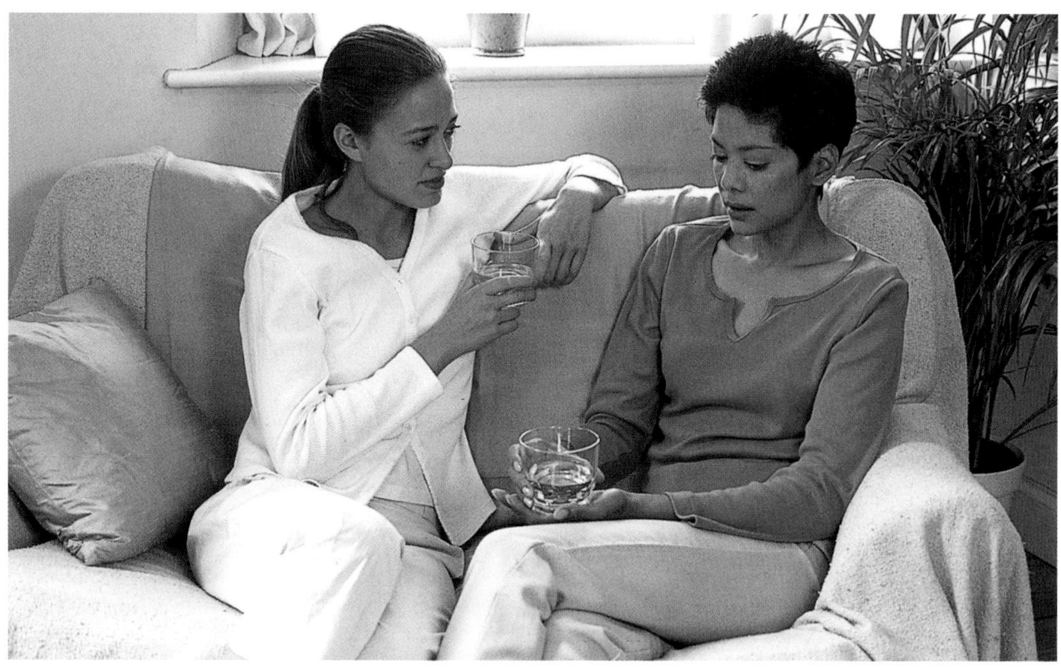

massage treatment for anxiety

To create trust in your partner, your touch will need to be particularly firm and confident. This will help your partner feel that it is safe to relax and let go. You should be able to build on the trust you established during your chat at the beginning of the session. For this massage, as for many others, your openness and empathy are as important as your physical skill.

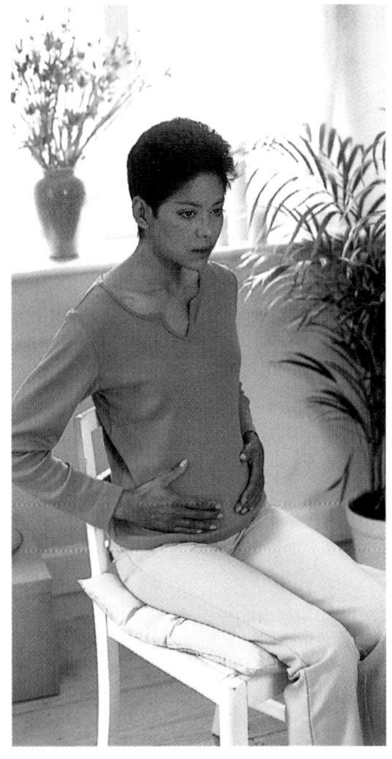

△ **1** Ask your partner to put their hands on their belly and to take a deep breath in to that area, feeling their belly expand outwards as they do so. On the out breath, their belly should contract and their hands move inwards. Repeat this sequence several times. You can do it with them to show them and to support them. Abdominal breathing will help your partner to relax and slow down. It will also help to move the focus of attention away from the anxiety. Once they have done this a few times you should be able to sense when the time is right to begin working on the massage sequence.

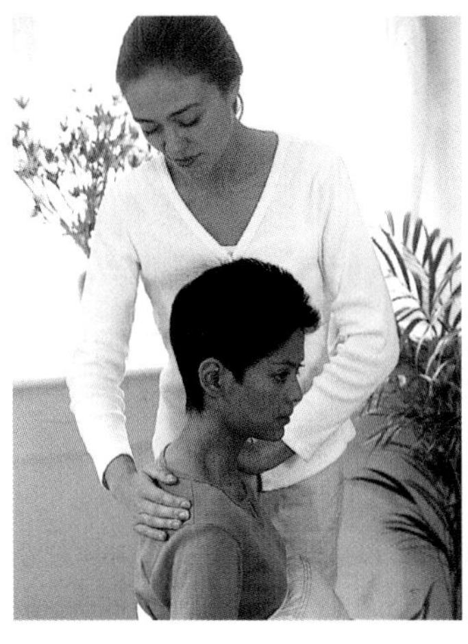

△ **2** Stand to the left of your partner and gently but firmly support their left shoulder with your left hand. With the fingers of your right hand close together, rub in a zigzag motion across their right shoulder. Work rhythmically and firmly over the shoulder, around the shoulder blade and into the upper back. Repeat three times. Repeat on the other side. Work briskly upwards along the edge of the shoulder blade three times, making circular strokes with your thumbs.

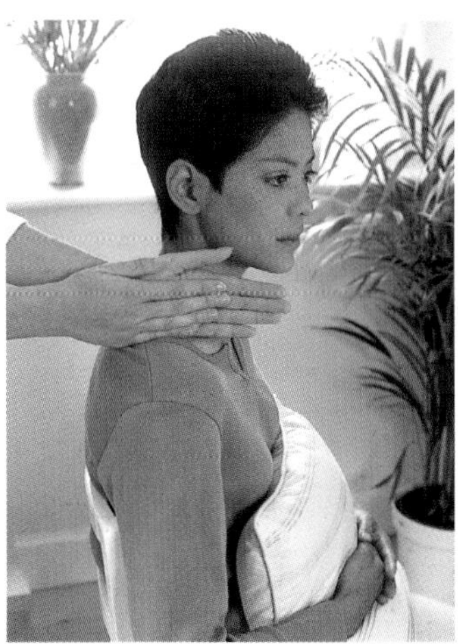

△ **3** Stand behind your partner. With your hands in prayer position, put them side-on at the base of your partner's neck. Applying pressure, rub your hands together in a sawing action and work swiftly across the top of the shoulder to the outer edge of the upper arm and then back again, building up speed as you get into a rhythm. Repeat three times and change to the other side. Use your fingers to firmly sweep out across the shoulders and down the back a few times.

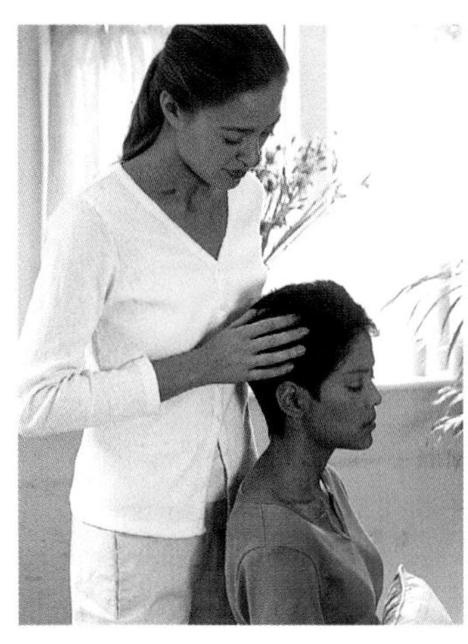

△ **4** Slide your hands up to your partner's head and put one on top of the other with your fingers pointing forwards. Slide the bottom hand away from the top, spread out your fingers and draw them down through the hair using a raking zigzag motion. As you come to the bottom of the head, let the top hand continue the stroke, raking down over another part of the head. Continue for the whole head. Repeat three times. Follow with soothing stroking.

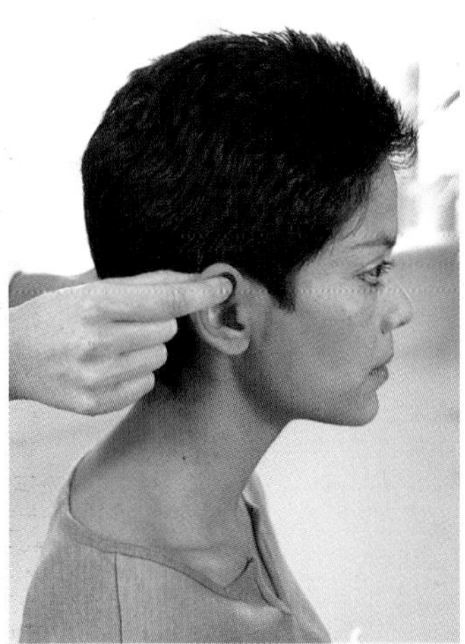

△ **5** An acupressure point for relieving anxiety is located near the front of the earlobe. Holding each ear between your fingers and thumbs, exert gentle pressure at this point for a few seconds and release. Then gently massage this point, moving upwards. Repeat three times on each ear. Use the same grip to squeeze and roll down the outside edge of each ear from top to bottom. Repeat three times. Finish by gently stroking and pulling the earlobes.

Headache relief

There are many different types of headache, such as cluster headaches and migraines. However, the vast majority of headaches are caused by muscular tension, with the pain ranging from mild to severe. Before rushing for the painkillers, try using a little head massage, as it is a very effective treatment for tension headaches. It not only eases the pain, but can also help re-educate the body so that it has a more relaxed response to stress and does not automatically tense up.

There are many reasons why muscular tension builds up, and tension headaches usually have a mixture of physical and psychological components. They often disappear once the stress trigger has gone. Where the trigger is ongoing however, the headaches can become chronic, with muscles locked in a state of contraction.

reflexology point for headaches

The pressure points that are most useful for headache treatments are those located at the base of the skull and the top of the spine. Make sure that when you are working on these points remain aware of how sensitive they are. Only apply very gentle pressure, and do not carry on if there is any pain or discomfort.

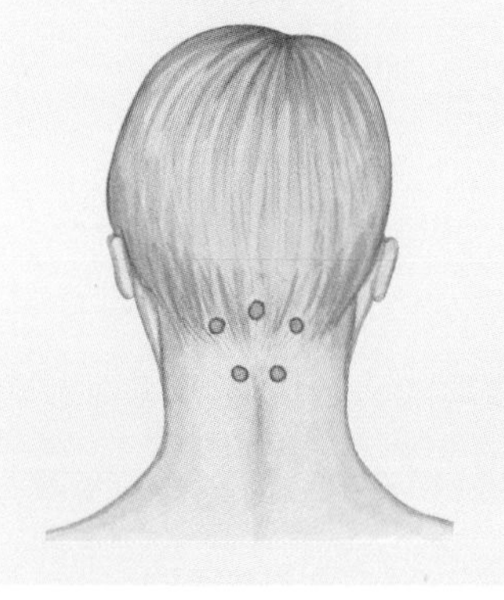

self-massage

The following strokes can be very effective for instant headache relief. They can be done almost anywhere. Leaning your elbows on the table and using your arms to provide support for your head makes the massage more effective.

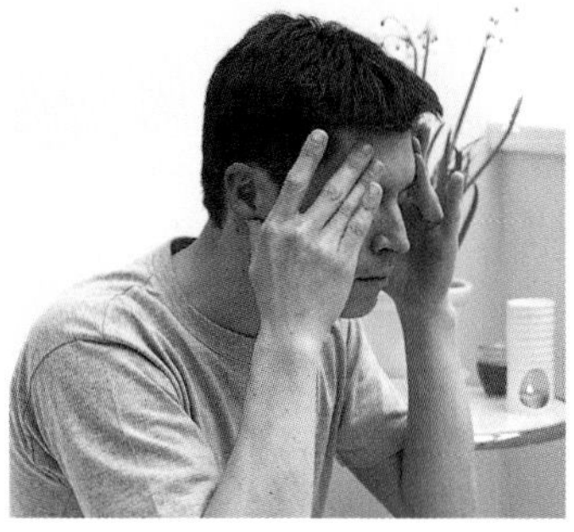

△ **1** Use the pads of your middle fingers to smooth out your forehead. Begin at the bottom of the brow area and work outwards, pressing and smoothing out towards the hairline. Then move your fingers up a little and work across the next section, continuing in this way until you have covered the whole forehead. Repeat twice more.

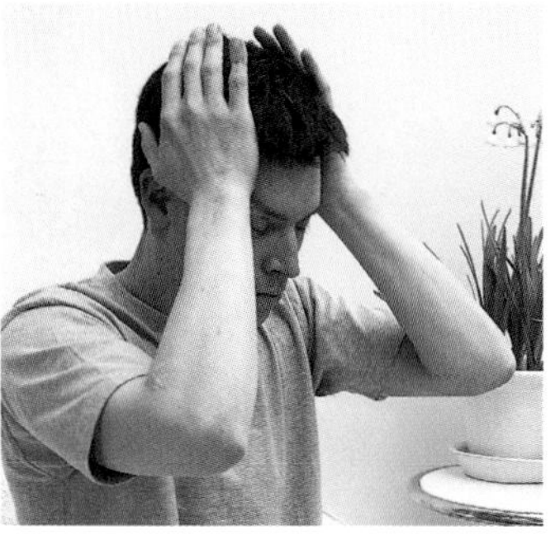

△ **2** Place your hands over your temples and press inwards with the heel of your hands (or use your palms if you prefer). Using a circling action, work six times in a clockwise direction and, reversing the movement, six times anti-clockwise.

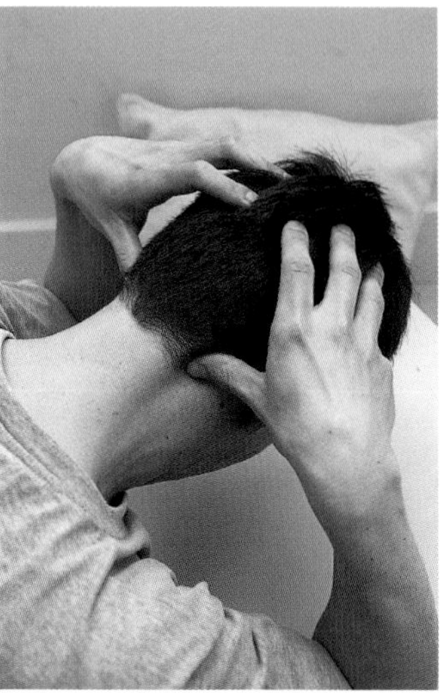

△ **3** Place your thumbs on the bony ridge behind your ears. Using a firm pressure, press and release. Continue with this action, working along the base of the skull until you get to the middle. Repeat three times. If you find any particularly tight spots, these are likely to be trigger points for the headache. Take a deep breath in, and on the out breath press more deeply, holding for a count of seven.

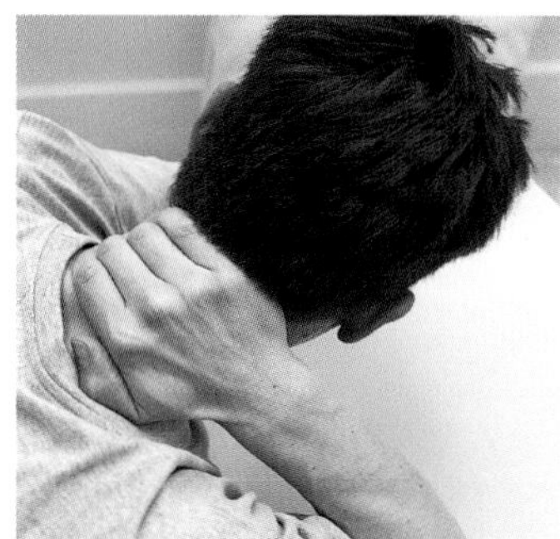

△ **4** Bend your head slightly forwards and support it with one hand. Use your other hand to clasp the back of your neck and squeeze it. Press as hard as you can and hold the pressure as you breathe out. Repeat so that the whole neck is worked over three times.

▷ To help your partner switch off and unwind, make sure the space you will be working in is relaxing and protective. You should both feel comfortable and at ease.

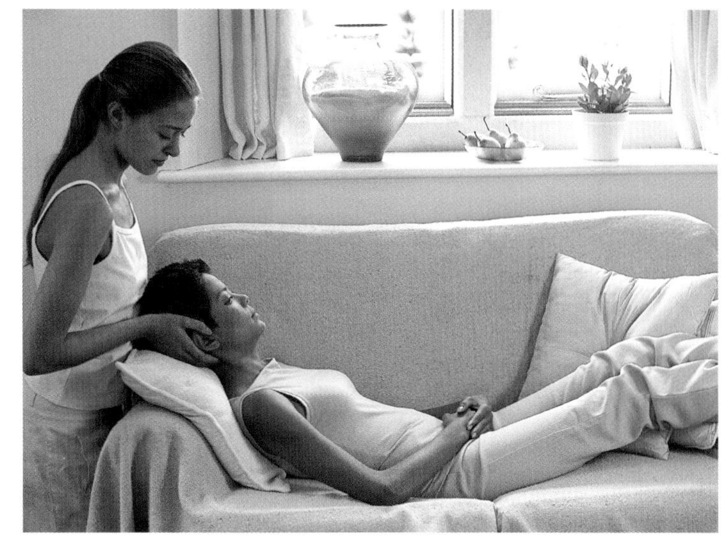

massage with a partner

Head massage can help ease the pain of a tension headache. Where the headaches are chronic, regular treatments can also help dissolve deep-seated muscular tension and play a key role in ongoing stress management. Headache treatments are best done with your partner lying down so that their head is completely supported and the neck muscles have a chance to relax and let go. Make sure that your partner drinks plenty of water before and afterwards to encourage the elimination of toxins.

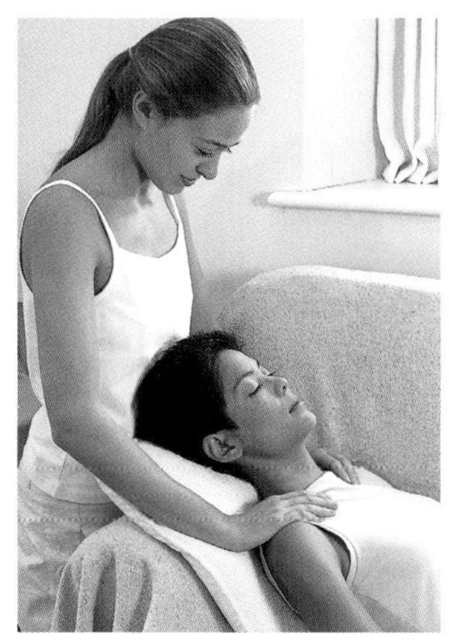

△ **1** Kneel at your partner's head and rest your hands over their shoulders. Ask your partner to take a deep breath in and out. On the out breath, gently press down on the shoulders, using both your hands. Repeat three times. This movement helps to relax tension in the shoulders, as well as releasing the muscles of the neck.

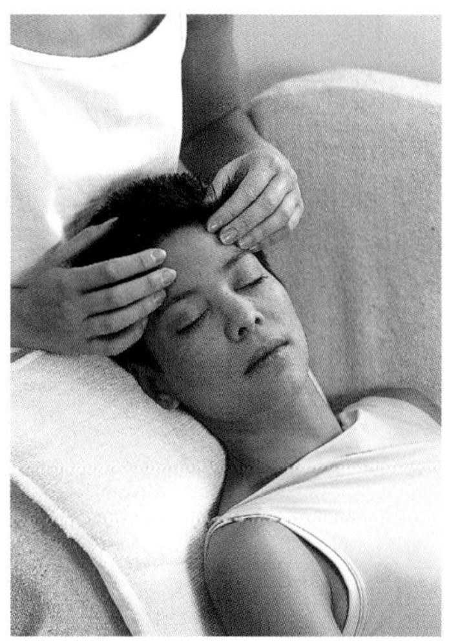

△ **2** Move your fingers to the middle of your partner's forehead. Keeping your fingers together, use smoothing strokes, working from the centre out towards the temples. Repeat several times. This relaxing movement helps to release tension in the tight muscles across the forehead.

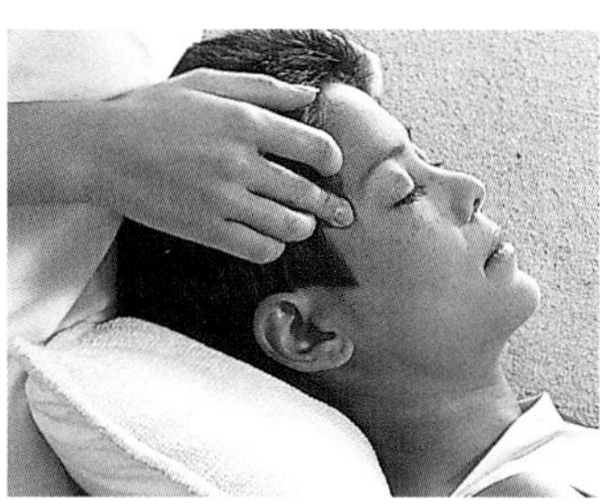

△ **3** With your hands positioned over your partner's temples, make small circular strokes with your fingertips. Check how much pressure feels good for your partner. If the headache is intense, a light touch is usually best. Move your fingers down and back slightly to continue the movement at the side of the skull just above the ears.

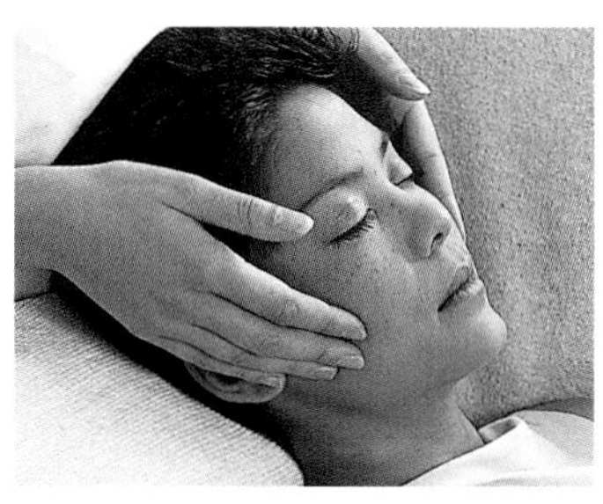

△ **4** Slide your hands down to the jaw hinge and continue to fingertip massage, using small circular strokes. Continue down the jaw line. The jaw holds a lot of tension and these strokes help it to release.

contraindications

Do not treat the following types of headaches with head massage: migraines and cluster headaches; those brought on by environmental factors such as noise or pollution, or by dehydration or exhaustion; and those associated with fever, illness, hangovers or infection.

Sinus decongestion

Sore sinuses can be extremely painful. They often follow in the wake of a cold or flu, but allergic conditions such as hay fever can also bring them on. The problem is caused by a build-up of mucus in the sinus cavities, which restricts the opening of the sinus into the nose. If the mucus membranes are inflamed or infected, the sinus area becomes very sore, and may give rise to headaches or facial pain. This condition is usually known as sinusitis. For mild cases or at the onset of an attack, massage can be extremely helpful in helping the mucus disperse and in relieving this distressing condition.

steam inhalations

A steam inhalation can work wonders, particularly after a massage when the mucus has been loosened. You need a towel, a bowl of hot water and maybe one or two essential oils. Eucalyptus and peppermint have anti-viral, cleansing and head-clearing properties, while lavender is anti-viral and a relaxant. Add 2–3 drops of oil to the hot water. Use the towel to make a tent over your head and the bowl, close your eyes and breathe in the steam. If you suffer from asthma, steam inhalations are best avoided.

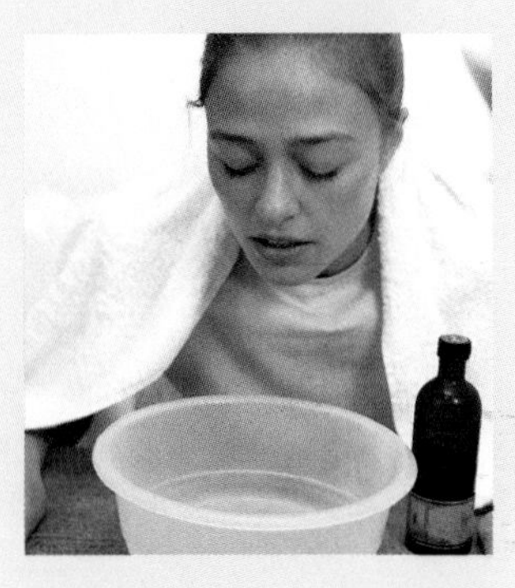

mucus production

The production of mucus is a primary response of the body's auto immune system. It is one of the body's first defences against pathogens (disease-causing agents), and is produced to destroy these hostile invaders. An increase in mucus could be in response to a virus, as in the case of coughs and colds. Or it could be an allergic reaction to substances such as tobacco smoke, pollen, chemicals, animal fur or certain foods. If an allergy is involved, it is advisable to try and identify the trigger and to eliminate it as far as possible.

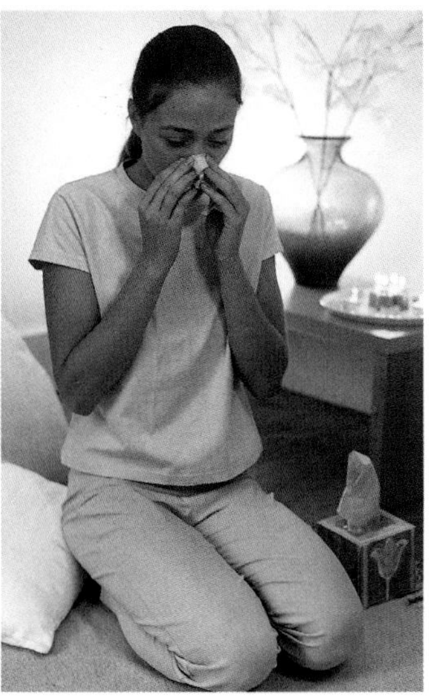

△ If you are suffering from congestion try to eliminate dairy products, sugar and wheat from your diet as these foods are all mucus forming. Increasing your fluid intake by drinking more water, herbal teas or hot ginger and lemon will also help the body to flush out congestion.

▷ When facial sinus points are too sensitive or painful to touch, the sides of the fingertips provide an alternative place to exert gentle pressure, using your thumb and index finger.

acupressure points for sinus pain

Applying pressure to these acupressure points on the face and neck will help relieve sinus pain. If the area feels tender, only use the gentlest pressure.

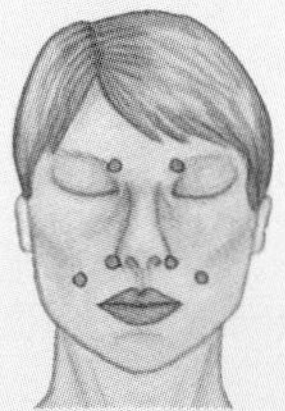

△ Use your ring fingers of both hands for these points on the face. Hold in position for a few seconds at a time.

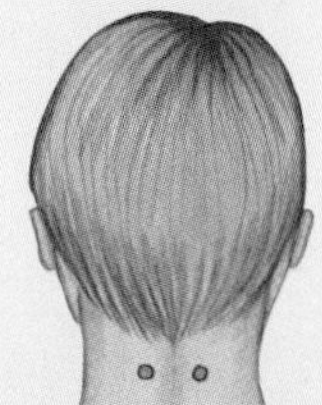

△ Acupressure points on the muscle either side of the spine just below the skull can help relieve congestion in the head. Apply gentle pressure on them with your thumbs.

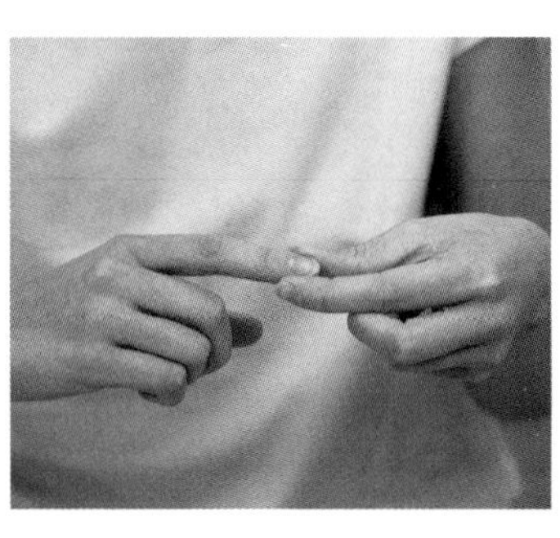

self-massage for sinus relief

Congested sinuses are often painful to touch, so working on yourself allows you to regulate the level of pressure. This routine can be done a number of times through the day to help clear congestion and assist breathing. Ideally, this massage should be followed by a steam inhalation with essential oils to help flush out the mobilized congestion.

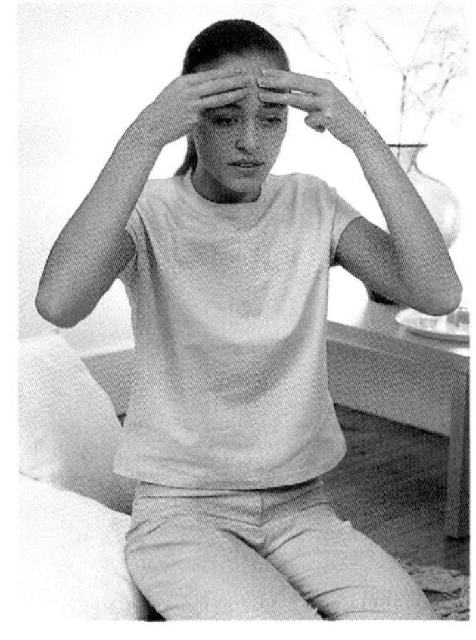

△ **1** Sit in a comfortable position and place your hands just above the mid-point between the eyebrows. Work your way across the forehead, making small circles with your fingertips. Anchor your thumbs at the temples and stretch your fingers to meet in the middle of the forehead. Then sweep your fingers out and across the forehead, imagining your sinuses clearing out as you do so. Use whatever pressure is comfortable.

contraindication

Massage is contraindicated in sinus conditions that are accompanied by a fever, green or yellow mucus, or that have been going on for more than three days. In these cases you should seek medical advice.

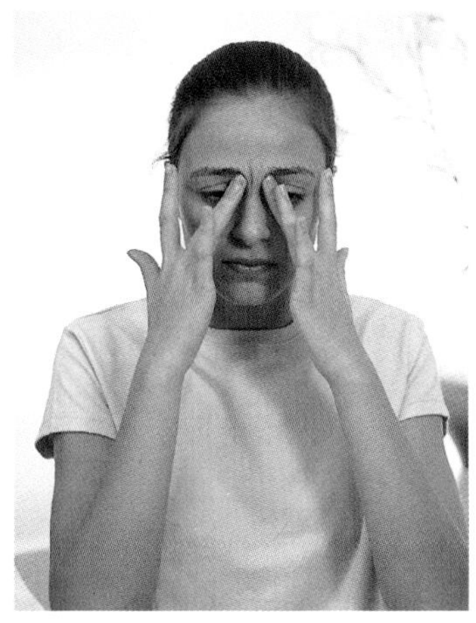

△ **2** Place your middle fingers in the spot on either side of the nose where it meets the underside of the eyebrows. Take a breath in, and on the out breath, press firmly for a few seconds and then release. Repeat three times. This is a crucial pressure point for the sinuses and may feel tender to touch. Continue along the underside of both eyebrows for about 2.5cm (1in), exerting similar pressure. The sequence is press, hold, release, repeat and move on. Complete by using a pinch-and-lift movement on the eyebrows, working your way along to the outside edge. Repeat a few times.

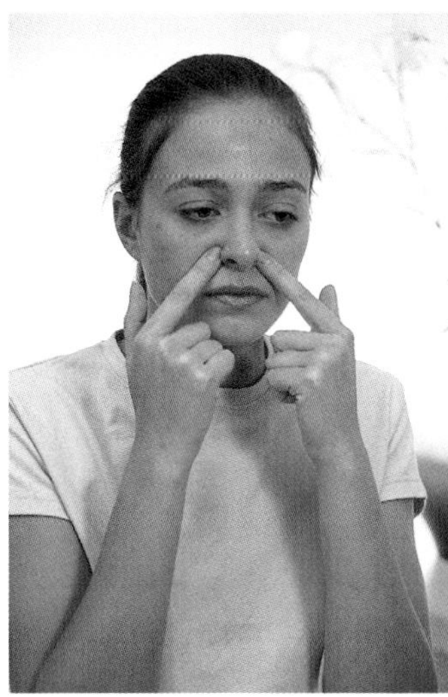

△ **3** Position your index fingers on either side at the base of the nose and apply pressure, holding and then releasing. Repeat three times. This is another important pressure point for opening up the sinuses.

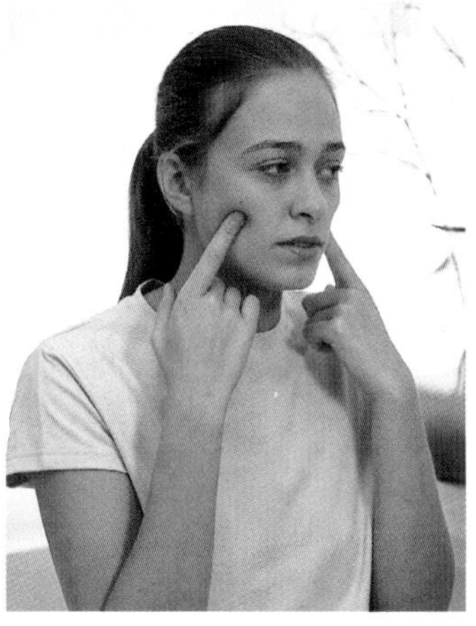

△ **4** Draw your fingers out along the underside of the cheekbones and use pressure strokes along its edge. A sinus drainage tube runs along this area. There are more drainage points underneath the jawbone, running from the middle of the chin to the ear. Use your thumbs to make small circular movements along this line. Finish with some smooth sliding strokes that will help to drain away the congestion.

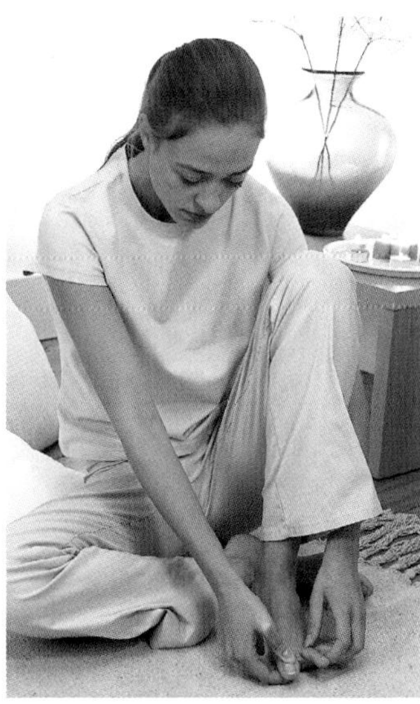

△**5** For maximum effect, or if the sinus areas are too painful, you can work with foot pressure points. Squeeze and press the tips of your toes and press and slide down their sides to the pads beneath. Continue doing this, paying particular attention to the big toes. To relieve a frontal sinus headache, apply pressure to just below the nail of the big toe.

Head massage for insomnia and illness

Massage can give comfort to someone who is unwell and accelerate the healing process, and for sleep-related problems it can relax the body and help the mind to switch off. These very different situations require different approaches.

treating insomnia

For chronic sleeplessness the underlying causes need to be investigated, but generally most sleep problems are linked to stress and tension. When you're lying in bed and can't get to sleep, you can use head massage to ease body tension and hopefully induce calm and peaceful slumber. The strokes are suitable for both partner and self-massage.

To prepare yourself breathe deeply in and out from your belly, perhaps letting out a sigh or a yawn on the out breath. Then let your jaw drop so that your mouth is partly open and your tongue rests softly in it. Roll up a small ball of saliva in your mouth and keep it there – higher levels of body fluid are associated with deeper states of relaxation. Keep your eyes gently closed, making sure that your eye sockets remain soft. Keep your mouth moist with saliva.

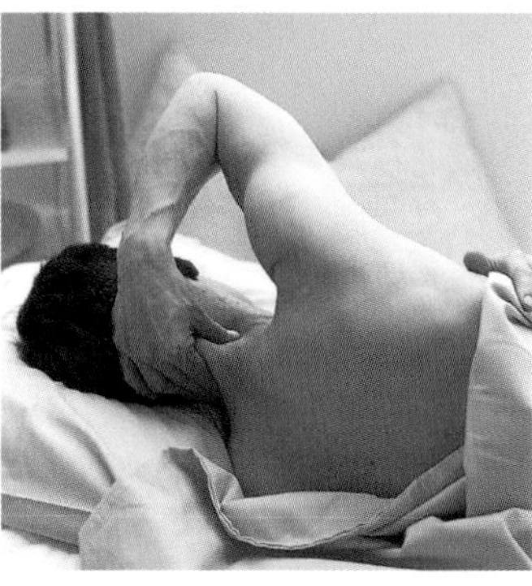

△ **1** As you breathe out, firmly squeeze the middle back of your neck with one hand. Hold the pressure for 15 seconds and slowly release. Repeat at the top and bottom of your neck. Cover the neck area three times and repeat on other side.

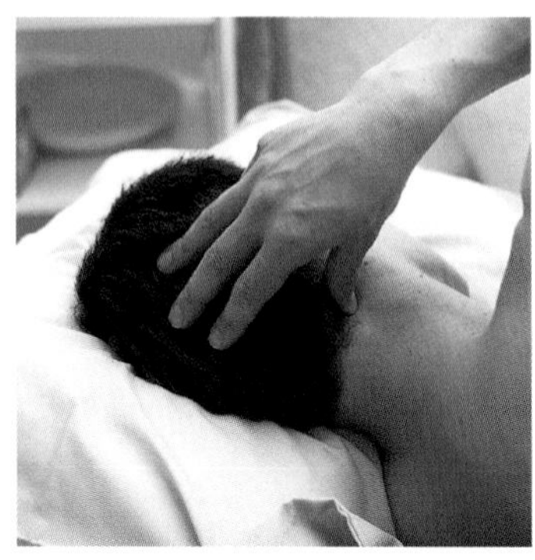

△ **2** Still lying on your side, use your thumb to press into the base of the skull in the area just behind the ear. Continue pressing, moving down along the skull's ridge to the hollow in the middle of its base. Stay longer in any particularly tight or painful spots. You can also make circular strokes here with your thumbs. There are many pressure points along this area that can help to promote restful sleep. Turn your head and repeat on the other side.

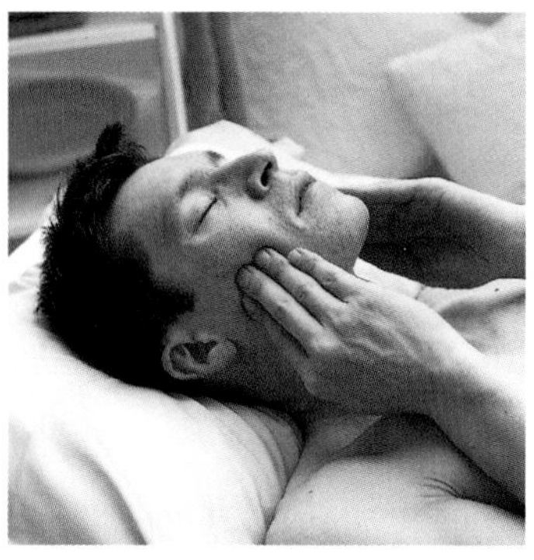

△ **3** Now lie on your back, and use your fingers to make circling strokes around the jaw area, paying particular attention to the jaw socket. Use stronger pressure here if you wish. As the jaw benefits from repetitive work, keep this action going for a few minutes. As you massage you can listen to the soothing sound of your breath. Alternatively, breathe in through your nose and out through your mouth to encourage repetitive, sleep-inducing yawning.

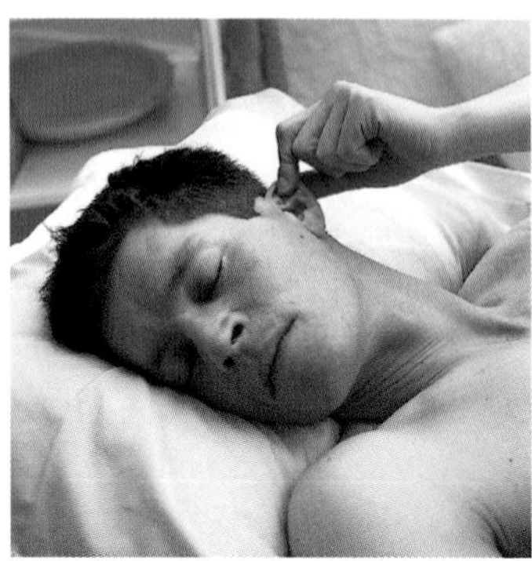

△ **4** Turning your head slightly, place your index finger at the top of your upper ear. Slide it down to just below the ear's top outer ridge and across to the edge of the dimple in this ridge. Position your thumb so that it is resting on the underside of the ear's ridge, just behind your index finger. Press firmly and use your finger to massage in a circular movement for about 30 seconds. This special pressure point is associated with calming the mind. Repeat on the other ear.

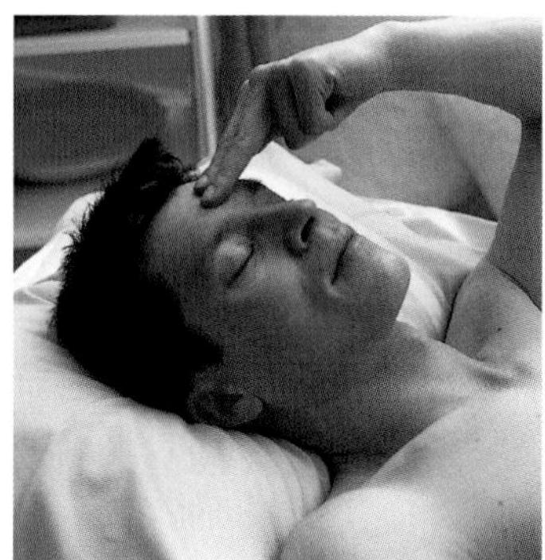

△ **5** With your head back to centre, place your first two fingers in the middle of your forehead and make slow circular strokes using a light pressure. Continue with this circling action and work out towards your right temple, making the circles bigger as you go. Circle over the temple area and then use connecting circular strokes to move to the left temple. Repeat once or twice more. This stroke also calms the mind and slows down thinking processes.

▷ **A soothing presence of touch can be very reassuring and pleasurable to receive when feeling unwell and can help accelerate healing.**

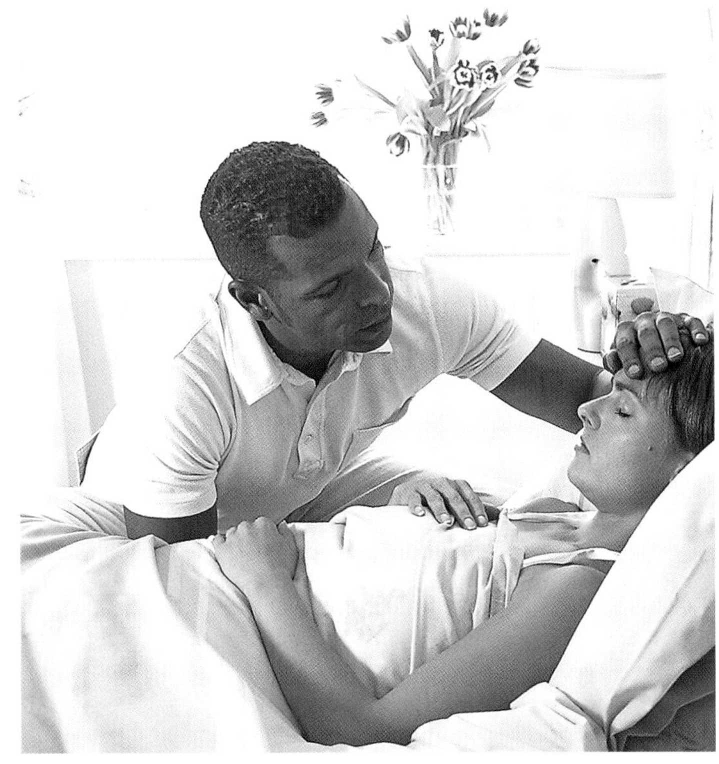

head massage and illness

During illness, a traditional style head massage would be over-stimulating and could feel invasive. The body's energies are taken up with trying to get well and in these situations a different kind of approach is called for. A gentle hand massage that uses light and tender strokes, however, can be healing and soothing to receive and also speed up recovery. This type of massage can be used during convalescence but not during acute conditions. Before massaging anyone who is unwell, observe the usual contraindications; if you have any doubt then check with a qualified medical practitioner. As a general guide, remember to keep your touch light and gentle and avoid firm pressure. The strokes should be fluid, smooth and flowing and stop when your partner has had enough.

hand massage

A light hand massage can promote healing and relaxation throughout the body's systems without being too vigorous. Pressure points on the hand have physiological correspondences to the rest of the body, there are also nerve receptors located here which will send messages of relaxation to the brain.

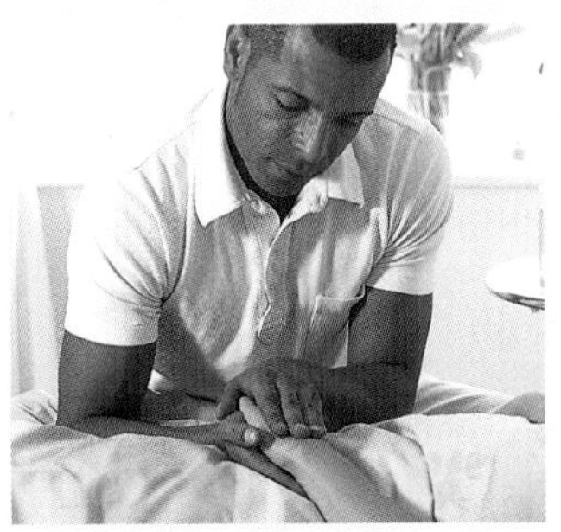

△ **1** Gently sandwich your partner's hand in between your hands and then use your top hand to stroke downwards in the direction of the fingertips. Next, take each finger at a time and stroke down to the fingertip. Repeat on each finger three times. Repeat on the other hand.

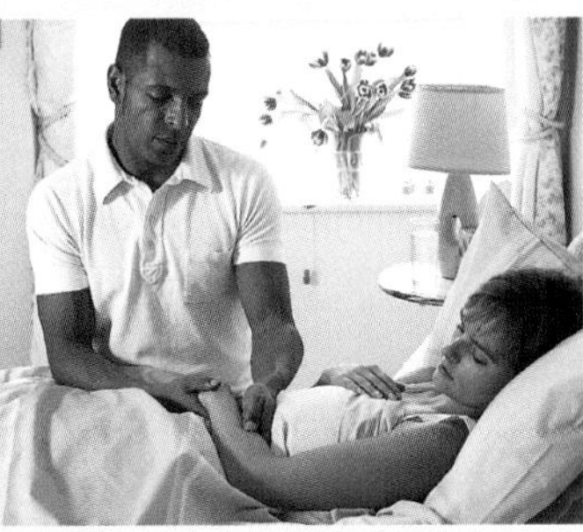

△ **2** Next, move your hands to the arm and make circling actions with your thumbs, working round the muscles of the arm, then the joints of the wrist and hand. Make your touch increasingly light as you move down the arm. Do this three times and then change to the other arm.

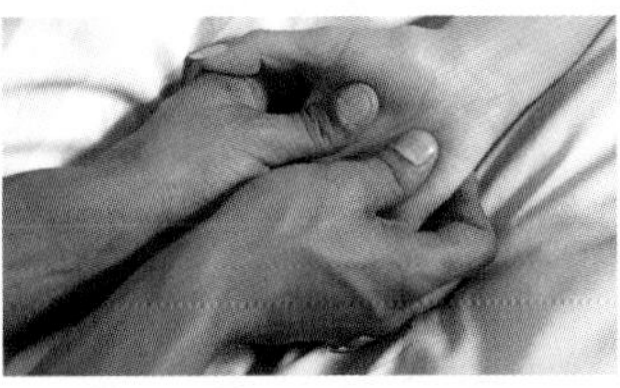

△ **3** Using your thumb pads, make small circular strokes across the whole palm at least three times, including the wrist area if you wish.

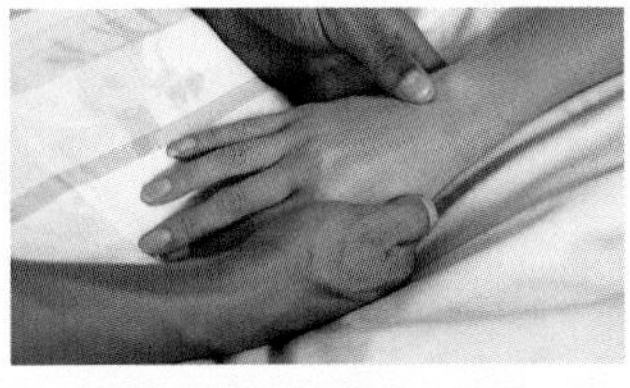

△ **4** Make light circular strokes over the front of the hand, working gently into the wrist and smoothing between the fingers. Finish with gentle stroking and a hold. Repeat on the other hand.

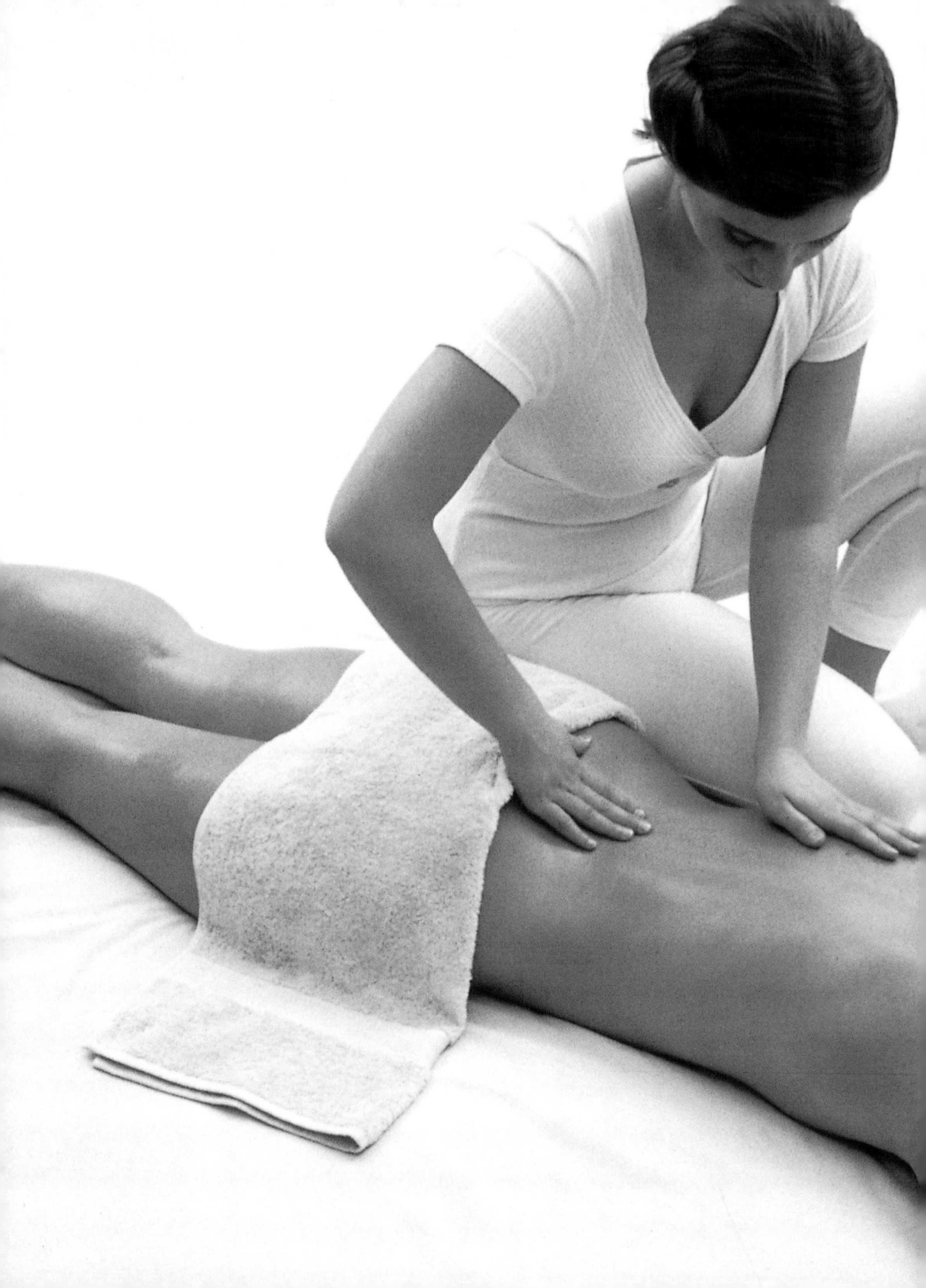

Part Three
Body Massage

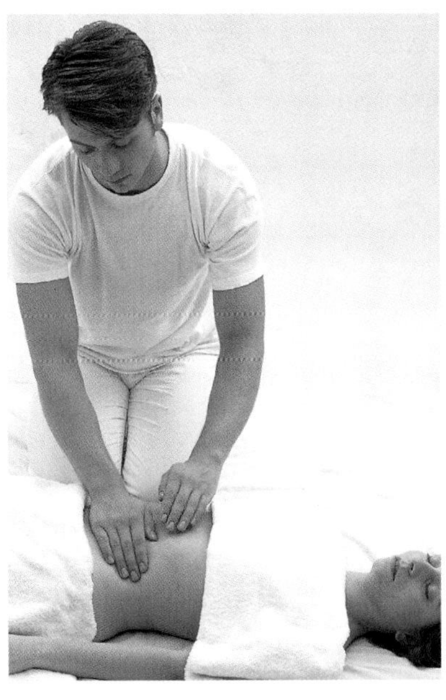

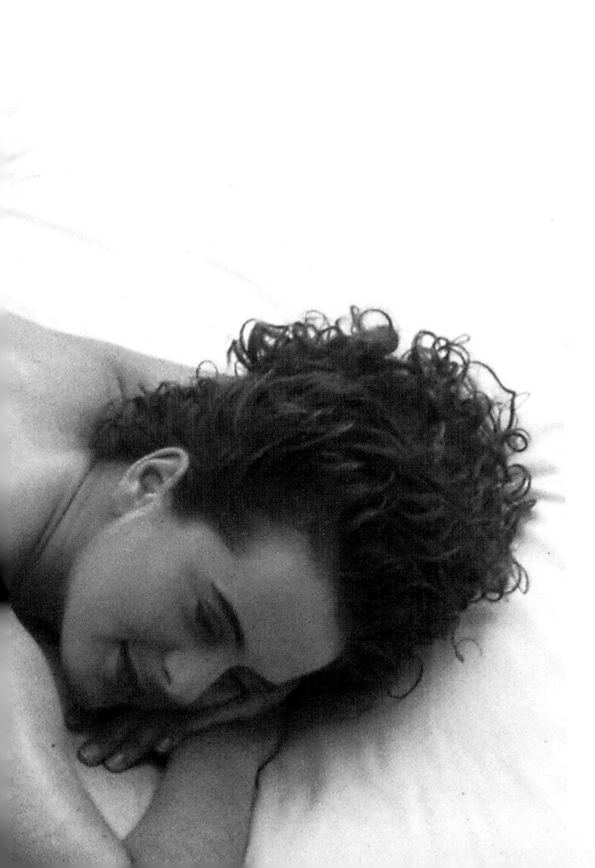

Introduction

The fast pace of modern life, combined with a sedentary lifestyle and an emphasis on mental activity, puts the body under a great strain. We can help to reduce body stress by practising certain stress-busting techniques and adopting healthy lifestyle habits. Because mind, body and spirit are part of one whole system, reducing stress in one area has a knock-on effect elsewhere. So techniques to relax the body also help the mind to unwind, while releasing pent-up emotions can help the body to relax.

a typical body profile

Many of us have a stressed body profile, with a "tension triangle" running from the top of the neck and down across the shoulders. The shoulders are often raised and hunched forward and the arms are gripped in tightly. This constricts the lungs and leads to shallow or restricted breathing. Poor posture throws the head out of alignment so that some muscles have to provide extra support for the skull's weight. As the back tightens this exerts pressure on the skull, pulling on the muscles at the base of the neck and around the head. This tightness is the most common cause of headaches and eyestrain, as well as neck and shoulder pain. Tension may also show up in the lower back as the muscles there get shortened through lack of movement and poor posture.

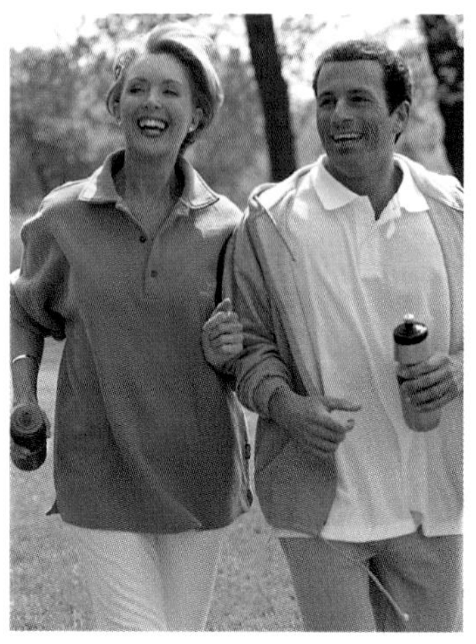

△ **Regular exercise and movement, especially when done in the fresh air, is fundamental to a healthy, flexible, resilient body and to feeling and looking good.**

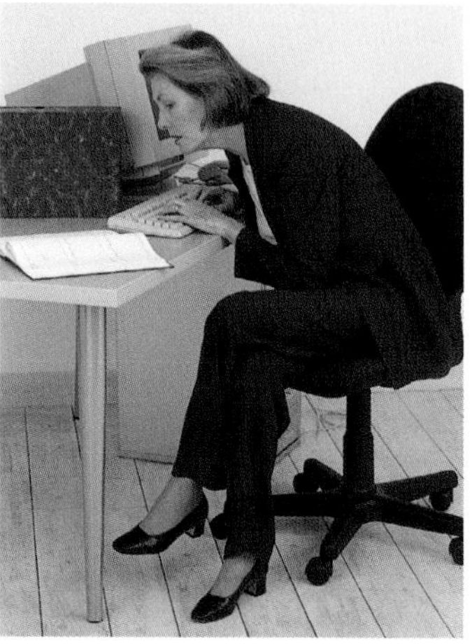

△ **Sitting for long periods of time with your head turned to one side, such as when looking at a computer screen, or clipping the phone between your shoulder and ear, creates body stress.**

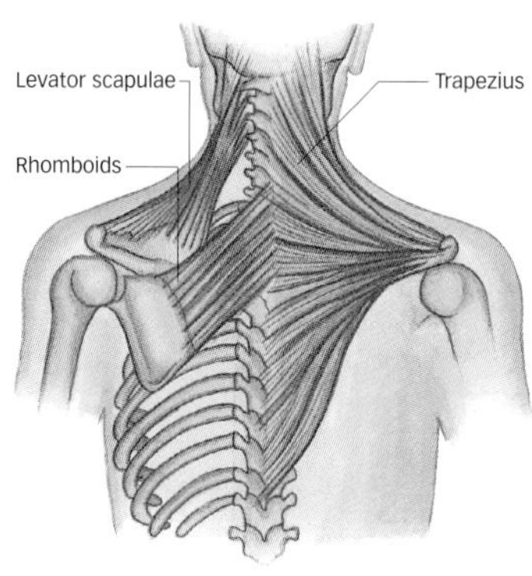

△ **Massage works effectively to reduce tightness and tension in the muscles of the body that accumulates over time, especially when a person is under stress or has a sedentary lifestyle.**

using our muscles

Our muscles give the body strength and movement. To work effectively, they need a good balance between movement, exercise and relaxation. Holding the muscles in the same position for extended periods of time, such as when working at a computer terminal, makes them contract and shorten, impeding the circulation and flow of nutrients through the muscle fibre. This leads to muscle spasm and stiffness. Tired and contracted muscles are also more prone to injury, which is probably why conditions such as repetitive strain injury (RSI) and Carpal Tunnel Syndrome are becoming increasingly common.

To avoid overusing certain muscle groups at the expense of others, take a tip from yoga, where movements one way are always balanced by a counter movement. So if you enjoy gardening, for example, intersperse bending over tasks, such as digging, with tasks that are performed standing up straight, like sweeping, or stretching up jobs, such as pruning tree branches.

Taking regular exercise is also one of the best stress-busting techniques. It relaxes your muscles, deepens your breathing, clears the mind and promotes restful sleep. Also, because it raises your endorphin levels (the "feel-good" chemical in the brain), it can lift your spirits and promote well-being. Find something that you enjoy, such as going to the gym, power walking, dancing, cycling or swimming. Even gentle stretching movements will help to discharge tension, keep the muscles toned and flexible and increase the body's range of movement.

emotional and mental stress

It is not only physical stress that impacts on the body. Emotional and mental pressures also contribute to body stress. When we are

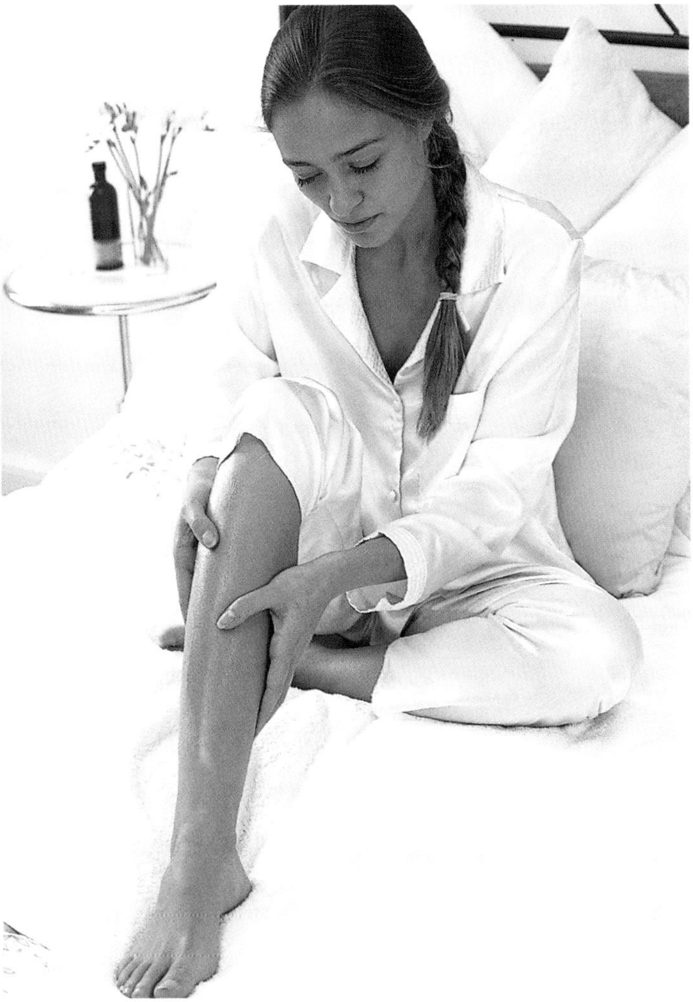

◁ **Taking time out to relax is essential for maintaining good health and well-being. Self-massage is a nurturing way to do this, requiring you to sit down quietly.**

faced with a stressful situation, the body's instinctive reaction is to prepare for immediate "fight or flight" by pumping out adrenalin. This is nature's way of increasing our levels of alertness and ability to respond to danger – whether real or perceived – and causes physiological changes, such as rapid breathing, increased heartbeat, sweating and muscle tension. If the adrenalin that has been produced is not then utilized or discharged in some way, it remains in the body, leading to high levels of anxiety and frustration, as well as disturbances in thought processes and perception.

It can take a long time for the body to return to normal after having been aroused in this way, and ongoing stress can result in exhaustion. At this stage, we may be continually tired and experience a range of unpleasant and frustrating physical and psychological symptoms.

relaxation and sleep

Being able to relax and enjoy a good night's sleep is one of nature's best stress cures. While we are under stress we need more sleep, but this is when we are most likely to experience sleep problems. Pursuits such as singing or painting, enjoying a long, warm aromatic bath, or eating delicious food, are all good ways of switching off in the evening. Massage is also excellent for relaxing body and mind. During a massage the brain waves can slow down to such an extent that you may enter a very deep state of relaxation, akin to meditation, in which mind, body and soul are recharged.

food and drink

Our diet can either help or hinder our ability to cope with stress. Stimulants such as caffeine, alcohol and smoking deplete our nutritional store and contribute to stress levels. Sugary snacks and most processed foods stimulate the release of the stress hormone cortisol, leading to swings in blood sugar and energy levels. Opt instead for "slow release" energy found in whole foods – fresh fruits, vegetables, pulses and grains, seeds and nuts. Substitute herbal teas for tea and coffee and drink plenty of water to keep the body hydrated. Under stress the body uses up its nutrients more quickly, particularly the B vitamins, vitamin C, calcium and magnesium, so it's worth considering a multi-vitamin and mineral supplement to correct any deficiencies.

▽ **Eating raw foods and drinking water helps reduce stressful thought patterns and is the best way to keep your body and skin hydrated.**

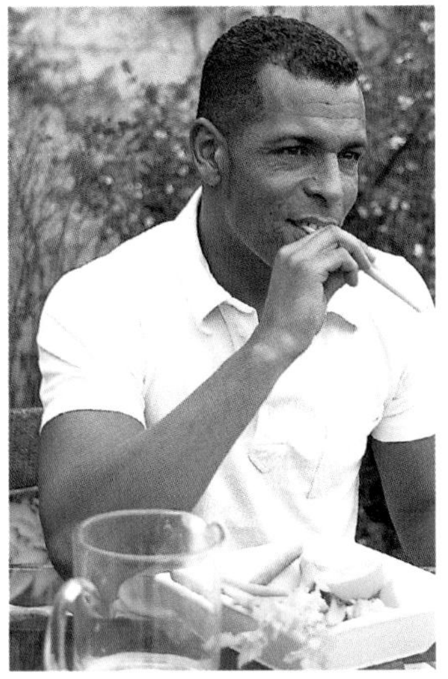

Body work

Holistic body massage uses the basic strokes of Swedish massage but tends to work in a softer and slower way, with emphasis on relaxing the client psychologically and emotionally as well as physically. The focus on relaxation applies to the practitioner as well, so that the experience has a calm and meditative quality for both people concerned. While the strokes and techniques remain important to the treatment, the caring and loving quality of the touch is fundamental to the holistic principle.

the art of massage

Correct breathing and posture are crucial in massage. It is essential to know how to relax your own body in order to pass the same vital message on to another person through the medium of your strokes. An awareness of breathing and posture helps you to remain energized and comfortable while giving a massage, so that the massage experience is wholly beneficial for both you and your partner. Particularly when massaging larger areas of the body, it will help you to perform fluid strokes and allow you to remain relaxed throughout the session, without tiring yourself or straining your own body. The following sequences introduce you to the fundamental techniques of good posture and full and easy breathing.

posture

A good posture, the way you hold and move your body, enables the whole physical structure to achieve graceful and flexible motion. This ease and grace within you will be imparted through your hands, carrying the message of relaxation to the person on whom you are working.

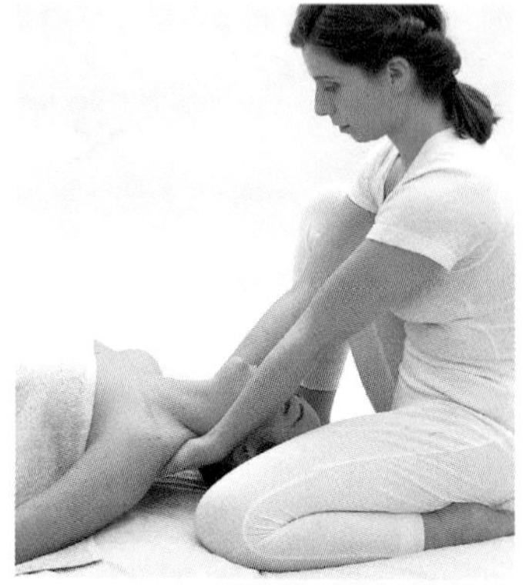

△ **While massaging at floor level, kneel with one foot on the ground so you can ease your body back and forth with the longer strokes. This will allow movement from the lower body, so your torso, spine, neck, and head remain relaxed.**

coordinating breathing and movement

This simple exercise helps you to deepen your breathing and to synchronize it with your movement, with each breath lasting for the length of each movement. This practice will allow you to remain calm but energized while giving a massage, increasing the vitality in your hands and bringing fluidity to your strokes. Repeat the cycle of movement and breathing up to ten times.

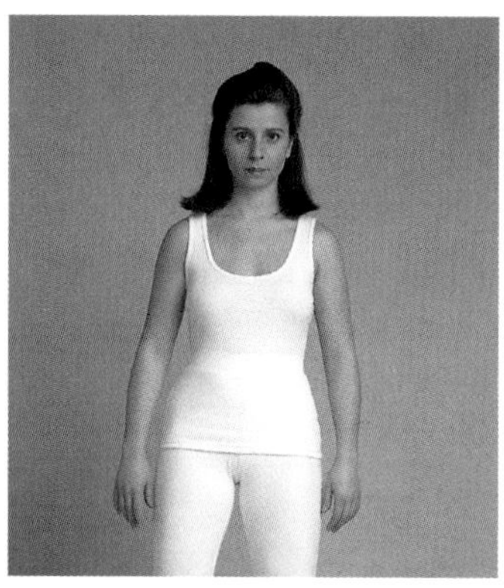

△ **1** Stand with your feet parallel and a hip-width apart, your knees slightly bent and arms loose. Lengthen your spine, keeping neck and head balanced lightly above it and away from your shoulders.

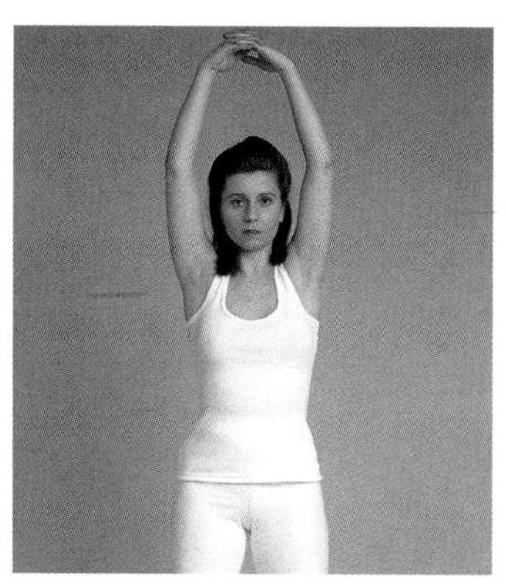

△ **2** As you inhale, let both arms float smoothly out from the sides of your body. Raise them slowly until they meet above your head, then clasp your fingers lightly together.

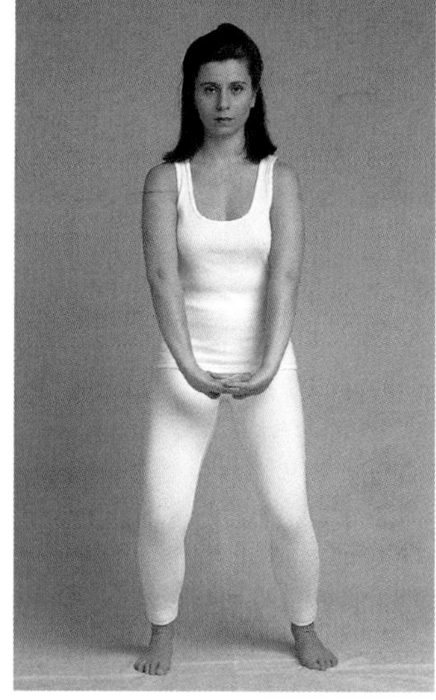

△ **3** As you slowly exhale, press your palms down towards the floor until your arms are straight. Unlock your fingers, and repeat the cycle of breathing and movement.

There are several main points to remember about posture while giving a massage. Always establish a good, firm contact with the ground, whether you are kneeling or standing during a session. This means letting the lower half of your body, your pelvis, legs, and feet, support your weight and movement. Ease your body back and forth with your strokes by using your leg muscles. Keep your knees flexed and tip forward from your hips, so that your spine is straight and extended upwards. Try to keep your neck and head in line with your spine so they don't hang forward.

Constantly remind yourself to relax your shoulders so there is width in your chest, and let your arms hang loosely downwards so that your shoulders, elbows, and wrists are flexible at all times. Keep a space between your arms and your body to avoid hunching in your shoulders. Each time your hands apply strokes to ease tension from a certain part of your partner's body, check that the same area is relaxed in your own body.

breath

Deep and easy breathing assists in bringing oxygen to the cells of your body and allows tense muscles to open and relax. Breath is the basic fuel of your vital life force, and will constantly replenish your energy. Full and easy breathing will allow you to be more present and attentive in your massage, bringing a vitality to your hands and your strokes. It will also enable you to be more connected with your feelings, thereby enhancing the loving quality of your touch.

Synchronizing your breath with your strokes will deepen the effects of the massage, so that it flows over the body like a wave of energy. The ease of your breathing and the relaxed vitality that it brings to you will transmit itself to your partner, enabling the release of tensions, and fuller, deeper breathing.

breathing and stamina

This exercise is more complex than the previous one and is adapted from the Chinese martial art form chi kung. It helps you to build up stamina and vital energy, while controlling and deepening your flow of breath. It also brings you in contact with your *ki*, the source of vital life energy in your belly, which is the centre of gravity in your body. Practice will help you to maintain a relaxed strength while giving a massage.

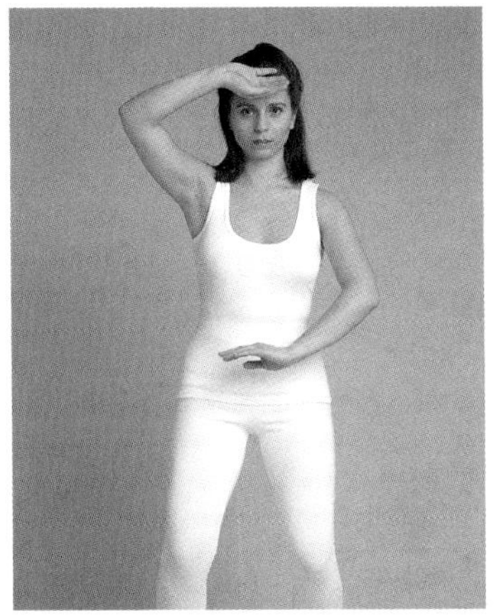

△ **1** Begin with the basic stance, but place one hand, palm facing outwards, at the front of your forehead, and the other hand, palm facing downwards, in front of your navel. Let both hands remain relaxed.

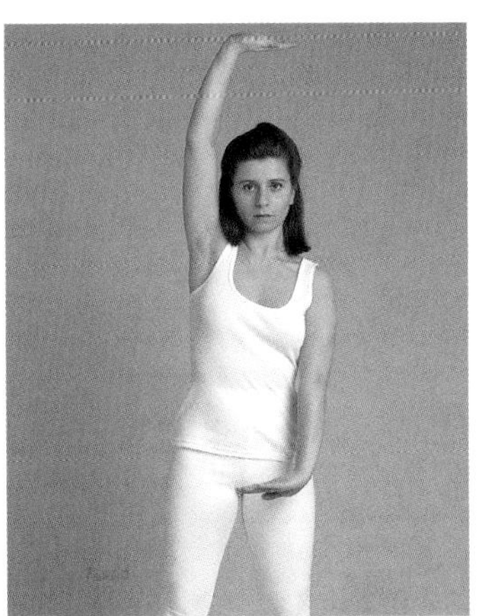

△ **2** As you breathe in, straighten your knees and push up with one hand and down with the other hand, until both arms are vertical to the body.

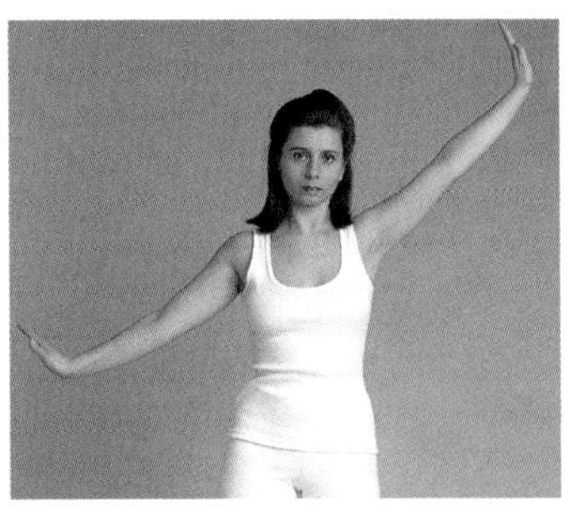

△ **3** Continue with this long inhalation of breath as you rotate your arms like a windmill to move into the opposite direction.

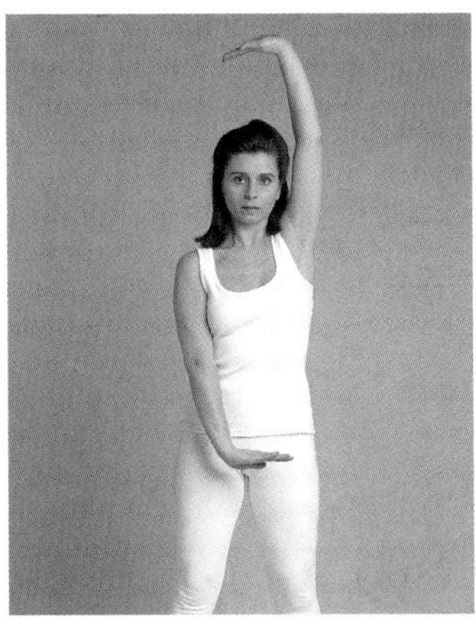

△ **4** Once you have switched the positions of your arms, flex your wrists and flatten your palms, pushing one hand up towards the sky, and the other hand down towards the ground.

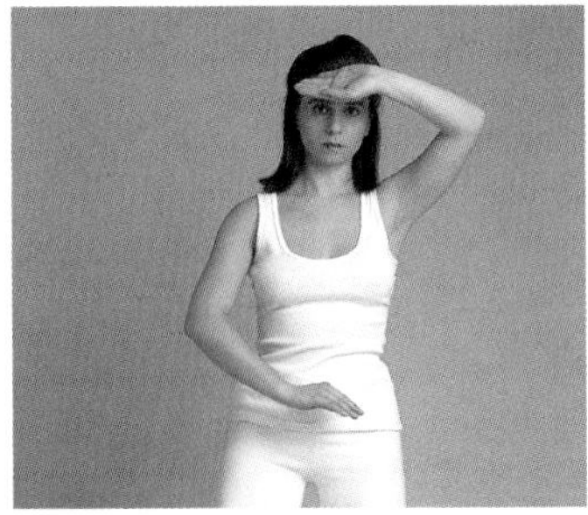

△ **5** Now slowly release your breath and sink your weight down into your knees, while bending your arms at the elbows so that, once again, one hand is in front of the forehead and the other is in front of the navel.

Body Massage Techniques

There are many different schools of body work and massage, but holistic body massage has become one of the most popular. At its core is the idea that caring touch in itself is a powerful agent for the healing process. When combined with skills and techniques drawn from both ancient and more modern approaches to the science of massage, it can bring about many beneficial changes within the body, mind and spirit of the whole person.

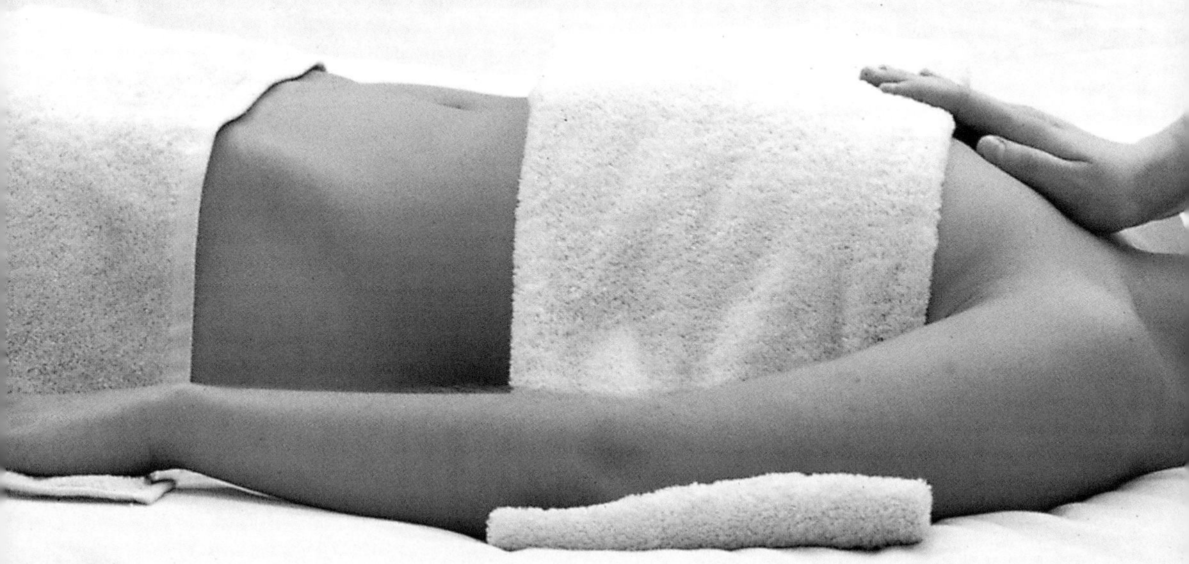

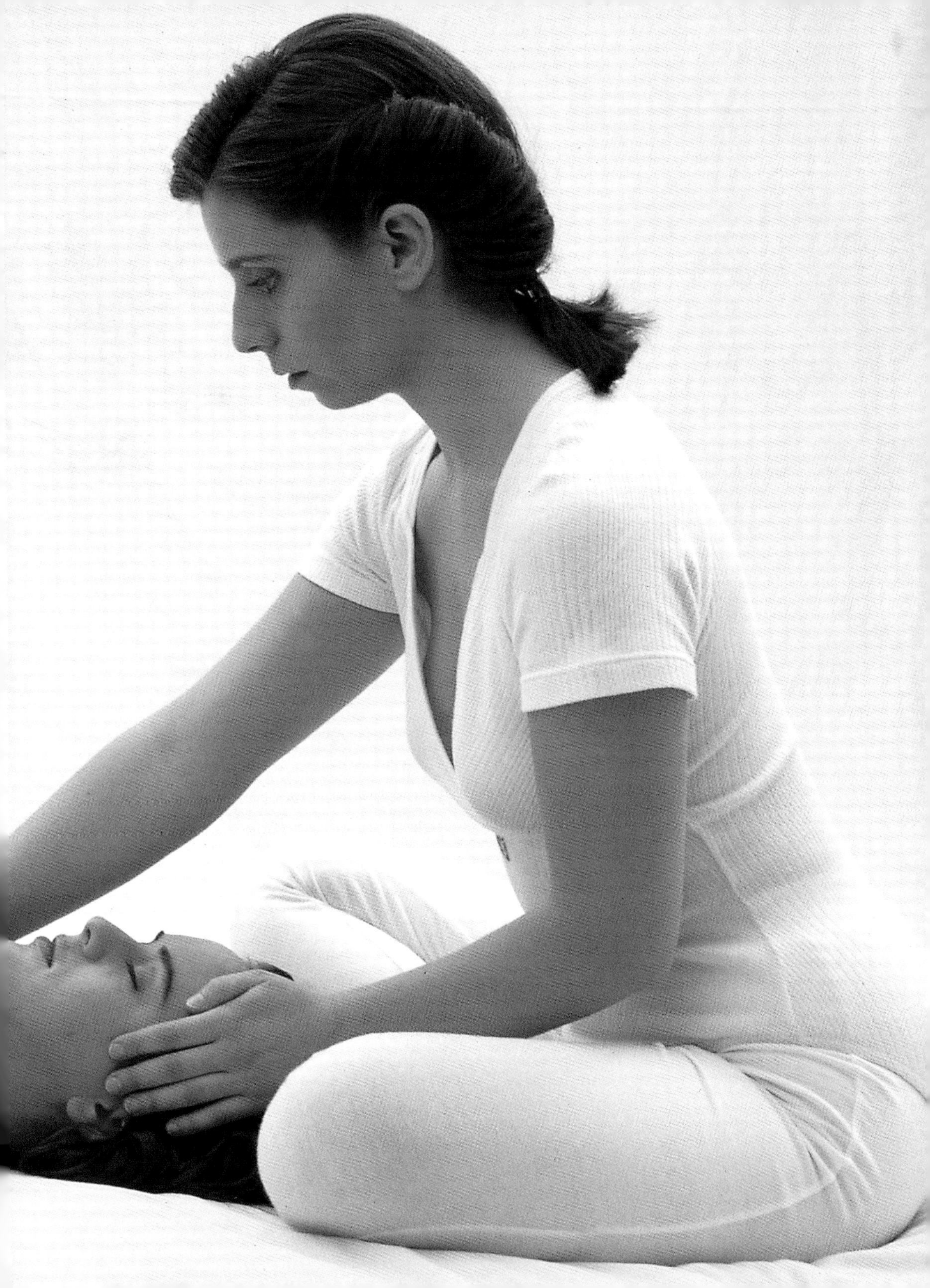

Body massage basics

The following sequence introduces the basic techniques of body massage, which will help you to build up a flowing sequence of strokes to bring harmony, relaxation and invigoration to your partner. From soothing effleurage strokes to more invigorating friction and pressure strokes, these basic sequences can be practised and combined together to achieve an effective massage.

effleurage

The first and main stroke of massage, effleurage prepares the body's soft tissues and warms the muscles for all deeper movements. It is also used to follow up more vigorous strokes such as kneading and friction, in order to soothe and relax an area that has just been massaged. Effleurage simply means "stroking", and is a free-flowing, continuous movement made with the flat of one or, more usually, both hands at a steady pressure.

Effleurage strokes have a calming and almost hypnotic effect on the body, allowing a sense of trust to develop so that the recipient can relax both physically and psychologically. The strokes can be applied with a light to medium pressure, with the whole hand in contact with the skin. When applied in a movement up towards the heart these strokes benefit the cardiovascular system (the heart and blood vessels) and the lymphatic system (the lymph vessels) by boosting the circulation of blood and lymph around the body. A lighter movement has a calming effect on the function of the nervous system.

The hands should be completely relaxed while making the strokes, so that they mould into the body's contours and define its shape and structure.

▷ **Effleurage strokes have a soothing, fluid quality, and are an important stroke to master because they begin, and punctuate, a massage sequence. These relaxing strokes flow smoothly around the body and never finish abruptly.**

preparation

The opening massage strokes are a flowing, continuous sequence of motions to define the contours of the area you intend to massage and also to warm the muscles and prepare them for subsequent massage techniques.

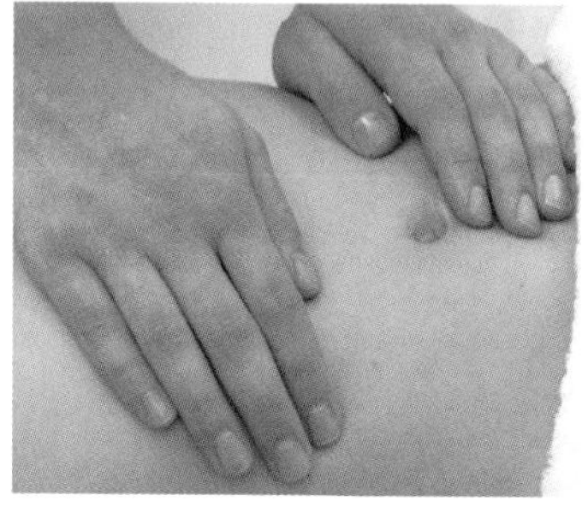

△ **1** Rub a little of the oil into the palms of your hands and spread it over the area you intend to massage with the flat of the hands, in smooth, flowing motions. This is the best method of spreading oil on any part of the body.

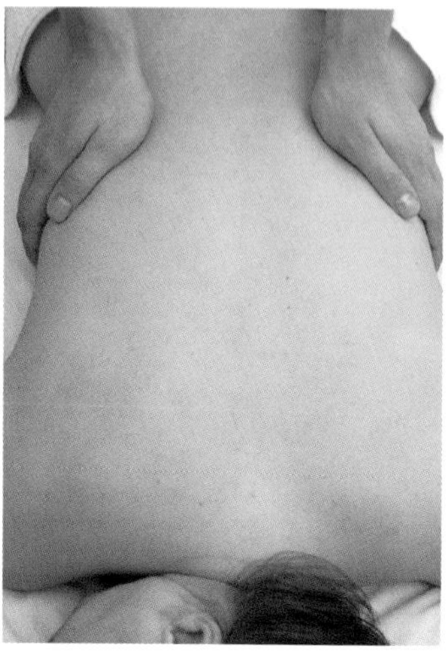

△ **2** It is important with effleurage to let your hands mould into the contours of the body shape. When applied as a preparatory, or integration, stroke it should be repeated three to five times for full effect.

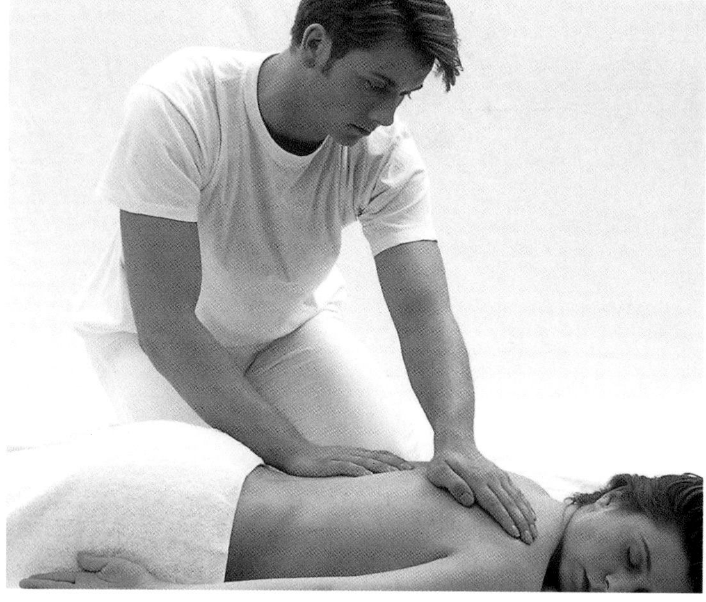

fanning

Fanning is an effleurage motion that can be applied to many areas of the body, including the back, chest, legs, and arms. It is an excellent stroke to follow on from larger preparatory movements and can be used to stretch and manipulate tension away from the muscles. Fanning can be applied either as a series of shorter movements for remedial benefit or in larger, more flowing motions for sensual and soothing effects.

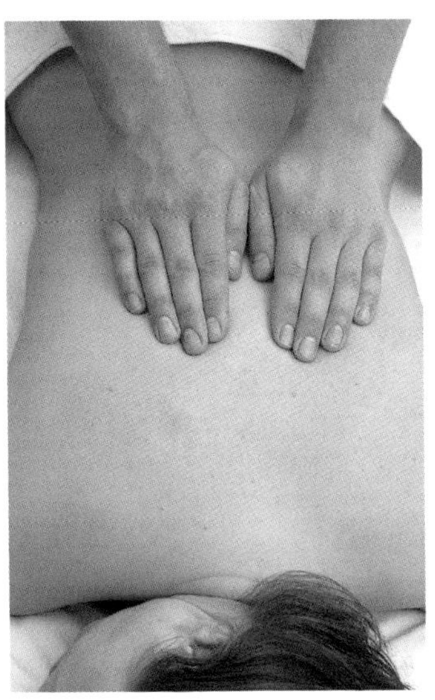

△ **1** Place the hands flat on either side of the spine, with the fingers close together and pointing towards the head. Stroke with an even pressure for about 15cm/6in up the back.

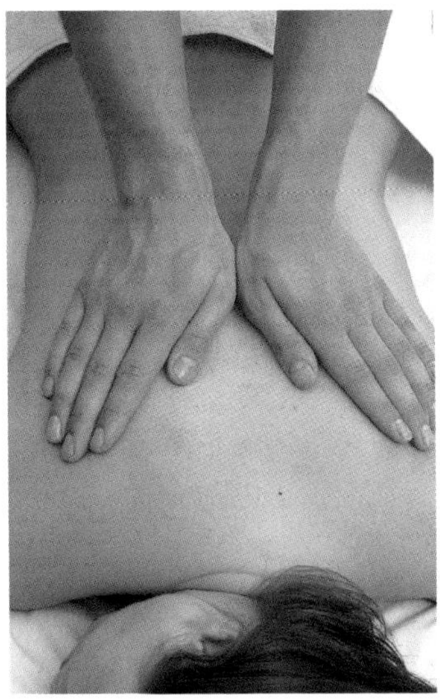

△ **2** Let your hands flow outwards in a fanning motion, moving towards the sides of the ribcage.

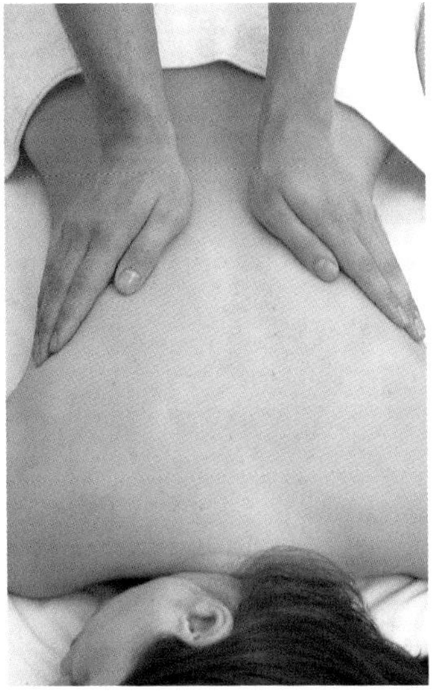

△ **3** Shape your hands to the sides of the body, then draw the hands down before sliding them lightly around and towards their original position alongside the spine. Now stroke further up the back.

continuous circle strokes

Continuous circle strokes add a sensual, relaxing, and soporific element to the massage. If applied at a more vigorous pace and with slightly firmer pressure, they are excellent for warming the superficial layer of tissue and for releasing tension. These effleurage strokes can be used on any broad expanse of the body, such as the sides of the ribcage, the back, and the thighs, when they are applied in a flowing unbroken motion. Continuous circle strokes also form the main preparatory stroke on the abdomen.

△ **1** Lay both hands parallel to each other and flat on the surface of the area you intend to massage. The hands should be both flexible and soft enough to mould into the body's contours. Begin to slide both hands in a circular motion.

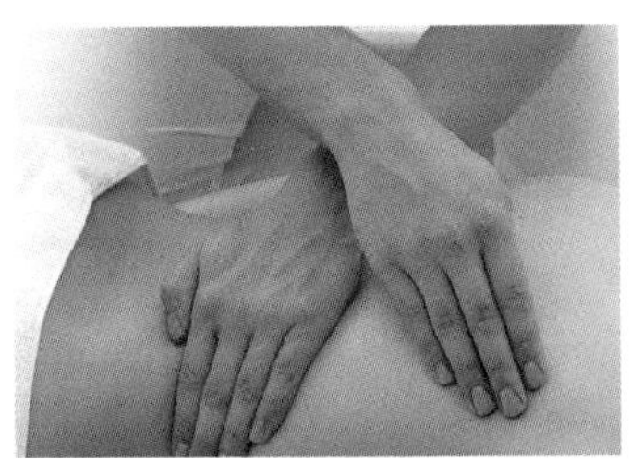

◁ **2** While your left hand continues to move full circle, the right hand lifts and passes over the moving left hand.

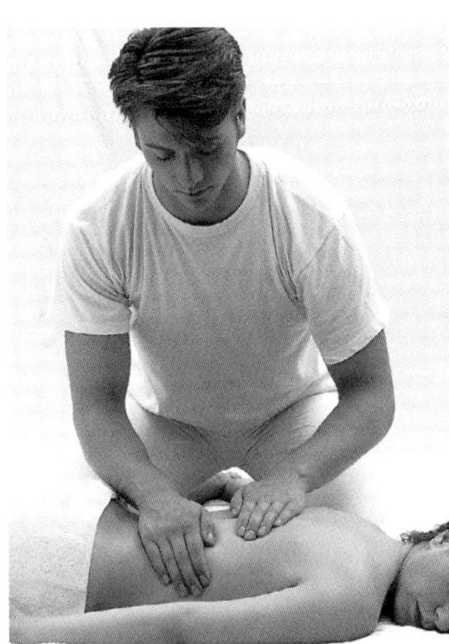

△ **3** The right hand returns to the body to perform a half-circle stroke before lifting off again to let the left hand complete the next full circular motion.

kneading

One of the most satisfying strokes in massage both to give and receive, kneading takes hold of the muscle and moves it about, creating greater flexibility and suppleness. To knead well the hands should be dextrous and pliable; the motion is similar to the action of a baker kneading dough. Kneading is a lifting, squeezing, and rolling movement that passes the flesh from one hand to the other. It has a rhythmic, circular motion and should be applied with the wrists and shoulders relaxed, and the arms held at a distance from the body.

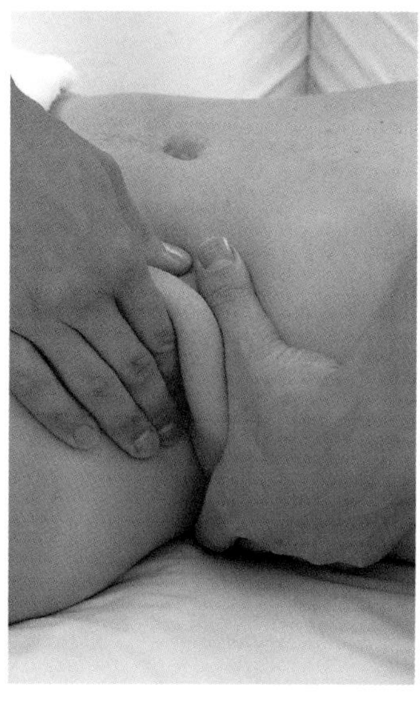

△ Kneading is an effective stroke to apply on muscular and fleshy areas such as the calves, thighs, buttocks, and waist. This stroke should be applied after the muscles have been relaxed and warmed by a sequence of effleurage strokes. It benefits the muscles by releasing underlying tension, breaking down fat deposits and toxins trapped in the tissues, and aiding the exchange of tissue fluids. Always follow up kneading strokes with further effleurage sequences to soothe the area and boost the blood and lymph circulation so that releasing toxins can be properly eliminated.

friction and pressure strokes

A pressure stroke is made by leaning your weight into a particular part of your hand or arm in order to sink into muscle or connective tissue (tissue that holds organs and other structures in place). The heel of the hand, thumb pads, finger pads, knuckles, and forearm can all be used. Always apply and release pressure slowly and sensitively. The grinding or stretching action can be a firm, sliding motion, circles, or a series of alternating circular motions. These deep strokes push the tissue down towards the bone and stretch it, causing friction between muscle and bone and releasing tension. Apply after kneading on fleshy areas, or after effleurage where the bone is close to the skin's surface, such as on hands, feet, face, or beside the spine.

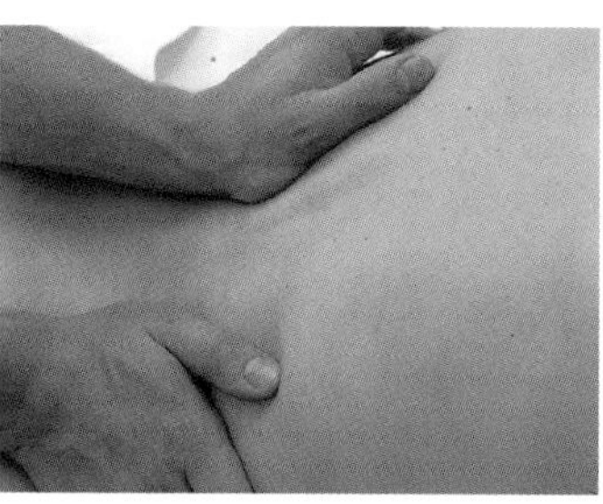

△ **1** The heel of the hand gives a broad surface to add pressure. Shift the weight in the hands to the heels and make circular motions – one hand after the other in a continuous flow. Apply pressure in the upward and outward half of the slide but lessen it in the last half, as the hands glide softly to repeat the stroke.

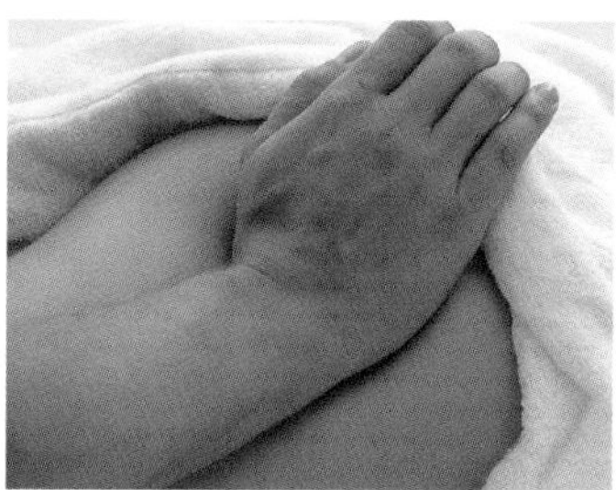

△ **2** By keeping the whole hand relaxed, but by applying direct pressure into the heel of the hand, these circular motions will ease tension from the muscles of the buttocks. These friction and pressure strokes are particularly effective in stretching and draining muscle in tight areas such as the lower back and thighs.

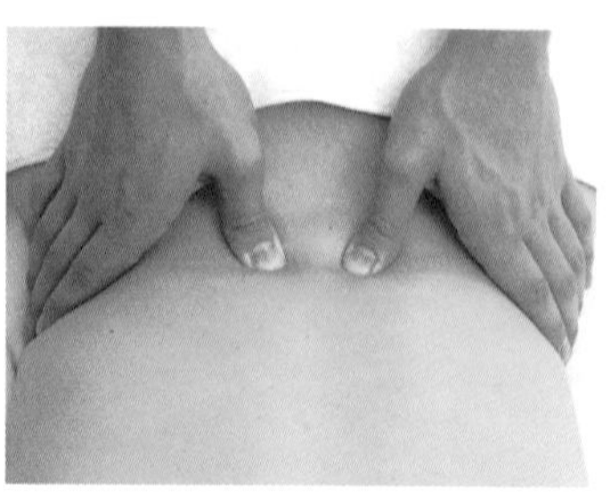

△ **3** The small surfaces of the thumb pads can penetrate areas where muscles and tendons are attached to bone, for example beside the spine. Tight spots can be eased by leaning weight into the thumbs with the hands relaxed, and then making a firm sliding motion up each side of the spine.

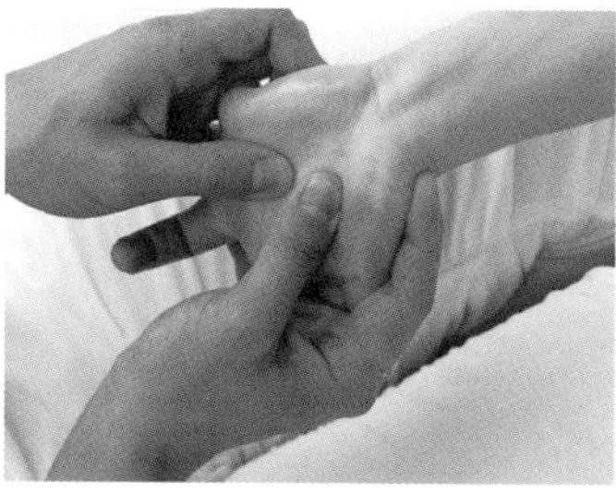

△ **4** Support the back of your partner's hand with your fingers, and use small and continuously alternating thumb circles over the palms and wrists to remove stiffness. To achieve the correct movement you must rotate the thumbs from their base joint.

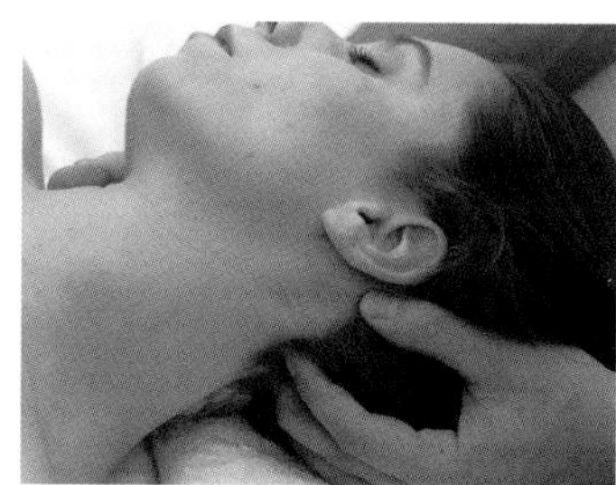

△ **5** Finger pad pressure can be applied in order to release tension from under bone, such as the ridge of the skull. The pressure should be applied gently and slowly to allow your partner time to relax. Slowly rotate your fingertips on one small area at a time. Then release the pressure gradually before moving to the next spot.

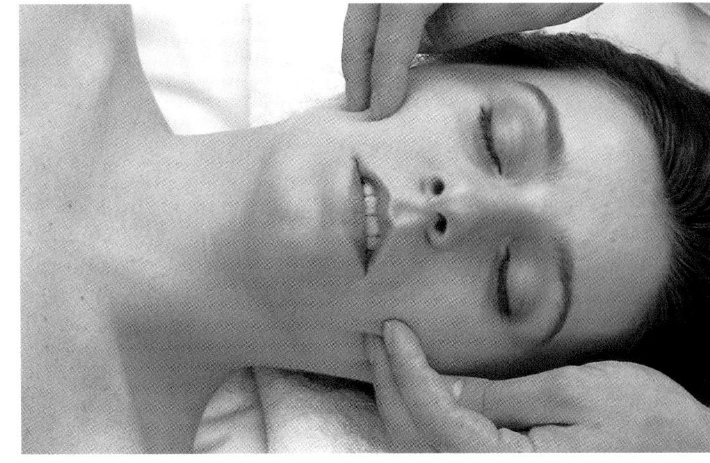

vibrating

This stroke helps to free muscle from a habitual pattern of tension. Vibration is particularly effective on small muscles such as in the cheeks of the face or those alongside the spine.

▷ Sink the fingertips into the fleshy area of the cheeks of the face and vibrate with rapid movements. Move to another spot and vibrate again. This will help the mouth and jaw to relax.

percussion

This includes a variety of invigorating movements that briskly strike fleshy and muscular areas of the body to produce a toning and stimulating effect on the skin. Percussion strokes are performed with one hand following the other in a series of rapid and rhythmic movements, helping to draw the blood towards the skin's surface and leaving it with a warm and healthy glow. The rapid action also dispels tension and rids the tissues of excess fluid and fatty deposits. To achieve the best results, keep your shoulders, wrists, and hands relaxed, and bounce your hands immediately back off the skin the moment they make contact.

The invigorating effects of percussion help to enliven the body after the euphoric effects of other massage strokes, but they may not be suitable to use if your partner is in a particularly sensitive or vulnerable mood. Percussion strokes should never be applied over varicose veins or directly on top of bone.

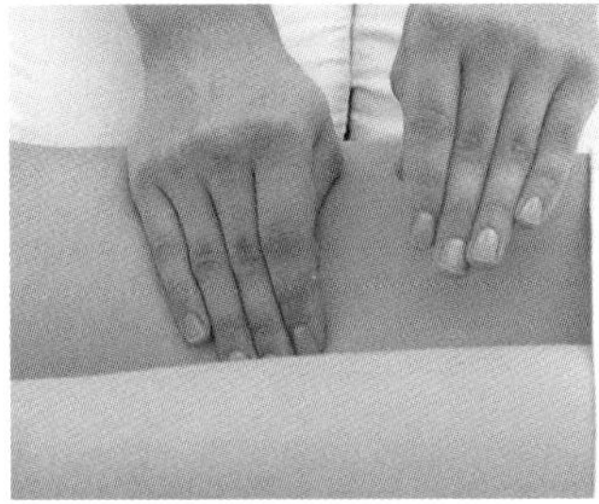

▷ To perform the cupping movement, form both hands into a softly cupped shape by keeping your fingers straight but bent at the lower knuckles; at the same time draw the thumbs close into the palms. This should create an airtight vacuum in the centre of your palms, which works as a suction on the skin during the rapid cupping action. Using the palms to make contact, briskly strike and flick off the skin, one hand following the other in quick succession over fleshy areas.

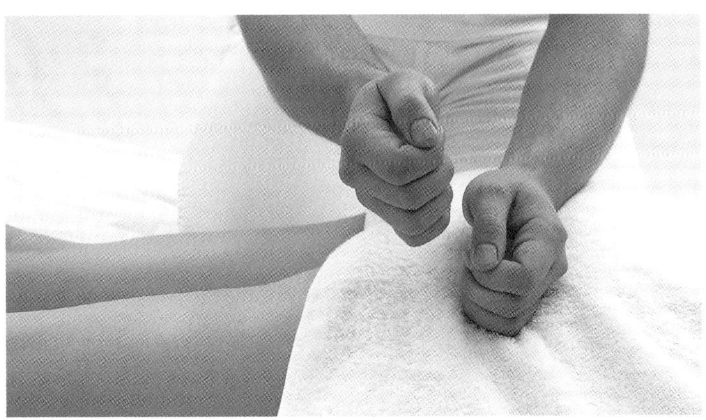

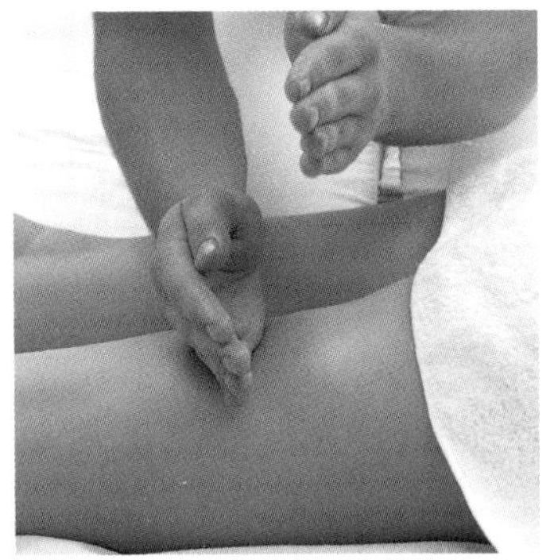

◁ Hacking uses the same fast rhythmic motion as cupping, but contact with the skin is made from the sides of the hands, one following the other in quick succession. The wrists and fingers should be relaxed, and the palms of each hand should face each other with only about 25mm/1in distance between them. Hacking tones and stimulates all fleshy areas, and works particularly well on the buttocks, thighs, and tops of the shoulders.

△ For the pummelling stroke, keep your shoulders and wrists relaxed and make loose fists in order to pummel over the fleshy parts of your partner's body. Contact with the skin is made with the sides of the hands. Apply the stroke in the same brisk fashion as the previous percussion strokes, letting one hand after the other pummel over the area. This stroke, applied to the thighs and buttocks, is excellent for helping to break down cellulite.

applying the correct sequence of strokes

The following sequence of strokes on the calf muscles of the leg show the order in which the basic techniques of massage should be applied to create a relaxing and invigorating effect. This sequence can be used, as appropriate, on any part of the body.

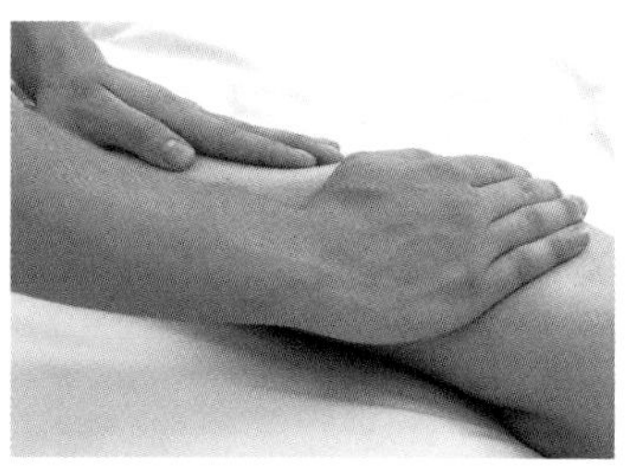

△ **1** Effleurage: Soothing strokes made with the flat of the hands will warm and loosen tense calf muscles and prepare them for deeper strokes.

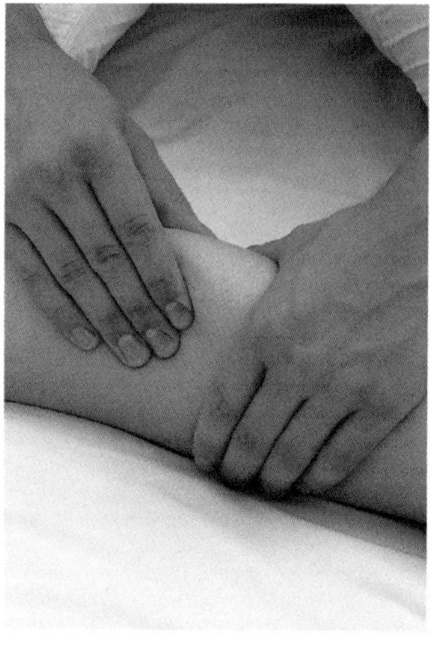

△ **2** Kneading: Knead the calf muscles to invigorate and aid the muscles to contract. Follow up with some soft strokes.

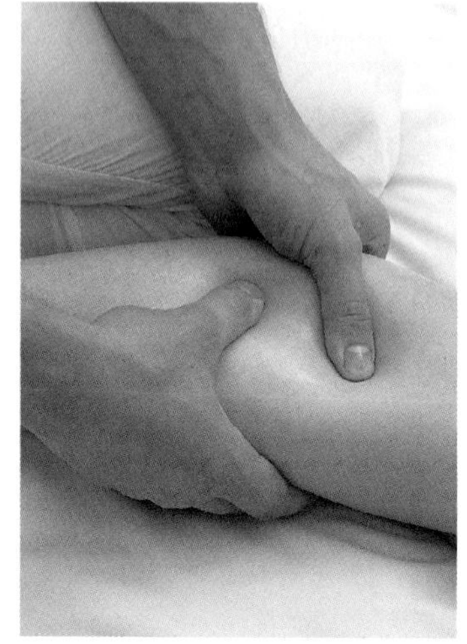

△ **3** Friction: Press your thumb pads sensitively into the muscle tissue using alternating thumb circle friction strokes. This will stretch and release a deeper level of tension. Work thoroughly over the whole area.

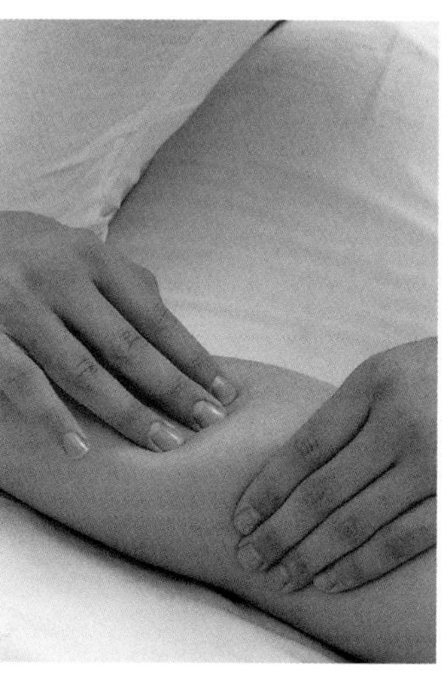

△ **4** Vibrating: Gently sink your finger tips into the calf muscle and vibrate it rapidly. Let your hands mould into the shape of the lower leg as you follow the vibrating action with flowing effleurage.

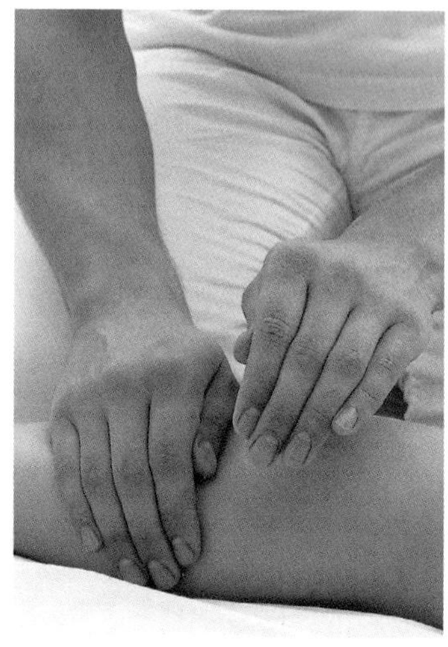

△ **5** Cupping: Cup the calf briskly to stimulate the blood circulation and tone the skin and muscles. Apply the cupping motion up and down the lower leg several times.

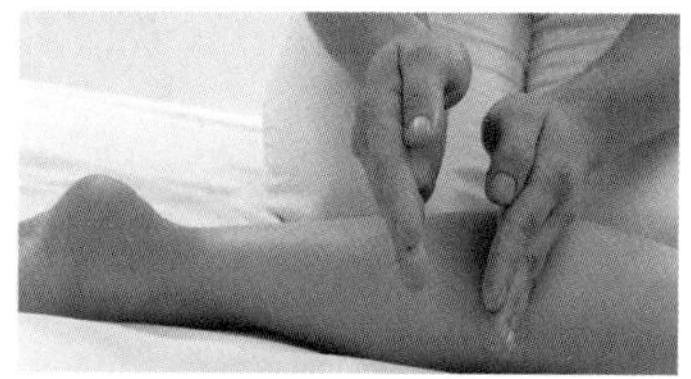

△ **6** Hacking: Use this stroke over the bulk of the calf muscles for further toning, and to aid elimination of excess tissue fluids. Do not strike the back of the knee.

▽ **7** Stroking: Gently stroke over the calf to harmonize the previous massage movements and to boost both the blood and lymph circulation towards the heart.

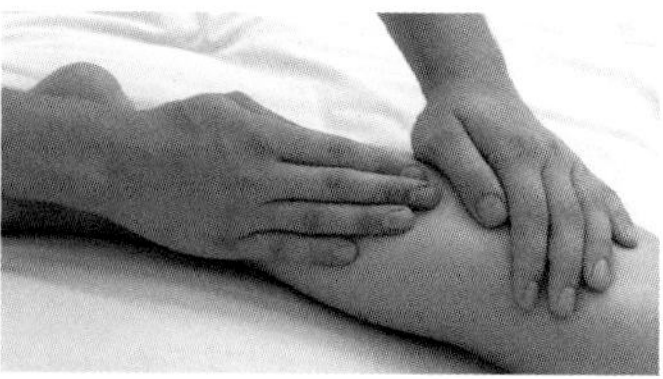

use of towels

Use warmed, fresh clean towels to cover your partner during massage. The towels are important because they prevent the loss of body heat once the oil has been applied and the person is lying still. They also ensure your partner's modesty. Move the towels as needed while applying your strokes, leaving uncovered only the area on which you are working during the massage.

▽ **1** Ideally you should use one large bath towel to cover the whole body, and two medium-sized towels to add further warmth to the upper body and the feet. Tuck the towel snugly around both feet.

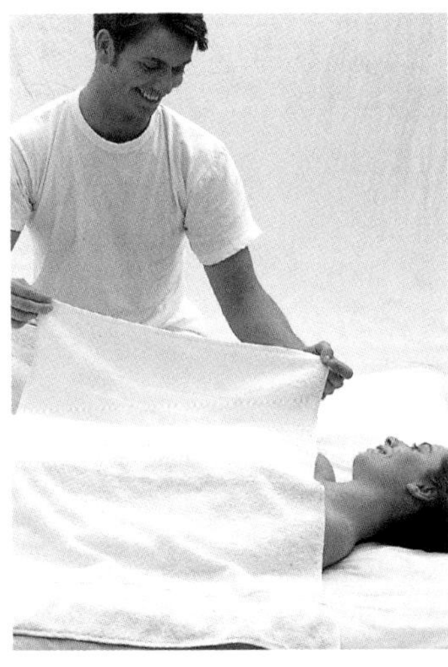

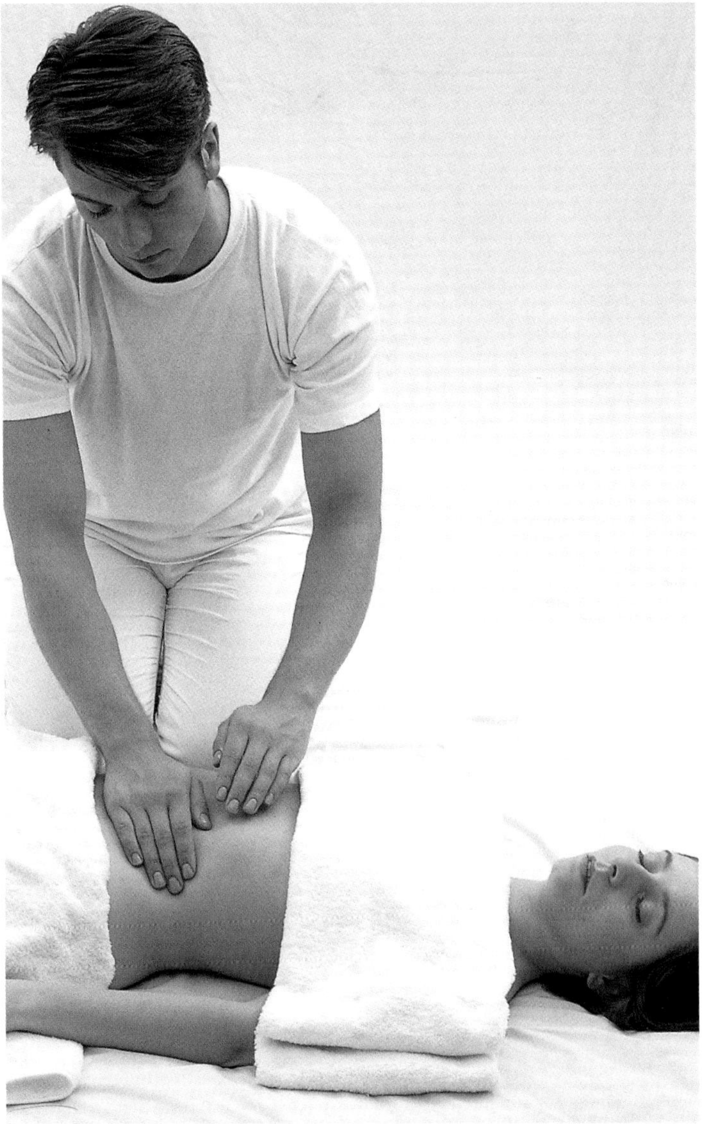

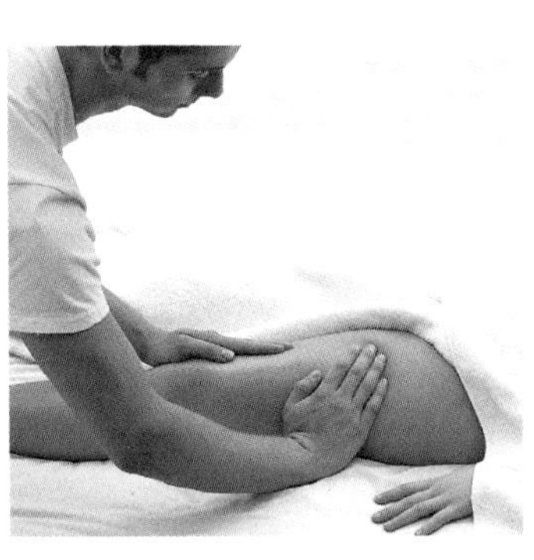

△ **2** When massaging the abdomen, peel back the large towel and cover the chest with a folded towel. Do not leave the chest exposed.

◁ **3** Once you are working on the legs, ensure that the upper body stays warm by covering it with an extra towel. Fold the large towel over so that only the leg on which you are working remains exposed.

▷ **4** When your partner turns over, hold the towel up between you both, and then let it drop softly down to cover the other side of the body.

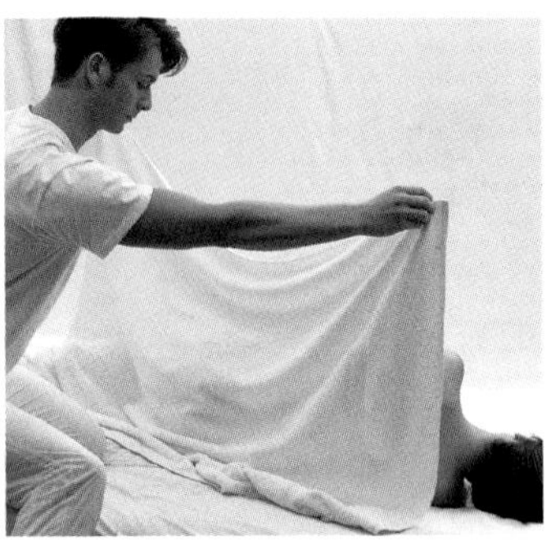

Using oils in body massage

The nurturing touch of a massage is considerably enhanced by the aroma of essential oils. A selection of blends appropriate to everyday circumstances is given below. These few suggestions are to be used as a guide. If you are already familiar with some of the essential oils and have a favourite blend, there is no reason why you should not use it.

carrier oil basics

Choosing the right vegetable carrier oil is vital. Essential oils dissolve easily in a carrier oil to make a blend that makes it easier to move the hands continuously on the skin without dragging or slipping. Some oils, such as olive oil, are too sticky for massage. Peach nut oil is good for delicate skin. Avocado oil has a distinctive fruity scent, so choose essential oils with complementary fragrances. Many carrier oils have health-giving, nutritious properties of their own, but will be much more effective if combined with a another richer carrier oil more suitable for massage.

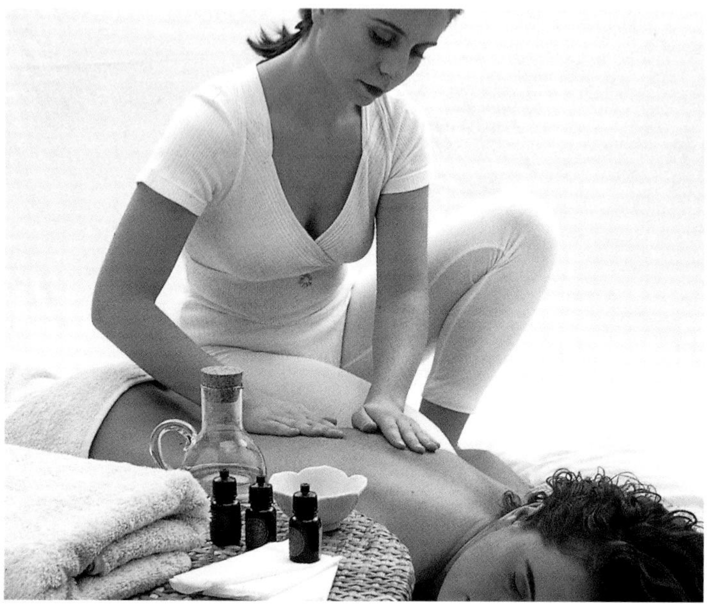

△ **The right oil blend enables the hands to move smoothly and continuously over the skin, and the sensual aroma of essential oils stimulates and soothes the body and the spirit.**

blending essential oils for massage

Experiment with different types of carrier oil to achieve the ideal blend for your massage style. Try adding a teaspoonful of another carrier oil as well as the essential oils for a highly personal mixture. It is worth remembering that even the weather affects the state of our skin, and in the winter central heating and cold temperatures will cause it to dry out. These variations can be accommodated by changing the exotic carrier oils used to enrich each blend.

Rub a little of the blend between the palms of your hands to warm it, then test the fragrance before beginning the massage. It may require slight adjustment before you are happy with the result.

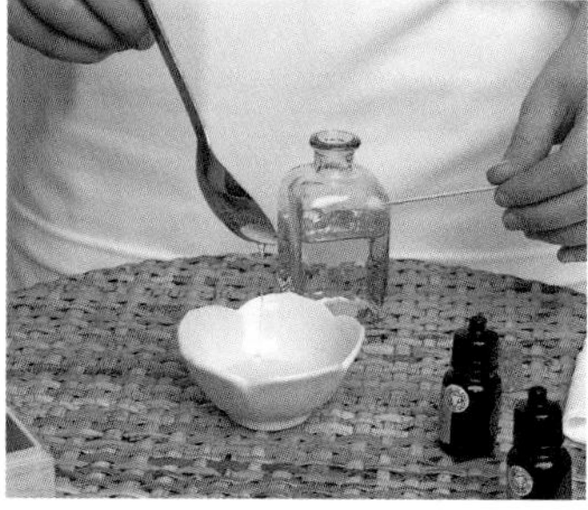

△ **1** Before you begin blending the oils, wash and dry your hands and make sure that you have all the bowls and bottles you need, and that all your utensils are clean and dry. Have your essential oils at the ready, but leave the lids on the bottles until they are required. Carefully measure out approximately 10ml (2 tsp) of your chosen carrier oil, and gently pour it into your blending bowl.

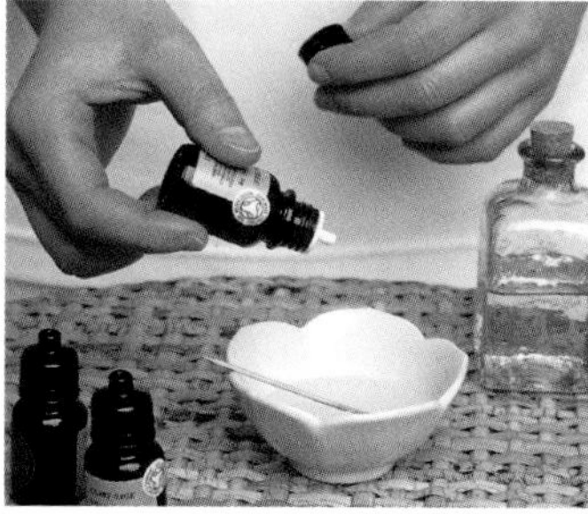

△ **2** Bearing in mind the correct ratio of essential oil to carrier oil (generally 10ml (2 tsp) base oil to 5 drops of essential oil), and the combination of top, middle, and base notes required, add the first essential oil a drop at a time. Add remaining oils a drop at a time and mix gently with a clean, dry cocktail stick or toothpick, to blend.

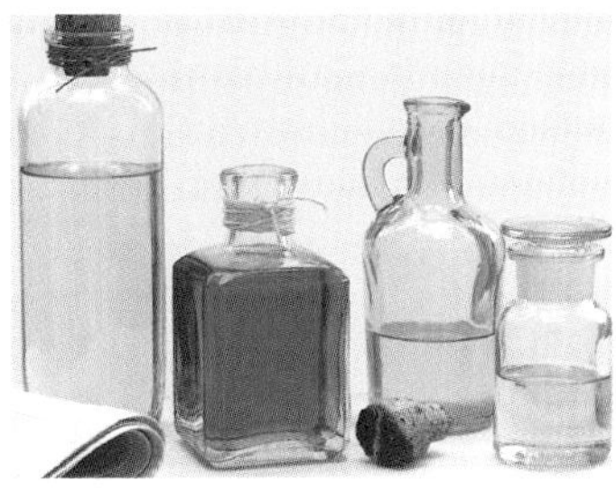

◁ Many of the vegetable carrier oils are suitable for massage, but they all have different qualities, so it is important to choose the right one.

some useful blends for body massage

Choose up to four oils to add to a carrier oil to create a blend suitable for your needs.

a blend to aid relaxation Relaxation is particularly important following a stressful day at work. A massage with a blend of the following oils is an effective way to encourage relaxation: bergamot, German chamomile, clary sage, lavender, rosewood, or sandalwood. To add an uplifting note choose one of the other citrus oils, which will produce a blend that is relaxing and uplifting at the same time.

an energizing blend When everything seems grey and depressing, an enlivening massage with a blend of the invigorating oils could help turn the day around from one of gloom and despair to a more energetic one. Try a blend of three or four of the following oils: black pepper, cypress, eucalyptus, fennel, ginger, grapefruit, jasmine, juniper, lemon, nutmeg, peppermint, rosemary, tea tree.

a blend for stiff muscles Everyone suffers from minor muscular aches and pains from time to time. They may be brought on by unusual physical exercise – from gardening or dancing to sporting activities – or simply by remaining in an uncomfortable position too long. At such times the warming oils that bring blood back into the aching muscles are the most helpful. Choose your oils from the following list: benzoin, black pepper, clary sage, eucalyptus, ginger, grapefruit, jasmine, juniper, lavender, lemon, marjoram, nutmeg, orange, peppermint, or rosemary.

a hangover remedy If you have over-indulged in alcoholic drinks, try to drink several glasses of water before sleeping, in order to help alleviate the dehydration caused by an excess of alcohol. Drink plenty of water and orange juice at breakfast to help detoxification and, if possible, eat some wholemeal toast with a yeast spread. A gentle massage, using three or four of the following oils, may help restore normal good health after eating or drinking too much: black pepper, fennel, geranium, ginger, juniper, orange, or peppermint.

a blend for raising the spirits For the days when the ordinary activities of life seem too difficult there are a number of oils that can help raise the spirits: benzoin, bergamot, cedarwood, clary sage, frankincense, geranium, grapefruit, jasmine, mandarin, nutmeg, orange, rose, rosewood, or ylang ylang. A blend of three or four from this list, and a soothing massage, can give you back a zest for life.

a warming blend After struggling with bitter winds and the cold of winter the idea of undressing for a massage may seem foolish. However, there are some warming and comforting essential oils that can be very nourishing when you are feeling emotionally, as well as physically, cold. Blend benzoin, ginger, orange, and rosewood, together, and allow them to envelop your body in their special aroma.

a sensual blend In a long-term relationship the intimate physical bond between partners may weaken or cease to exist. A long illness, overwork, or emotional crises can also lead to a lack of sexual interest. At such times the non-sexual but loving touch of massage can play an important part in rekindling the sexual intimacy that has been missing. Essential oils that may be helpful are: black pepper, cedarwood, clary sage, fennel, frankincense, ginger, jasmine, rose, and sandalwood. This is an area where it is particularly important to bear in mind each individual's personal preferences.

seasonal blends For a festive mood, use the essences of Christmas: frankincense, ginger, and mandarin. You could also try blending with benzoin, neroli, and orange. Easter, occurring at the time of renewal and refreshment, is a good time to try a blend of geranium, palmarosa, and rosewood.

a pre-wedding blend There is only one blend for a pre-wedding massage: jasmine and rose, respectively the king and queen of fragrances, and neroli, to calm the nerves. A luxurious blend to bring the essence of calm to the beginning of married life.

a blend to calm Frankincense, sandalwood, neroli, and ylang ylang blend together to create a rich perfume of peace. This blend can bring feelings of tranquillity and reduce feelings of fragmentation. It can be valuable in helping to reconnect someone to their strong inner core. Give or receive a massage with this mixture, and help yourself regain peace in your life.

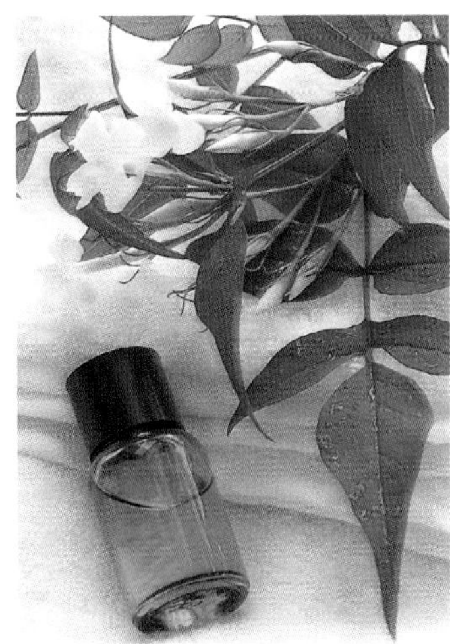

△ Jasmine, known as the king of flower oils, has a strong scent that can produce feelings of optimism, euphoria and confidence.

Getting started

In order to ensure your massage has maximum effectiveness it is important to make sure that you and your partner are in the right frame of mind. Preliminaries include making sure your equipment is ready, setting the scene and preparing yourself and your partner for treatment.

setting the mood

Creating an atmosphere of confidence and trust is an important element in giving a successful body massage. It will help your massage partner relax if it is clear that you are carefully prepared and in control. Make sure that the room is heated and all of your equipment and oils are ready. Take time to compose yourself so that your whole attention is focused on the massage. Give your partner privacy to undress, and clear directions on how to lie down on the mattress. Use the towels correctly to cover the body, both to keep it warm and to protect modesty. By following these suggestions, your partner will immediately feel safe and secure in your hands.

working at a couch

While some people prefer to kneel and give a massage at ground level, working at a specially-designed couch increases your mobility, as you can use your feet and legs to move more freely around the body. This puts less stress on your posture, enabling you to bring length to your spine and neck and a relaxed width to your shoulders. In common with the kneeling position, your movement at the couch should come from the lower half of your body, to prevent strain on your back.

▷ A massage couch with adjustable legs allows people of various heights to use it successfully. The height can also be adjusted to suit the type of massage you are giving. In a deep tissue massage a greater degree of pressure is applied to the strokes, and so a lower height is required than would be the case for soft tissue massage.

establishing contact and applying oils

Before you begin, suggest your partner takes a moment to settle comfortably on to the mattress.

▷ **1** Establish contact with your partner by placing your hands gently on the body, so that one hand rests on the top of the spine and the other at its base.

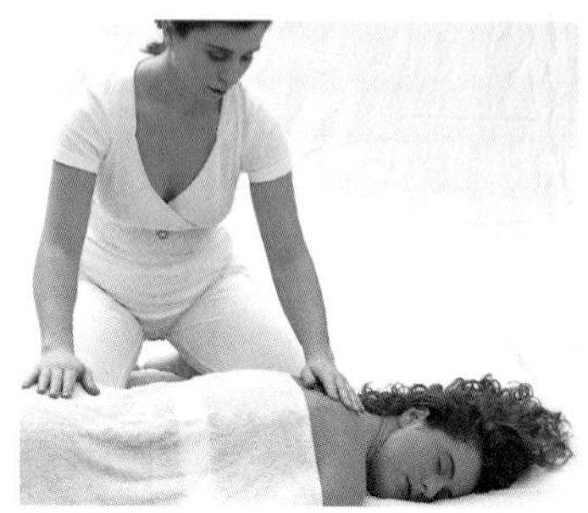

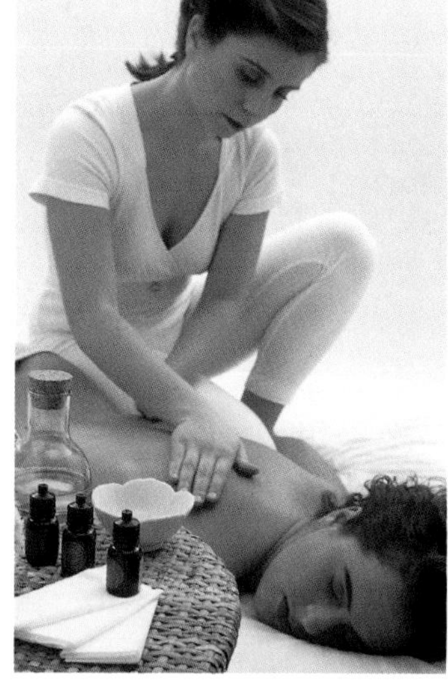

◁ **2** Fold the top towel over the lower half of the body. Pour 2.5ml (½ tsp) of blended oils into the palm of one hand, then rub your hands together to warm the oil. Apply more oil as appropriate. Using smooth and flowing effleurage strokes, spread the oil over the back. Relax your hands so they become pliable and are able to mould into the body's curves.

the body massage

The body massage usually starts on the back of the body, with special focus on main areas of tension. Once your partner has turned over, the massage moves up the entire front of the body.

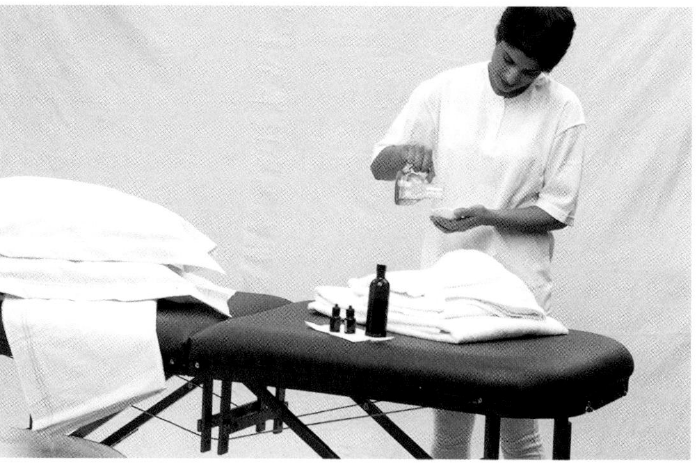

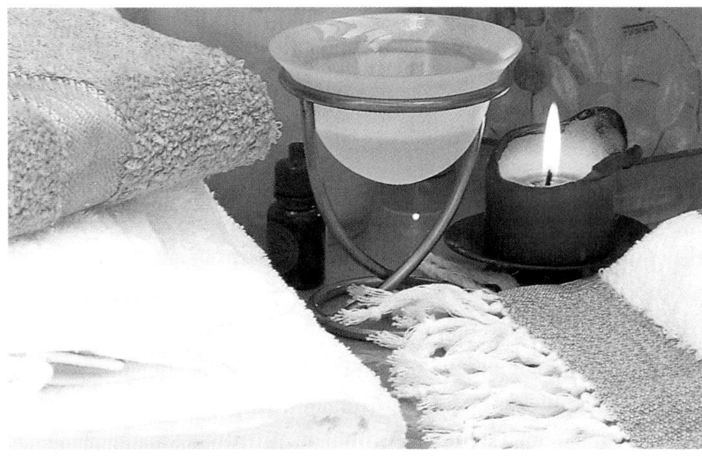

◁ **When preparing for a massage it is a good idea to make sure that the room is warm and that you have all the equipment that you need to hand. It is disruptive for your partner if you have to break off half way through to replenish your massage oil blend, adjust the heating or fetch a cushion or a warm towel.**

using pillows and towels to ease body tension

Postural tension remains in the body even when a person is lying down and appears to be relaxed. In fact, a prolonged period of resting on a flat surface can even exacerbate physical strain, particularly in the major joints of the body. The more you massage, the more you will be able to detect where someone is holding their tension. Once you have worked out where the problem is pillows and towels can be used effectively to support key areas of the body in order to ease tension.

△ Lower back pain may be caused by a curve in the base of the spine, or a chronic pattern of tension in the pelvic region. A pillow placed under the abdomen can redress this imbalance during a massage, helping the lumbar region to relax under your touch.

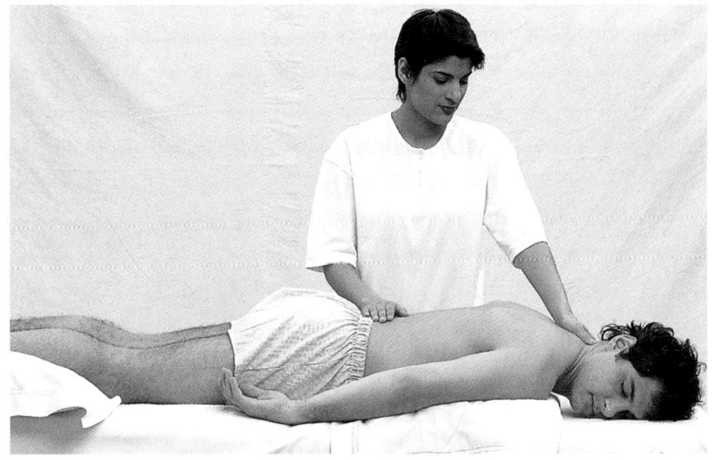

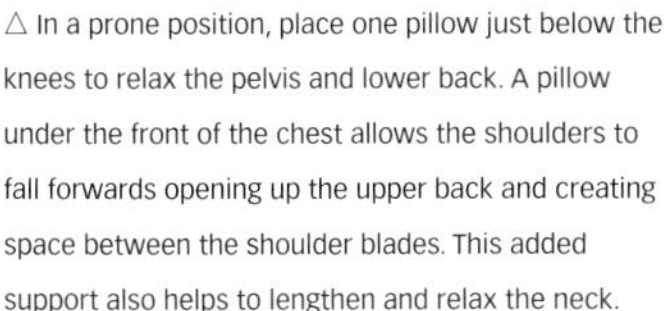

△ In a prone position, place one pillow just below the knees to relax the pelvis and lower back. A pillow under the front of the chest allows the shoulders to fall forwards opening up the upper back and creating space between the shoulder blades. This added support also helps to lengthen and relax the neck.

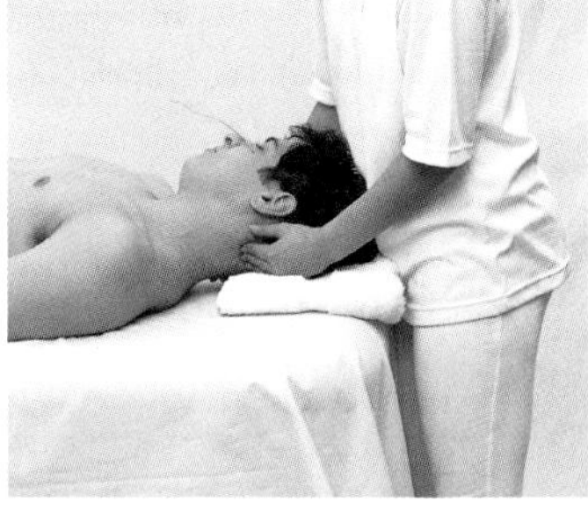

▷ Constriction in the muscles at the base of the skull will shorten the neck muscles, causing the head to contract backwards. Place a thin, folded towel under the skull to lift the head upwards to relieve this.

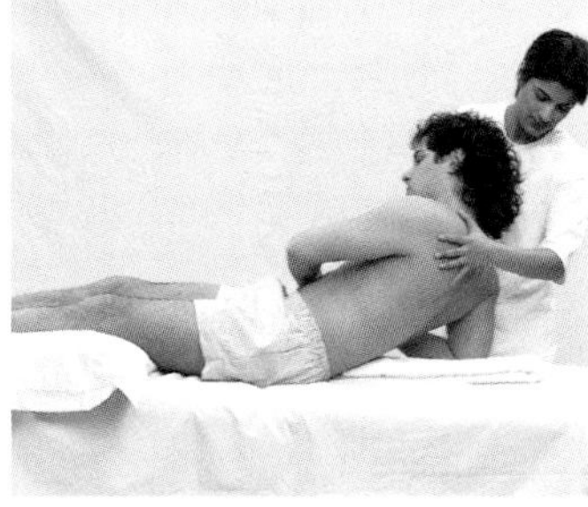

△ Tension in the chest and ribs can cause muscles to contract, pulling the shoulders forward so that they cannot rest on the table. Ease this posture by placing a towel, folded into a thin strip, under and along the spine. This helps the chest expand and the shoulders to fall back. Help your partner into position so that the towel remains in the correct place.

The Body Massages

The massage basics can be applied to soothe and relax the whole body. This chapter takes you step-by-step through the sequence of strokes that is needed to give a satisfying and effective body massage. Starting with the upper and lower back, which are especially prone to tension, it moves on through clearly defined and punctuated stages to the front of the body, and finally the arms and hands. A self-massage sequence and a sensual massage are also included.

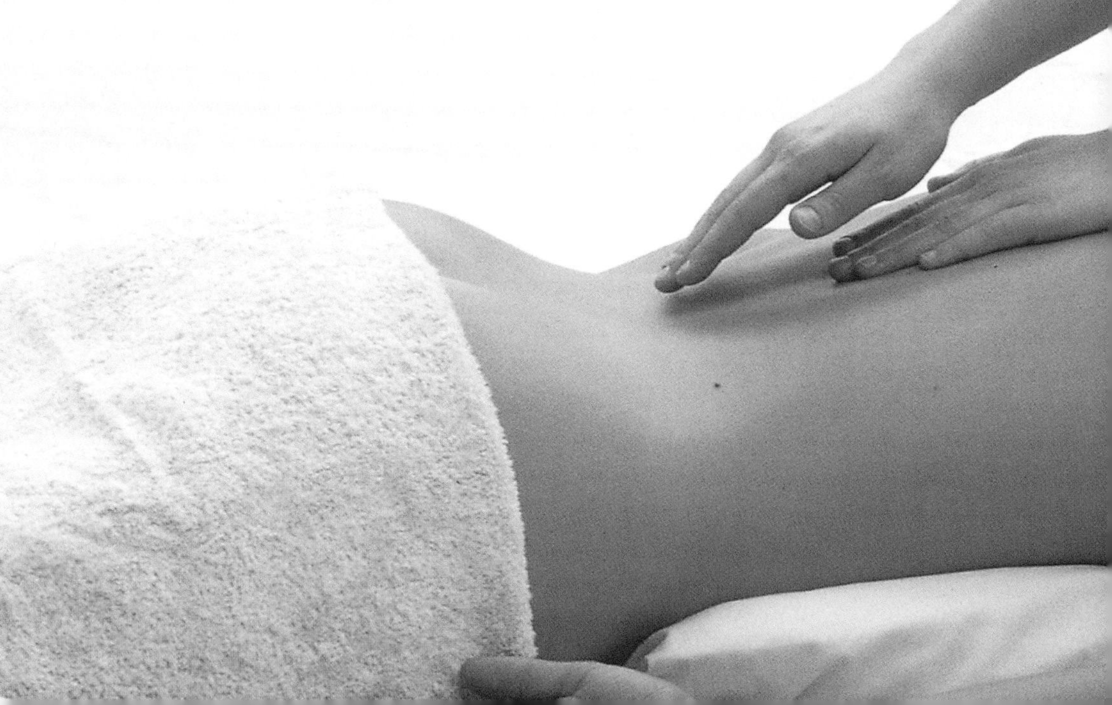

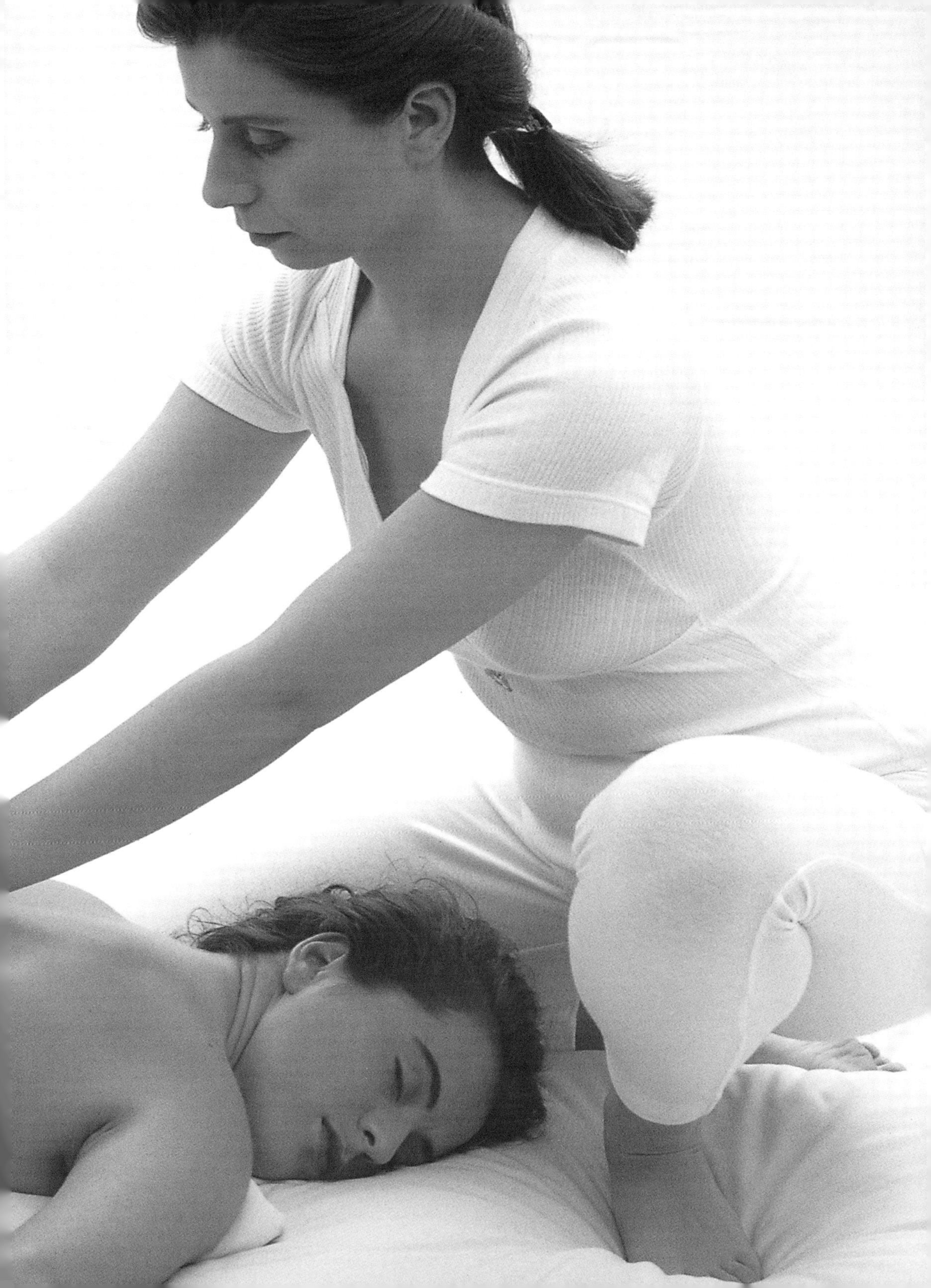

Massaging the back

There are several good reasons for beginning a body massage on the back. Some people need time to relax sufficiently to allow the process of massage to work properly, and the back presents a broad surface that does not feel as immediately intimate or as vulnerable to touch as, for example, the chest or stomach. At the same time, the muscles of the back are especially prone to tension resulting from stress, uncomfortable posture, and injury.

A thorough back massage can take the strain out of the whole body. Combine your strokes to prepare, soothe, warm, and relax the back, while working therapeutically on all the main areas of tension, such as the spine, the lower back, and the shoulders.

relaxing the spine

The first stage of the back massage focuses on relaxing the spine and the muscles that support it. Begin from a position behind your partner's head so that you can carry out a series of soothing effleurage strokes over the whole back, followed by some deeper pressure strokes to release tension from alongside the spine.

caution

During a back massage you should never apply pressure directly on the spine. The focus should be on releasing tension from the muscles alongside the spine.

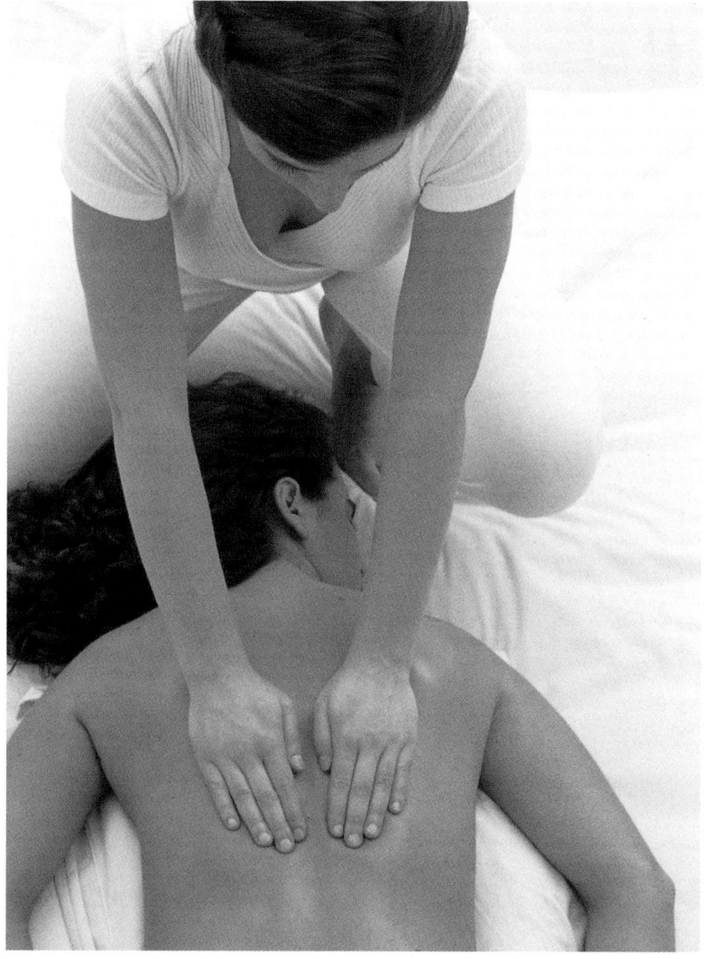

the initial integration stroke

This initial main effleurage movement embraces the whole shape of the back, warming the muscles and tissues. It can be applied up to five times as the preparatory stroke in a continuous sequence of motions.

◁ **1** To start, place your hands flat on each side of the spine, fingers pointing towards the lower back. Lean your weight into your hands and slide them steadily downwards to stretch the long muscles beside the spine.

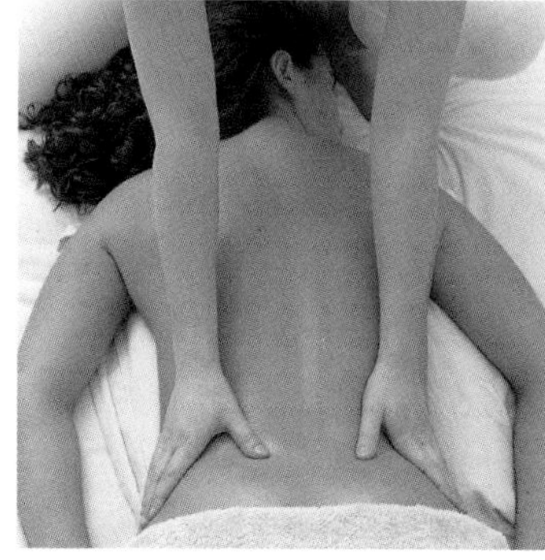

△ **2** As your hands reach the lower back, swing them out and around the hips to enfold the sides of the body. Your fingers should slip slightly under the front of the body.

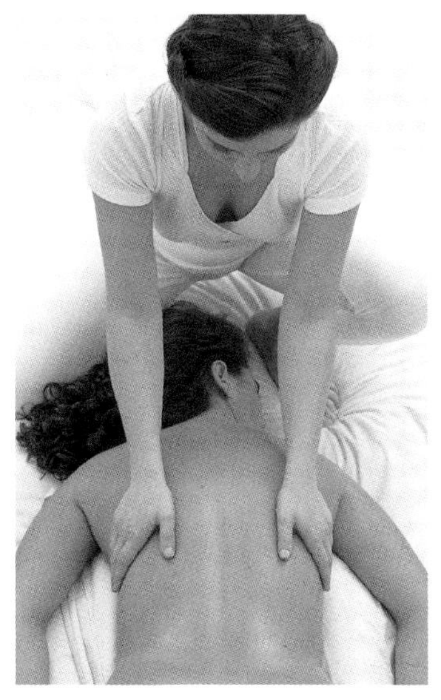

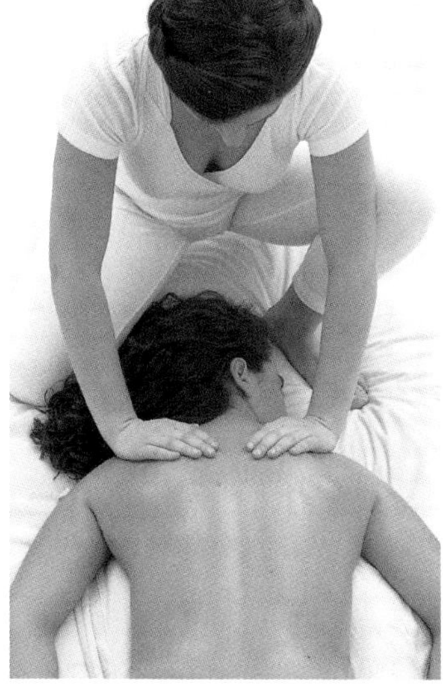

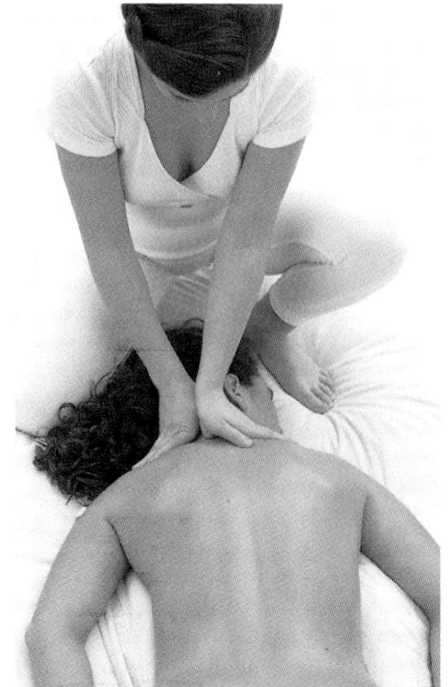

△ **3** Draw your hands gently but firmly up along the sides of the waist and ribcage until they reach the shoulder blades. Turn your wrists so that your hands glide in and around the edges of the shoulder blades.

△ **4** As your hands draw out across the top of the shoulders, shift the pressure into their heels to give a good stretch to tense shoulder muscles.

△ **5** Slip your hands softly around the shoulder joints and swivel your wrists to glide them lightly back in across the top of the shoulders. Take the stroke up the back of the neck and out through the head and hair.

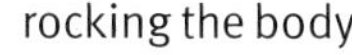

rocking the body

Some variation can be added to the above stroke to bring extra vitality and movement to the body. Complete both rocking sequences with a sweep around the shoulders, drawing your hands towards the neck and up over the head.

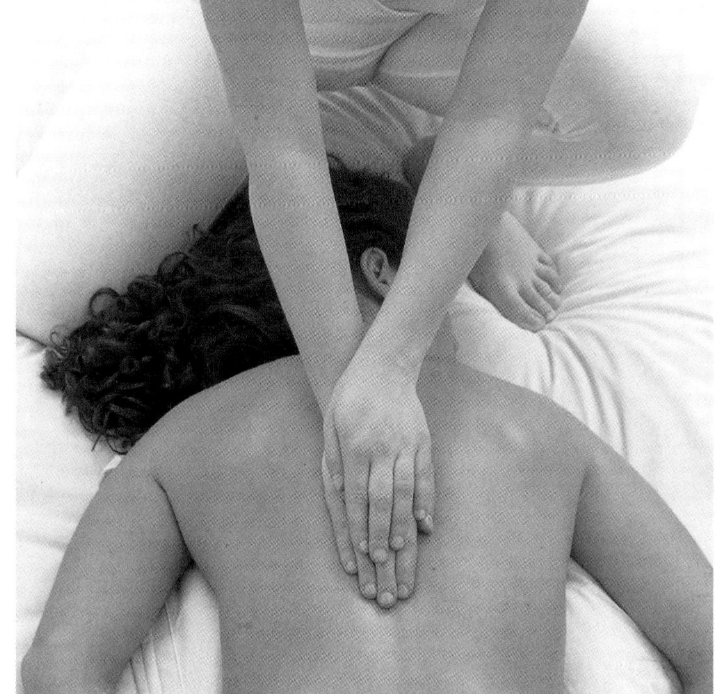

◁ **1** After your hands have curved around the sides of the lower back, draw them in towards the base of the spine. Slip your left hand on top of your right hand to add support. Slightly cup your right hand to create a suction effect and rock gently and rhythmically up over the length of the spine.

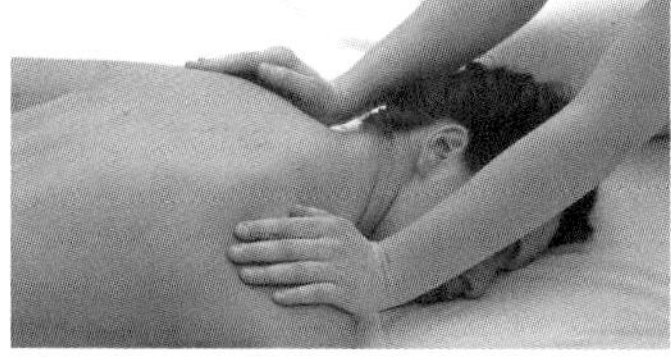

△ **2** Separate your hands at the top of the spine. Put pressure into the heel of each hand to create an alternating press-and-release movement, which works out towards the shoulders. This rocking motion is similar to the way in which a cat kneads a soft surface with its paws.

fanning

To enhance the overall relaxation of the back, perform three sequences of fanning strokes. Massage towards the lower back, and then return your hands by sweeping them out and up along the sides of the body in the same manner as the initial effleurage stroke.

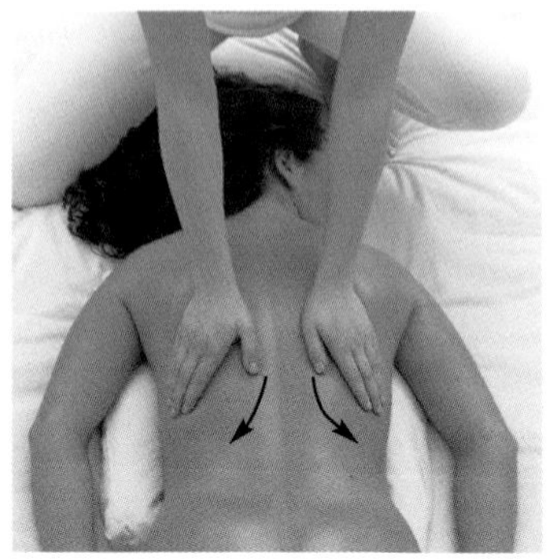

△ **1** Place your hands flat on each side of the spine at the top of the back, fingers pointing downwards. Stroke down below the shoulder blades before sliding your hands out to the sides of the body.

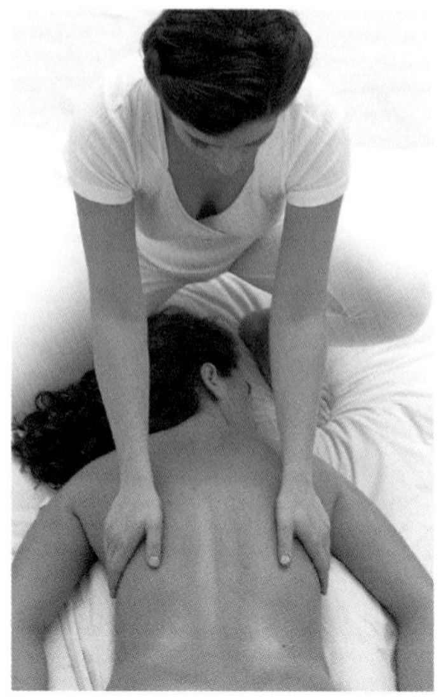

△ **2** Mould your hands to the sides of the body, gliding them up the ribcage for a short distance before flexing your wrists to draw them very lightly towards the centre of the back.

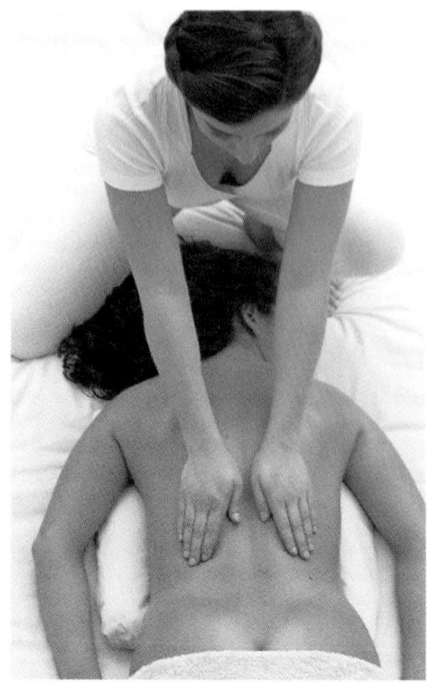

△ **3** Turn your hands so they are once again lying flat against each side of the spine, fingers pointing to the lower back. Stroke down another hand's length to repeat the fanning motion.

double stretch stroke

This stroke focuses on the long muscles, or erector spinae, which give support to the spine and help it extend and rotate the trunk of the body. Its stretching and rubbing effect releases tension and brings heat to the muscles, creating greater flexibility and movement in the back.

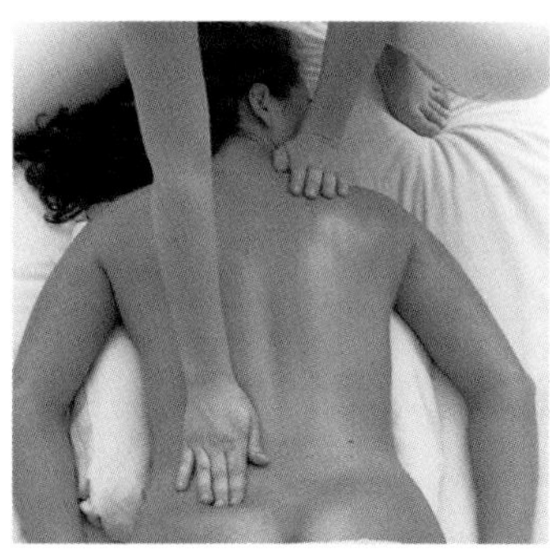

△ **1** Place both hands over the top of the shoulders and close to the spine, fingers pointing down the back. Using a firm and steady pressure, slide the right hand down over the long muscles while keeping the left hand in its original position.

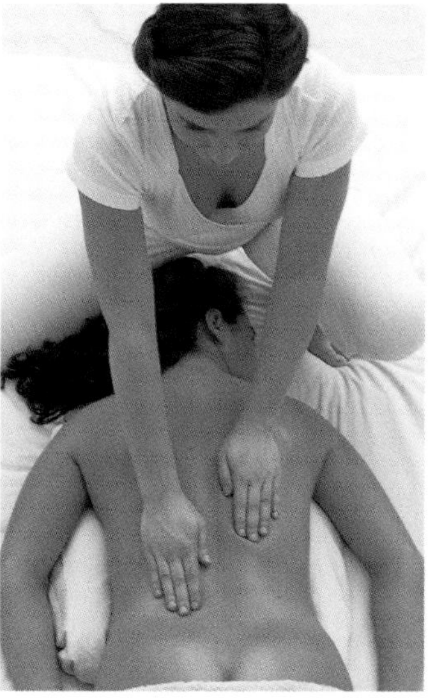

△ **2** When the right hand reaches the small of the back, curve it around the hip and back to the base of the spine, before drawing it back up the long muscle on the left side of the spinal column. At the same time, slide your left hand down to repeat the motion on the right side of the spine.

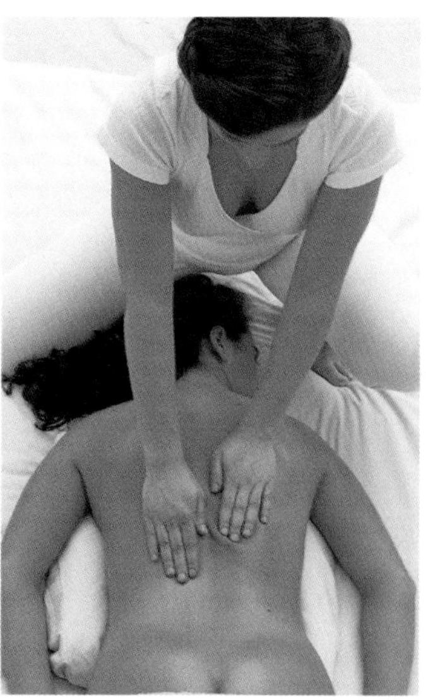

△ **3** Continue to move both hands back and forth over the long muscles for up to five sequences. Increase the speed and pressure to create a heat-producing friction and rippling effect in the tissue as the hands pass each other. Complete the stroke with both hands resting by the shoulders.

pressure strokes along the spine

Now is the time to increase the pressure of your strokes along the spine in order to ease tight spots and bring relief. Sink the weight slowly into the muscle tissue at the top of the shoulders before starting the stroke, remaining sensitive to your partner's response to the pressure. Keep the strokes close to the spine, but avoid pressing directly on the bone. Once your stroke has reached the base of the spine, open out your hands to sweep them around and up the sides of the body so that each sequence can be repeated.

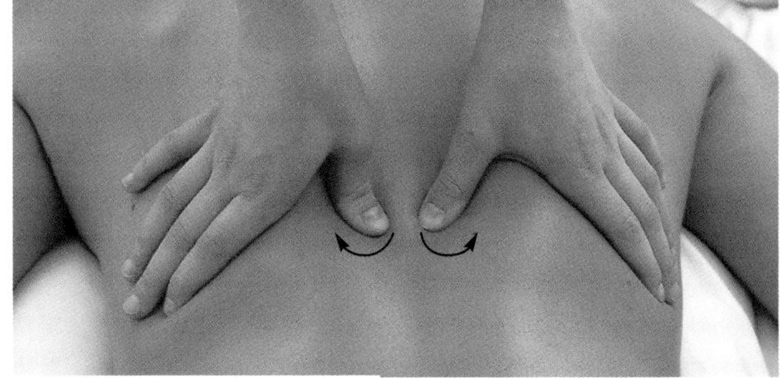

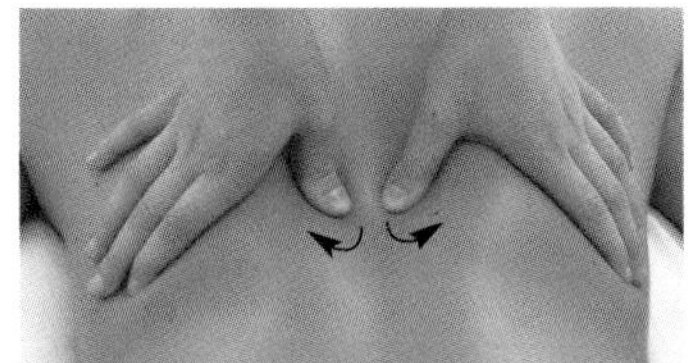

◁ **1** Starting at the top of the back, place your thumb pads on either side of the spine. It is important to remember not to apply pressure directly to the spine. Shift the weight into your thumbs while your fingers rest on the body. Massage in small circular motions close to the edge of the bone.

△ **2** Deepen the pressure as your thumbs rotate towards and away from the spine in the first half of the circle, and release the pressure to glide softly back and around. Work down the length of the spine in a spiralling motion. Repeat the stroke, increasing the pressure.

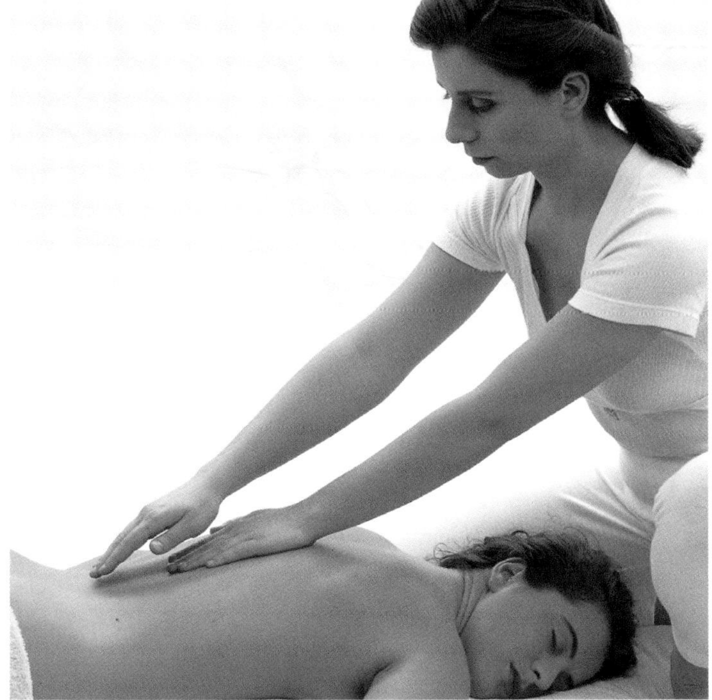

overlapping strokes

Following the double stretch and pressure strokes on the long muscles, soothe the areas with soft, gentle movements.

△ Carry out a series of strokes up over the spine, with one hand following the other in short, overlapping motions, with the fingers relaxed and spread apart.

knuckle stretch

To complete this stage of the back massage, carry out an invigorating knuckle stretch.

▽ Starting at the lower back, use loose knuckles, crossing your thumbs over each other for support, to work up either side of the spine. Wait until your knuckles have settled comfortably into a deeper level of tissue, and slide them slowly and steadily down the spine again to give a good stretch. Repeat this twice, remaining aware of your partner's breathing. To integrate the different strokes and to complete the spine massage, make several large effleurage strokes to encompass the back, and finish by placing your hands softly over the spine for several moments.

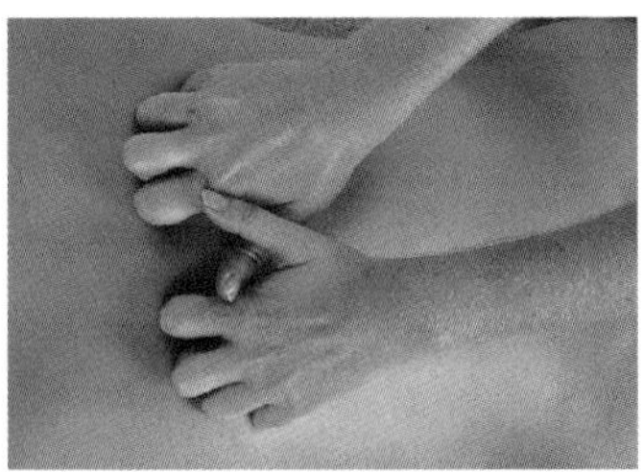

focus on the lumbar region

Change your position so that you are kneeling beside the hip and facing towards the head. Spread a little more oil on the skin if necessary. Your focus is now on relaxing the lower half of the back, known as the lumbar region. This area is particularly prone to aches and pains which are the result of compression and strain caused by uncomfortable posture, awkward movement or prolonged sitting. Many of the following strokes also benefit those muscles that cross over the sides of the body from the abdomen to the back. These muscles, known as abdominus obliques, support abdominal organs and flex the spine.

soothing with effleurage

Start with a series of relaxing effleurage movements over the whole back before working specifically on the muscles between the pelvic girdle and the shoulder blades. To avoid twisting in your own posture, you can straddle your partner's body while doing these strokes. Keep one foot on the mattress, and use your leg muscles to lever yourself back and forth, and to support your own weight. Ensure that you remain at some physical distance from your partner.

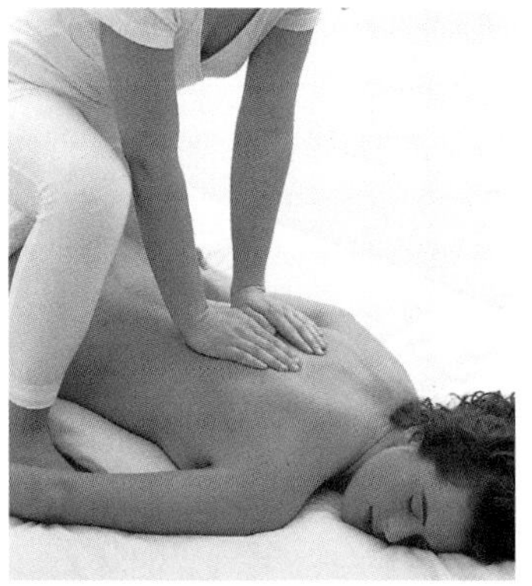

△ **1** Begin a large effleurage stroke from the lower back. Place both hands flat beside the spine, fingers towards the head. Lean into your hands, stroking up the back towards the head with a steady pressure.

△ **2** As your hands reach the top of the back, fan them out towards the shoulders in a continuous flow of motion.

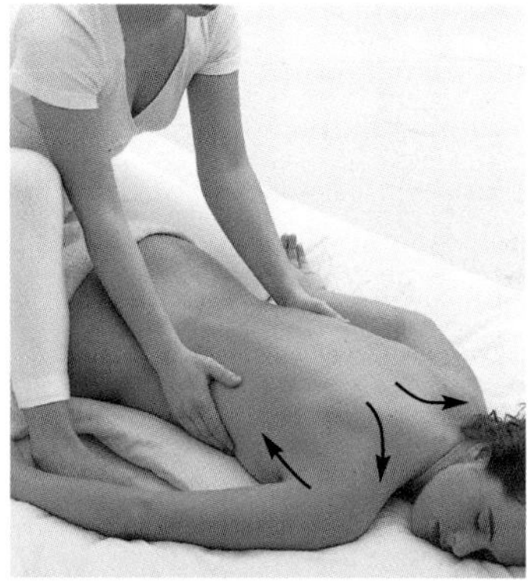

△ **3** Moulding your hands to the body, glide them over the shoulders, down the sides of the ribcage and waist as far as the lower back.

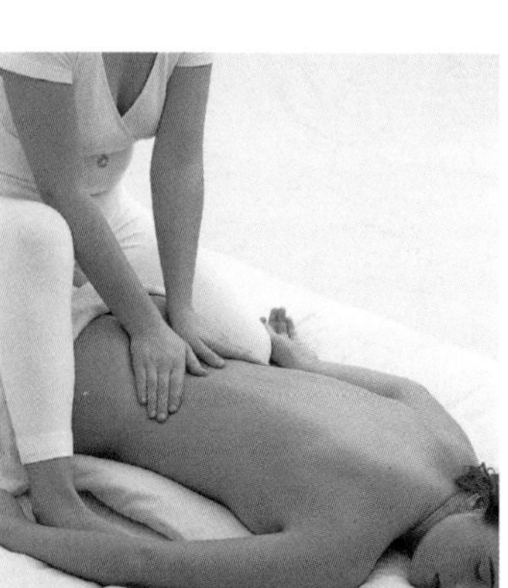

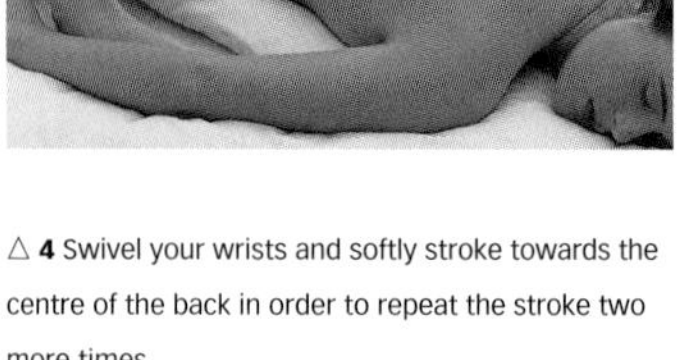

△ **4** Swivel your wrists and softly stroke towards the centre of the back in order to repeat the stroke two more times.

fanning upwards

A firm fanning motion towards the heart can give a boost to the blood circulation. Massage with smaller fanning motions, moving up the back until your hands reach the shoulder blades, and then adapt the stroke to encompass the broad surface of the upper back before gliding back down the sides of the body.

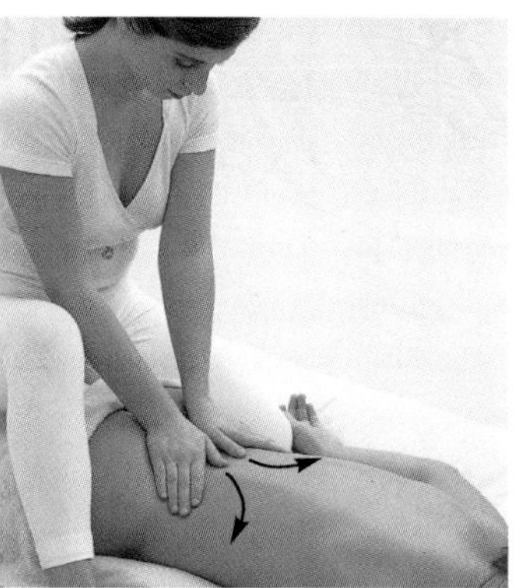

△ **1** Place your hands on each side of the spine, fingers pointing to the head. Stroke upwards with a steady pressure before fanning your hands outwards.

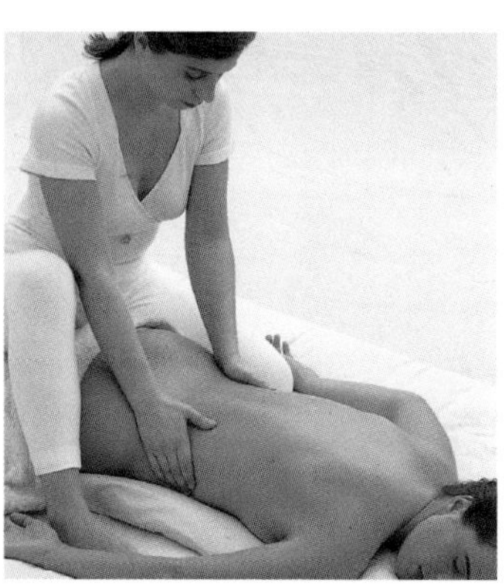

△ **2** Sculpting the sides of the body, pull softly but firmly downwards. Flex your wrists to stroke very lightly back into the body.

pressure circles on the lower back

Pressure circles are excellent strokes for removing tension from a tight lumbar region. Start the stroke softly, and as the tissue warms, increase the pressure into the heels of your hands. Build up speed to massage vigorously on the small of the back. Use firm pressure on the upward and outward half of the circle, flexing your wrists to glide your hands very lightly around to the start of the stroke. Complete the sequence with a full and soothing effleurage stroke over the back.

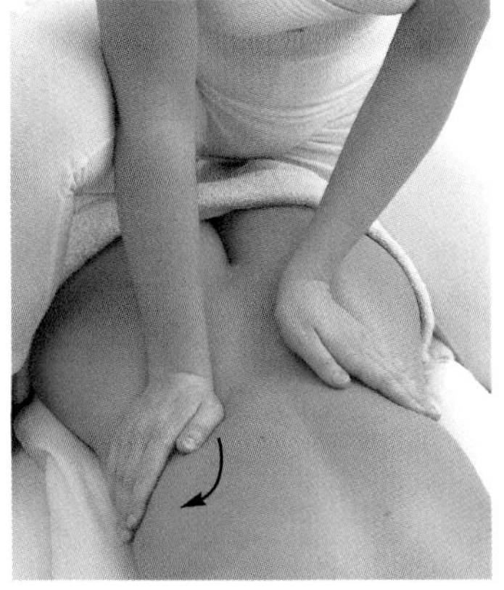

△ **1** Place both hands flat on each side of the base of the spine, with the fingers slightly tilted towards the sides of the body. Stroke your right hand up a short distance, fanning it outwards into a circular motion.

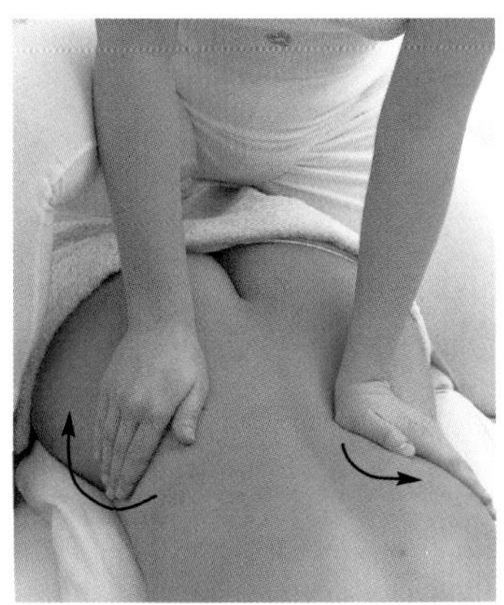

△ **2** At this point the left hand begins to stroke upwards. As the right hand decreases pressure and glides lightly back in a circular motion towards the start of the stroke, the left hand fans up and downwards.

soft circle strokes

To accomplish the next series of strokes, turn to face into the back. Once you have finished the sequence, change position to repeat the whole sequence from the opposite side of the body. Flow from stroke to stroke without breaking the movement of your hands.

Soft circle strokes feel wonderful on the skin, with their overlapping and fluid motion easing and stretching tension out of the body's soft tissue. They are a perfect stroke for the broad yet rounded dimensions of the back. Begin circle stroking up the side of the body opposite to you, spiralling from the hip to the edge of the shoulder blade. Without breaking the flow, swing the stroke out to cover the spine and massage down towards the sacrum. Repeat three times.

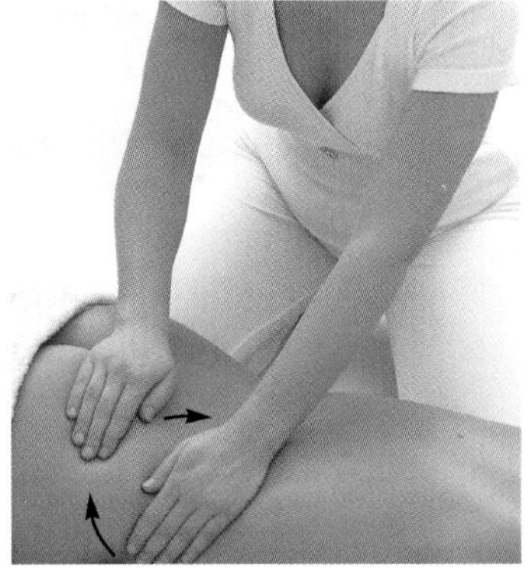

△ **1** Lay your hands over the opposite side to you, keeping the hands about 10cm/4in apart. Circle both hands in a clockwise motion.

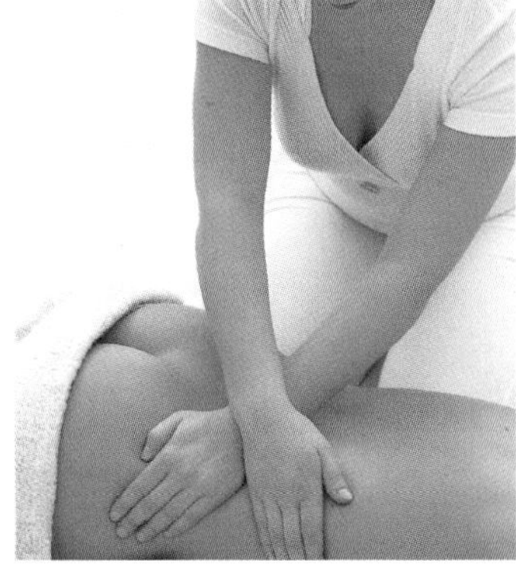

△ **3** As the left hand continues to circle over the side of the body, cross the right hand over it, dropping it lightly back on to the skin.

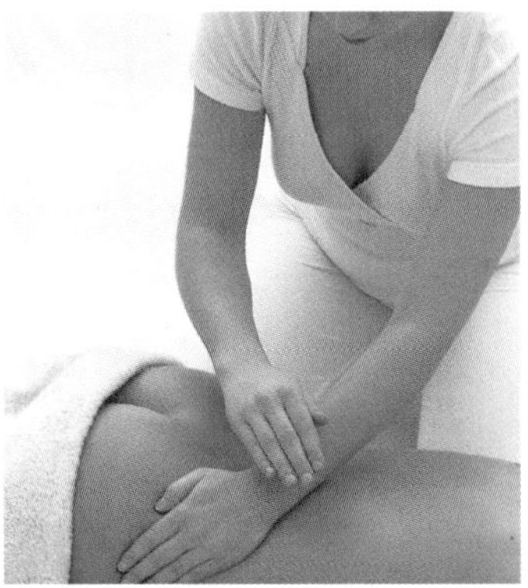

△ **2** Lift up the right hand as it completes the first half-circle to allow the left hand to pass underneath it in an unbroken motion.

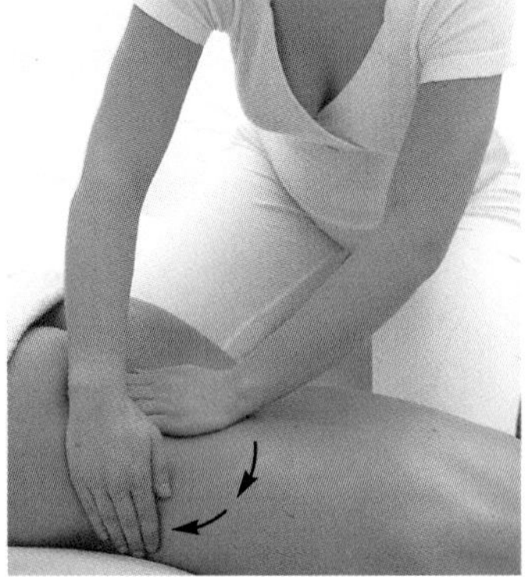

△ **4** Let the right hand form another half-circle stroke before lifting off as the left hand completes the full circle, spiralling upwards.

wringing the back

The wringing action on the lower back is done by crossing your hands from side to side, creating a warm friction on the muscle fibres. Work the stroke across the back, from the hips to the shoulder blades, and down again three times, always making sure that your hands fully encompass both sides of the body. Increase the speed and pressure of the wringing for an invigorating effect, and then slow it down for a soothing finish.

▽ **1** Place your right hand over the hip opposite to you, with your fingers wrapped slightly under the belly, the left hand cupped over the hip closest to you. Slide your hands towards each other with enough pressure to lift and roll the flesh on the sides of the body.

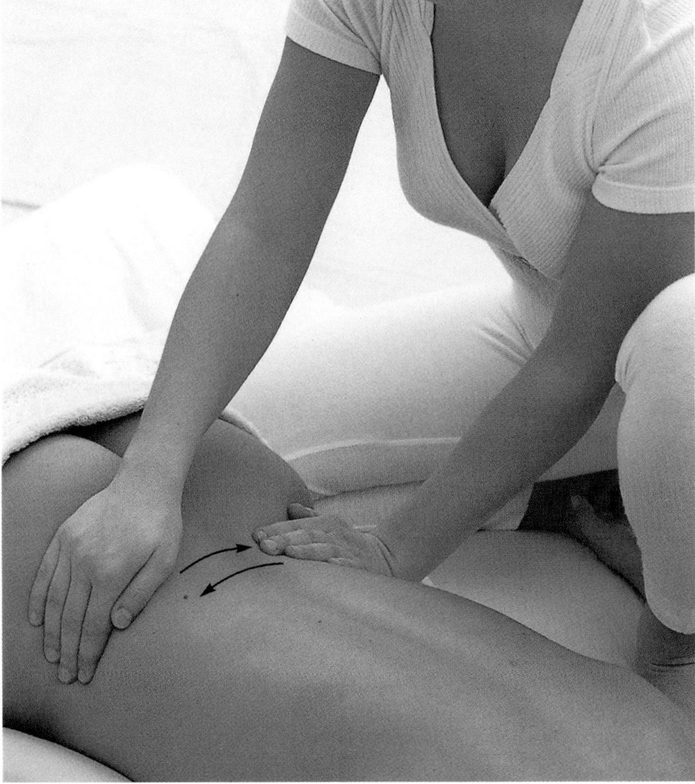

▽ **2** Decrease the pressure as you stroke across the back, hands passing each other to the opposite sides of the body. Without stopping, immediately begin to slide them back. Continuously stroke your hands back and forth while you wring up and down the lumbar region.

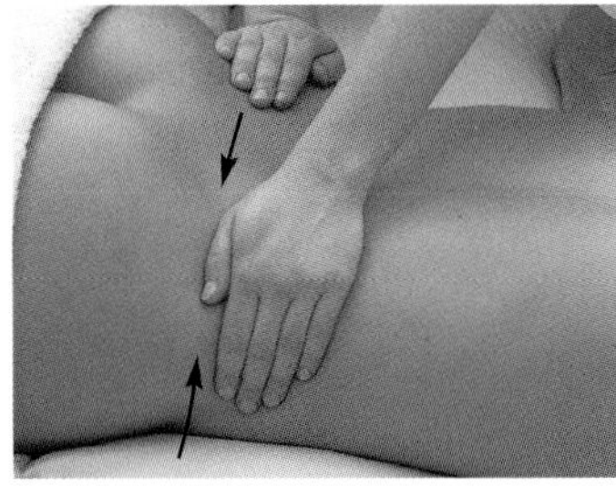

kneading

Invigorating kneading on the buttocks, hips, and along the flank of the body will help to release weight and tension from the back, bringing relief to the whole area. Scoop, squeeze, and roll the flesh with your right hand and then roll it towards the left hand. Without breaking the motion, repeat the action with the left hand so that it passes the flesh back. Keep the stroke moving back and forth in a rhythmic and circular manner. Take care to relax your own shoulders, wrists, and hands. Knead thoroughly from the hip to just below the arm and back down again. Repeat once more.

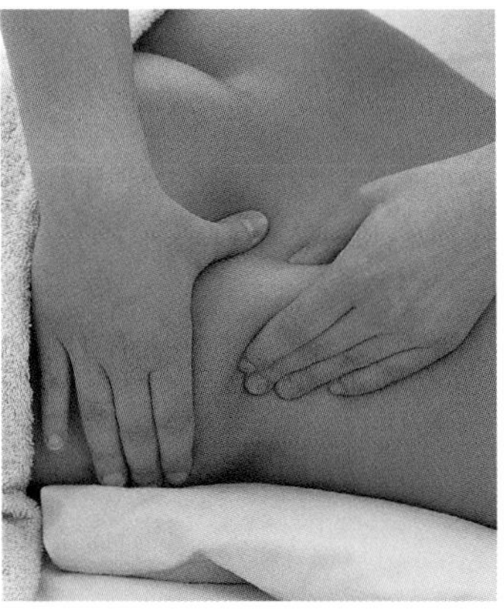

△ **1** Knead over the top of the buttock and beside the hip on the side of the body opposite to you. Work the kneading stroke up alongside the waist and rib cage. The amount of flesh on this area varies considerably from person to person.

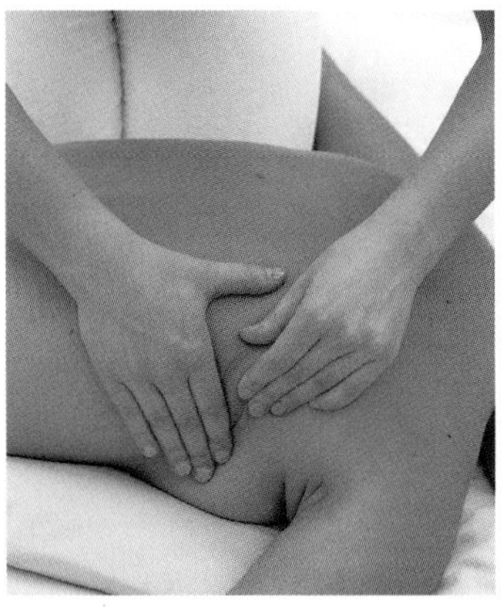

△ **2** Thorough kneading beside the shoulder blade will help the upper back to relax and the shoulder to drop.

hip, shoulder and spine stretch

This stretch stroke brings a pleasing sense of integration to the body as the hands move diagonally from the hip to the opposite shoulder, fan around and over the shoulder blade several times and then finish with a soft stretch over the length of the spine.

▷ **1** Place your hands close together, fingers pointing towards the opposite shoulder, over the hip nearest to you. Stroke across the body to make a sweeping diagonal stretch.

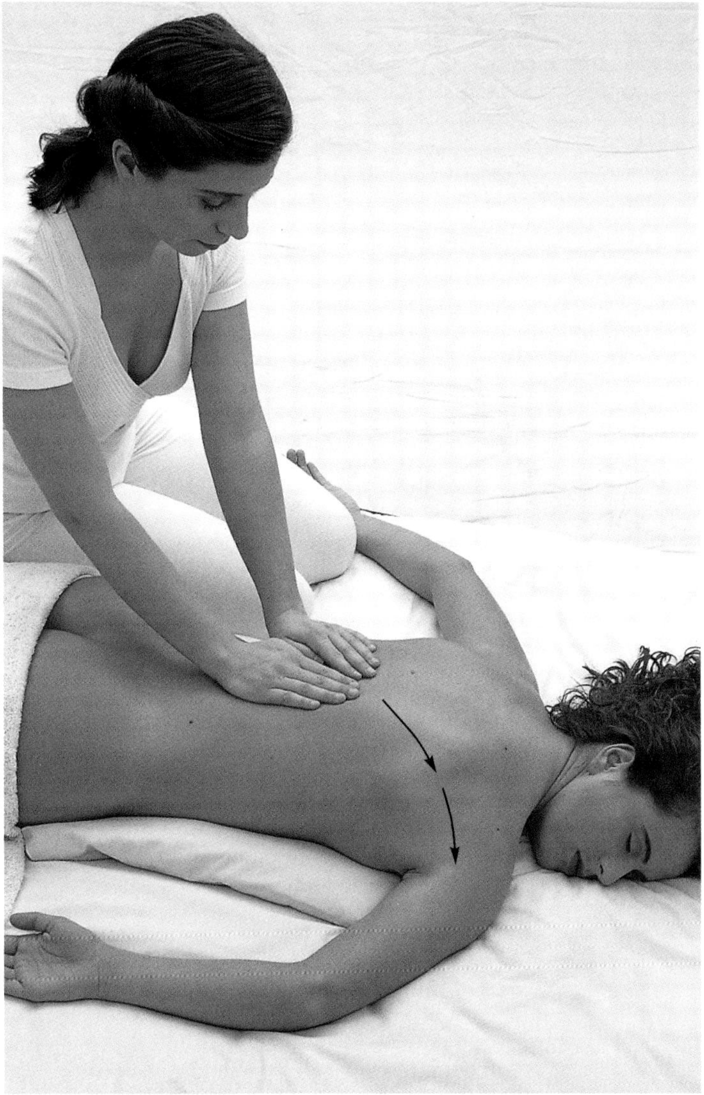

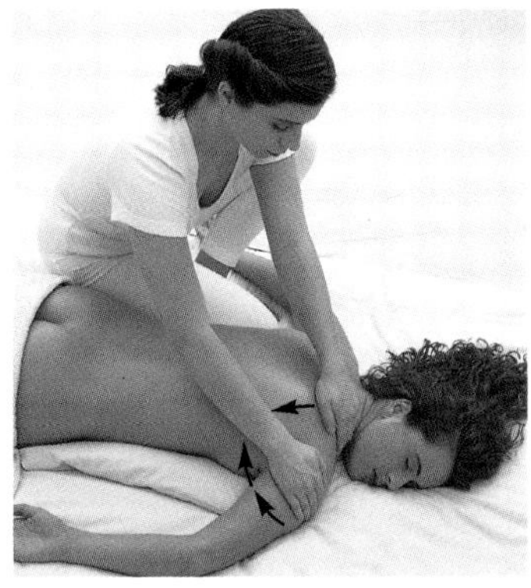

△ **2** When your fingers reach the tip of the opposite shoulder joint, mould them to curve into the shape of the shoulder blade. Draw your hands outwards to surround its circumference until the fingers of both hands meet at the centre of its inner ridge.

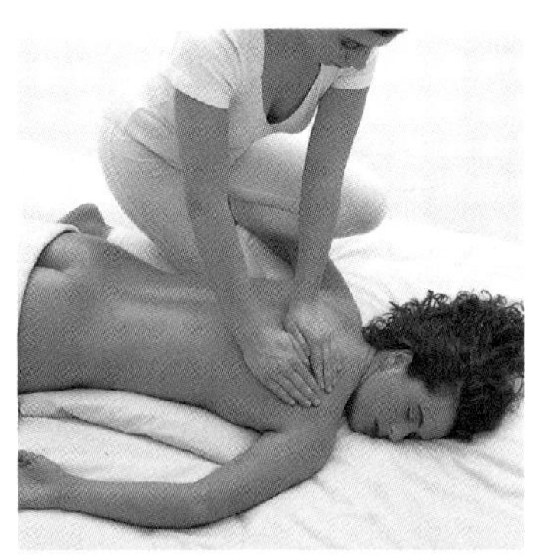

◁ **3** Sweep your hands several times over and around the bone, keeping your hands supple and wrists loose in order to fully enfold its flat triangular shape. Feel the muscles warm up beneath your touch.

▷ **4** Now pull both hands back towards the spine and draw your hands in opposite directions over the vertebrae, one towards the neck and the other towards the lower back. Stop briefly to rest your hands in a calm, still hold over each end of the spine. Move to the other side of your partner and repeat these strokes, following up with harmonious effleurage strokes to cover the whole surface of the back.

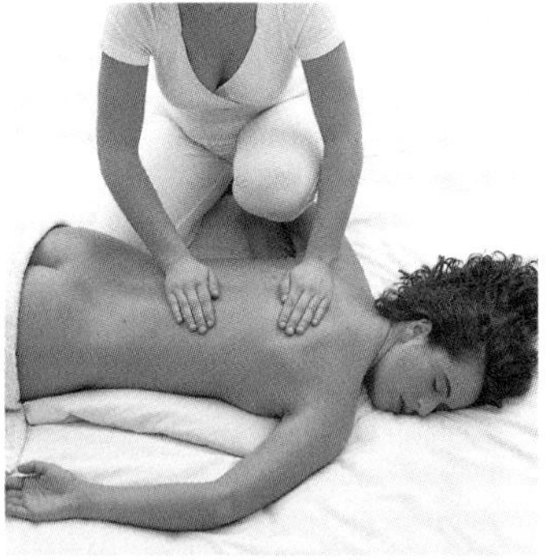

focus on the upper back

The upper back tightens under stress, and most people welcome the therapeutic touch in this region. The following strokes will help to disperse the tension, allowing a greater sense of freedom and vitality.

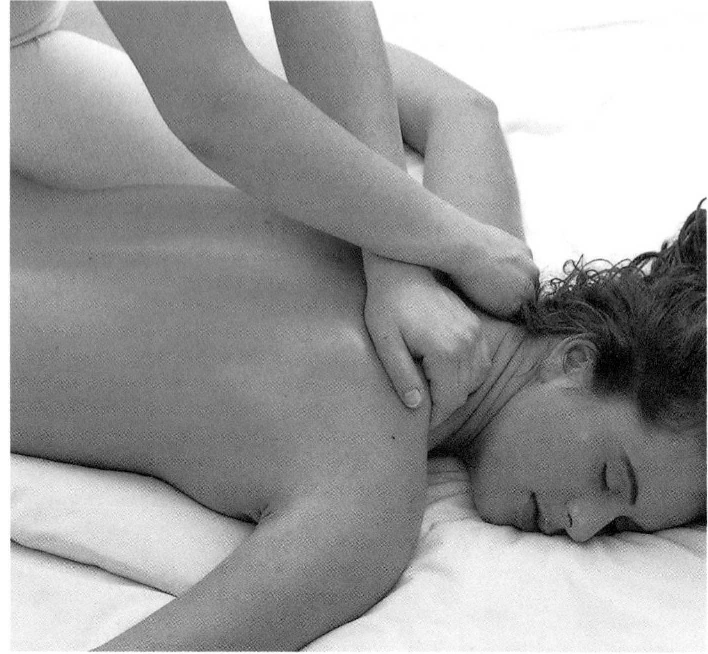

criss-cross and squeeze

This criss-cross stroke requires coordinated movement. It combines effleurage with a squeezing action and follows the line of the diamond-shaped trapezius muscle that lifts and lowers the shoulder girdle and helps to raise the head.

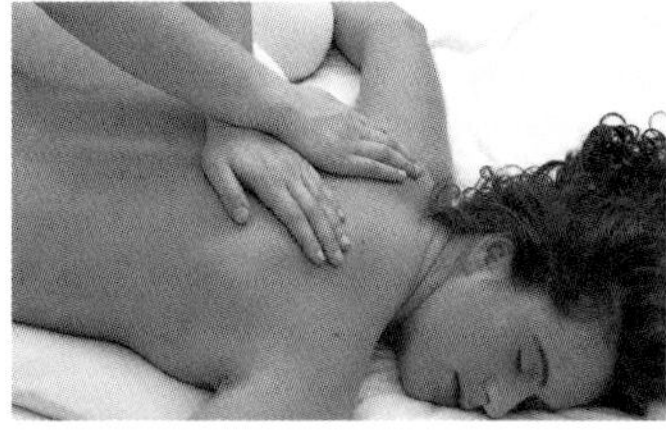

△ **1** Place your hands over the spine at the mid-point of the back. Both hands should be slightly angled towards each other, with the fingers of your right hand resting lightly over the fingers of the left hand. Stroke both hands directly out towards the opposite shoulders in a cross-over action.

△ **2** Without breaking the motion, wrap your fingers slightly over the front of the shoulders, then, adding pressure to both your fingers and the heels of the hands, lift, roll, and squeeze the flesh. Release the pressure and pull your hands back towards the mid-point so that your arms are no longer crossed.

▽ **3** Now glide your hands out again to the shoulders, so that the hands form a V-shape. Again let your fingers wrap over the top of the shoulder, but this time slide your hands back without squeezing the muscles. Repeat at least two more times.

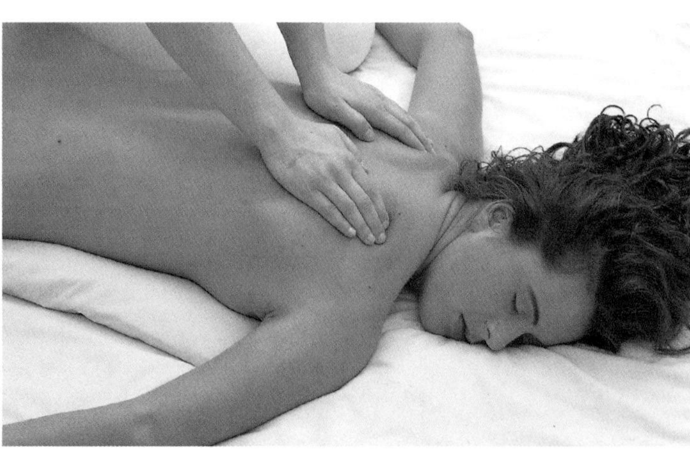

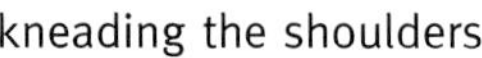

kneading the shoulders

Use a kneading action to roll and squeeze the muscles between the thumbs and fingers in order to ease tight spots at the base of the neck and over the shoulder.

▽ Work on the shoulder opposite you and ask your partner to turn her head to you so that the shoulder's surface is fully exposed.

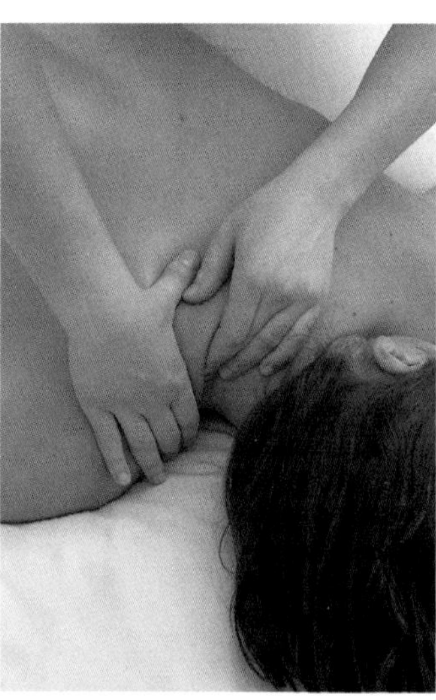

friction strokes

Friction strokes act to release tension from the upper back by pushing the tissue down towards the bone, then stretching it. Apply these strokes after kneading in fleshy areas, or after effleurage in areas where the bone is close to the skin.

easing the vertebrae

The thumbs and fingers are the perfect massage tools with which to penetrate deeper tissue around the shoulder blades and spine. The following friction strokes will bring help to bring relief to sore, constricted muscles.

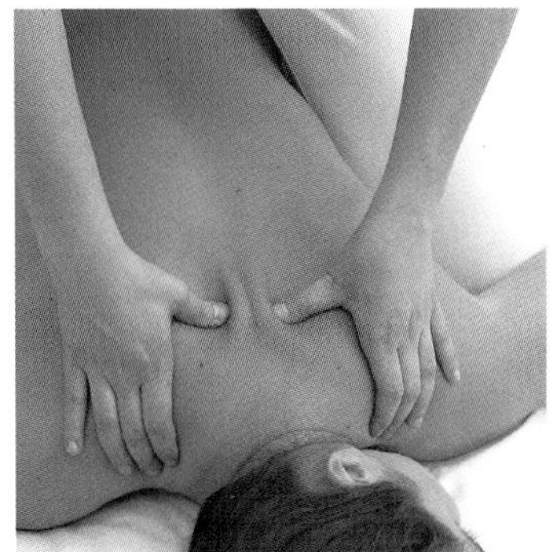

△ **1** Anchor your fingers gently but securely in front of the shoulders, placing your palms on either side of the spine. Apply pressure into your thumbs and sink them into the tissue alongside the vertebrae. Begin to slide firmly up towards the top of the shoulders.

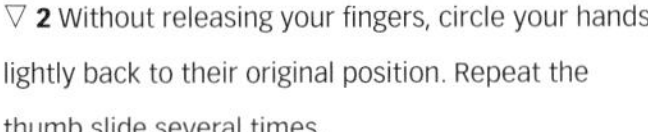

▽ **2** Without releasing your fingers, circle your hands lightly back to their original position. Repeat the thumb slide several times.

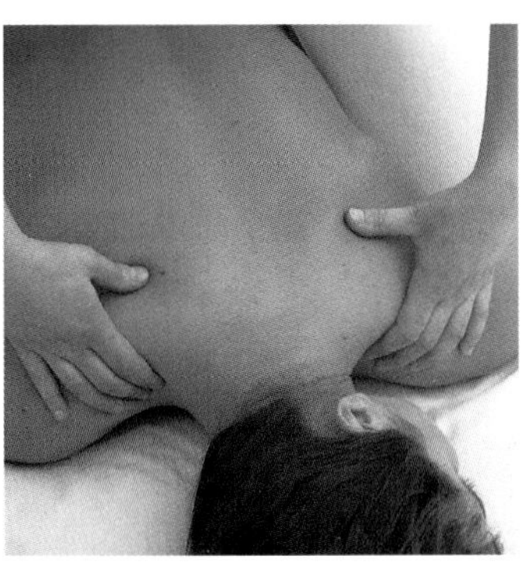

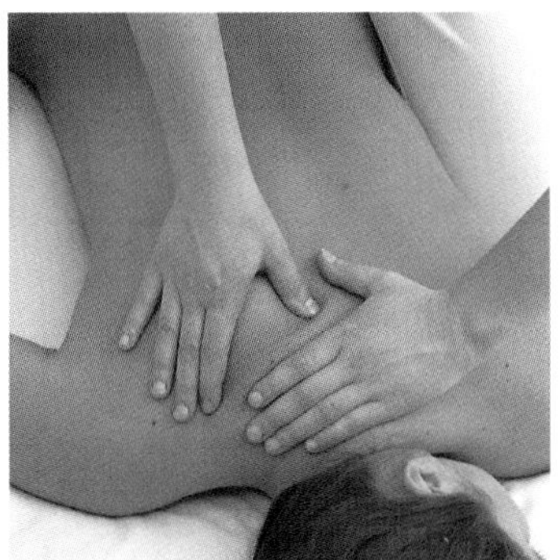

△ **3** A further deep friction stroke can be achieved by using the thumb pad to press tissue against the bone, helping to dispel toxic build-up in muscle fibres. Using one hand to push the muscle towards the stroke, make a sequence of short slides with the other hand, using the thumb pad to stretch and relieve tense areas. Always remember to sink into and release pressure slowly and gently from a friction stroke.

calming holds

Mark the end of each of the body massages with soothing strokes and a calming hold.

Bring a restful sense of completion to this section of the back massage by doing three full integration strokes. Then place your hands on the neck and the base of the spine before moving on to the next sequence.

a soothing finish

The deeper tissue work of kneading and friction strokes should now be followed by a series of soft and soothing effleurage strokes to bring a sense of overall relaxation and integration to the upper back.

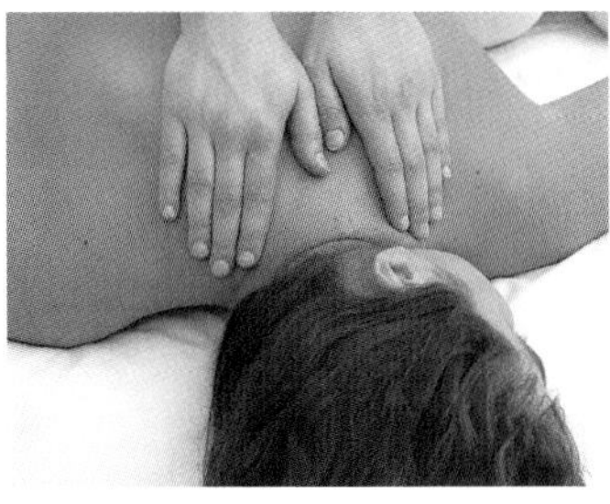

△ **1** Place your hands on the mid-back, flat against each side of the spine with the fingers pointing towards the head. Sweep your hands up towards the top of the shoulders.

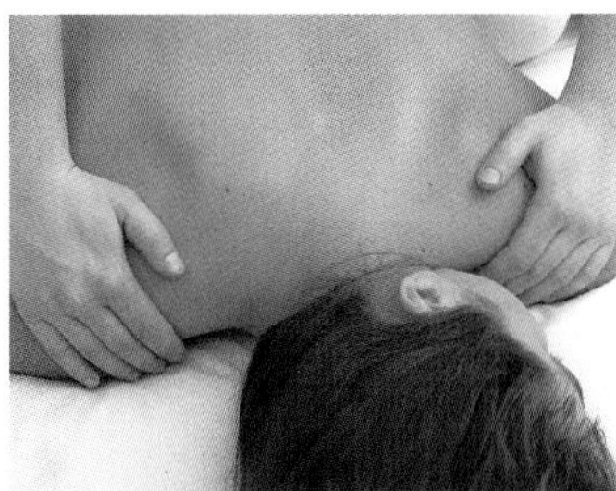

△ **2** Using your hands to mould perfectly to the curve of the body, spread them out to the edge of the shoulders, and in a flowing movement glide them soothingly around the joints.

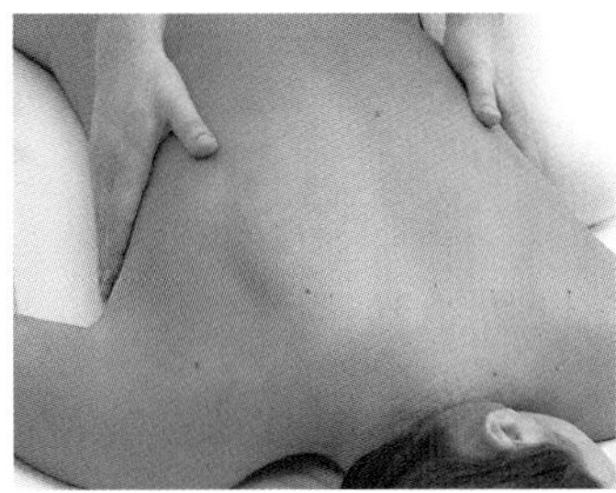

△ **3** Draw your hands down the sides of the ribcage until they are once again on the mid-back. Turn your hands so they can slide lightly to the centre of the back and repeat the effleurage stroke two more times.

Massaging the backs of the legs

The following sequence of massage strokes focuses on the lower half of the body – the legs and buttocks. This is an area of primary importance to the body's posture, weight, and locomotion. By combining the techniques of effleurage, kneading, friction, percussion, and passive movements, this programme of massage will help to warm and stretch the muscles, improve the circulation of blood and lymph, ease tension from the large strong muscles, and free contracted joints. Begin the massage on the left leg before repeating all the strokes on the right side of the body.

preliminary strokes

These opening strokes are important because they prepare the leg's soft tissues and warm the muscles for all deeper massage movements.

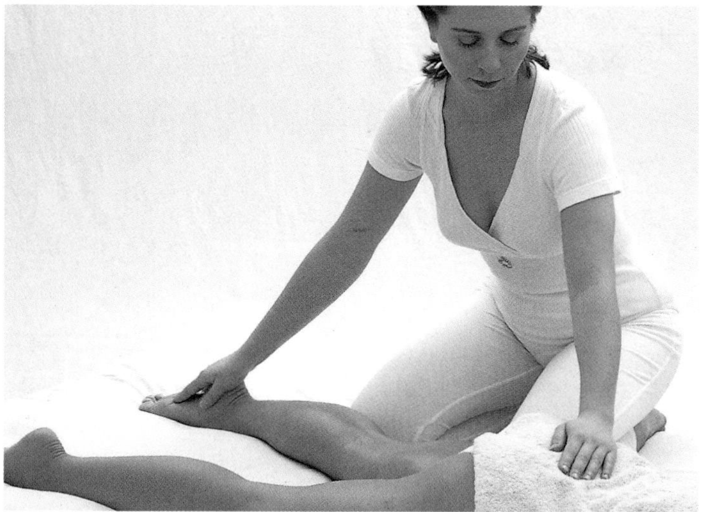

△ **1** Connecting the leg and back: Bring your partner's awareness to the leg with a connecting hold on the sacrum and foot. The gentle pressure of your hands begins the process of relaxation.

▷ **2** Integration stroke on the leg: Spread the oil smoothly down the whole leg, from the buttocks to the foot, then begin with the initial integration stroke. Repeat the stroke three times, increasing the pressure with each upward movement. Be sure to mould your hands to the shape of the leg and to adopt a posture that enables you to stroke upwards and pull back with ease. Place one foot on the mattress ahead of your body to lever your position back and forth.

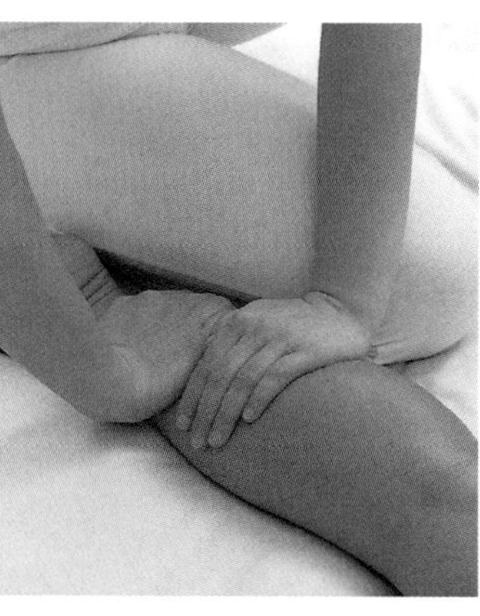

gentle leg stretch

For this stroke, start on the left leg, wrap both hands over the back of the ankle, little fingers leading, with your left hand in the top position.

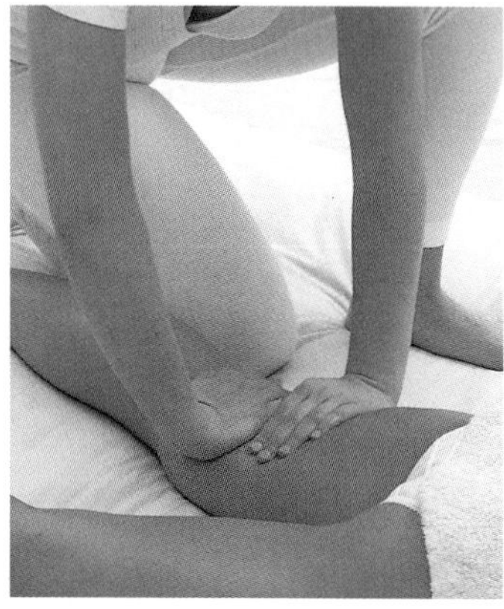

△ **1** Slide with a steady pressure up over the calf. Continue to stroke both hands towards the thigh, sliding lightly over the back of the knee. Then use enough pressure to create a ripple in the strong thigh muscles.

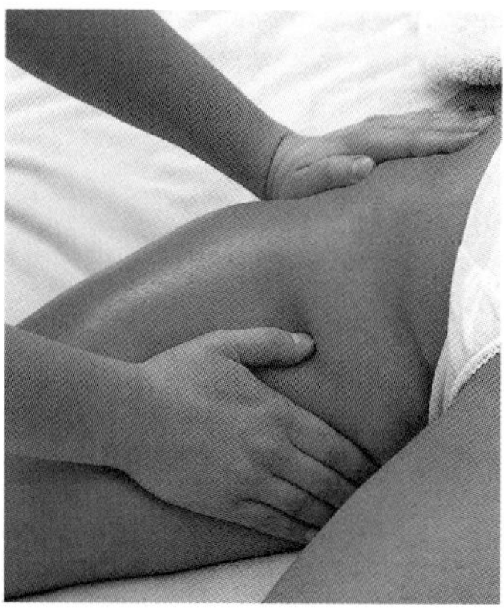

△ **2** As your hands approach the top of the leg, glide the lower one on to the inside of the thigh to rest for some moments while stroking the upper hand over the buttock and out around the hip joint.

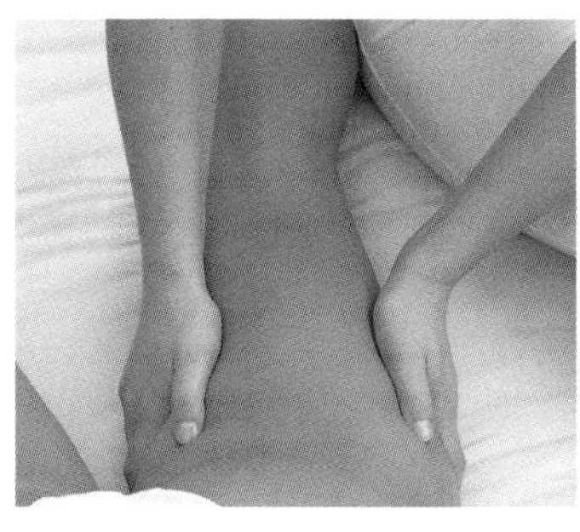

△ **3** When the moving hand descends to the outer thigh and is parallel with the waiting hand, slip your fingers slightly under the front of the leg so that you are holding it securely.

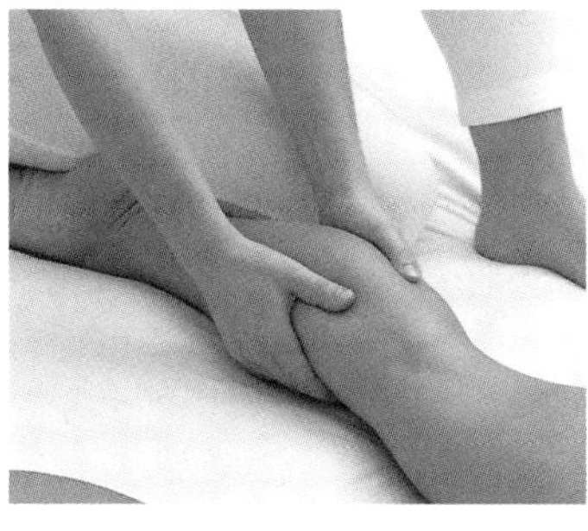

△ **4** Moulding both hands to the leg, lean the weight of your body backwards, returning the stroke steadily towards the ankle in an unbroken motion. This gentle stretch brings a feeling of length and release.

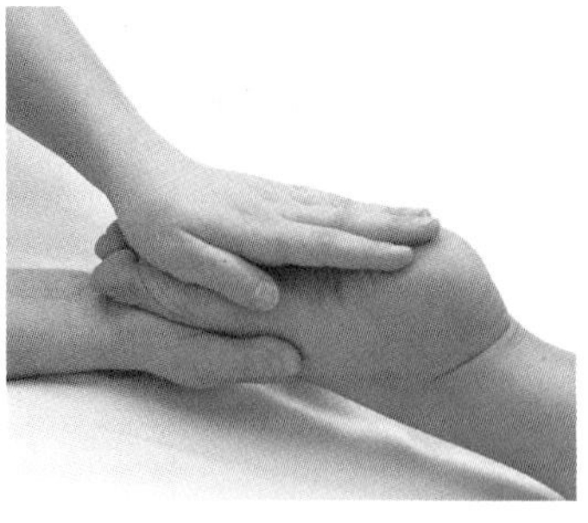

△ **5** As your hands reach the ankle, slip the hand on the outside of the leg over the back of the heel of the foot and, lifting the foot slightly, pass the other hand over the instep. Stroke out over both sides of the foot.

focus on the calf

The function of the calf muscles is to flex the knee and ankle joints, while the Achilles tendon flexes the foot and provides leverage for body movement. Keeping this area supple is important for general health. Muscle stiffness causes a sluggish blood circulation and poor lymphatic drainage, which results in low energy levels. The purpose of this sequence of strokes is to bring relief and relaxation to sore calf muscles.

Begin the sequence with some integrating effleurage strokes, which cover the lower leg from the ankle to just below the back of the knee.

fanning to the knee

Perform a series of fanning motions on the lower leg, moving up from the ankle to just behind the knee. Then glide your hands back down the sides of the leg and repeat the sequence.

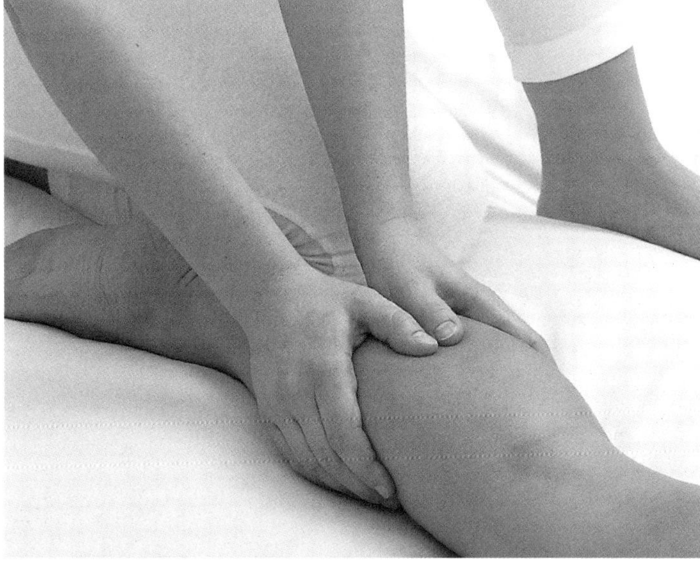

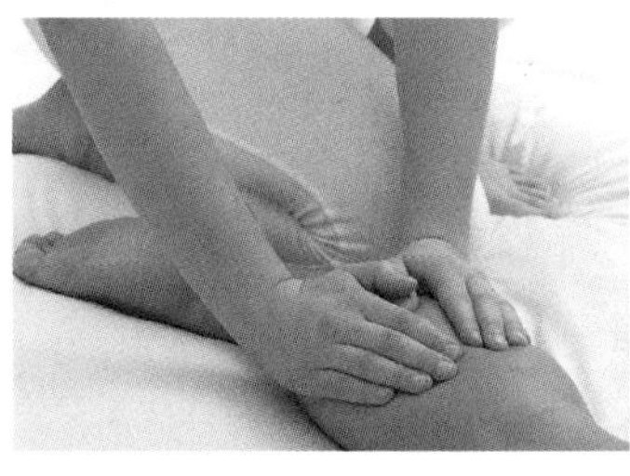

△ **1** Softening your hands to the shape of the leg, place them side by side so that the fingers tilt towards each other but point to the back of the knee. Stroke a hand's length up over the calf muscles.

△ **2** Fan both hands out to wrap around the sides and front of the leg, before sliding down and back towards the original position. Stroke further up over the calf to repeat the motion.

relaxing the achilles tendon

Cup your fingers under the front of the ankle, with the heels of both hands snugly on each side of the heel, and your thumbs on the lower calf.

▷ Flex your wrists to rotate your hands in steady circular motions, soothing away strain from the heel and the Achilles tendon.

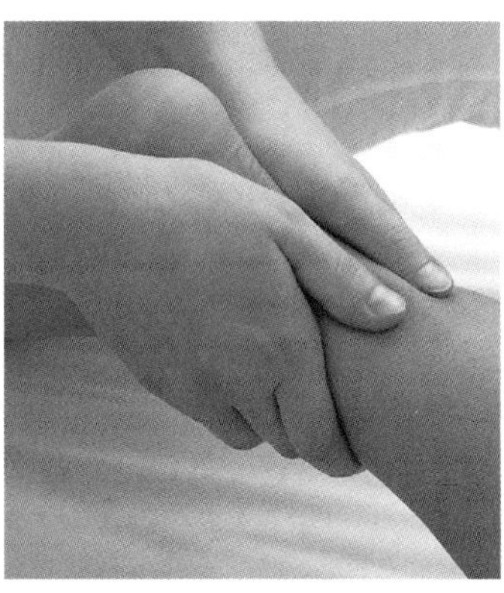

draining the lower leg

This stroke drains blood and lymph from the extremity of the body. It also creates a long, firm stretch on the lower leg muscles.

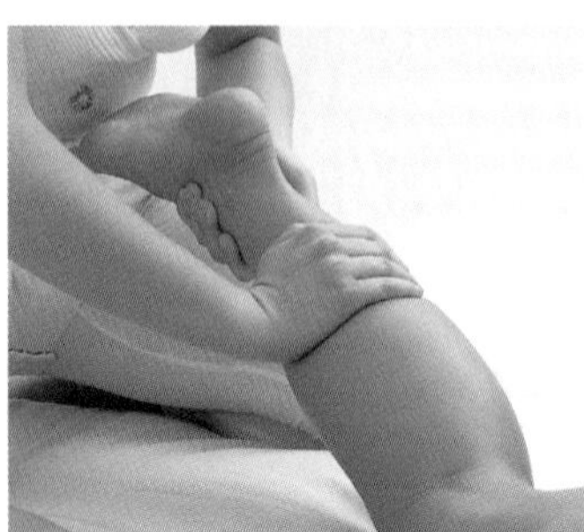

△ **1** Raise the foot and lower leg off the mattress by lifting and supporting the front of the ankle with your left hand. Wrap your right hand over the back of the ankle so that the palm and heel of the hand folds over the inner half of the leg.

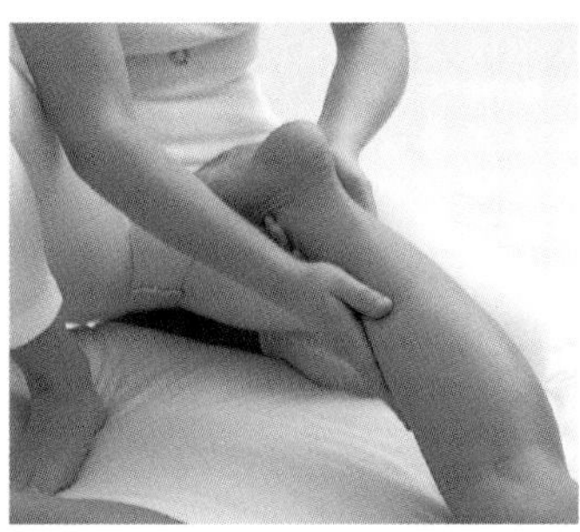

△ **2** Stroke with a firm and steady pressure up the leg towards the back of the knee. Swing the hand to glide down the front of the leg to the ankle.

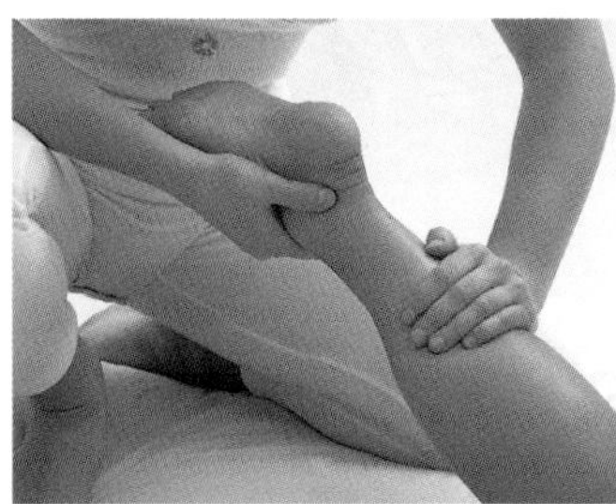

△ **3** Pass the leg to the right hand and repeat the motion with the left hand up over the outer half of the leg; return the stroke to the ankle. Repeat the sequence two more times.

kneading the calf

Kneading strokes will revive fatigued or aching calf muscles resulting from poor circulation, prolonged standing, or excessive exertion. Position yourself to face the calf and knead thoroughly from the ankle to just below the back of the knee and down again. Follow up with effleurage strokes.

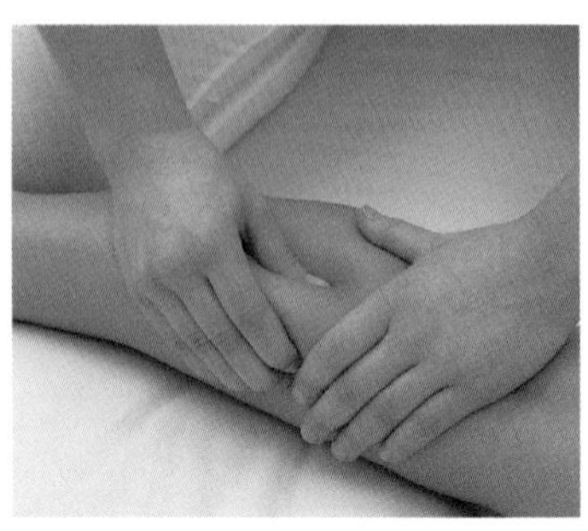

△ **1** Keeping both hands slightly apart, place them over the leg with the thumbs angled away from the fingers. Scoop, lift, and squeeze the muscle by applying pressure between the thumb, heel, and fingers and push it towards the left hand.

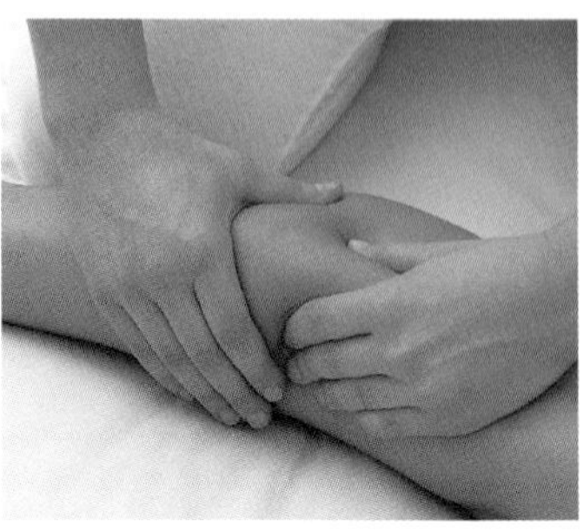

△ **2** Pick up and squeeze the flesh with the left hand and push it back to the right hand. Keeping both hands on the leg, pass the muscle back and forth in a rhythmic and circular movement.

deep friction

These deep friction strokes use the thumbs to penetrate and stretch a deeper level of muscle tissue, freeing it from underlying tension. Sink into the muscle slowly, always remaining aware of your partner's response to the pressure. Both strokes are achieved by rotating the thumbs from their base joints. Once your hands have reached to just below the knee, glide them back down the sides of the leg and repeat the sequence.

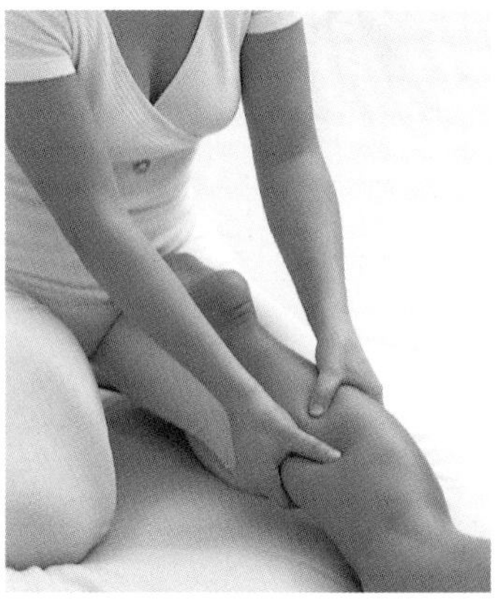

△ **1** Clasp the front of the leg with your fingers and stroke one thumb after the other up over the calf. Using short sliding movements, press firmly into the upward movement and then swing each thumb out and glide lightly back to perform the next upward stroke. At the same time gently roll the leg from hand to hand, squeezing the sides of the calf muscles with the heels of your hands.

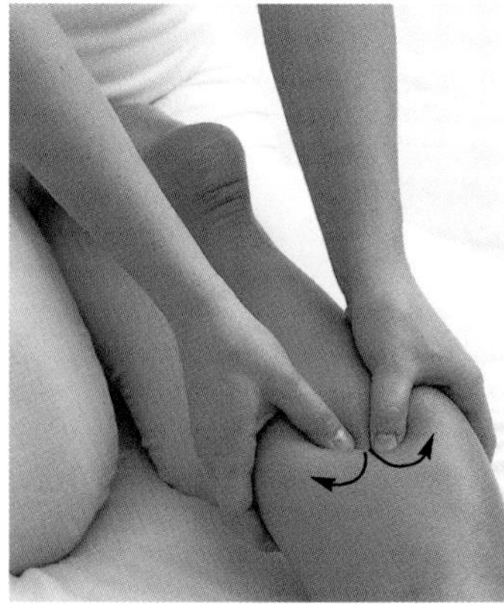

△ **2** Focus the pressure into your thumb pads, and rotate them in alternate and tiny outward flowing circles. Soften the stroke on the last half of the circle. Move up over the calf in three separate lines from above the back of the ankle to just below the knee. Follow up with several flowing integration strokes to cover the whole leg from the ankle to the top of the thigh.

focus on the thigh

A thorough massage of the thighs brings relief to this ample area of powerful body muscle, which provides essential support to the body's posture and mobility.

fanning and soft circle strokes

These flowing, relaxing strokes warm and soothe the leg, from the back of the knee to just below the buttock.

▷ **1** Glide your hands down the sides of the leg, swivelling around on to the back of the knee. Repeat the fanning sequence two more times.

▽ **2** Turn your body so that you face into the thigh and cover the top of the leg with continuous circle strokes to relax and soften the tissue. Pay special attention to the inner thigh muscles, which draw the leg towards the centre of the body.

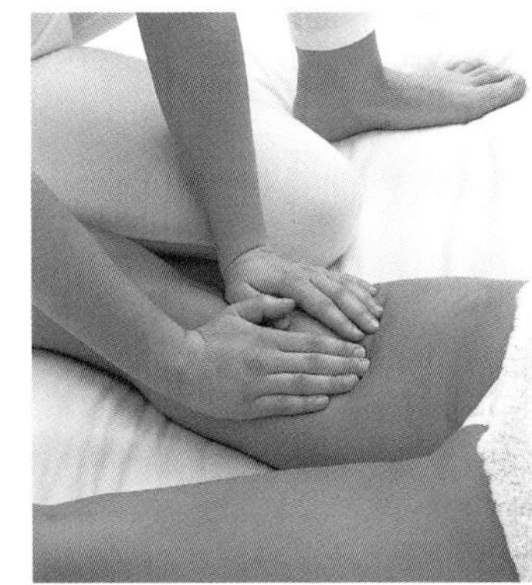

wringing the thigh

This wringing action massages across the bulk of muscle fibres and connective tissue that surrounds them on the thigh.

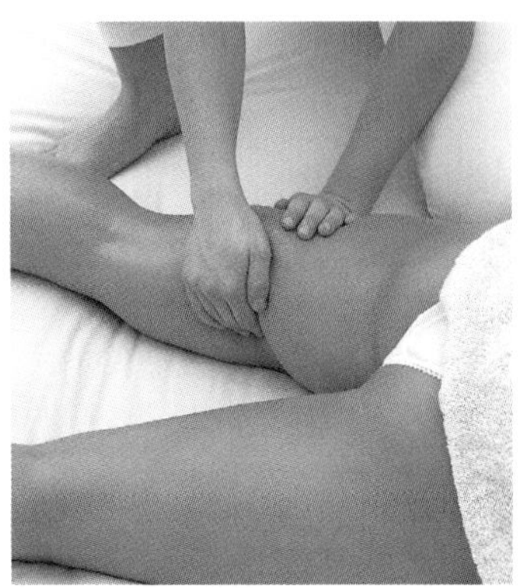

△ **1** Wrap your right hand over the inner edge of the thigh so that your fingers slip slightly under the leg. Place your left hand over the outer side of the leg so that the fingers rest on the thigh. Pull firmly to scoop up the flesh before crossing your hands over the top of the thigh to the opposite sides.

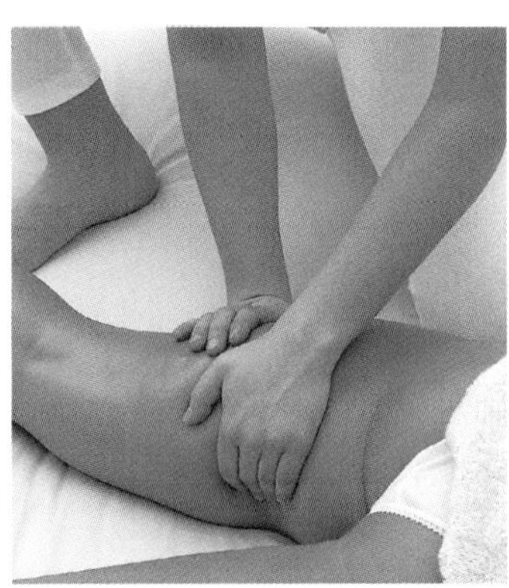

△ **2** Continue to pass your hands rhythmically back and forth over the thigh, creating a slight twist in the movement to produce a wringing effect in the muscles. Stroke from above the knee to the top of the leg and back down again. Repeat once.

draining and kneading the thigh

These strokes help to break down excess fat deposits and boost the exchange of tissue fluids. With the soothing effleurage strokes, this boosts the lymph drainage and blood circulation in the thigh.

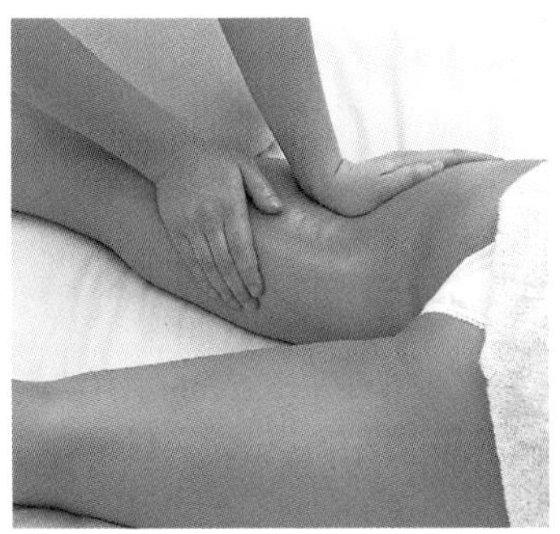

△ **1** Lean your weight into the heels of both hands for a series of firm, alternating pressure circles, one hand following the other. Lessen the pressure of the stroke as each hand fans out to the sides of the leg and glides back and around.

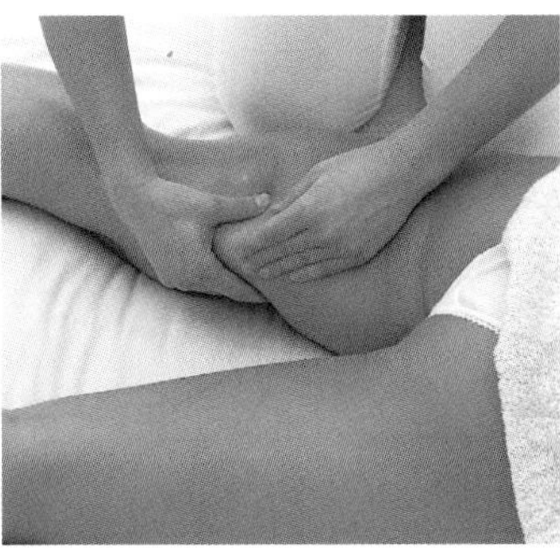

△ **2** Vigorous kneading of the thigh muscles will enliven the upper leg. Lift, squeeze, and roll the flesh from hand to hand, working first up along the inner thigh and over the bulk of the muscles. Follow up with soothing fanning motions and other effleurage strokes.

final strokes for massaging the backs of the legs

The powerful buttock muscles help to elevate the body and move the thighs. Massage aids a relaxed posture so the body's weight is supported by the lower half of the body, taking strain off the lower back. After massaging the thigh, focus on the buttock on the same side.

focus on the buttocks

Begin with some flowing integration strokes that cover and connect the thigh and buttock and mould into its contours. The strokes below are shown on the right side of the body for clearer instruction.

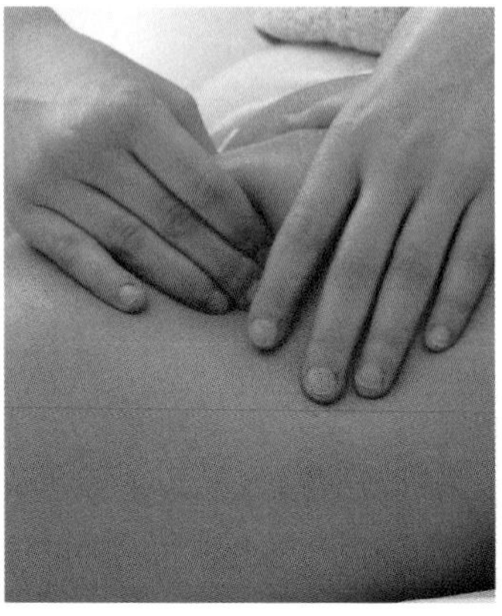

△ **1** Release tension from the buttocks by thoroughly kneading this fleshy area. You may find it easier to knead from a position on the opposite side of the body; stretching your arms will enhance the squeezing and rolling action of the stroke.

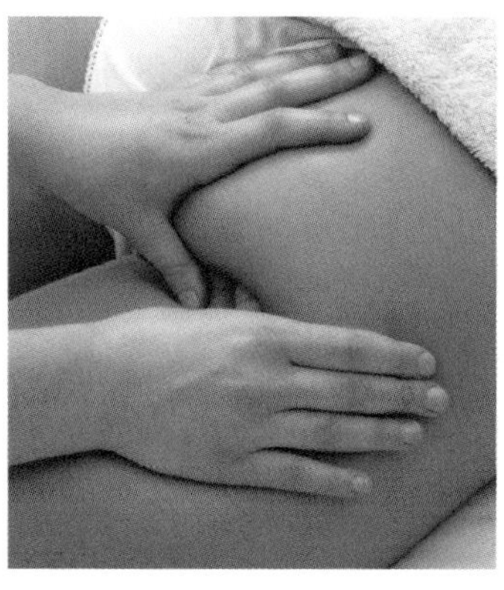

△ **2** Continue the massage from the left side of the body, and use your thumbs to work around and under the bones at the base of the pelvic girdle. Placing both hands over the buttocks for support, roll one thumb after another in short firm slides into the crease at the juncture of the buttocks and thigh.

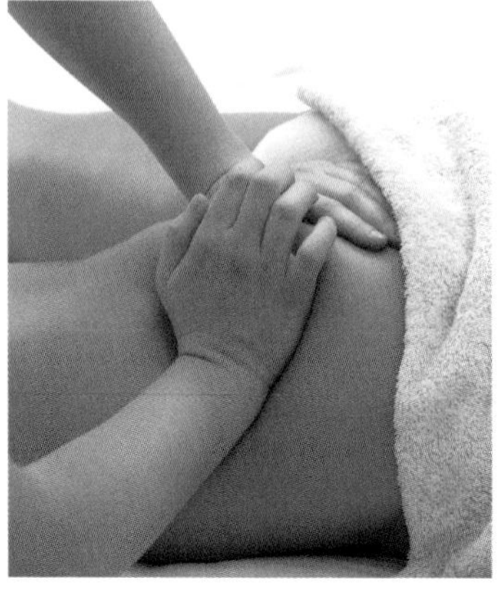

△ **3** To press deeper into the muscle, sink the heel of your hand into the buttock and rotate. Lean your weight into the first half of the circular motion and release the pressure on the return. Place your other hand close to the stroke and push the muscle towards the action. Apply these heel-pressure rotations over the whole area.

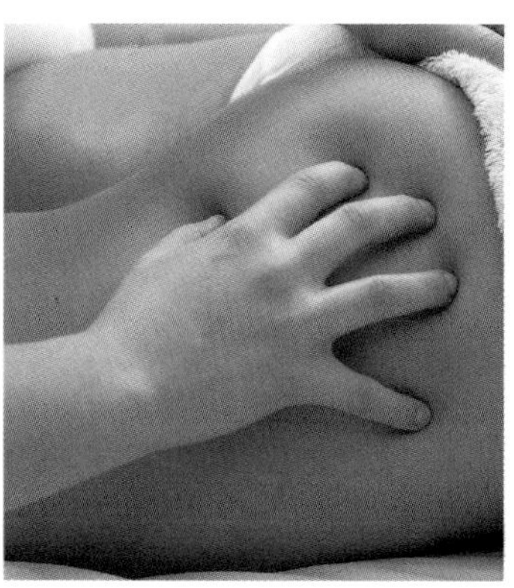

△ **4** Shaking the buttocks can loosen any remaining stiffness and tension in the muscles. Place one hand softly over the sacrum to add support. Sink the fingers of the other hand into the muscle and vibrate rhythmically.

stimulating the whole leg

After applying the strokes on the leg and buttocks, return to a position by the ankle and repeat the initial integration stroke several times. Now begin a series of percussion strokes on the leg to enliven the skin and tone the muscles.

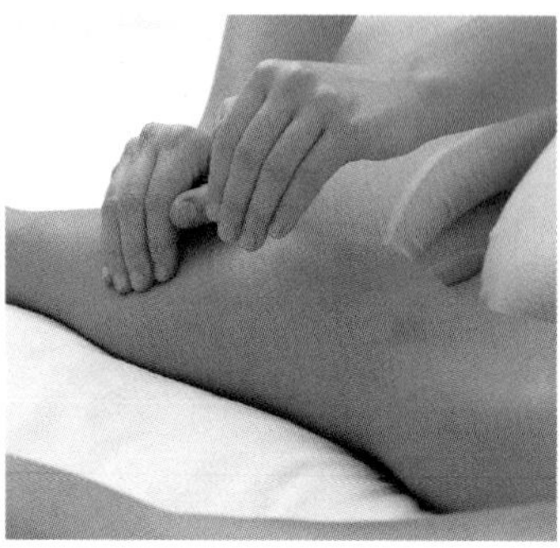

△ **1** Turn to face into the leg and briskly cup it, working from the calf up to the thigh, one hand following the other in rapid succession. Form a vacuum in the palms of your hands by bending the base knuckles and holding the fingers straight and close together while pulling the thumb in tight to the palm. As the hands cup the leg, flick them off the skin at the moment of contact. This creates a suction of air, drawing the blood supply up to the surface of the skin and leaving it with a healthy glow.

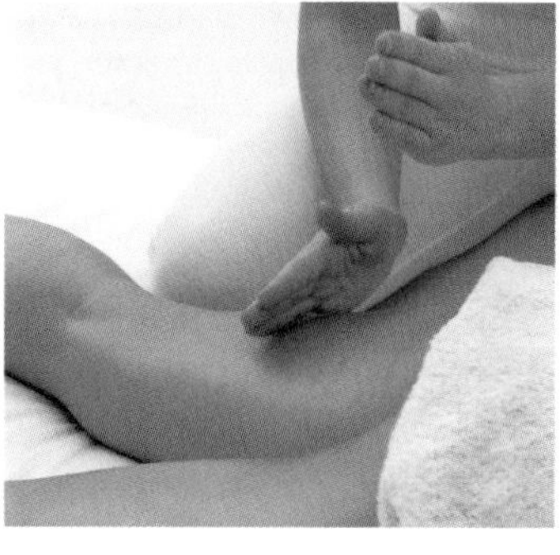

△ **2** Now use the hacking stroke, moving up the leg from the calf to the thigh, but taking care not to strike the delicate area on the back of the knee. Keeping your shoulders and wrists relaxed, hold your hands straight with the palms facing. Briskly strike the flesh with the sides of your hands, one hand following the other in quick, rhythmic succession so that they bounce off the skin immediately.

passive movements on the leg

Once the leg muscles are relaxed, you can introduce passive movements to gently stretch and ease tension from the joints, ligaments, and tendons. The most important thing to remember while making passive movements is never to move a part of the body beyond its point of resistance, and always to work within its natural range of movement. Your hands should impart sufficient confidence to encourage your partner to relax completely and allow you to lift, move, and stretch that part of the body.

enlivening the skin

Complete the percussion strokes by stimulating the skin with soft feather touches.

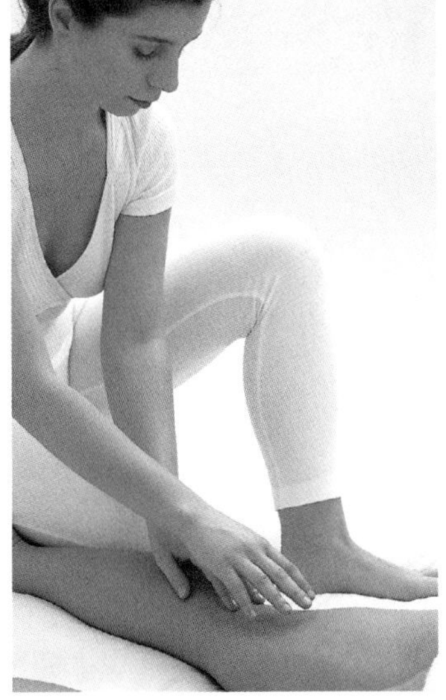

△ Starting at the top of the thigh, use your fingertips to brush down the leg in short strokes with one hand at a time. Lift each hand off the leg to cross above the other in a stream of downward overlapping motions.

gentle hip and knee stretch

This passive movement helps to stretch the muscle attachments around the hip and knee joints by gently pushing the lower leg towards the thigh.

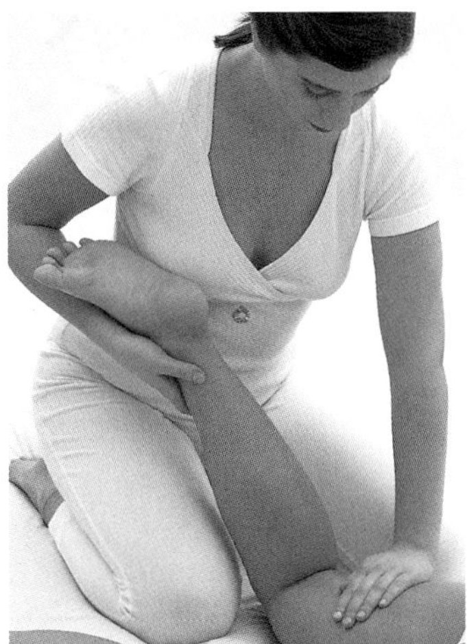

△ **1** Kneel alongside the foot and slip your right hand under the ankle so that you will be able to support the leg. As you are sliding your right hand under the ankle, place your left hand just above the back of the knee. Slowly begin to raise the lower leg off the mattress so that the knee is flexed.

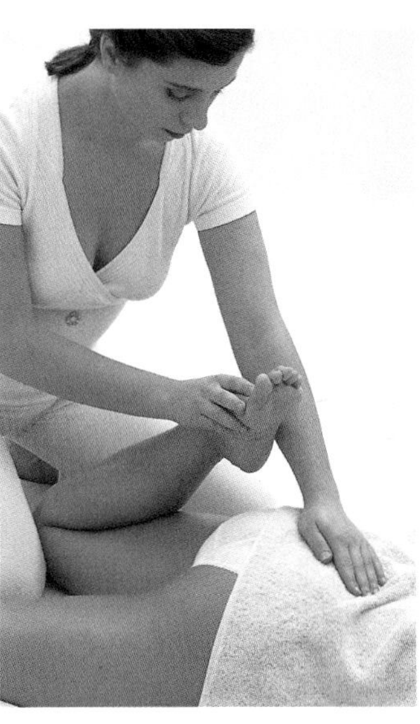

△ **2** Move your left hand to rest securely on the sacrum and lean forward to ease the raised part of the leg down towards the top of the thigh. Bounce the lower leg in tiny movements, gently against the point of resistance, and then lower it slowly back down to the mattress, keeping it in a straight line with the thigh.

lifting the leg

Take care of your own posture while doing this passive movement. Ensure that your back is straight, and elevate your own body from the muscles in your haunches during the upward lift. Do not attempt this movement if you have a weak back or the leg is too heavy.

▷ Raise the lower leg so the knee is flexed and then clasp the ankle firmly with both hands. Lift the leg slowly upwards to take the thigh slightly off the mattress. Bob the leg up and down a little before lowering the thigh.

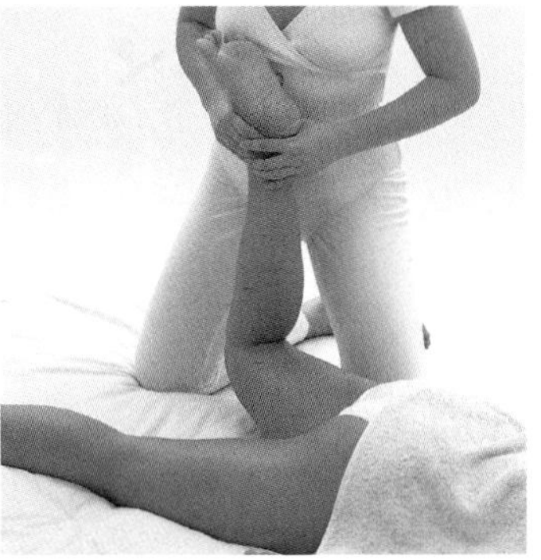

completing the first stage of the body massage

Once all the sequences of strokes have been carried out on the left and the right legs, lay your hands in a firm, but soothing hold on the back of the calves. This brief hold will bring a sense of balance and will also indicate to your partner that this initial stage of the body massage is now complete.

Massaging the front of the body

When your partner has turned over and you are ready to apply your strokes to the front of the body, take a few moments to compose yourself and relax your own body, so that you can focus your full attention on the massage. You will be touching the more vulnerable areas of the body, such as the face, chest, and belly, so you need to bring sensitivity, confidence, and care into your hands. Give your partner a few moments to settle into her new position, and reassure her with a calm and tender hold.

focus on the front of the leg

You will now begin working on the front of the body and continue the leg massage. Most strokes are similar to those used on the back of the legs. Specific strokes are required for the shin and knee as the bones are closer to the surface of the skin.

balance and joint release

These opening holds and stretches prepare the front of the legs for massage.

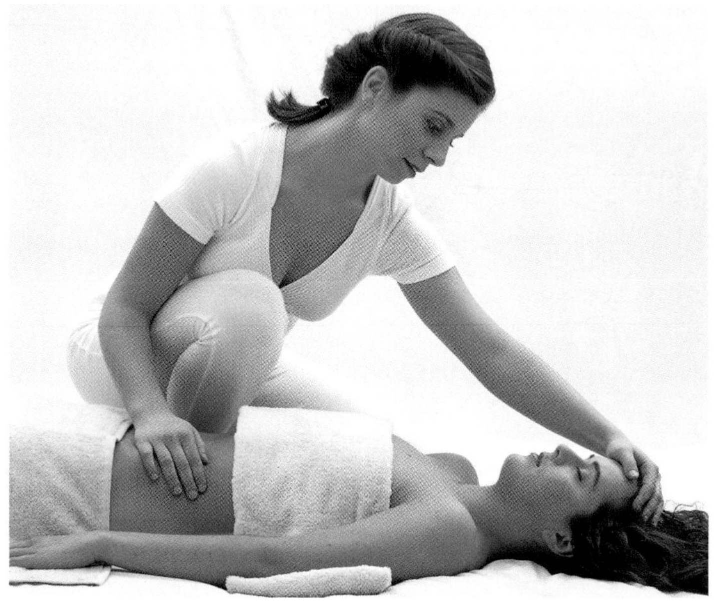

△ **A calm and tender hold signals the beginning of the next stage of the body massage.**

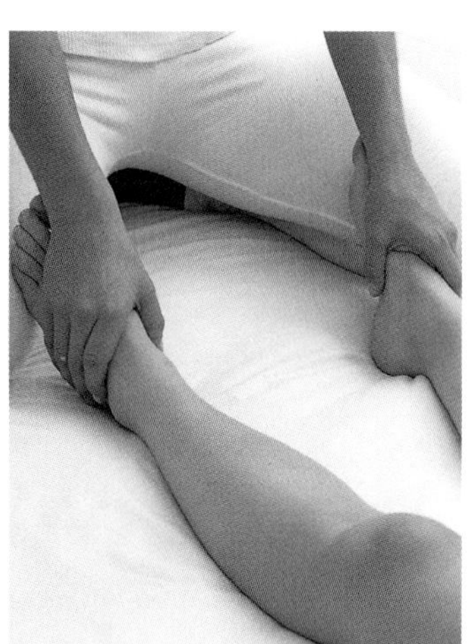

△ **1** Hold the feet for several moments to bring a sense of balance to both sides of the body. Then begin your massage on the left leg.

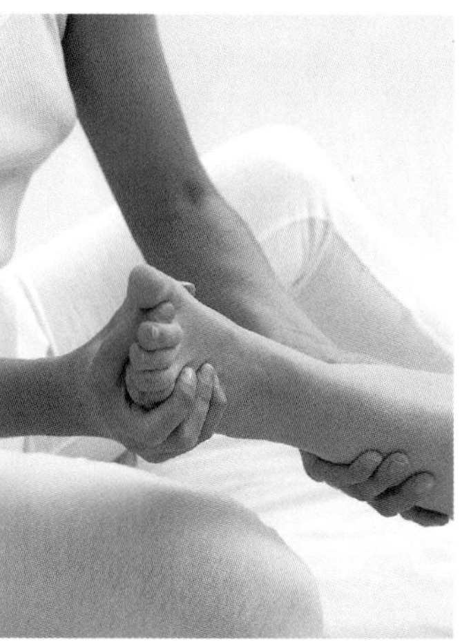

△ **2** Create space in the ankle joints with passive movements. Support the back of the lower leg with one hand, and place your other hand over the sole with your thumb and fingers lightly clasping the foot.

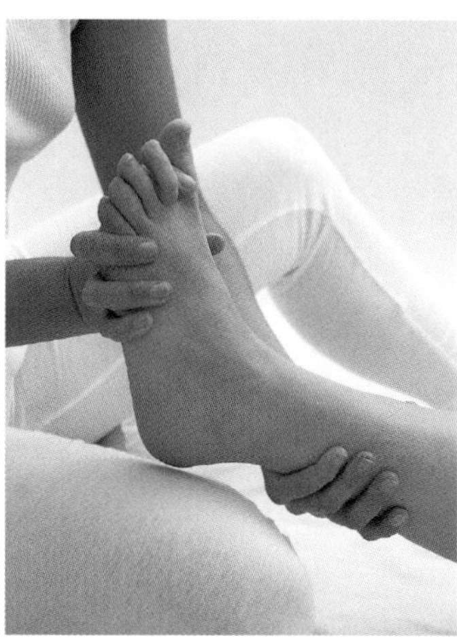

△ **3** Slip the index finger between the first and second toes to maintain a secure grip. Circle the ankle three times to the right and then three times to the left to rotate its joints.

the main integration stroke

Begin by using the same flowing effleurage motion that you applied to the back of the leg.

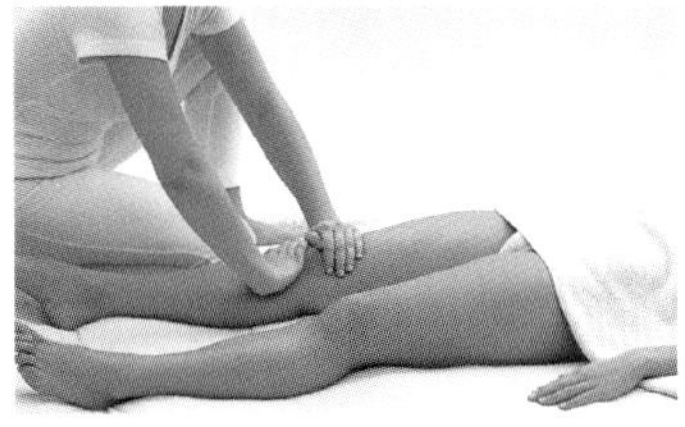

△ **1** Spread your essential oil on the front of the leg, stroking it down the length of the leg from the hip to the foot. Glide gently over the knee before taking the stroke up to the thigh.

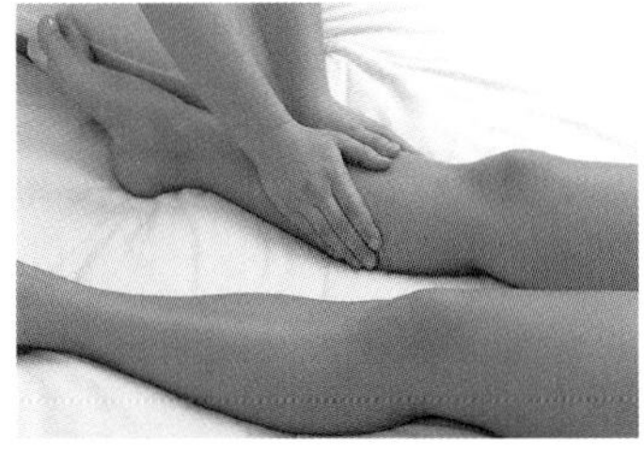

△ **2** Warm and stretch the muscles that cover the shin with a series of fanning strokes, moving up from the ankle to just below the knee before gliding your hands back down to the lower leg.

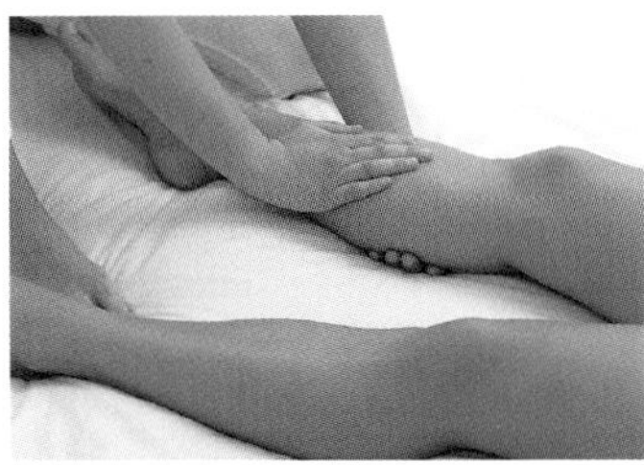

△ **3** Glide one hand after the other over the shin in a series of alternating fanning motions, slipping your fingers under the leg on the return movement to stroke back down over the calf.

a long stretch

This friction stroke stretches and eases the tissue between the two long bones that form the shin.

▷ Secure the back of the leg with your left hand and pull gently on the leg to create a slight traction. Wrapping your right hand over the inside of the lower leg, sink the right thumb sensitively between the two bones at the point where they join the front of the ankle. Slide the thumb slowly and steadily along the edge of the large bone until your hand reaches the knee. Lighten the pressure and glide your hand around the kneecap and back down the side of the leg. Follow this deep stretch with some effleurage.

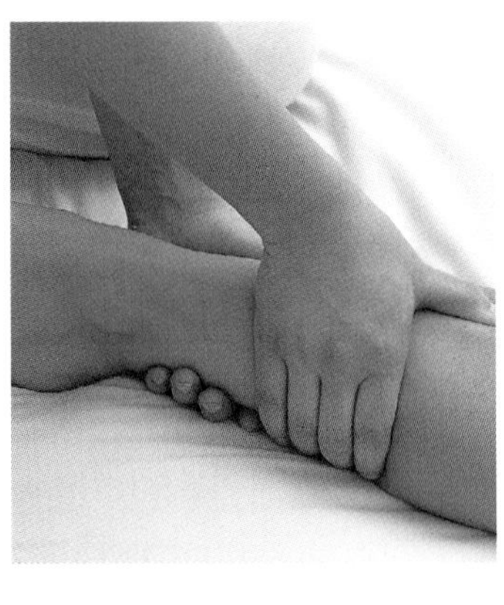

relaxing the knee

The knee, like the ankle, plays an important part in the support and mobility of the body's weight and structure. The kneecap itself is bound by tendons and ligaments, which attach to the muscles and long bones in the thigh and lower leg. Strain and injury in the knee are common complaints, and it is important to include this area in your massage strokes to help keep it flexible. When working on and around the kneecap, settle your fingers beneath the knee to give it support.

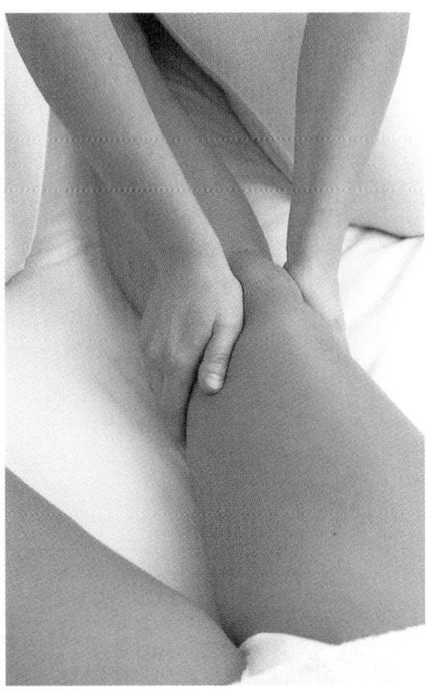

△ **1** Using the heels of both hands at the same time, rotate them firmly around the sides and above the top of the kneecap.

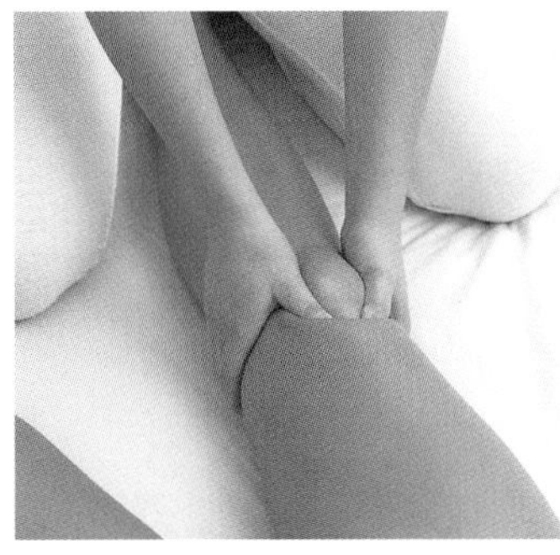

△ **2** Place both thumbs, one above the other, across the base of the knee. Slide them over the bone and then draw them out in opposite directions to encircle the edge of the kneecap until they return to their first position. Repeat the stroke several times as a continuous motion.

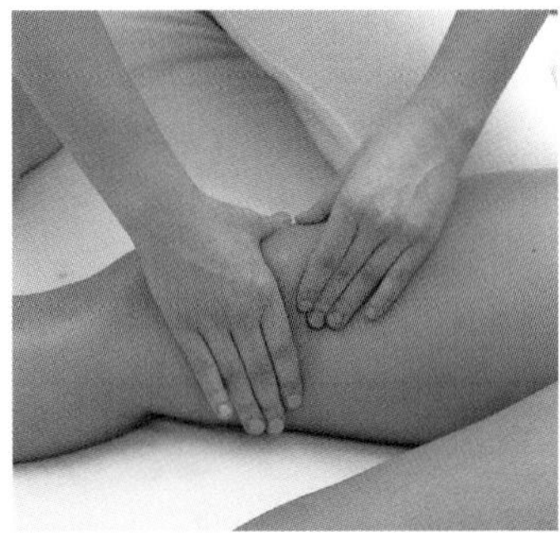

△ **3** Face towards the leg and knead thoroughly just above the knee. This will increase suppleness and circulation to the ligaments, tendons, and the muscles that attach to the joint.

the front of the thigh

The fanning, wringing, and kneading strokes applied to the back of the thigh can now be used on the front of the leg.

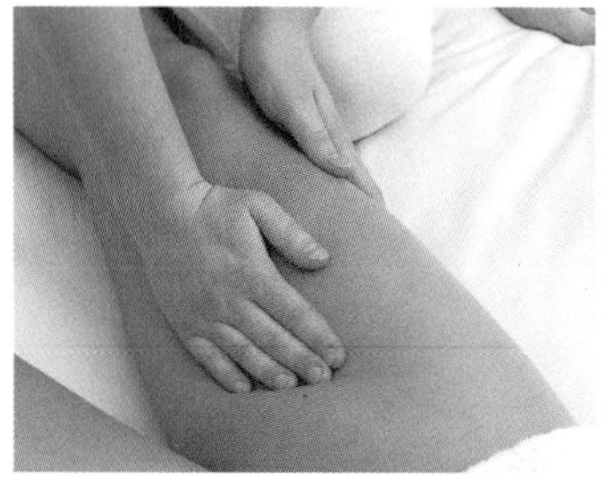

△ **1** Use a firm pressure to fan each hand alternately up over the thigh muscles.

▽ **2** Ask your partner to bend her knee so that the foot supports the weight of her leg. While the thigh is in a raised position, add some strokes to drain the blood flow towards the heart, followed by some deep tissue stretches on both sides of the leg. Wrap your hands around the leg so that your thumbs rest on the centre of the thigh. Firmly slide the heels of your hands and the thumbs a short distance up the thigh before drawing them out to the sides of the leg. Glide your hands down and around to their original position before taking the stroke further up the thigh.

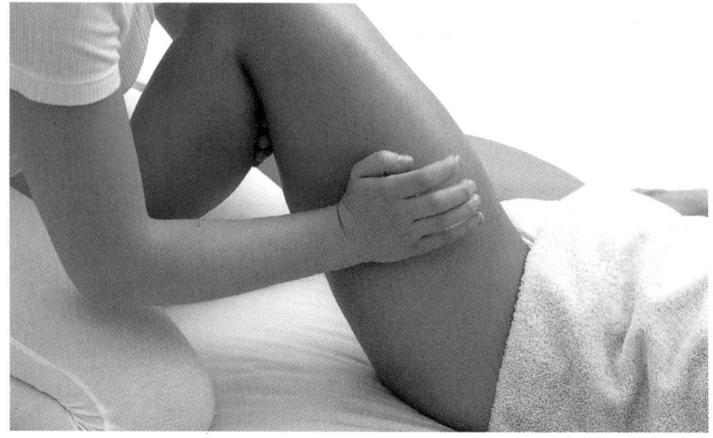

△ **3** Hold the lower leg with one hand, using the heel pressure of the other hand to make a steady stretch up along the band of connective tissue that runs from the knee to the hip.

▽ **4** Continue the stretching stroke by sliding the heel of your hand around the hip socket before gliding your hand back down the leg.

▽ **5** Lean the leg outwards into the support of one hand, using the heel of the other hand to make a similar long, deep stretch down the inner thigh muscles stopping just below the groin. Then slide your hand around and back to the knee. Lower the leg gently on to the mattress and follow up with a sequence of stimulating percussion strokes to the thigh.

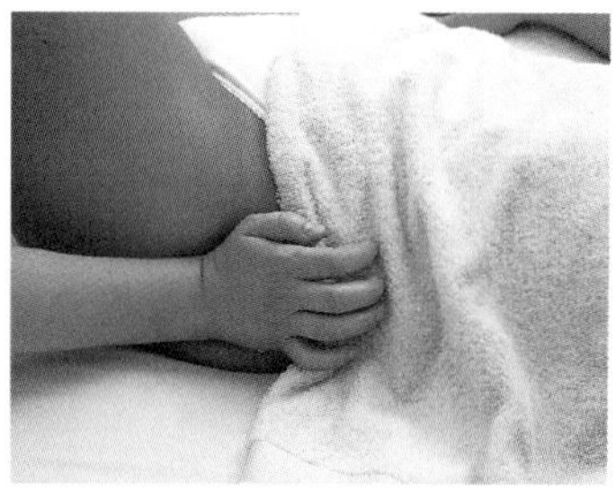

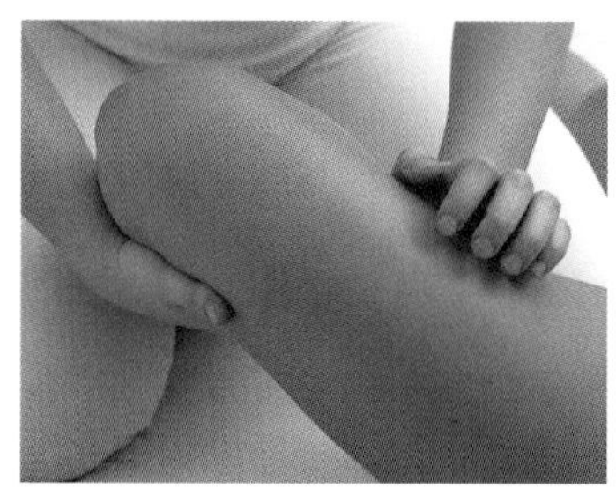

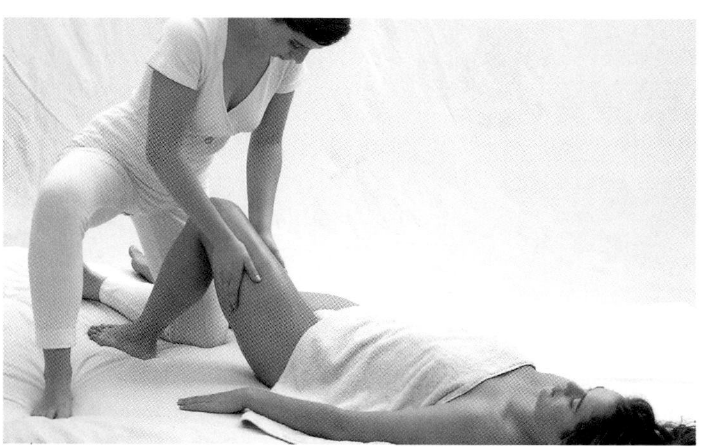

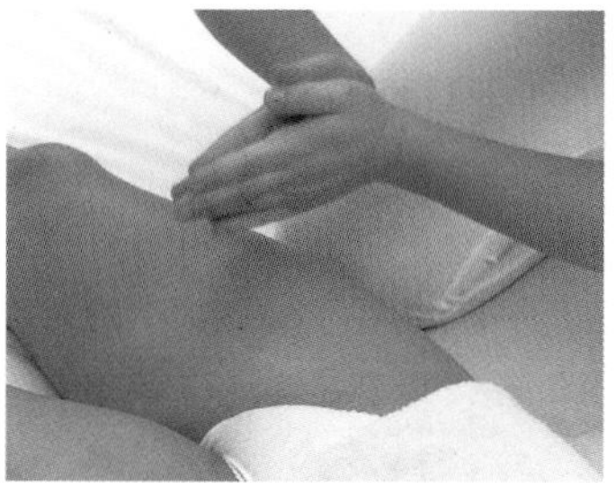

△ **6** Hack briskly to tone the muscles. Bring both palms together and strike the skin rapidly with the sides of the hands. End the leg massage with several full-length effleurage strokes, and repeat the whole sequence of massage strokes on the other leg.

focus on the abdomen

Massage on the abdomen can relieve symptoms of stress, deepen breathing, and help dissolve tensions formed when strong emotional feelings are retained. The abdomen is an extremely sensitive area containing many vital organs that are unprotected by skeletal structure. Before applying your strokes, take a few moments to allow the abdomen to relax under the caring touch of your hands.

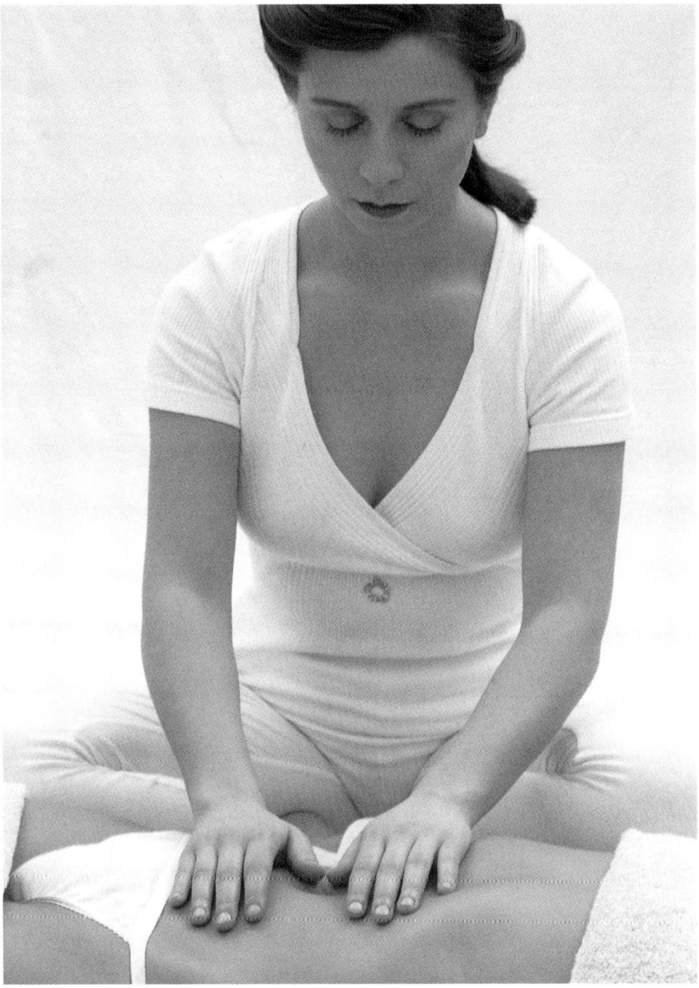

the integration stroke

Rub a little essential oil into the palms to warm them, and spread the oil gently over the abdomen. Kneel on the right side of your partner, and begin with an integration stroke that flows over the abdomen from the pubic bone to the ribcage. Continue the stroke by gliding under the back to the spine and then out above the hips. Repeat three times in a continuous movement.

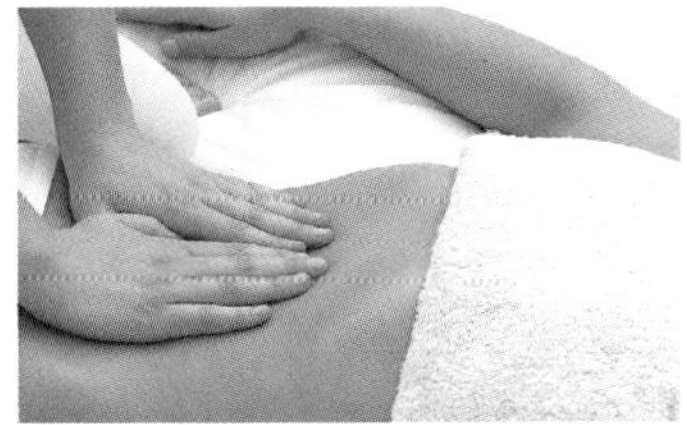

△ **1** Place both hands flat over the centre of the lower abdomen, fingers pointing towards the head. Stroke softly up to the base of the breast bone.

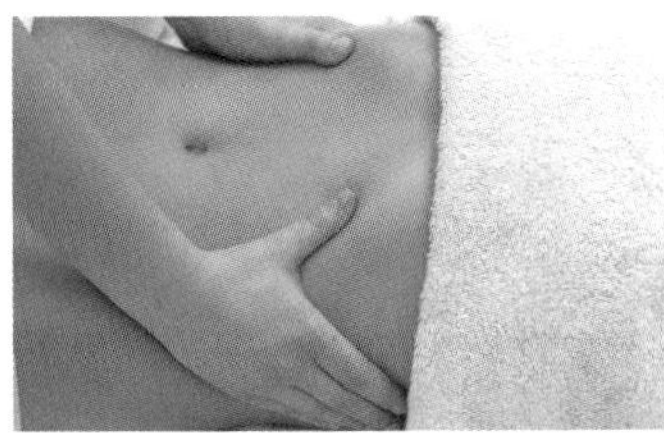

△ **2** Continue the stroke by fanning both hands out to either side of the ribcage and gliding under the back of the body.

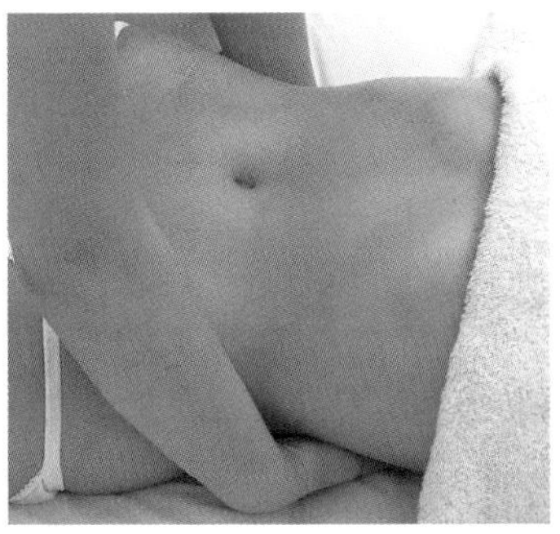

△ **3** Let the fingers of both hands slide under the back to meet at the spine. Lift the body slightly to arch the back before pulling your hands out towards the hips.

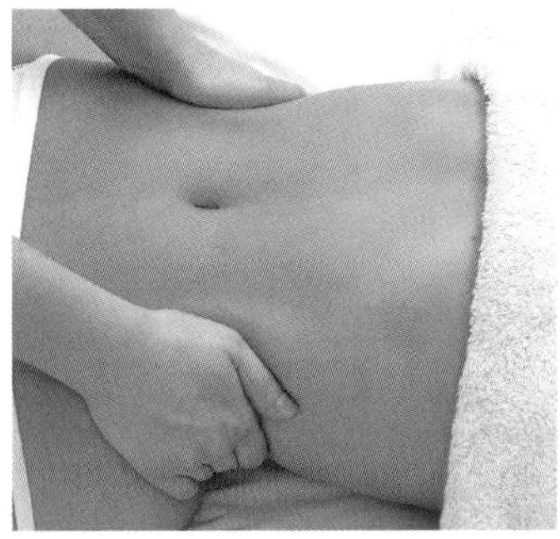

△ **4** Firmly draw your hands over the waist and then glide them back to their original position to repeat the stroke.

circling the abdomen

These circle strokes act to soothe and relax the abdomen. They flow over the area and fit perfectly to its shape.

▷ **1** Repeat continuous circles with the whole surfaces of your hands, moving in a clockwise direction until you feel the abdomen becoming soft and warm.

▽ **2** As the abdominal muscles relax, sensitively shift the pressure into your fingertips as you make the circular strokes. Decrease the circle so that you are stroking around the navel, then widen the circular movement outwards to cover the abdomen, shifting the weight back into the full surface of your hands.

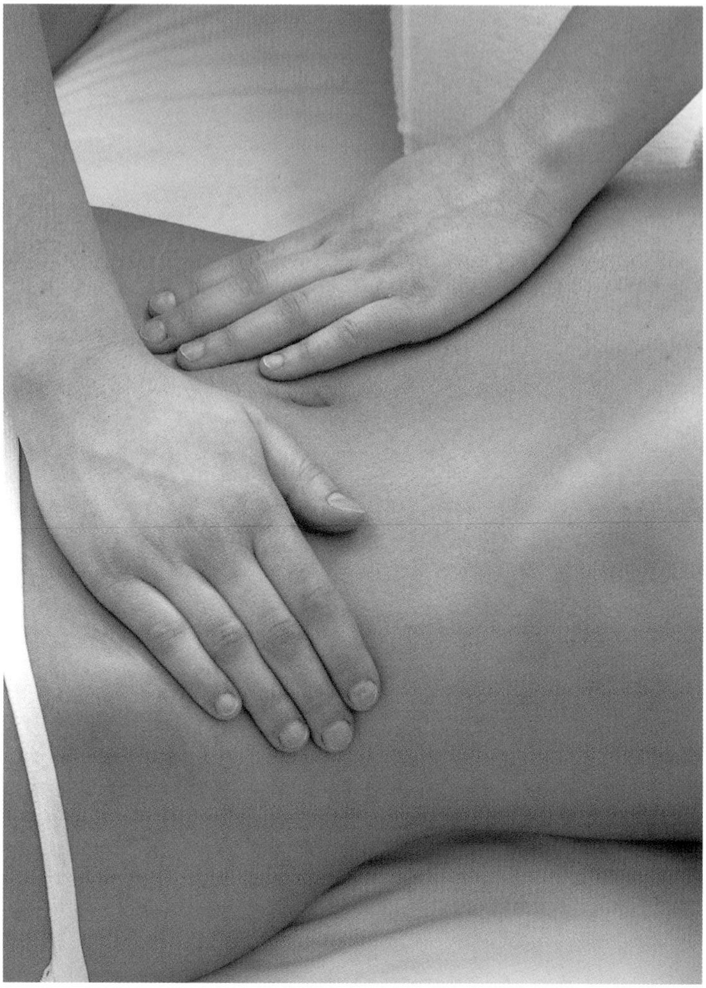

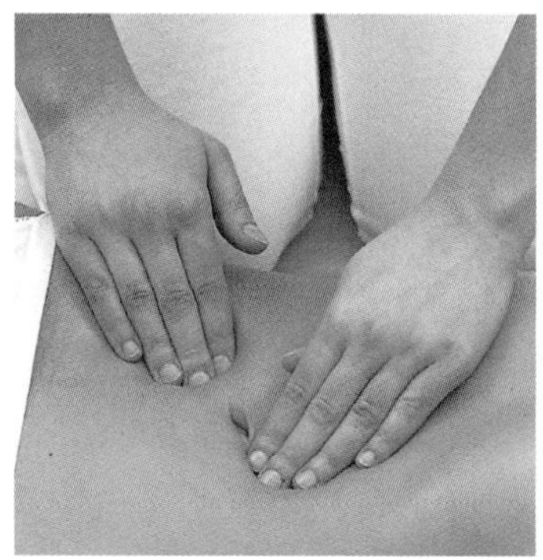

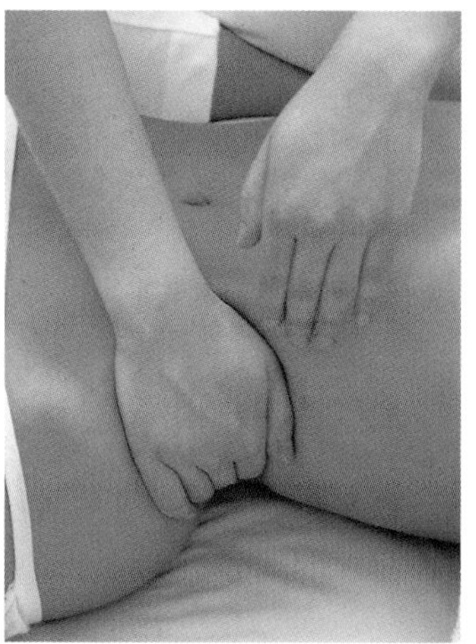

relaxing the sides of the abdomen

The muscles that cross from the back of the body to the front of the abdomen help to support the vital organs and rotate the spine. Make the following milking and kneading strokes on both sides of the body to increase suppleness.

◁ **1** Using one hand after the other in a milking action, pull firmly over the sides of the abdomen from just under the back. Glide lightly to the centre of the abdomen before lifting the hand off to repeat the stroke. Stroke in this way from the hip to the ribcage.

▷ **2** Lift, squeeze, and roll the flesh from hand to hand in a kneading stroke along the sides of the abdomen from the hip to the base of the ribcage.

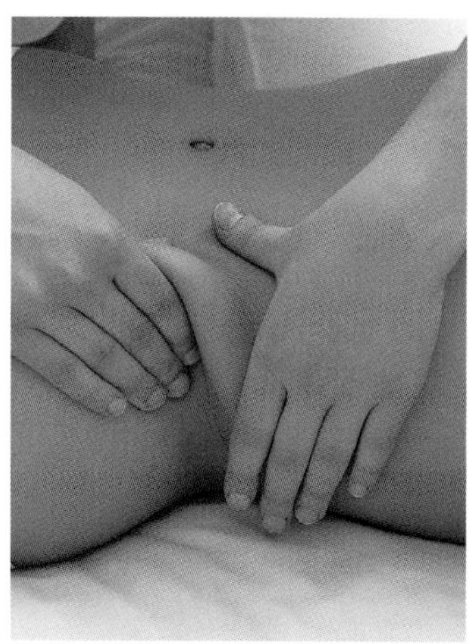

deeper strokes for the abdomen

If your partner is responding well to this massage and the area is relaxing, you can begin to apply the deeper abdominal strokes. Be very sensitive and alert to your partner's responses, applying and releasing pressure slowly, ensuring that any deeper strokes are appropriate.

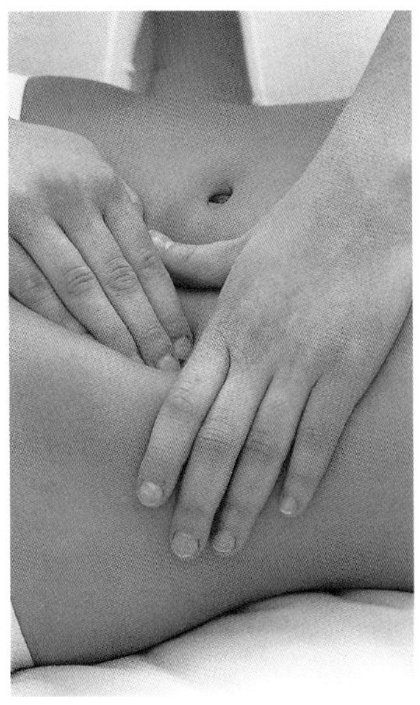

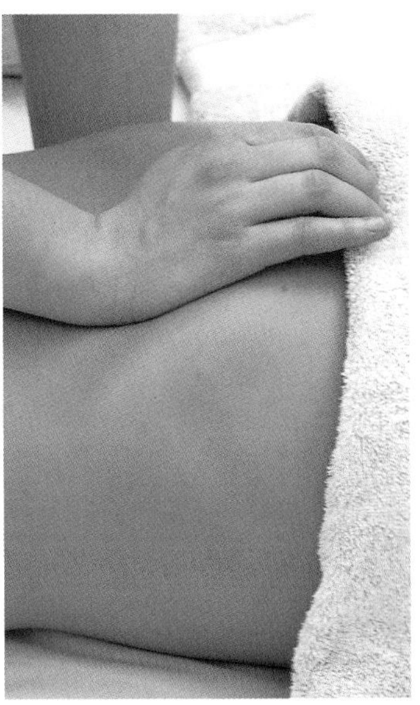

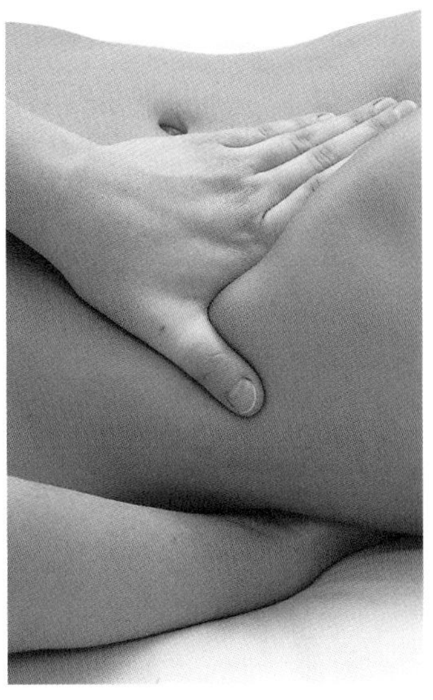

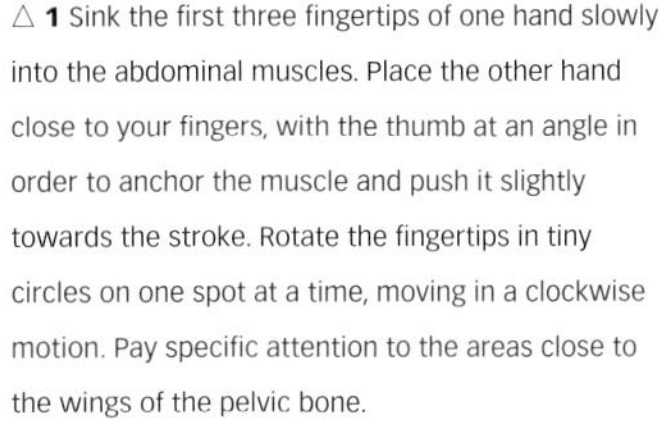

△ **1** Sink the first three fingertips of one hand slowly into the abdominal muscles. Place the other hand close to your fingers, with the thumb at an angle in order to anchor the muscle and push it slightly towards the stroke. Rotate the fingertips in tiny circles on one spot at a time, moving in a clockwise motion. Pay specific attention to the areas close to the wings of the pelvic bone.

△ **2** The upper abdomen can be tense in times of stress, as the diaphragm muscle between the chest and abdomen tightens, and the solar plexus, a nerve centre, becomes hyperactive. Once the area has been relaxed by softer strokes, and the breath deepens, slip your left hand under the body to rest below the spine. This creates a sense of support as you use the heel of your right hand to massage gently, but with increased pressure, in circles around the base of the ribcage.

△ **3** Ease constriction from under the ribcage with a firm, steady slide of one hand, while the other hand rests parallel and just beneath the body for support. Keeping your fingers close together and your thumb at an angle, sink the side of the index finger and hand gently under the edge of the lower rib. Slowly slide your hand down to the side of the body, lightening the pressure towards the end of the stroke. Repeat this stroke on the other side of the body.

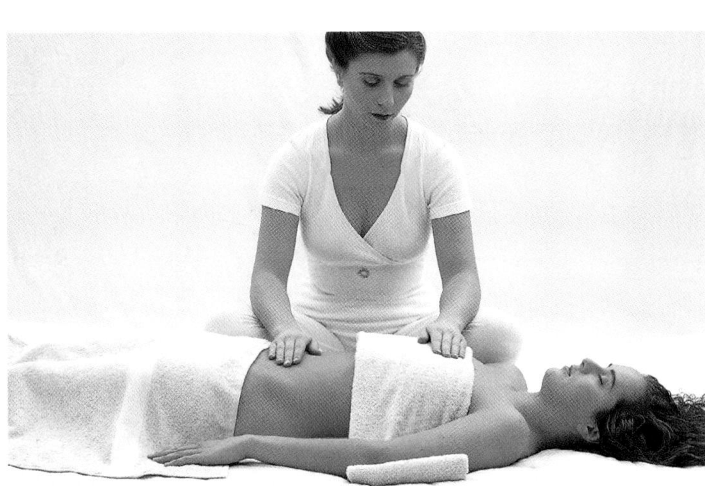

harmonious finish and hold

To bring a harmonious finish to the deeper sequences of strokes, repeat the flowing, soft, circular motions on the abdomen.

◁ To complete this part of the massage place one hand over the abdomen and the other on the chest so that it rests over the heart. Maintain this hold for a few moments to bring a calming sense of equilibrium and unity to the body.

Focus on the arms

Muscular tension forms in the arms and hands for a number of reasons. Poor posture can cause the shoulder girdle to stiffen and inhibit the flexibility of the upper limbs. Repetitive movements at work put strain, wear and tear on the muscles, tendons, and ligaments. On an emotional level, the arms and hands represent the ability to reach out and contact the outside world, or the means of expressing creativity. Arm and hand massage feels wonderfully relaxing, bringing relief and ease to the upper body and renewing vitality. Using the following strokes, work first on one arm and hand, and then on the other.

opening out

This first movement helps the upper chest and shoulders to open out to create freedom from contraction in the shoulder joint and a feeling of length in the arm. The oil remaining on your hands from the previous strokes should be sufficient for this opening stretch but, if necessary, add just a little more to your hands as you work.

▷ **1** Face in towards the shoulder to lift it, and slip the hand furthest from the body under the top of the back so that the fingers point towards the spine. Place the other hand across the top of the chest, fingers pointing towards the breast bone. As you feel the shoulder relaxing between your hands, pull firmly and steadily out towards its edge.

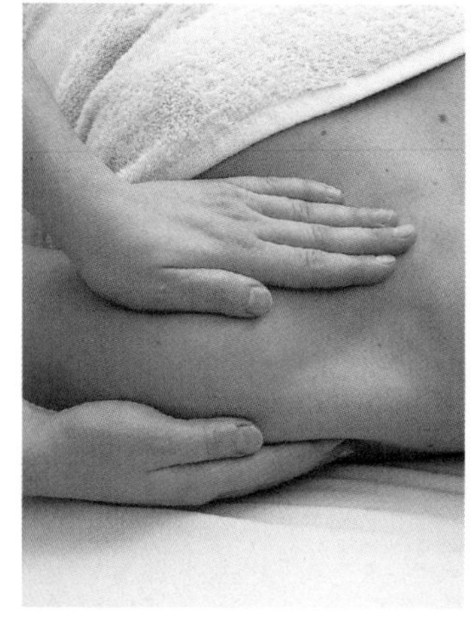

▽ **2** Keeping one foot on the mattress, manoeuvre your position so you are able to sandwich the top of the arm between both hands, and then pull steadily down its entire length to give a gentle stretch to the shoulder joint.

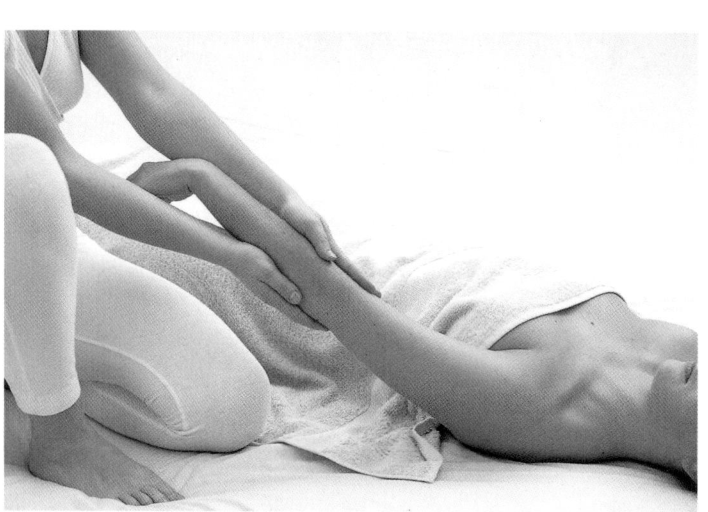

the integration stroke

Use oiled hands to mould the shape of the arm in overlapping strokes.

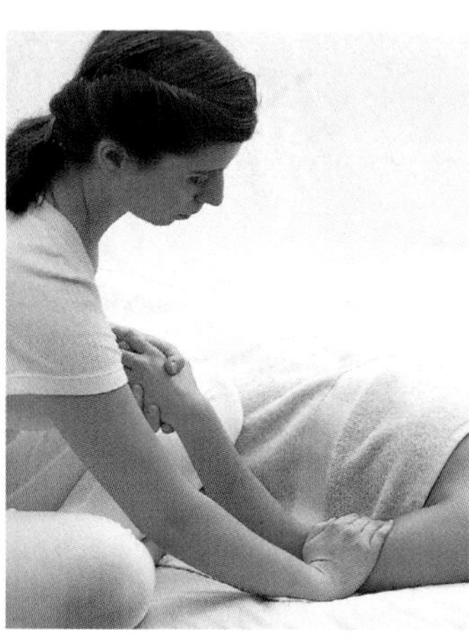

△ **1** Hold your partner's hand with the hand closest to the body. Wrap your other hand across the wrist, to lead the stroke with your little finger. Glide your hand firmly up the arm towards the shoulder.

▽ **2** Forming your hand to the curve over the shoulder, glide it around the joint.

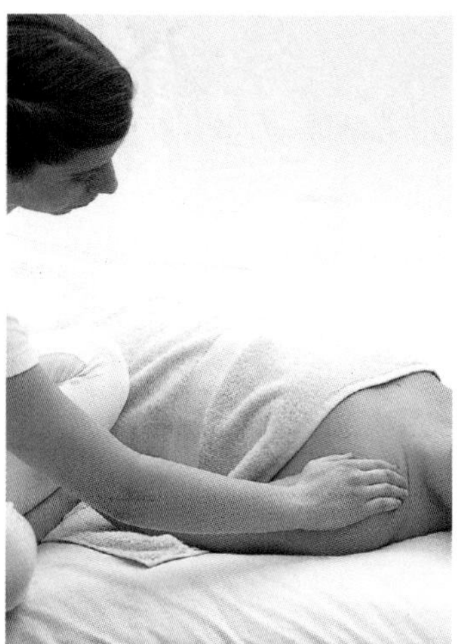

relaxing the forearm

Continue to relax the forearm with a series of alternating fanning motions. Fanning can be used to stretch and manipulate tension away from the muscles.

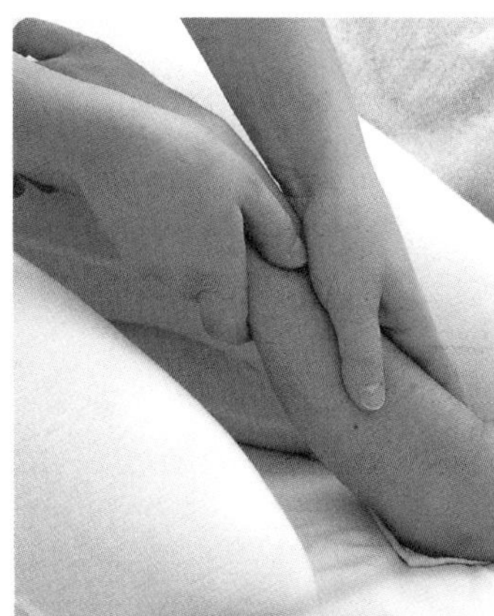

◁ **1** One hand following the other, move the fanning strokes up from the wrist to the elbow. Squeeze the muscles gently between the heel and fingers as the hand curves outwards, stroking firmly with your fingers on the underside of the arm as your hand glides back round. Slide your hands from the elbow back to the wrist to repeat the sequence again twice.

▽ **2** Secure the wrist with the hand closest to the body, and pull the arm gently to create a slight traction. Wrap the other hand around the outer forearm, sinking the thumb slowly into the groove where the long bones of the forearm join the wrist. Stroke firmly and slowly up the arm, between the bones, releasing the pressure at the elbow. Slip your hand around the joint and glide it back down to the wrist.

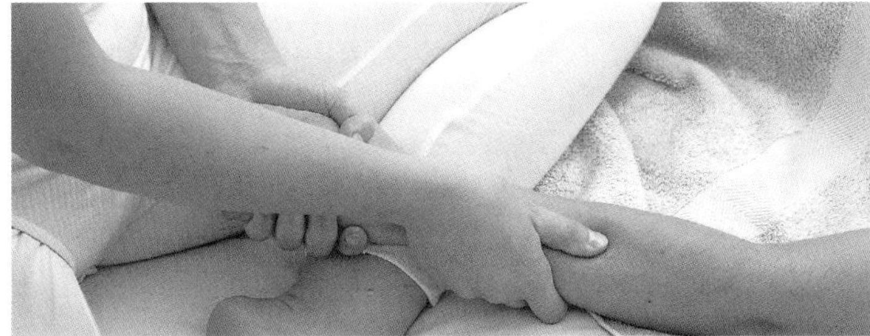

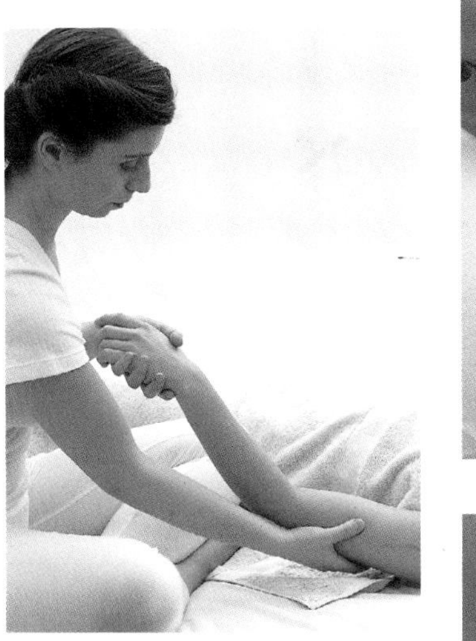

△ **3** Lifting the arm slightly off the mattress, stroke lightly down the back of the arm to the wrist.

▽ **4** Pass your partner's arm to your other hand and clasp it by the wrist. Stroke up along the inside of the arm with the hand closest to the body, the little finger leading. Swivel your hand around just below the armpit and glide it back down the arm. Repeat the sequence two more times.

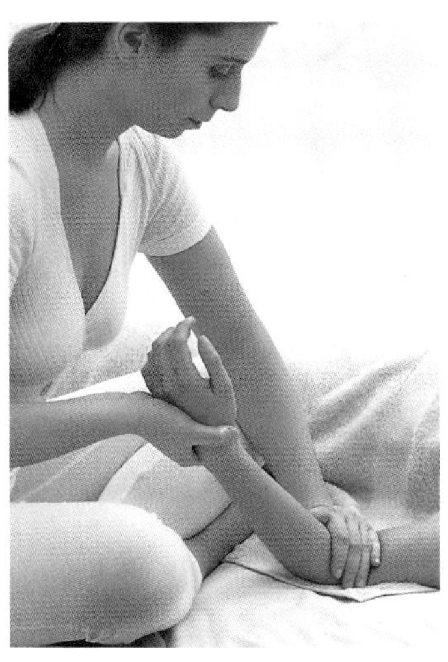

draining strokes

These strokes boost the circulation towards the heart and help to drain the lower arm.

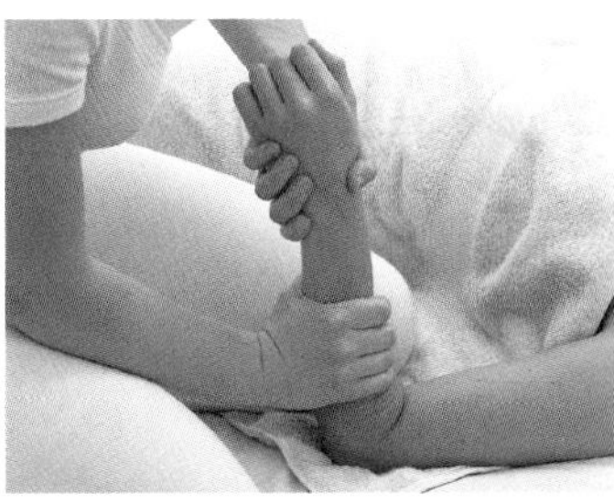

△ **1** Raise the forearm vertically so that it rests on the elbow. Clasp your partner's hand with your left hand and wrap your other hand around the top of the wrist, the little finger leading the stroke. Slide firmly down the arm as if to drain it. Open your hand to glide softly around the elbow joint and lightly back up the forearm.

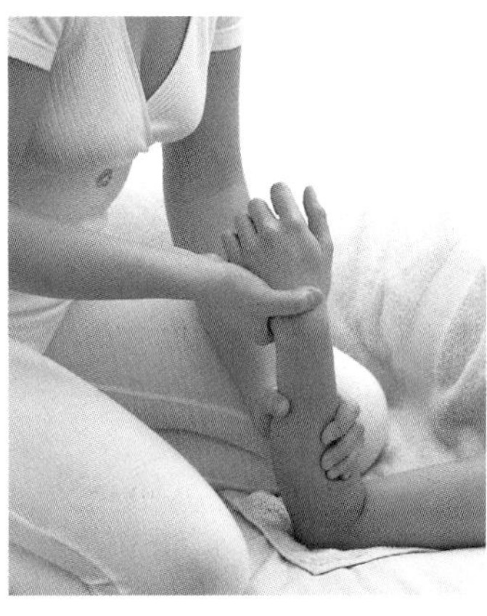

△ **2** Repeat the same draining motion on the inside of the arm, changing the position of your hands.

loosening the upper arm

The position and narrow structure of the arm can make the application of strokes more difficult than usual, so be sure that the limb is supported comfortably before massaging the upper half of the arm.

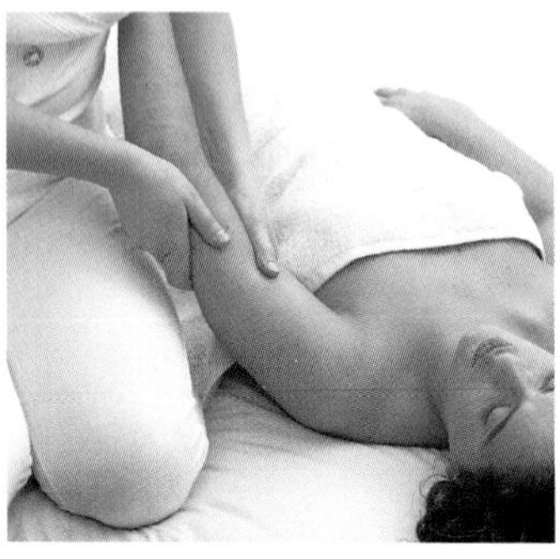

△ **1** Start with a series of alternating fanning motions, one hand following the other, from just above the elbow to the shoulder. Squeeze the muscles gently between your fingers and the heels of the hands as each hand fans outwards. When your hands reach the top of the arm, sweep them around and back down towards the elbow. Repeat once. To keep the arm in a raised position, secure its lower half between your own body and arm.

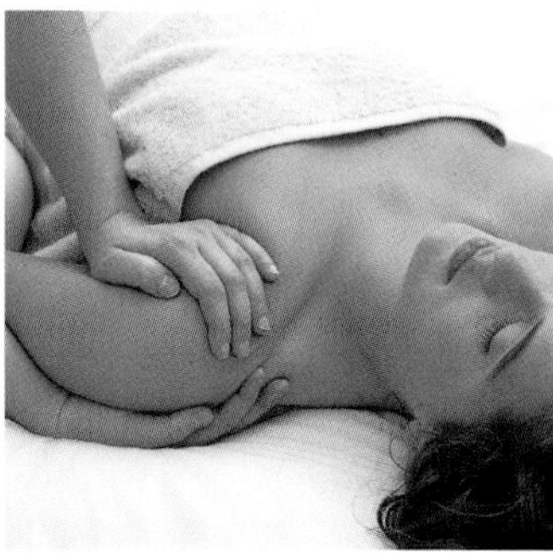

△ **2** Cradle the shoulder joint between both hands, placing the hand furthest from the body beneath the shoulder, and the hand closest to the body on top. Slide both hands back and forth over the top of the shoulder several times, making a see-saw motion for a warming effect.

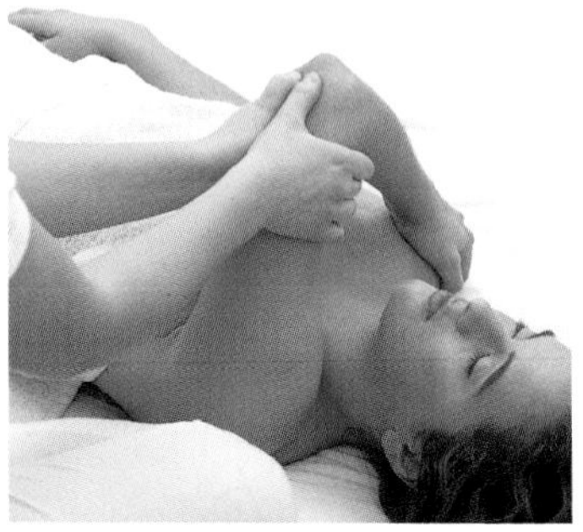

△ **3** Keeping the elbow flexed, lift the arm and place it across the body, asking your partner to clasp her other shoulder so that the upper arm remains steady and vertical. From this position, it is easy to apply your strokes. Holding the inside of the arm with your fingers, work around the back of the elbow joint with tiny alternating thumb circles.

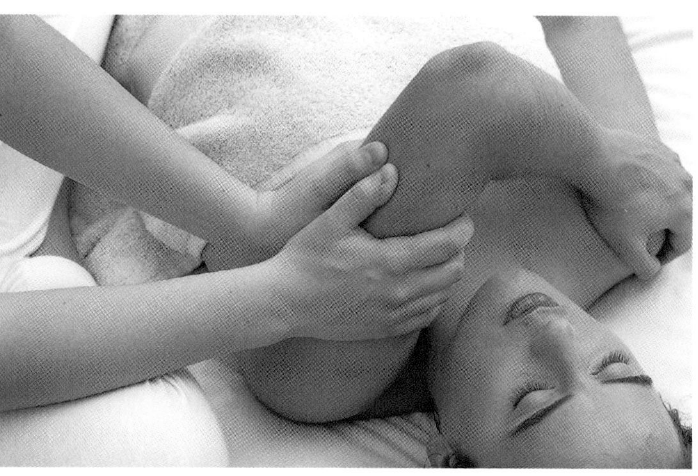

△ **4** Clasping the upper arm firmly with the thumbs placed centrally next to each other, slide both hands steadily downwards in a draining action. Complete by gliding the right hand softly around the back of the shoulder and then repeating the stroke.

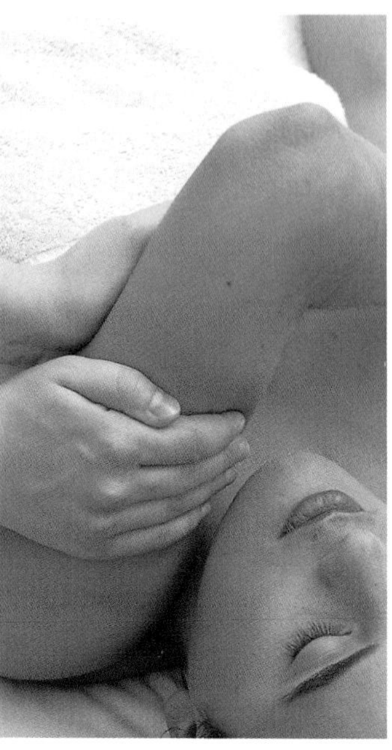

△ **5** Wrapping your fingers around the inside of the arm, squeeze and knead down the upper arm muscles with circular fanning motions, applying pressure from the heels of the hands as they move outwards, and then gliding them back around more lightly.

passive movements on the arm

These passive arm movements create a sense of length and space in the upper body and shoulder girdle by gently stretching the joints. Carry out these passive movements slowly and sensitively, working with the natural movement of the shoulder joint. Never force the arm or shoulder beyond its point of resistance or tension.

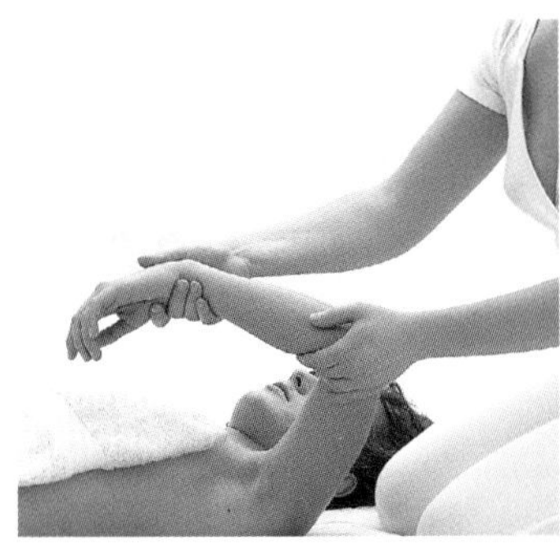

△ **1** Kneel behind the shoulder to remove the arm from its previous position. Support this movement by wrapping your right hand around the wrist and the left hand under the elbow. Begin to circle the arm slowly in a low arc-shaped motion, compatible with the movement of the shoulder joint, until it is stretched out behind your partner's head.

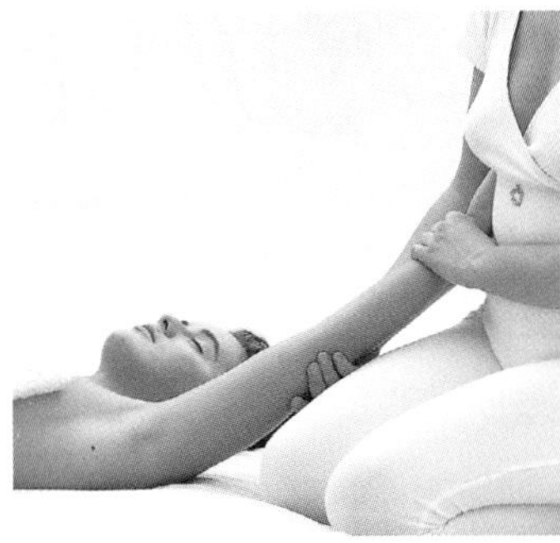

△ **2** Tuck the arm into the side of your body and change the position of your hands to support the elbow with your right hand. Pull very gently on the arm to create a slight traction.

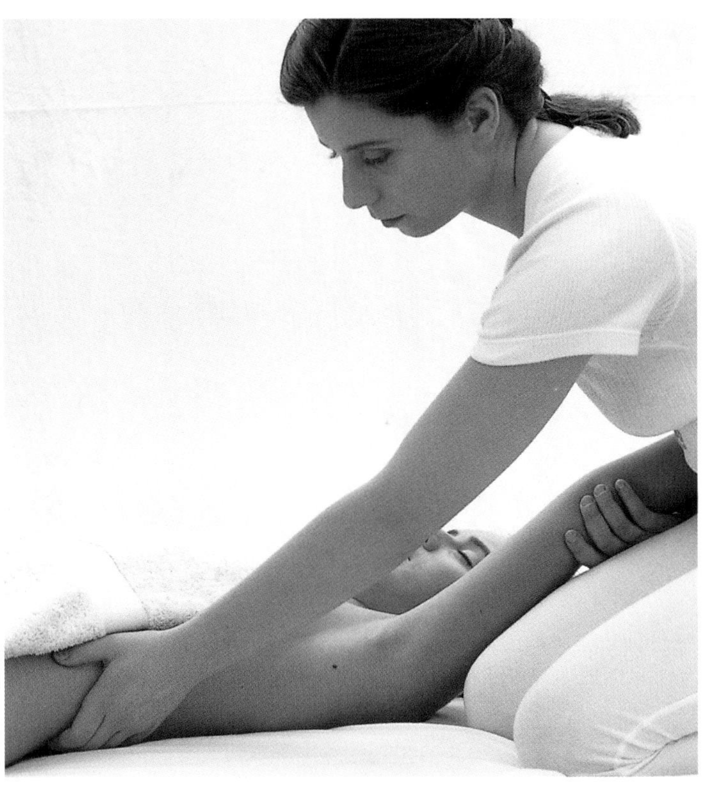

△ **3** Lean forward to mould your left hand to the waist, and then slide it firmly up along the side of the body and softly under the shoulder joint in a steady stretching motion, bringing the feeling of length to the upper body.

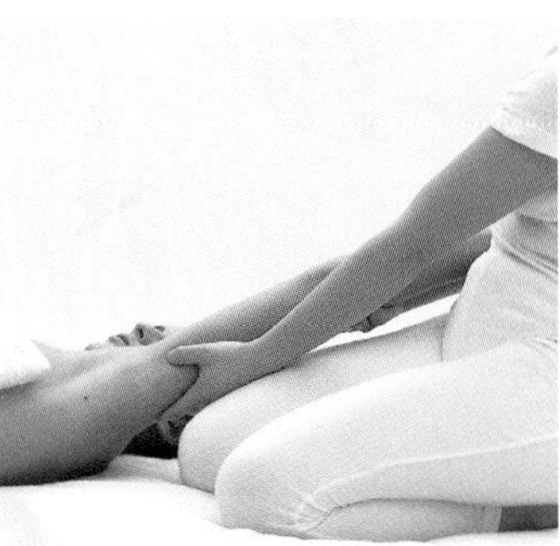

△ **4** Continue sliding your left hand up the back of the arm towards the elbow to increase the stretch in the shoulder joint. Now relax the shoulder and move yourself slowly back to the side of the body, taking the arm with you in a fluid arc-shaped movement. Ensure the arm is properly supported by your hands and the elbow stays flexed until the whole limb has relaxed back on to the mattress.

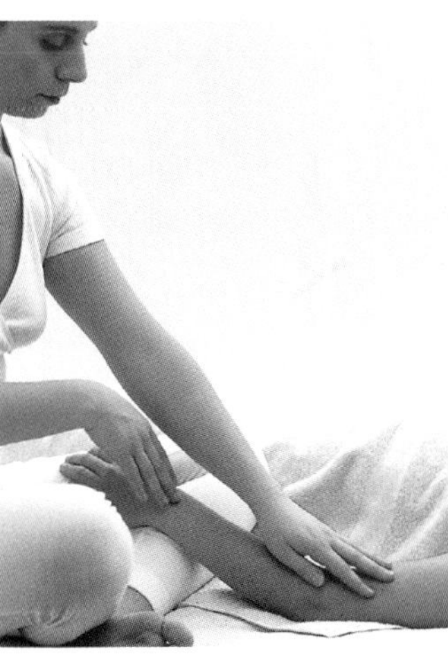

△ **5** Complete the passive arm movement with soft feathering touches, letting your fingertips sweep over the whole limb, one hand following the other in overlapping strokes.

Focus on the hands

Once the arm is relaxed, turn your attention to the hand. Your strokes will ease away tension from the tendons, muscles and bones to increase suppleness and dexterity. They will also stimulate the hand's many sensory nerve endings. A hand massage soothes away the stress of a day's activity: it is an essential part of a whole body massage, or can be done as a session in itself.

hand massage sequence

Kneel or sit below your partner's hand so that it can rest comfortably on your lap with the forearm slightly elevated. Change hands when necessary to complete the strokes on both sides of the hand. Use only a small amount of oil in order to secure a firm slide with your strokes.

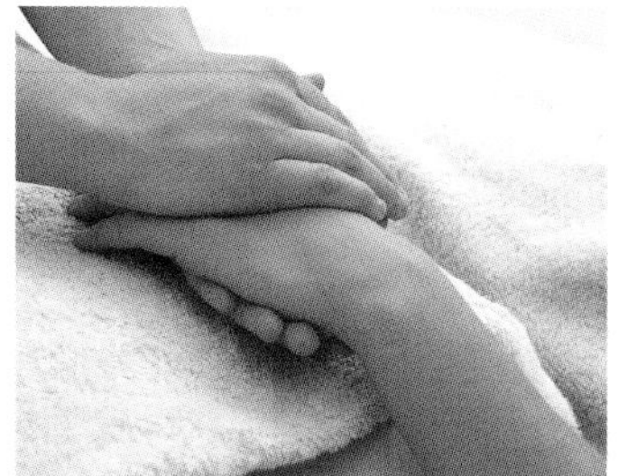

△ **1** Cradle the hand gently for several moments to allow the warmth radiating from your palms to melt away tensions. The stillness of this calming hand-to-hand hold will enhance the deep sense of connection between you.

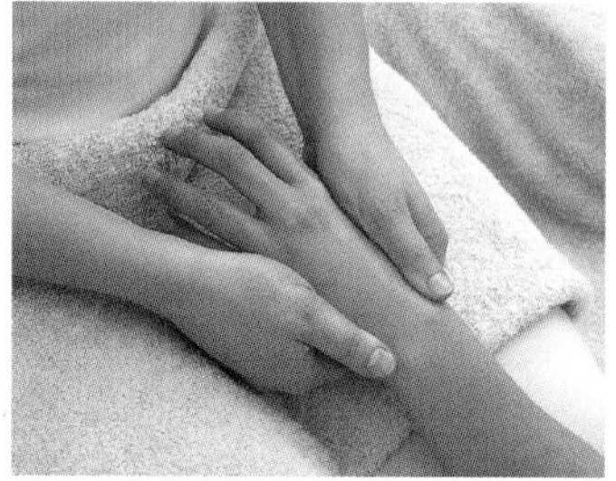

△ **2** Support the palm with your fingers and place your thumbs side-by-side over the centre of the top of the hand. Draw your heels and thumbs firmly out to the edges of the hand in a stretching motion, to create space between the bones and tendons. Repeat the stroke higher on the hand.

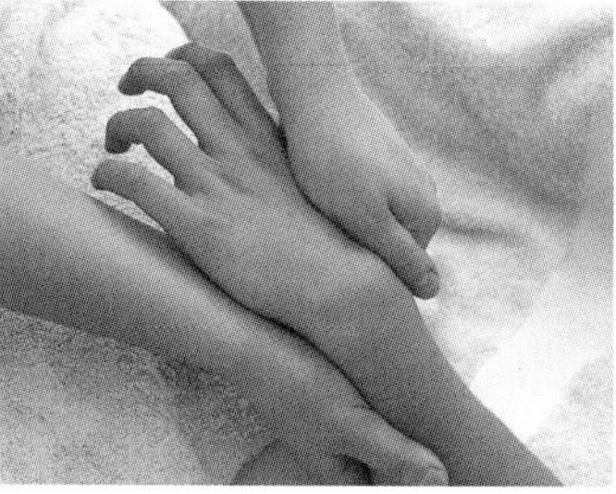

△ **3** Support your partner's palm and wrist with one hand, and use the heel of your other hand to make firm circular motions over the near-side of the top of the hand. Apply pressure in the heel on the outward fan of the circle, while stroking the palm firmly with your fingertips on the return slide. Perform the same stroke over the other half of the hand.

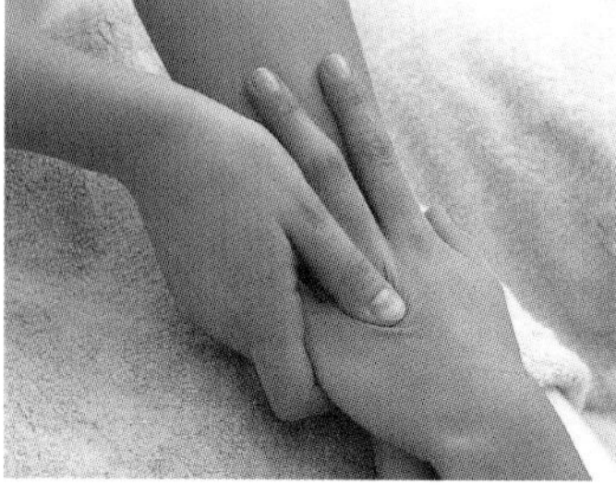

△ **4** Keep the hand supported and slide your thumb firmly in a straight line between each tendon and bone on the top of the hand, lightening the pressure as the stroke reaches close to the wrist.

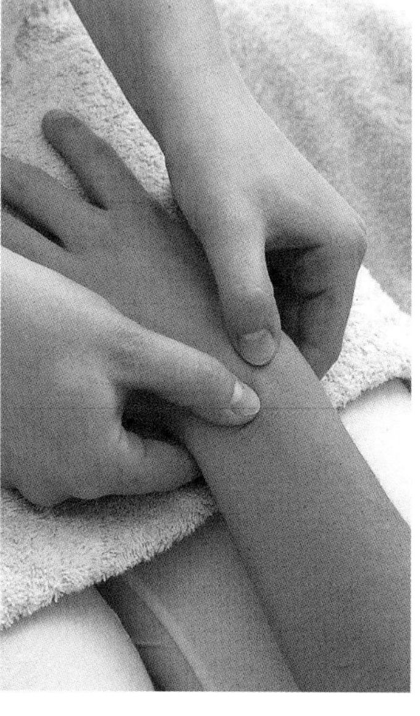

△ **5** Place your fingers under the wrist and make small, alternating thumb circles to ease the strain away from the tiny bones and surrounding ligaments on the top of the wrist joint.

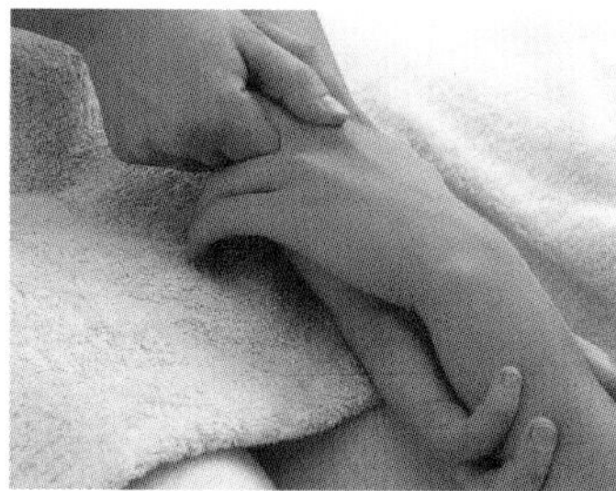

△ **6** Relax the fingers and thumb, starting with the little finger and working across the hand. Begin by massaging the base knuckle with gentle circular motions using your thumb and index finger.

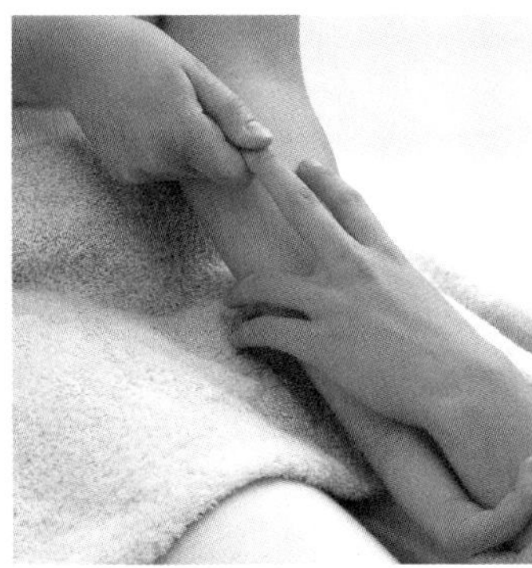

△ **7** Now pull firmly but gently along the top and bottom of each digit and out of its tip as if you are releasing tension away from the extremities of the body. Use smooth actions as the joints in the fingers are relatively delicate.

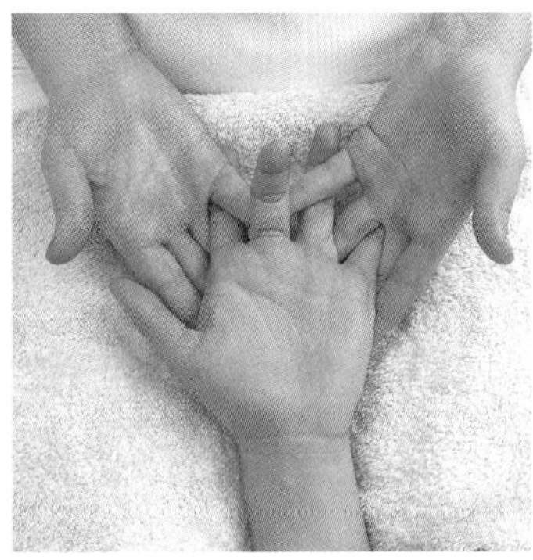

△ **8** Turn the hand so the palm is facing upwards. Interlock your fingers between those of your partner's hand, as shown, so that they rest against the back of the hand. Push them gently upwards, using enough pressure to open up and spread out the palm.

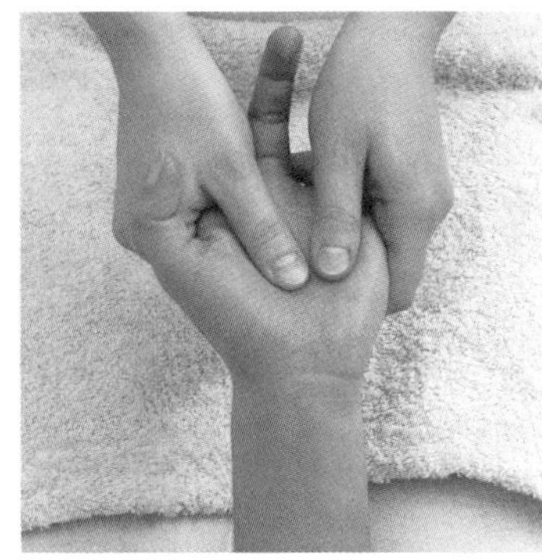

△ **9** Use both thumbs to make short, alternate sliding strokes over the surface of the palm to stretch and release tension from the muscles. Be sensitive to your partner's reactions.

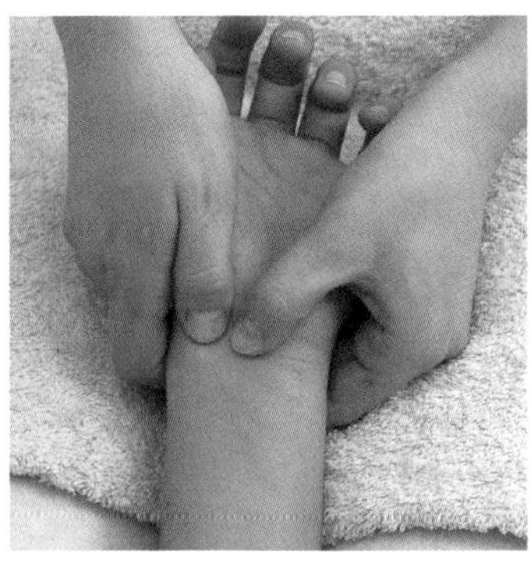

△ **10** Once the palm is relaxed, unlock your fingers and place them behind the back of the wrist. Massage over the inside of the wrist with small, alternating thumb circles.

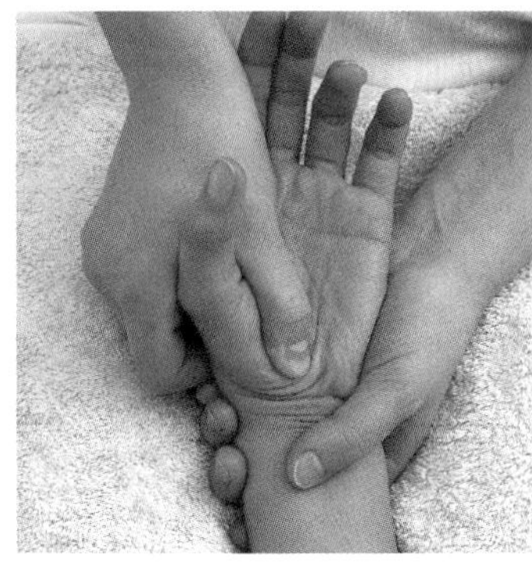

△ **11** To massage more vigorously on the palm, support the back of your partner's hand with your hand, and use your other thumb to apply stronger pressure circle strokes, working on one spot at a time. Focus particularly on the area at the base of the thumb.

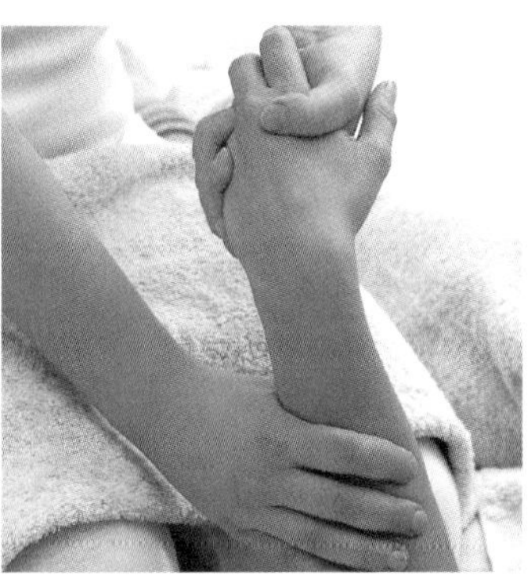

△ **12** Apply some passive movements to loosen the wrist joints. Raise the forearm by flexing the elbow and supporting it with one hand. Firmly clasp your partner's hand with your other hand. Rotate the wrist several times, first in one direction, and then in the other.

how to finish a body massage

To complete your body massage apply a restful and calming hold. Bring your full attention to your touch, allowing both of you time to assimilate the beneficial effects of the session and to bring it to a gentle close.

Once you have withdrawn your hands from your partner's body, stand silently for several minutes. Make sure the whole body is covered with a sheet or blanket, and allow time for a few moments of complete relaxation, while you go to wash your hands. When you are ready, offer assistance to get up from the mattress or couch and have a warm towel ready to wrap around the shoulders if necessary. Encourage stretching and moving around a little to allow for adjustment to the standing position.

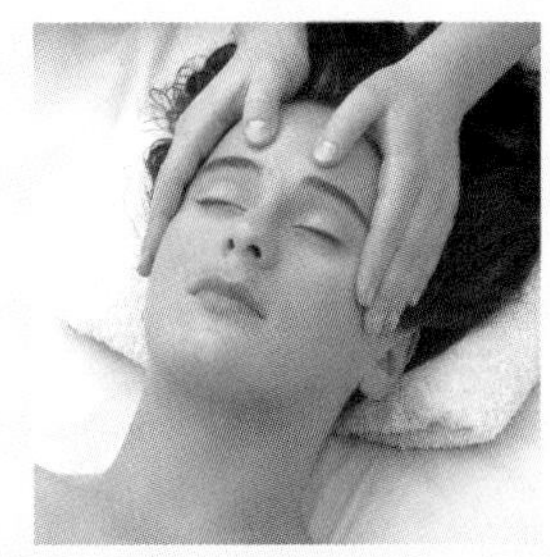

Self-massage programme

Tone up your body and give yourself an energy lift with a self-massage programme that uses a variety of strokes to relax tense muscles and stimulate the circulation. Self-massage is not only beneficial to your physical system; it also gives you a psychological boost when you are tired or under stress. It increases your awareness of your body, an essential part of learning how to help others become more conscious of their bodies through massage. Another benefit is that it helps you to practise the techniques and gain the confidence to apply them to a partner when you are carrying out a body massage.

wake-up programme

This self-massage programme is guaranteed to invigorate you when you wake up in the morning and need a energizing boost, or whenever you are feeling generally run-down. It is also an excellent programme to use prior to giving a massage, so that you can begin the session with a fresh mind and body. Both you and your massage partner will feel the benefit.

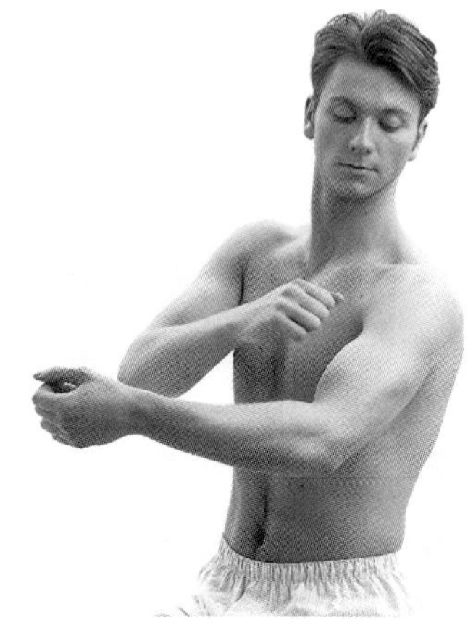

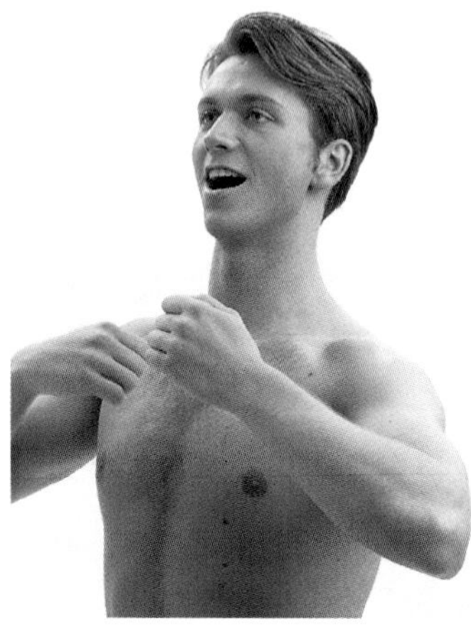

△▽ **2** Use your fist to pummel from the shoulder down the outside of the arm and hand. Feel how the skin begins to tingle. Turn the arm and, with the other fist, steadily pummel the inside of the hand and up the arm to the shoulder. Shake the whole arm to loosen up the joints. Then repeat steps 1 and 2 for the opposite side of the body.

△ **3** Use both hands to vigorously pummel your ribcage and pectoral muscles. Open your mouth and let out a roar to clear your throat and chest.

▽ **4** Warm up your abdominal muscles and boost your digestive processes with a brisk abdomen rub. Place one hand flat over the other and massage in a clockwise direction several times.

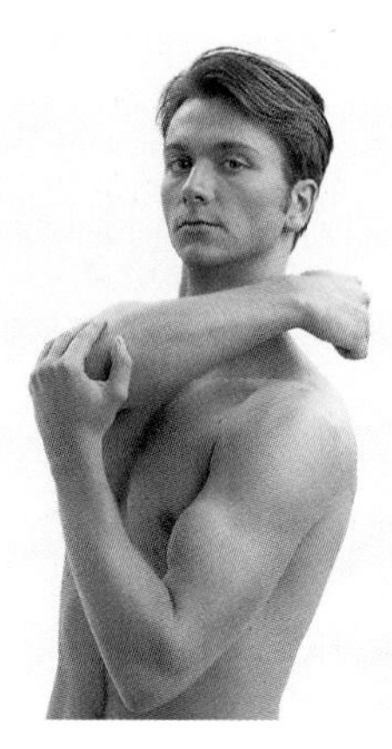

△ **1** To relax a stiff neck and shoulders, support your elbow with one hand and make a loose fist with the other hand. Use the flat edge of your knuckles to pummel the muscles on the opposite side of the body. Pound gently, but firmly, down the back of the neck towards the edge of the shoulder.

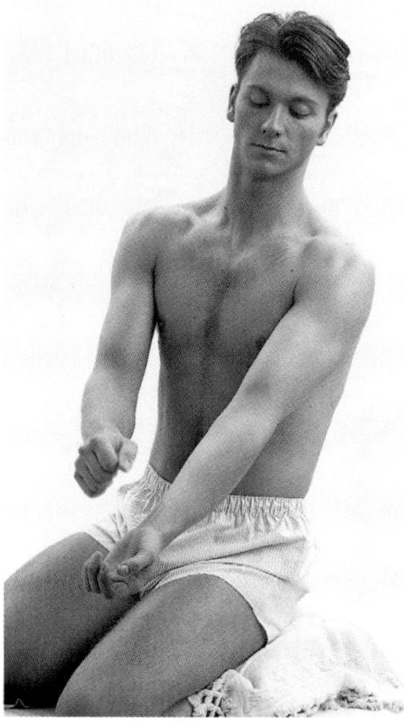

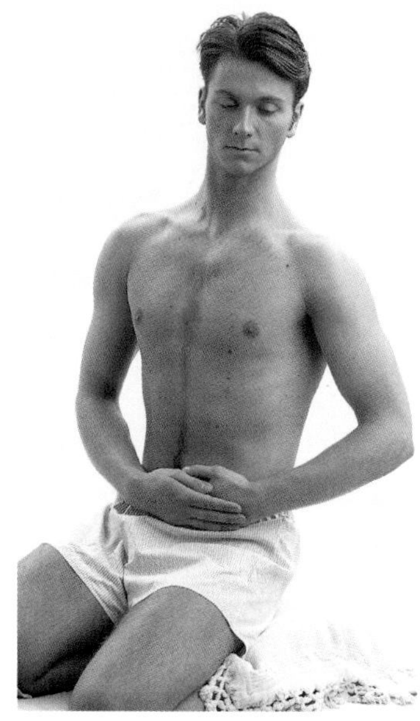

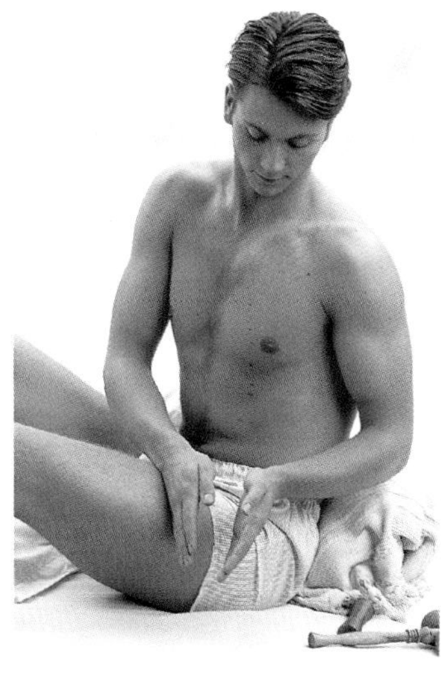

△ **5** Tone the muscles and stimulate the circulation in your legs using hacking strokes, repeatedly striking the skin with the sides of both hands.

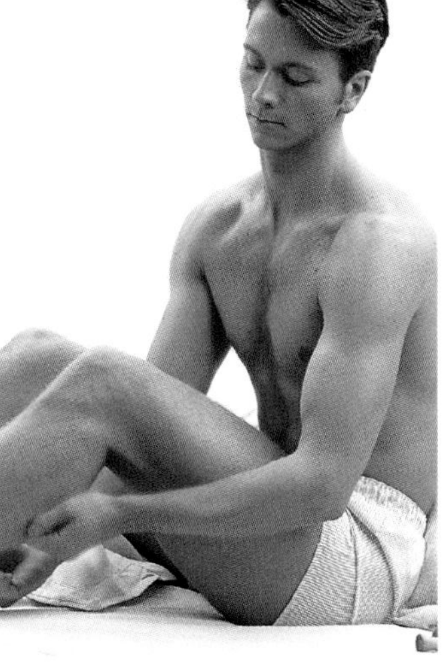

△ **6** Tight calf muscles can slow blood circulation. Use one hand after the other to pummel the lower leg to relieve tension and revitalize the system.

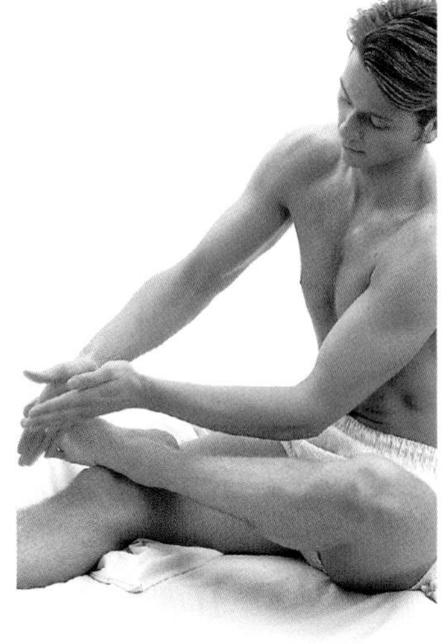

△ **7** Hack briskly, but gently, over the top and bottom of the foot to relieve stiffness in the muscles, joints, and tendons.

Repeat steps 5–7 for the opposite side of the body. When you have completed the Wake-up Programme, stand up and shake your whole body to release any remaining tension and loosen the joints. Then stand completely still so that you can appreciate the sensation of vitality it gives.

massage instruments

Nothing feels better than the touch of hands on the body, but massage instruments can be used successfully in self-massage to reach awkward areas. A two-ball roller, for example, is ideal for working on sore points on the back.

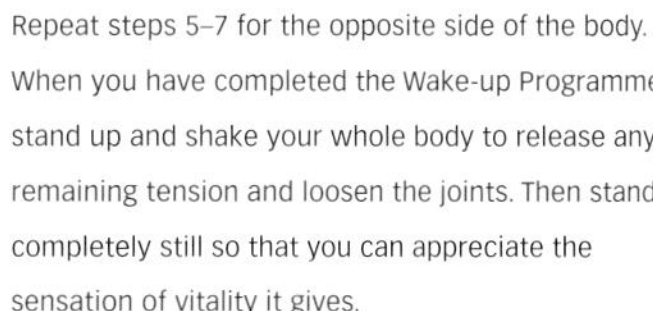

self-massage for the hands

Keeping your hands supple and relaxed is an important part of massage. While practising the strokes, you may find yourself using certain hand movements for the first time, so it is a good idea to exercise the hand joints frequently to increase their flexibility. Use one hand to gently squeeze all over the other. Repeat for the other hand. Rub the palms together briskly to increase warmth and vitality.

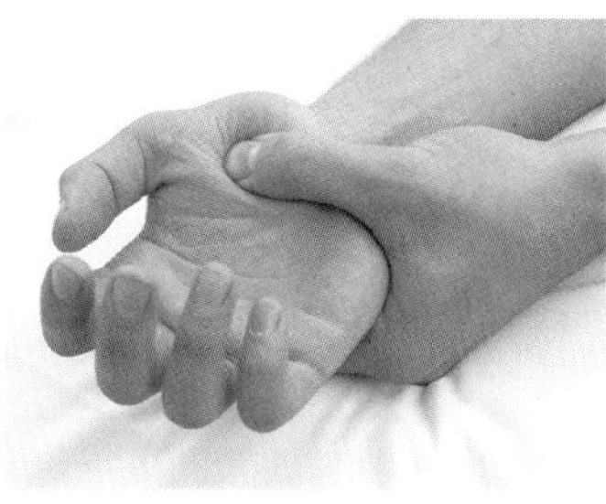

△ **1** Release tension in the muscular pad at the base of the thumb by pressing into it with the thumb of the other hand and then rotating it on one spot at a time. Support the back of the hand with the fingers. Work over the entire palm in a similar way.

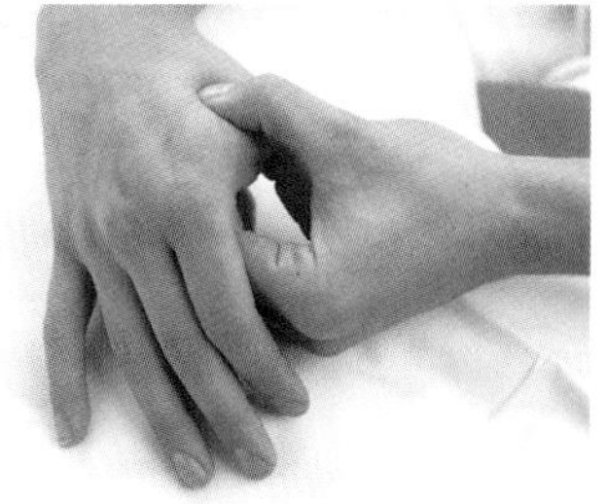

△ **2** Sink and rotate your thumb into the web between the thumb and index finger of the other hand. You will find a tender spot that can bring relief from toothache, headaches and digestive problems.

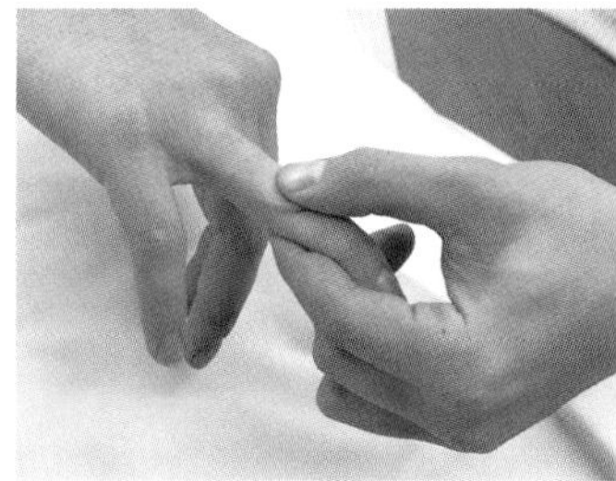

△ **3** Pinch the base of a finger on one hand between the thumb and index finger of the other hand, then pull the thumb and index finger in alternate short, firm slides along the length of the finger to its tip to stretch it. Repeat this movement on all the digits. Repeat the whole hand massage sequence for the other hand.

The sensual massage

Massage can become an integral part of a relationship, a means of communication, a way to show how much you care for each other. The skin is so sensitive that it is able to transmit and receive loving messages and feelings conveyed through the hands. Touch within a loving relationship has many dimensions. It can be therapeutic, playful, sensual or intimate. It is a beautiful way to explore, refresh and delight each other's bodies.

setting the mood

Set the mood for a sensual massage by lighting candles and making sure that the room is comfortably warm. Vaporize some of the essential oil blend you will be using for the massage, using a special burner, to fragrance the room.

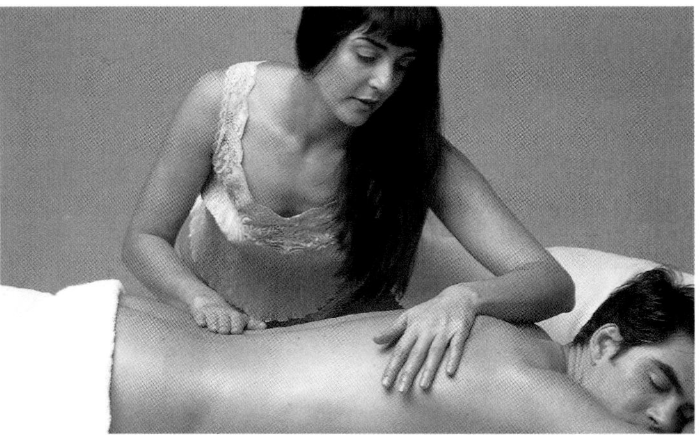

△ **1** Spread your chosen blend of essential oils over the back of your partner's body with soothing, languid and sensual strokes. Take plenty of time to allow the flowing movement of your hands to relax your partner both physically and emotionally before applying your strokes.

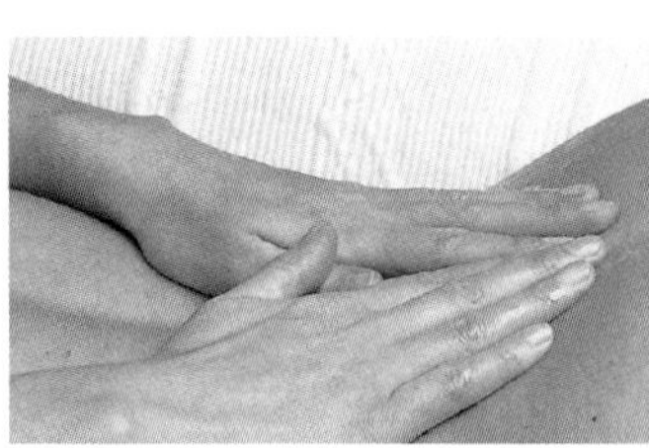

△ **2** As you ease tension from his back let your hands become soft and pliable, so that they mould and encompass the shapes and curves of the body.

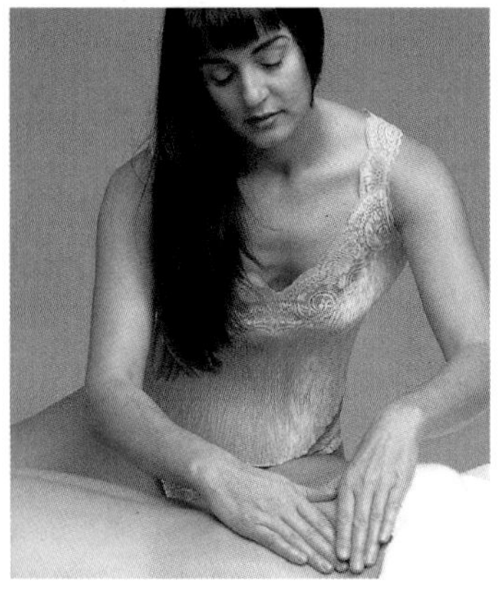

△ **3** Kneading on the buttocks not only brings a deep relief to the lower back area, but can also be a pleasurable and sensual experience.

massaging the chest

Relaxing the chest and ribcage with massage helps your partner to release tensions and breathe more fully. This will enable him to become more open and more able to connect with his feelings. Sit or kneel comfortably behind your partner so that his head is supported in your lap. Spread the oil over his ribcage, increasing the amount used if he has a lot of hair on his chest.

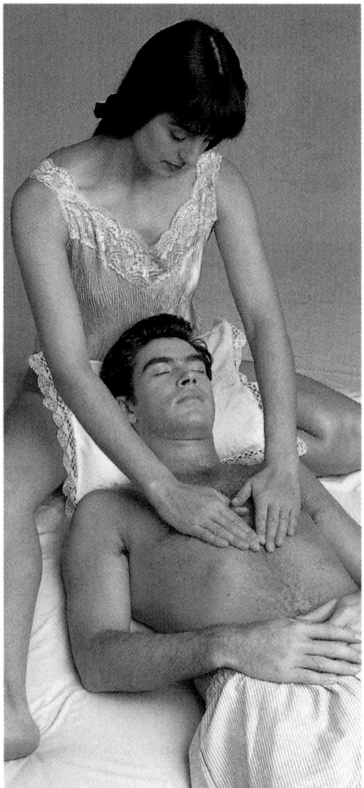

△ **1** Place both hands flat over the top of the breastbone so that your fingers point down the body. Stroke gently and steadily in a flowing movement down to the base of the chest.

△ **2** Without breaking the flow of motion, fan both hands out over the lower ribs, towards the sides of his body, so that your fingers slip slightly below the back. Moulding your hands to his ribcage, pull them up towards the edge of his armpits.

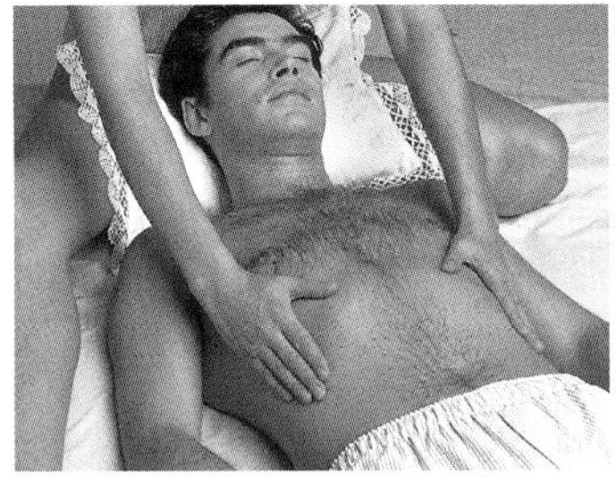

△ **3** Flex your wrists, gliding both hands into the body and out towards the edge of the shoulders, increasing the pressure slightly to open and stretch the top of the chest. Slip both hands softly around the shoulders and slide them lightly back over the pectoral muscles, towards the breast bone. Repeat this stroke several times.

soothing and caressing

Soft caressing is profoundly relaxing, especially on the face and jaw.

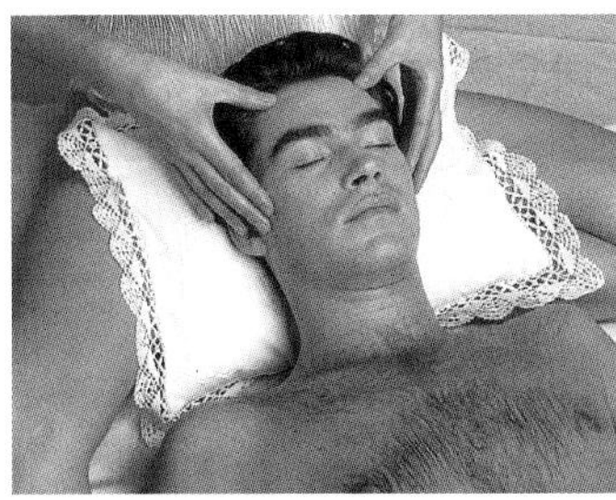

△ Stroke one hand after the other along the sides of the face. Then use gentle thumb strokes, circling the temples clockwise, to relax the forehead.

soft and flowing

A sensual massage can be made up entirely of soft, flowing effleurage strokes, using the flat of the hands to soothe the skin and relax the nervous system, while at the same time bringing tactile joy to the senses. This overlapping stroke, using the palms of the hands, creates the sensation of many hands caressing the body. It feels particularly good on the legs and arms.

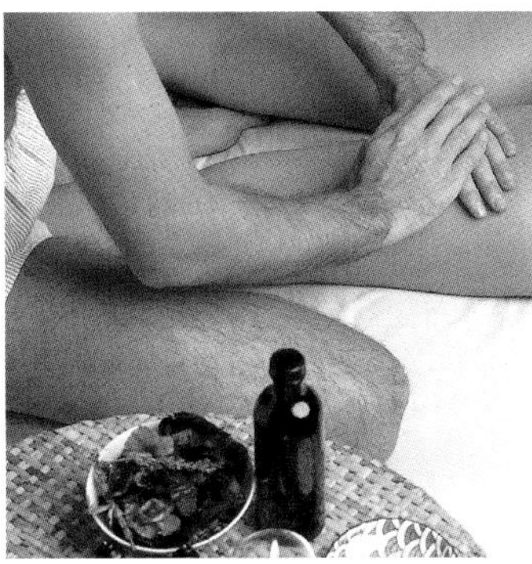

△ One hand follows the other in short, tender brushes to the limb, with the leading hand lifting away from the skin to loop over the following hand, ready to repeat the stroke.

feather touches

Delicate feather touches are playful and deliciously arousing to the nerve endings, bringing the skin alive with shivers of pleasure. Soft skin areas, such as the undersides of the arms, the inner thighs, and the nape of the neck, are most receptive to these teasing strokes.

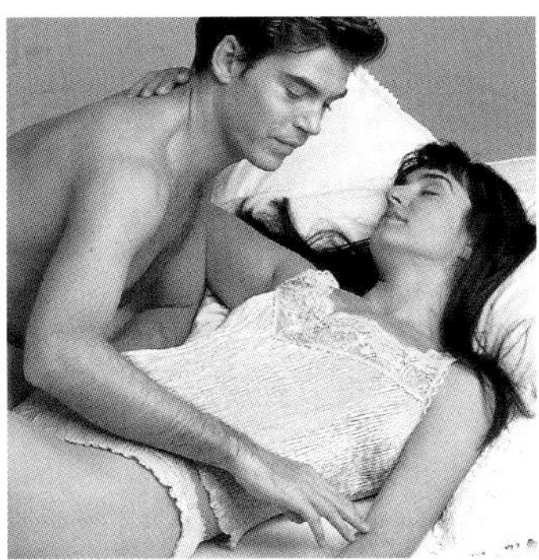

△ Using only the barest minimum of touch, slowly trail your fingertips down the highly sensitive skin on the underside of the arm.

sensual scents

Use aromatherapy recipes to help one another relax after a stressful day, or to replenish vitality when you are tired. By carefully selecting your essential oils you can enhance the sensual romantic mood created by your massage. Personal taste is an important factor in choosing oils for sensual massage, because it will not be a pleasurable experience if the person giving or receiving the massage finds the blend of oils unappealing. There are, however, a few oils that seem to have a universal appeal: jasmine, rose, rosewood, sandalwood and ylang ylang. These oils are the embodiment of luxury and indeed some of the most expensive to buy. They have a warming, and enveloping quality, freeing the mind from the mundane and opening it to the exotic and romantic. To add spice or stimulation to your chosen blend, add either black pepper or frankincense.

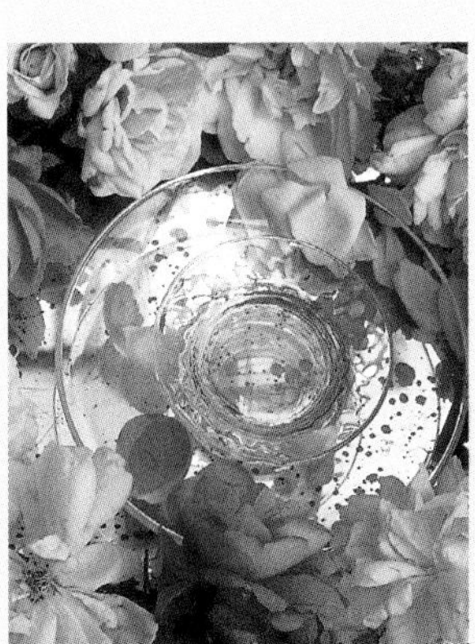

△ Massage oils scented with exotic essential oils are a sensual delight.

Therapeutic Body Treatments

Once you have mastered the basic massage skills you will want to broaden your knowledge and technique. The beauty of this healing art is the process of discovering how the body functions, and the way it responds to treatment. This section shows how oil blends can be combined with strokes to treat a whole range of conditions. Your enhanced skills will enable you to bring greater relief, relaxation, invigoration, and comfort.

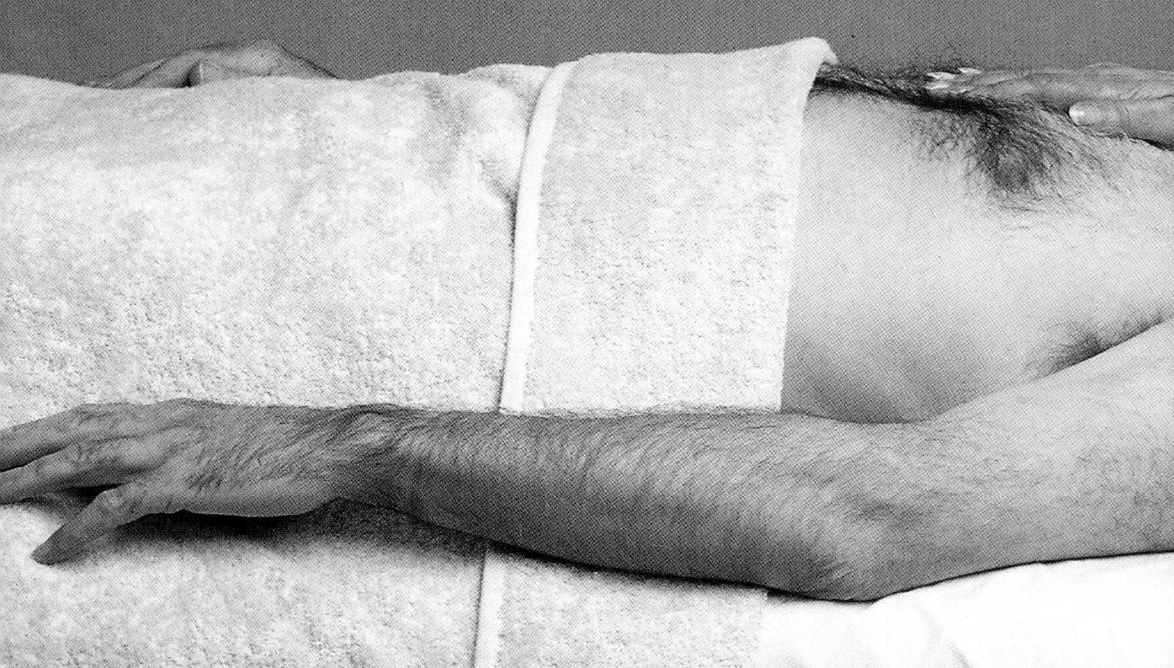

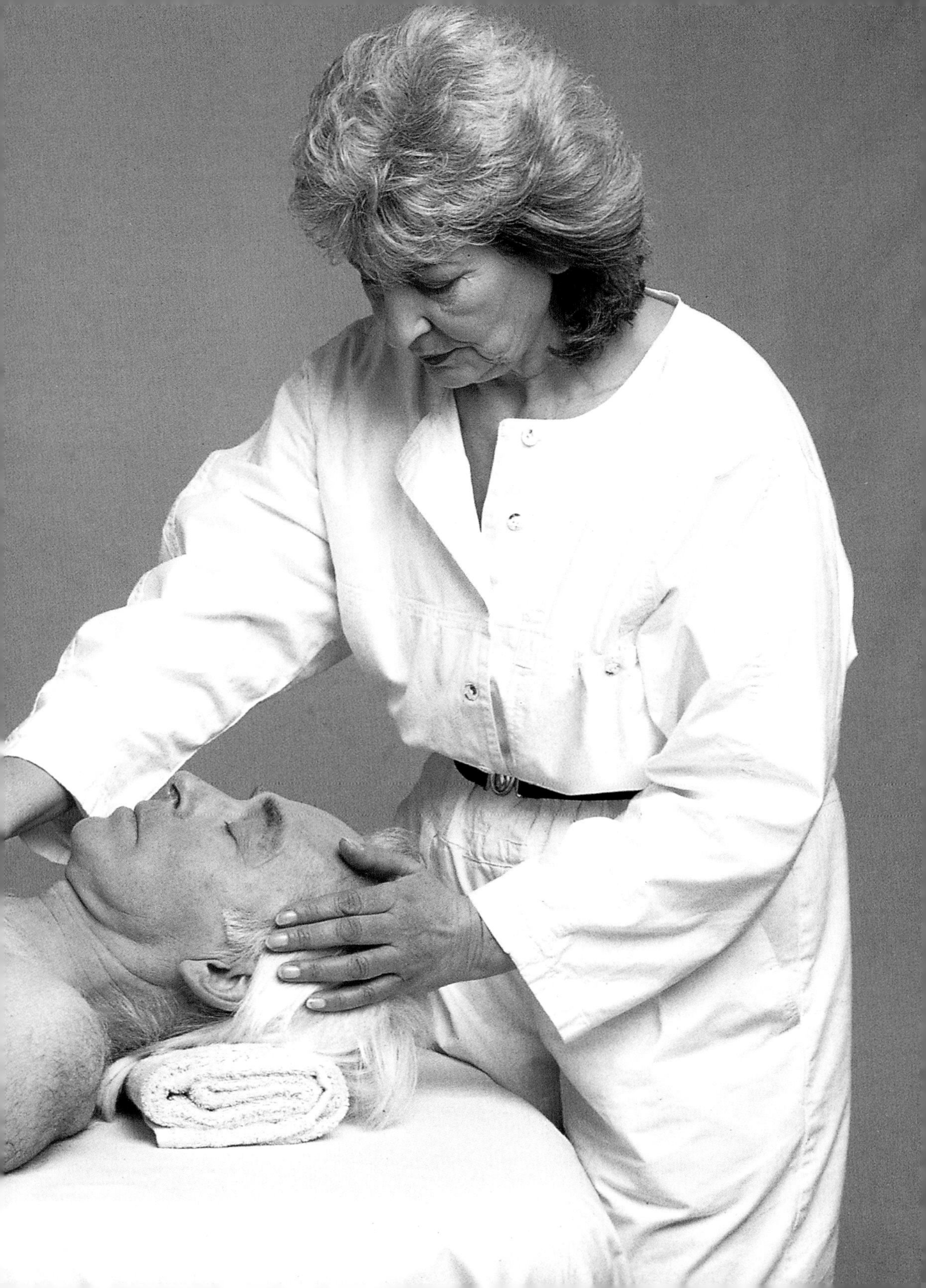

Strokes and oils for insomnia

Soothing, hypnotic strokes and sedative essential oils help to separate the activities of the day from the vital period of sleep and rest at night, and enable the insomniac to break the cycle of sleeplessness.

In cases of insomnia or bad dreams that lead to broken nights, it is important to reduce the intake of stimulating drinks such as tea and coffee, and to avoid eating late at night. It is also helpful to create a relaxing ritual to prepare for falling asleep. The suggested massage treatments, given here and for the treatment of anxiety, combined with a recommended blend of aromatherapy oils, will prove invaluable for this bed-time preparation.

soft and soothing strokes

This sequence of strokes should wash over the body in outward flowing motions, creating a gentle stream of movement that draws tension and anxiety away from the central core of the body. The soft, downward pulling strokes have a hypnotic and sedative effect, which will calm the emotions and quiet an over-active mind, thereby helping to induce relaxation and sleep.

As you apply the strokes, be aware of your breathing, drawing your hands down on the inhalation and pausing briefly on exhalation. This slight pause in the motion will create a wave-like feeling, rather than a straight pulling effect. Rub a little oil into your hands and mould them to the body, imparting a steady softness, and always begin the sequence on any limb from above the major joint, such as the shoulder or hip, in order to draw tension away from the constricted area.

Take the stroke right out of the head, hands, or feet, and beyond the actual physical body, as if you are emptying it of the stress and worries that may inhibit sleep. Each sequence should be performed up to five times on each part of the body. Begin by pulling your hands along the back of the neck to help to release tension.

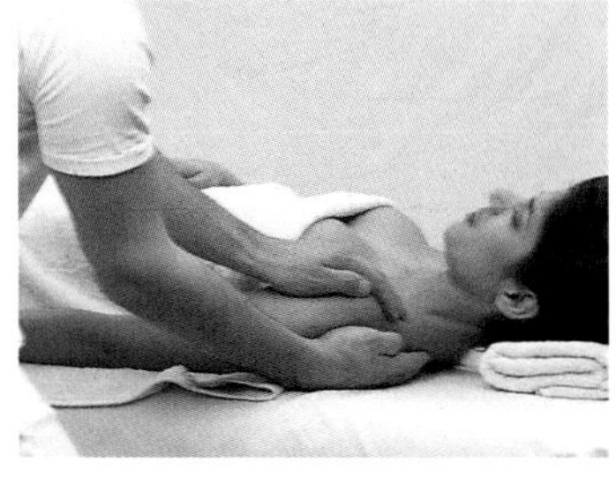

△ **1** Place one hand over the top of the chest, and the other over the muscles on the back of the shoulder, so that the fingers point towards the centre of the body. As you breathe in, pull your hands steadily outwards to the edge of the shoulder and down to just below the joint. Pause briefly as you exhale, letting your hands rest and lightly cradle the top of the arm.

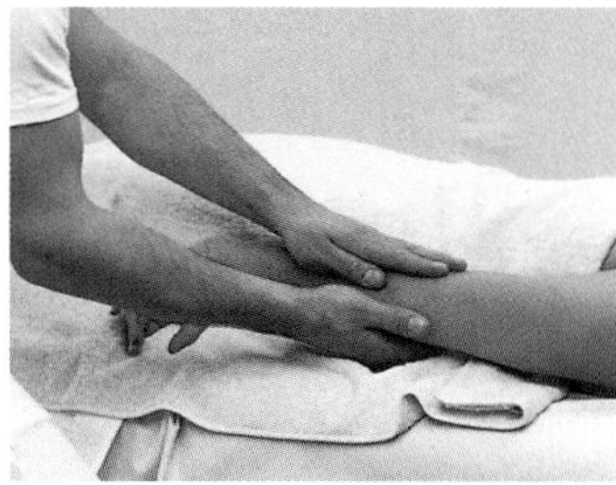

△ **2** Adjust your position so that you can continue the pulling motion down the arm. As you breathe in, pull both hands down to just below the elbow. Relax as you breathe out, and continue the slide down the forearm and below the wrist while inhaling.

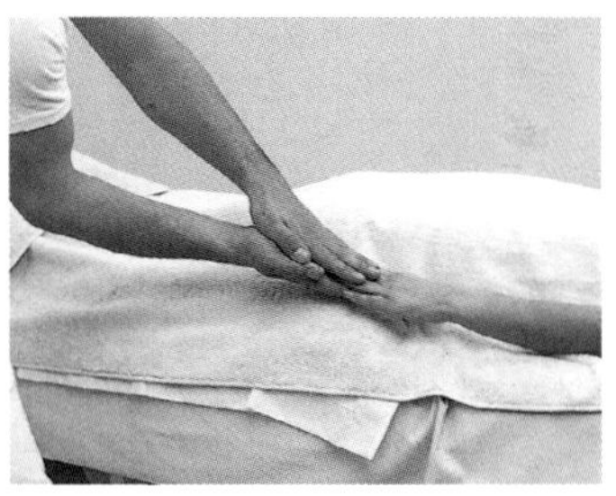

◁ **3** Draw your hands over both sides of your partner's hand and fingers, taking your stroke out as the hand settles back on to the mattress. Repeat steps 1 to 3 on the other side of the body.

releasing neck tension

Place both hands, fingers pointing down, on each side of the spine. Ask your partner to breathe deeply and to relax the neck and head into your hands. Pull your hands gently but firmly, with the fingertips slightly indented into the tissue, up the back of the neck and then out from under the head.

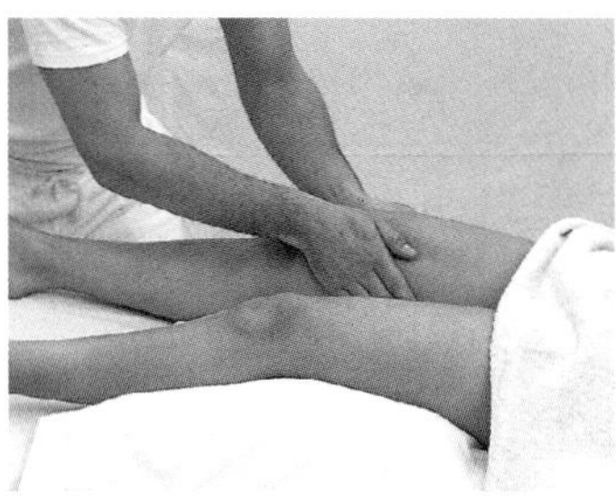

△ **4** Begin the hip, leg, and foot sequence by laying both hands just above the pelvic girdle to cradle the side of the body. Pull both hands down over the hip socket as you inhale, separating them as they reach the thigh in order to hold each side of the leg: rest briefly as you exhale. With the next inhalation, draw your hands down the leg to just below the knee.

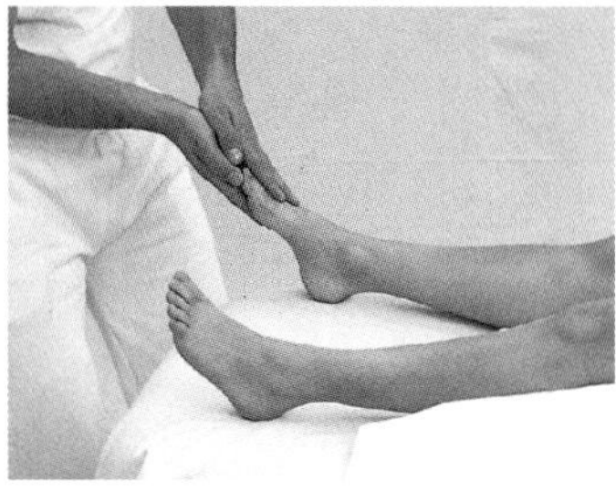

△ **5** Continue this wave-like motion down the lower leg to just below the ankle. Then slide one hand under the foot, with the other on top of the foot, pulling gently and steadily until your hands pass over the toes. Repeat the strokes on the other side of the body.

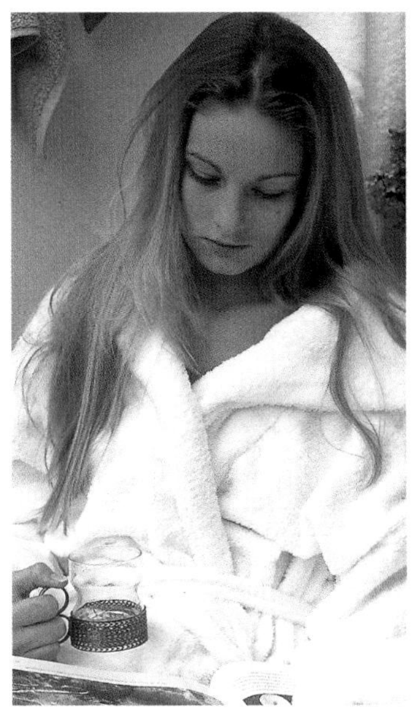

△ Sleeplessness is a very common response to stress. Learning to relax is vital, and massage can be extremely helpful. However, massage will need to be part of a daily routine that also includes a healthy diet and regular exercise.

sedating strokes on the legs and feet

Soft, soothing, downward-flowing strokes over both legs will further enhance the calming and sedative effect of your massage.

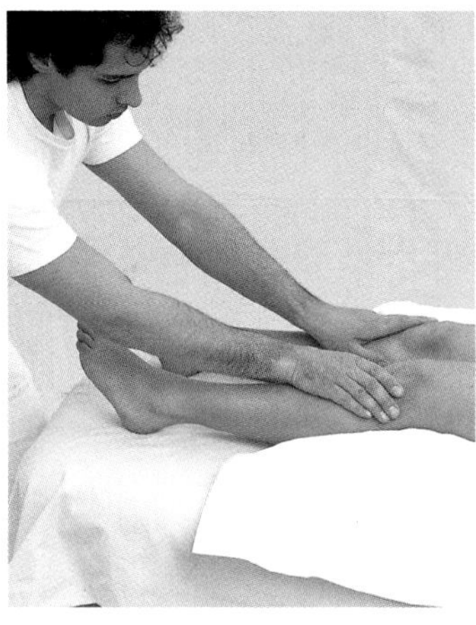

△ **1** Using the flat surface of both hands, softly stroke down the legs from the thighs until your hands pass over and out of the feet. Repeat the movement as many times as you like to allow your partner to relax.

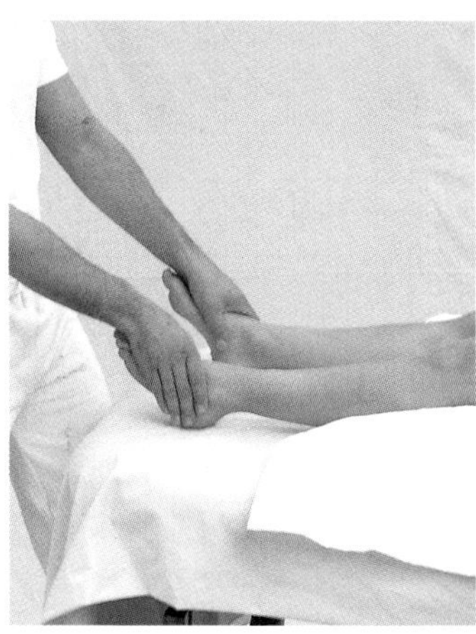

△ **2** To increase the sedative effect of your strokes, complete these sequences with a still, calm hold of your hands over the front of both feet. This will draw the energy down the body, bringing a sense of balance and peace.

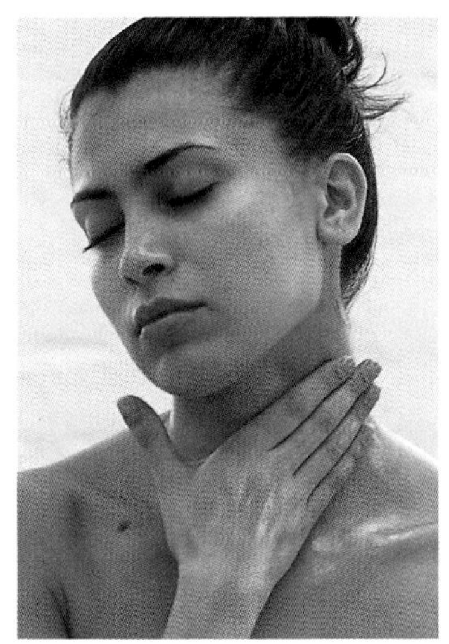

△ A soothing self-massage of the neck, shoulders and arms will relieve nervous tension and have a relaxing sedative effect. An ylang ylang oil massage blend can be particularly helpful for insomnia that has been caused by bad dreams.

useful essential oils

In cases of insomnia, all the relaxing, sedative oils are useful, these include: chamomile, clary sage, lavender, marjoram, mandarin, neroli, orange, rose, rosewood, and sandalwood. Use 2–3 drops of essential oil blended with 15ml (1 tbsp) of an appropriate carrier oil.

- frankincense or lemon blended with one of the oils listed above can help to calm and soothe.
- ylang ylang can be very helpful to relax and calm anxiety in cases of disturbed sleep following a bad dream.

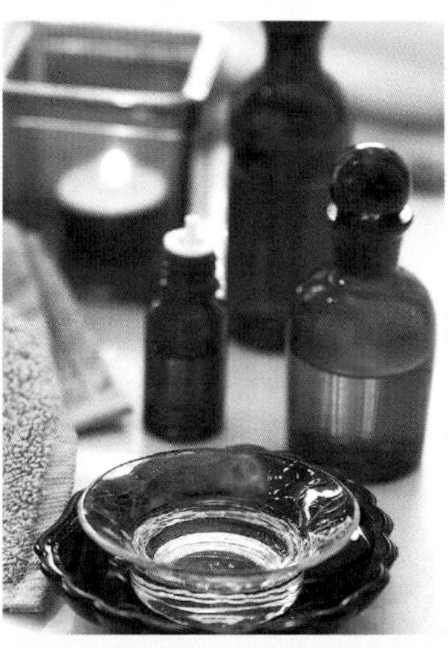

Massage for digestive disorders

When stress is manifested physically in the abdominal area, massage and touch can bring the sense of safety and comfort needed to relax and relieve mild digestive disorders and abdominal discomfort.

Emotional tension can cause us to tighten our abdominal muscles and reduce our breathing in order to avoid the experience of painful or uncomfortable feelings. If we are unable to assimilate those emotions, or express them appropriately, they can manifest themselves as physical disorders, particularly playing havoc with the digestive system. Massage helps to deepen breathing, allowing the muscles to soften and expand, and to restore harmony.

All the strokes shown on the abdomen in the Body Massage section are suitable when stress is felt in this area. Reflexology, shiatsu, hands-on breathing techniques, self-massage and passive movements can also bring relief to simple digestive disorders.

shiatsu elimination point

An important shiatsu point for the release of intestinal congestion is the one found on the web of skin between the thumb and index finger. The exact location is indicated by its tenderness to pressure. This point is known as Large Intestine 4, or in Chinese terms as "the Great Eliminator".

▽ Press gently on this point for up to five seconds, then release the pressure gradually.

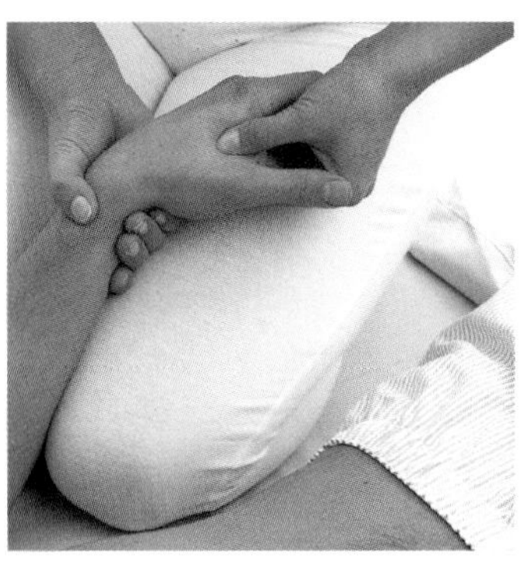

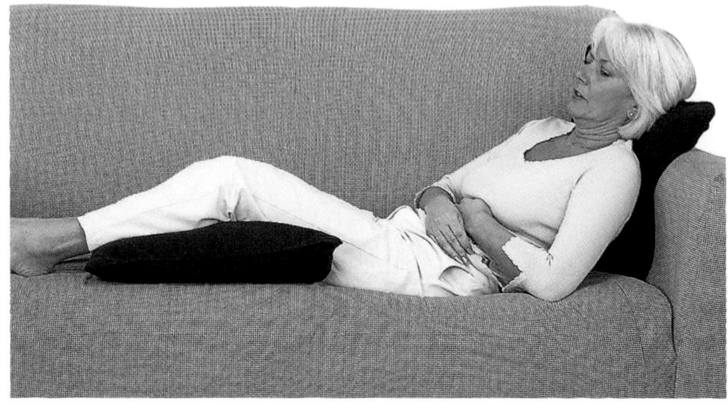

△ **Abdominal pain can be a warning that there is disorder in the system, so always consult a doctor if it is persistent.**

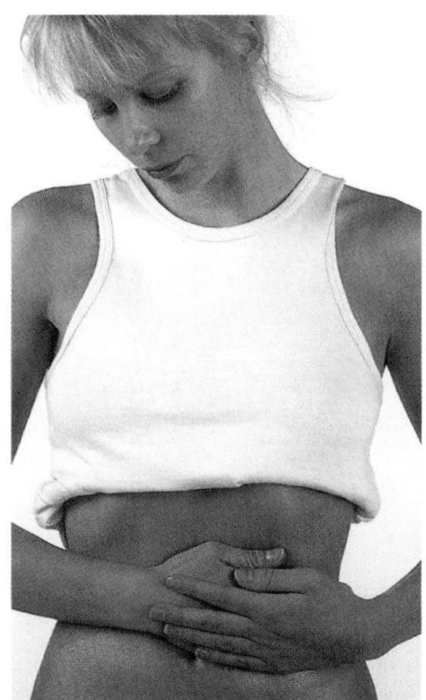

△ **Peppermint essential oil is particularly useful for digestive disorders. For self-massage place your hands on your abdomen and move your hands in a clockwise direction to encourage digestive and bowel action.**

holding and breathing

Still, calm holds over the abdominal area will encourage deeper breathing, allowing the release of pent-up emotions and stress. The following holds will all help to promote relaxation and eliminate tension, enabling the digestive tract to function properly.

▽ **1** If your partner is under extreme stress and is experiencing abdominal discomfort, the best position is to lie sideways with the knees drawn up slightly. Pillows under the head and between the knees will create a feeling of security. Place one hand over the lower back and the other on the belly, and encourage slow, deep breathing from the abdomen. When the abdominal muscles are relaxed, rub the abdomen with gentle clockwise strokes.

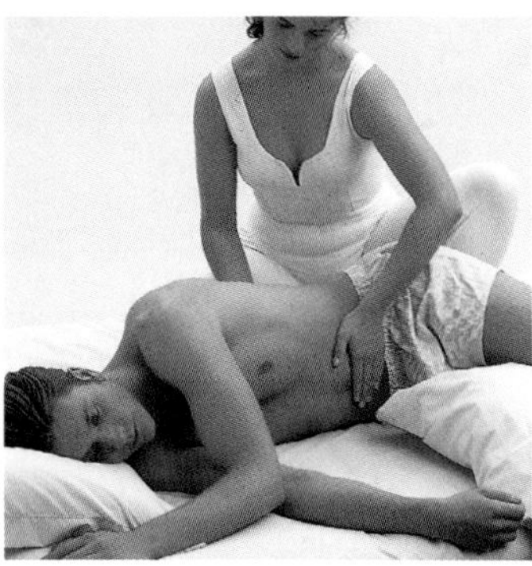

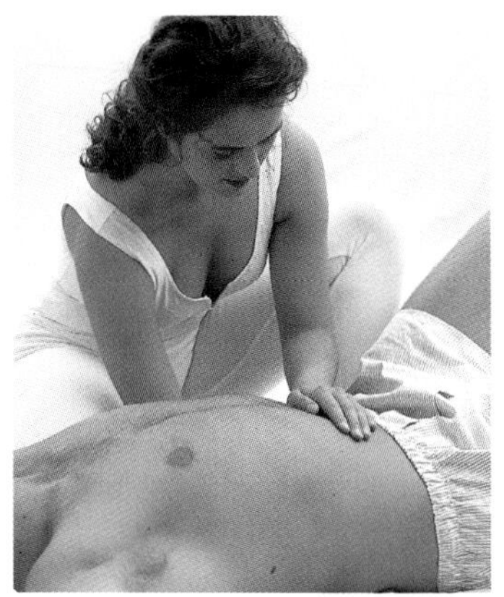

△ **2** With your partner lying down with knees raised, place one hand under the small of the back and ask that the weight of the pelvis be dropped towards your hand. Place your other hand over the abdomen so that its warmth helps to dissolve constriction in the muscles. Then ask your partner to direct breathing towards your hands and to imagine that each breath is helping the abdomen to expand and release tension. Keeping one hand under the pelvis, move your hand to hold different parts of the abdomen.

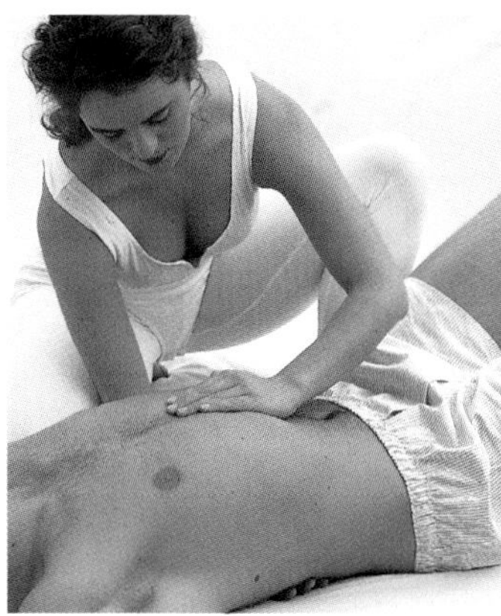

△ **3** Encourage deep but gentle breathing in the diaphragm and solar plexus region by placing one hand below the mid-back and the other over the top of the abdomen. This will encourage the release of tension that can lead to digestive problems. As the area relaxes, gently massage it with soft circular strokes of your palm.

useful essential oils

For specific digestive complaints the following essential oils and blends may be useful:

- *constipation and pain:* three drops each of ginger, orange, bergamot, and clary sage
- *sluggish digestion:* peppermint, juniper, rosemary
- *indigestion:* drop of peppermint, three drops each of ginger, lemon, bergamot
- *flatulence:* bergamot, fennel, ginger, lemon, marjoram, neroli, nutmeg, peppermint, rosemary
- *colicky pain:* bergamot, chamomile, clary sage, ginger, cypress, lemon, orange, peppermint, sandalwood
- *constipation:* fennel, ginger, marjoram, neroli, orange, peppermint, rose
- *diarrhoea:* cypress, chamomile, ginger, lemon, orange, peppermint

▽ **Rosemary has analgesic properties which will benefit headaches, painful digestion and muscular pain.**

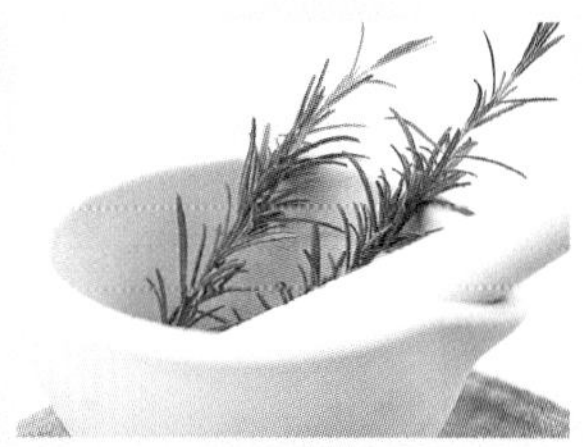

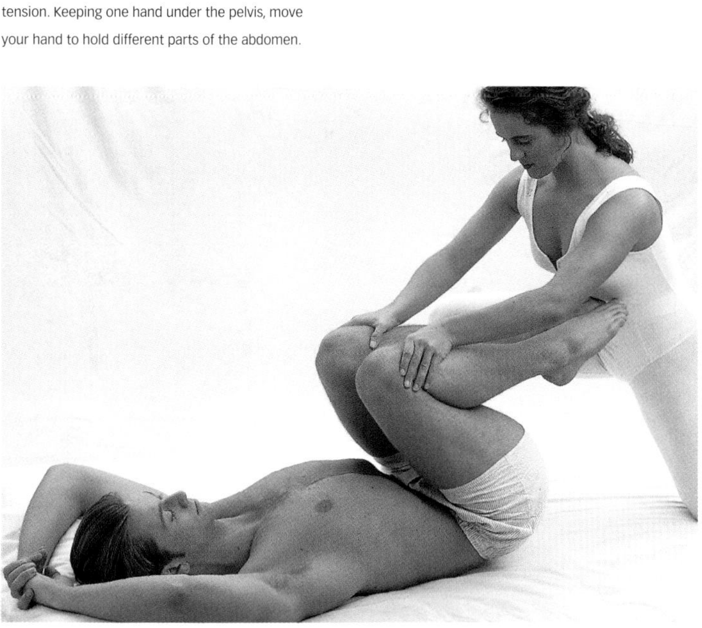

relieving abdominal cramp

Pushing the knees towards the abdomen can help to relieve tightness there. With your partner's knees bent so the feet are flat on the mattress, adjust your posture so that you can lean your weight forward as you perform this passive movement.

◁ Slowly push the knees towards the trunk of the body, taking care not to force them beyond their natural point of resistance. Help to lower your partner's feet to the mattress, then repeat the movement twice more.

Improving circulation

A healthy circulatory system is vital to the well-being of both mind and body. Massage, combined with a healthy diet and exercise, is an effective way to boost both blood and lymph circulation in order to promote health and vitality.

The circulatory system is divided into two parts: blood circulation that is pumped by the heart; and lymph fluid circulation that is moved by muscle action. The lymphatic system carries waste products to the lymph nodes, which act as filters to prevent harmful substances from entering the bloodstream, and is an important part of the body's immune defence system.

causes of poor circulation

Poor circulation may be caused by hereditary factors, but it can also be brought on by a sedentary lifestyle, smoking, an unhealthy diet, or emotional stress and tension. A sluggish circulation will cause a depletion of vital nutrients in the body leading to exhaustion, ill-health, and even depression as toxins build up and the elimination process is impeded.

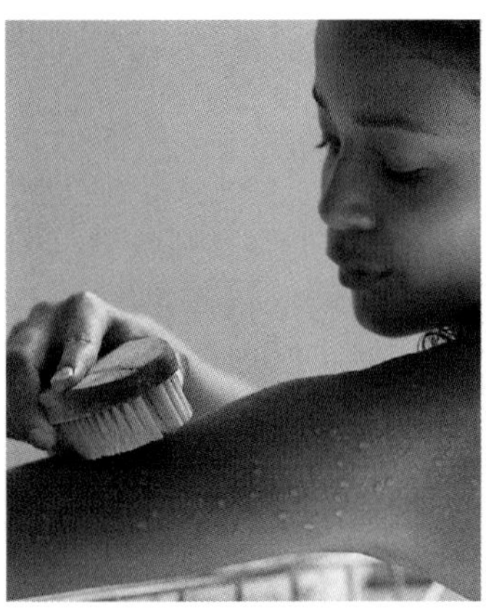

△ **Use a natural bristle brush for a stimulating body massage while you are bathing. This stimulates lymph circulation, which helps the body rid itself of waste products.**

boosting and draining

The signs of a sluggish circulation can be detected in pale, mottled, or blue-tinged skin, which is usually cold to the touch. The most common areas of poor circulation are the extremities of the body. Lift the limb and apply flowing strokes to boost and drain the blood supply on its return to the heart.

▽ **1** Cold arms, hands and fingers indicate poor circulation. To assist the return of blood to the heart, raise your partner's forearm and clasp the hand with whichever of your hands is closest. Wrap the other hand over the back of the wrist and drain firmly down the arm towards the elbow with a long steady stroke. Glide lightly around the elbow and back up to the wrist. Swap hands to repeat the movement on the inner forearm.

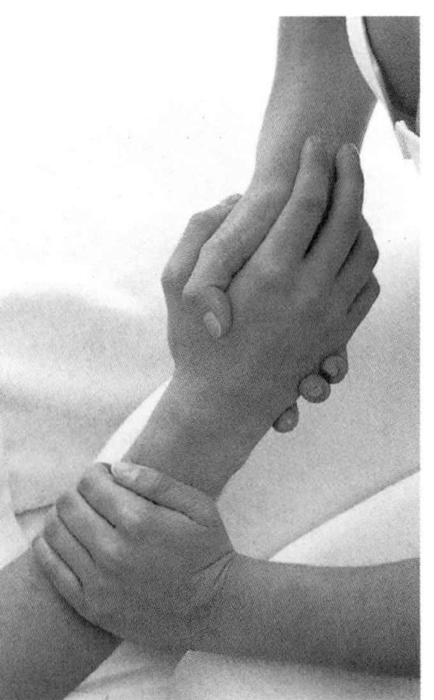

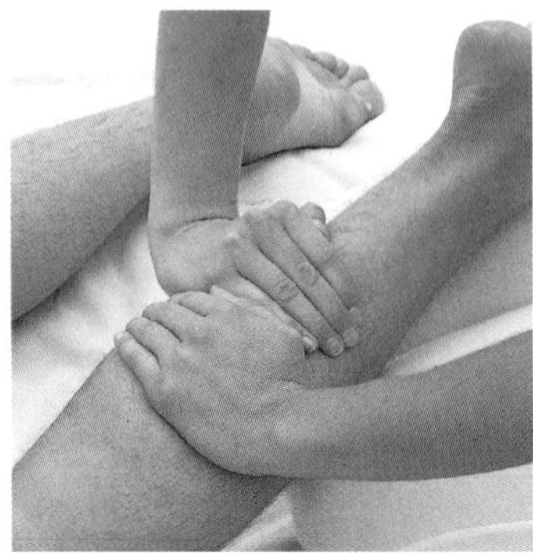

△ **2** Help to increase vitality in the legs and feet by first applying the basic effleurage stroke from the ankle to the back of the knee, with the lower leg in a raised position. Wrap both hands over the back of the ankle, little fingers leading, and firmly stroke up the calf. This position also helps to drain excess water from around puffy ankles.

▽ **3** Deeper drainage strokes can be achieved by using your thumbs to stroke, in alternating short slides, from the ankle to just below the back of the knee. Repeat several times.

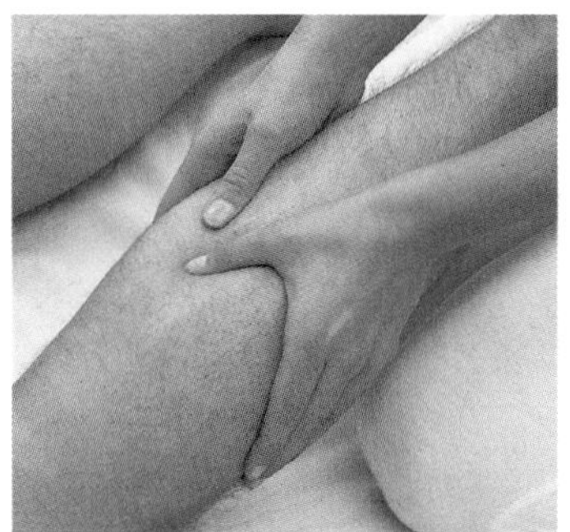

useful essential oils

The following essential oils aid circulation: cedarwood, cypress, eucalyptus, geranium, lemon, mandarin, neroli, rose, rosemary.

To address the problem more fully, create a blend that includes a detoxifying oil from the list of oils recommended for cellulite and one of the general tonic and stimulant oils.

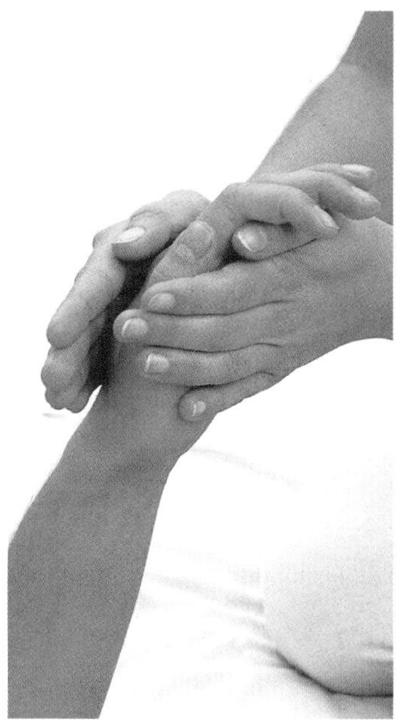

warming up

△ Hands and feet that are cold as a result of poor circulation can be warmed up by briskly rubbing them between both hands. The friction produces heat and stimulates the blood supply.

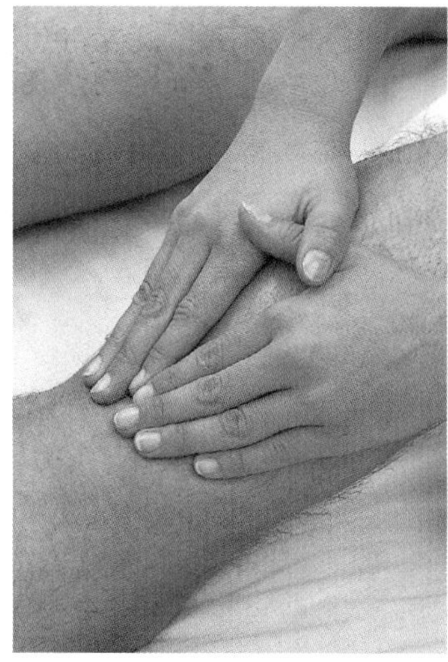

stroking towards lymph nodes

△ Lymphatic massage follows a specific procedure and requires the therapist to have a clear knowledge of the distribution of lymph vessels and nodes throughout the body. However, in a basic massage, gentle, upward effleurage strokes towards the major superficial lymph nodes – such as those in the back of the knee – can assist the lymphatic circulatory system to eliminate toxins from the body, particularly after kneading, friction, and deep tissue strokes.

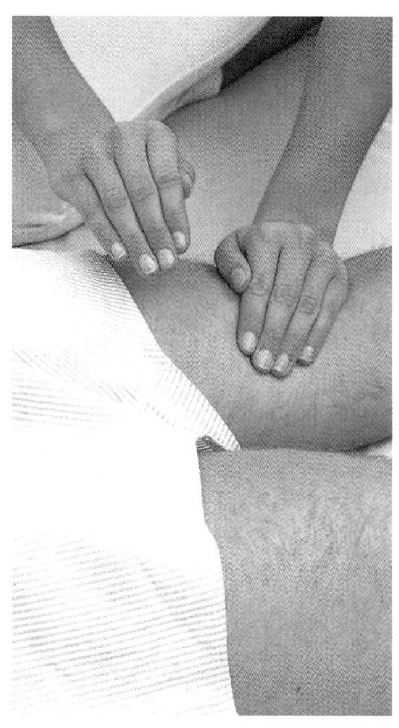

benefiting the skin

△ Pale, flaccid skin benefits from the stimulating effects of all percussion strokes. In particular, the suction effect of cupping draws the blood up towards the skin, bringing vital oxygen and nutrients to its peripheral nerve endings and underlying tissues.

self-massage for varicose veins

The return of de-oxygenated blood to the heart from the lower half of the body is against the pull of gravity, and so the veins have valves in them that open and close to prevent back-flow. When a valve is damaged the veins become dilated, causing the condition known as varicose veins. This condition can be exacerbated by pregnancy, obesity, or prolonged standing. It is not advisable to massage directly above or below a varicose vein, but gentle upward-flowing effleurage over the sides of the leg, or away from the damaged vein, will ensure that the area is not neglected during a massage.

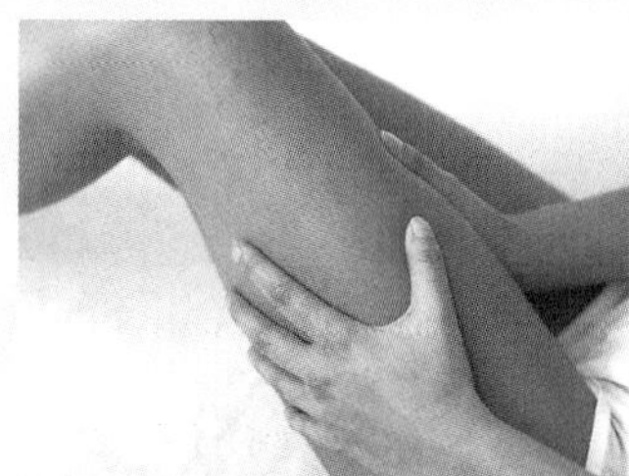

△ **1** Begin by smoothing the essential oil blend all over the leg. Then massage the upper half of the leg using upward movements. This helps to clear the valves so that blood passes more easily from the lower leg.

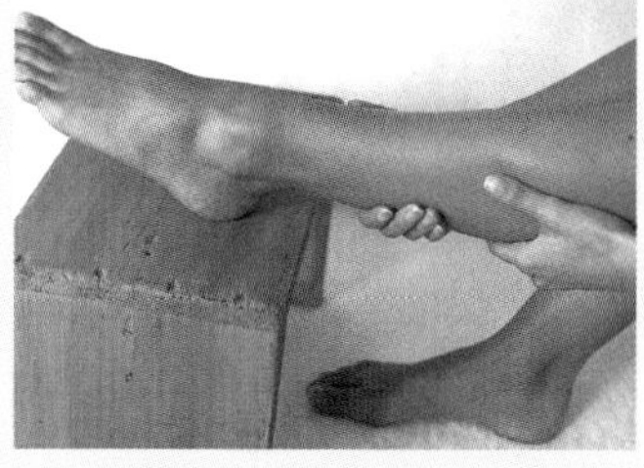

△ **2** Massage in an upward direction only, using the palms of both hands. Moving up the calf muscle, make long, firm strokes.

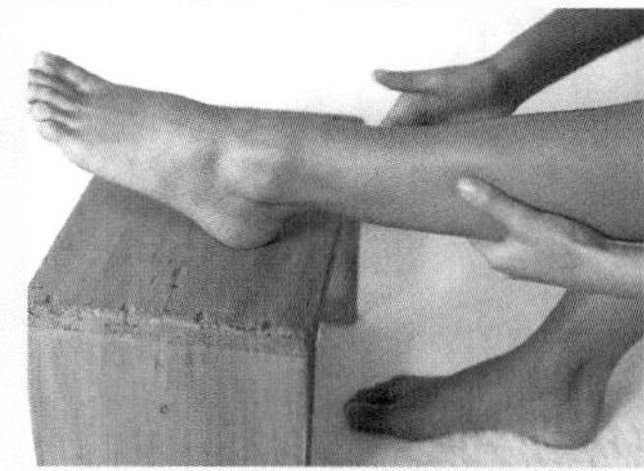

△ **3** Run the fingers of one hand up the calf muscle then repeat with the other hand. Finish by repeating step 2, then carry out the sequence on the other leg.

Convalescence and recuperation

After an illness or injury the body is left in a vulnerable condition, and a period of convalescence is vital to give the immune system time to rebuild its defences. Massage helps to promote this important transition.

healing holds

Gentle, hands-on holds are ideal for the first fragile stages of convalescence. The power of touch can be very useful because it can comfort the body, stimulating the nerves that replenish the vital organs, and return the body to a normal resting stage. As your partner recuperates, whole body massage will tone up the muscles, boosting circulation and increasing the body's overall vitality and sense of well-being.

Soothing holds help to balance the nervous system and increase the body's energy levels. Start at the head, gently placing your hands over the forehead, temples and cheeks, then work slowly and methodically down both sides of the body to the feet.

▷ The touch of your hands will calm and comfort the body. A gentle, hands-on hold is ideal in the early stages of convalescence, where massage would not be appropriate.

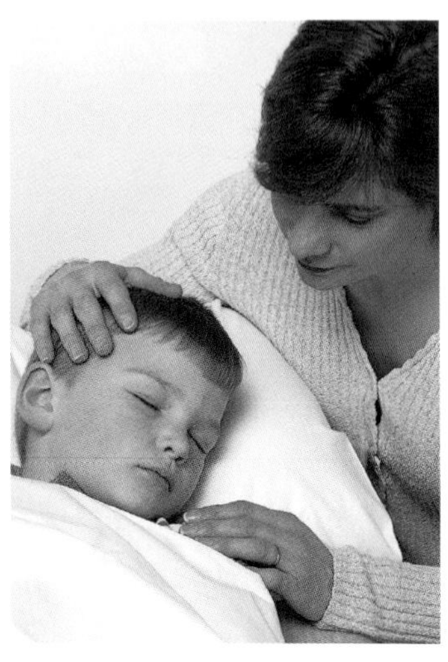

▽ If recovery from illness or injury involves being confined to bed for some time, massage can be invaluable. Initially it is helpful to soothe and calm the body, and later more gently invigorating treatments will speed the recuperation process.

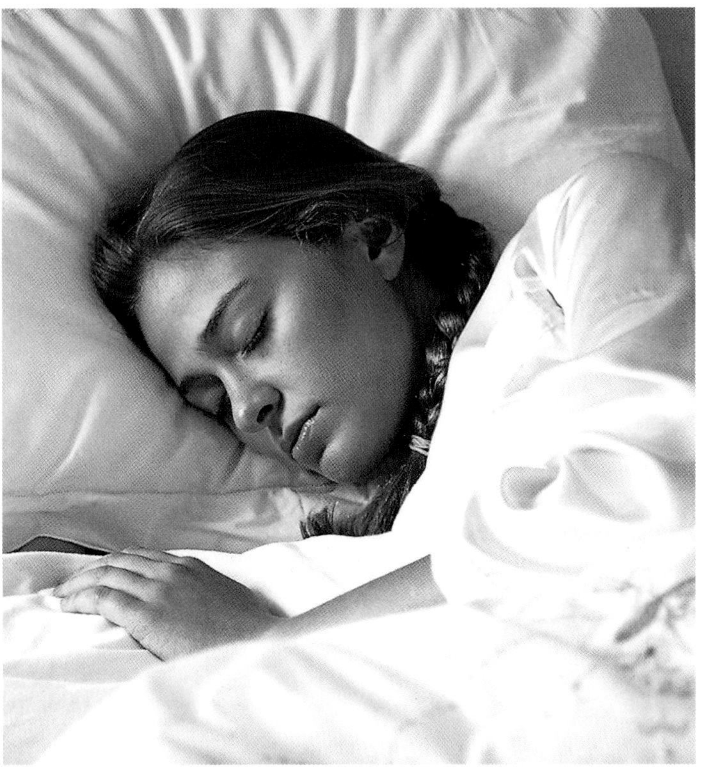

useful essential oils

The period of convalescence is often a time of physical and emotional change. The patient may experience bursts of energy, followed by fatigue when the spirits fall. The oils that are useful for convalescence include ginger and orange to stimulate the appetite, which may still be lacking at this time. The stimulating quality of eucalyptus and tea tree may help overcome lethargy. Orange and lavender both have an uplifting and comforting nature, and are more gentle, and these oils may be all that are needed to get over the last part of an illness. Also, during this recovery period the immune system needs boosting. The oils to choose for this are bergamot, frankincense, patchouli, lemon, rosewood, and tea tree. Mandarin is a relaxing tonic oil, and clary sage is also very useful. Cypress and juniper are helpful for inducing sleep.

reducing tension and clearing the head

The prolonged periods of inactivity in convalescence can cause the shoulder and neck muscles to tense up. This tension restricts the circulation which, in turn, leads to discomfort and headaches.

▷ Gentle kneading of the shoulders can help to reduce tension in the shoulder and neck muscles. If appropriate follow this with a relaxing neck, head and face massage.

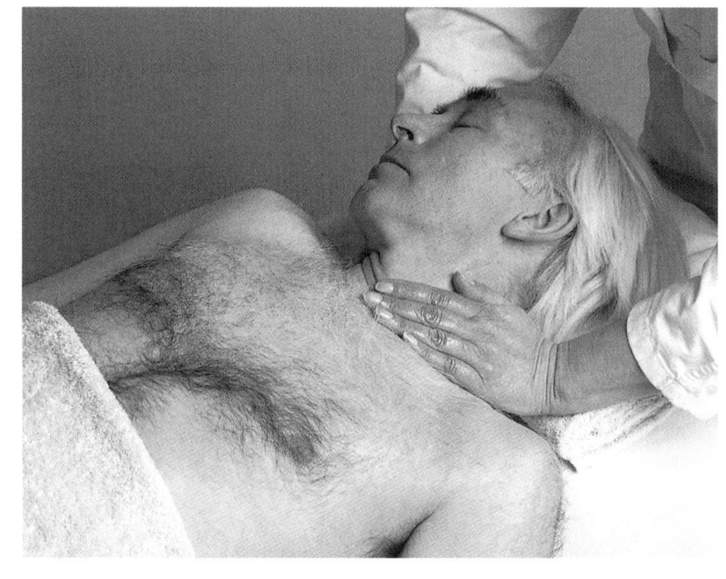

getting ready for action

As your partner recuperates and becomes stronger, the desire to resume normal activities grows. At this stage in convalescence, it is often useful to focus your massage on the feet and legs to boost a sluggish circulatory system, and massage the arms and hands to renew their strength and dexterity.

◁ **1** Begin the massage with a healing hold. Cup your left hand over your partner's temple and place your right hand over the heart area. This helps to encourage a sense of integration between mind and body.

▽ **2** Massage the hands and fingers to release tension and increase flexibility.

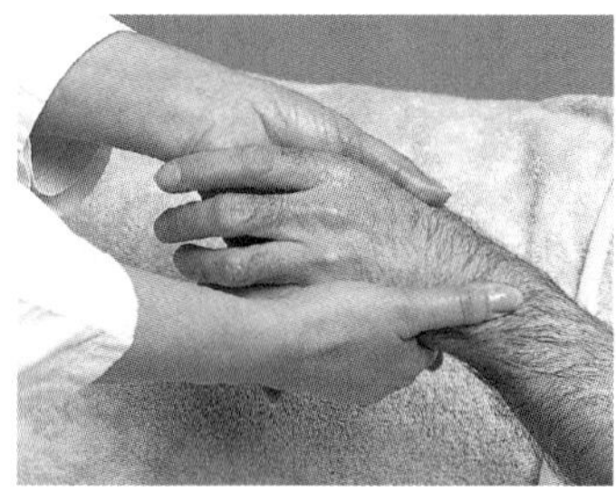

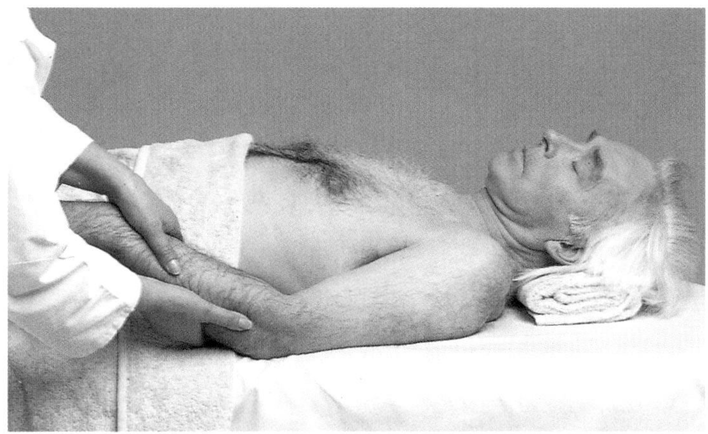

◁ **3** Now massage the forearms, using draining strokes to help the circulation flow back to the heart. To loosen and warm the muscles, use one hand after the other in a fanning motion, working from the wrist towards the elbow.

Anti-cellulite massage

Cellulite is detectable by the bumpy "orange peel" look of the skin on the fleshy areas of the body. It is caused by the accumulation of toxic deposits in the fatty tissues. Massage alone cannot rid the tissues of such deposits, but it can greatly assist the process.

Cellulite, which collects mostly on the hips, buttocks, and upper arms, is not specifically related to body weight and affects people of all sizes, especially women. It usually results from a sluggish circulation and poor elimination of toxins from the body, and in order to improve the condition it is necessary to use a combination of approaches. This includes a change of diet to cut down on the intake of toxins such as refined carbohydrates, caffeine, and alcohol. This should be combined with an increase in the daily intake of fresh vegetables and water. Regular exercise is also important, as it helps the lymphatic system rid the body of waste products.

The following massage programme, combined with the appropriate essential oils, should become part of a daily routine for six to eight weeks if you are to achieve a smooth and healthy skin. Mechanical massage instruments are also useful for this purpose.

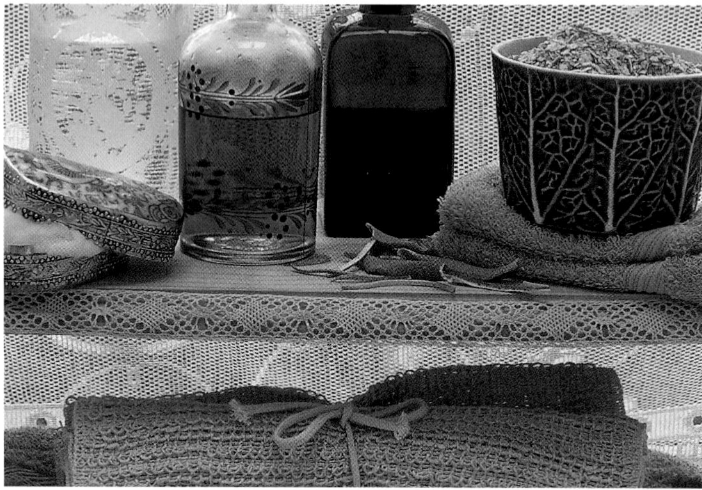

△ **Brisk rubbing with a rough cloth, or a loofah, before applying essential oils in a carrier lotion or oil, can help to disperse cellulite.**

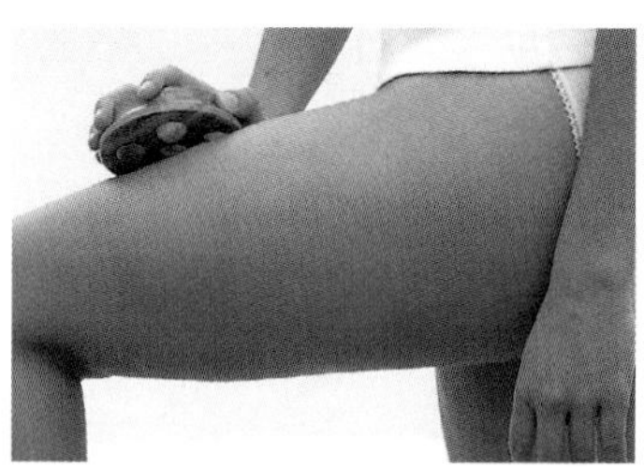

◁ **Hand-held massage instruments such as this wooden six-ball roller are ideal for making the circular pressure motions that help to smooth out cellulite spots on the thighs.**

self-help

A quick self-massage programme to stimulate the circulation and elimination process from fleshy cellulite areas can be carried out several times a day, such as when dressing and undressing, or after taking a bath or shower. Squeeze and knead the thighs and buttocks, and follow up with percussion movements.

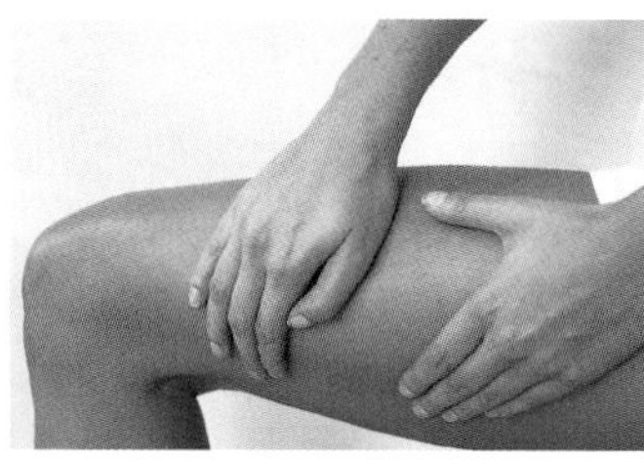

△ **1** After firmly rubbing in your prepared oil mix or lotion, move both hands alternately up the outside of the leg. Use a loofah or bristle brush if preferred.

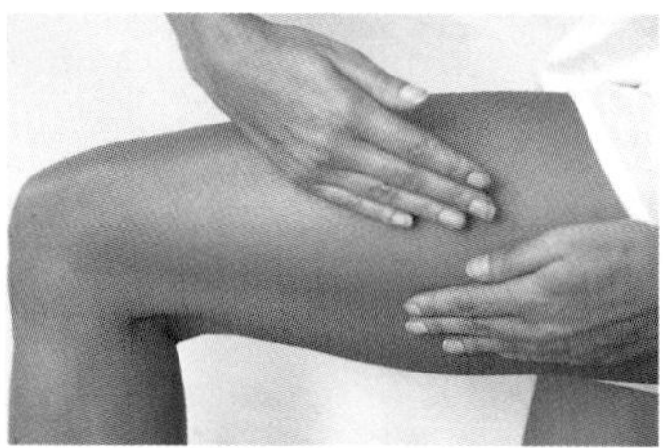

△ **2** Hack, cup, and pummel the thighs briskly to tone the area and revitalize the blood circulation. This stimulates the circulation and allows quicker penetration of the essential oils.

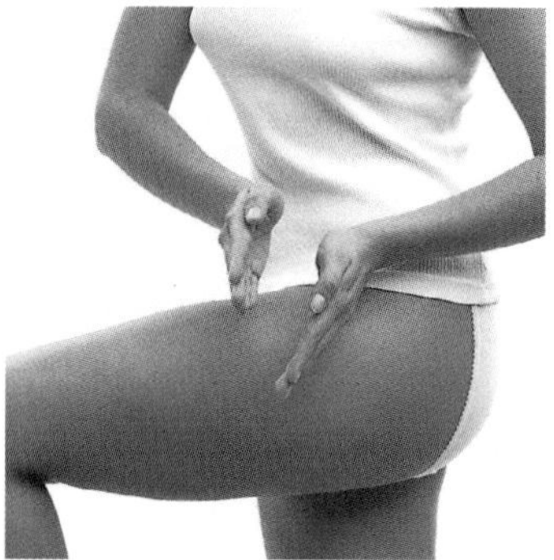

△ **3** Continue to work over the cellulite area using the heels of both hands alternately. Maintaining the firmness of the strokes, repeat step 1. Then repeat on the other leg.

cellulite reduction massage

If your partner is worried about cellulite, focus your attention on the problem areas of the thighs and buttocks during the massage. By using the correct sequence of basic massage strokes, you can soothe, tone, and stimulate the whole area, boosting the blood supply to the tissues and helping to increase the lymphatic drainage of waste products.

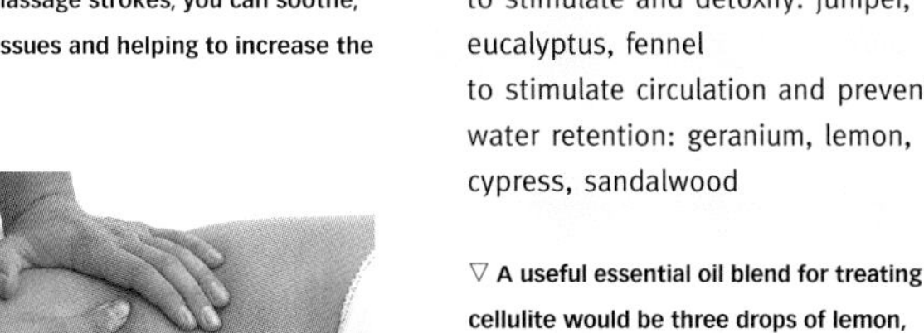

useful essential oils

to stimulate and detoxify: juniper, eucalyptus, fennel
to stimulate circulation and prevent water retention: geranium, lemon, cypress, sandalwood

▽ **A useful essential oil blend for treating cellulite would be three drops of lemon, two drops of geranium, two drops of fennel and one drop of cedarwood**

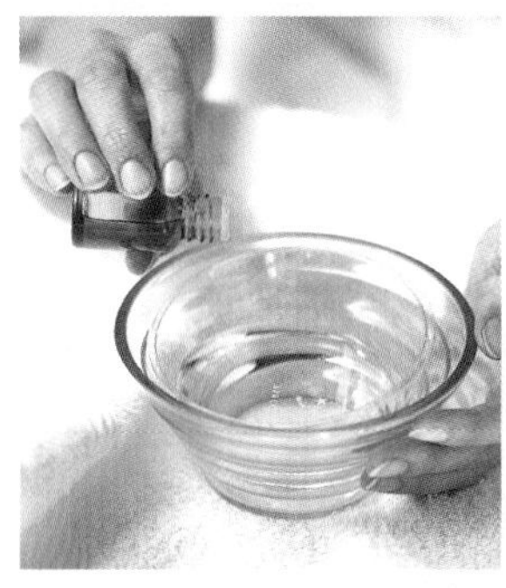

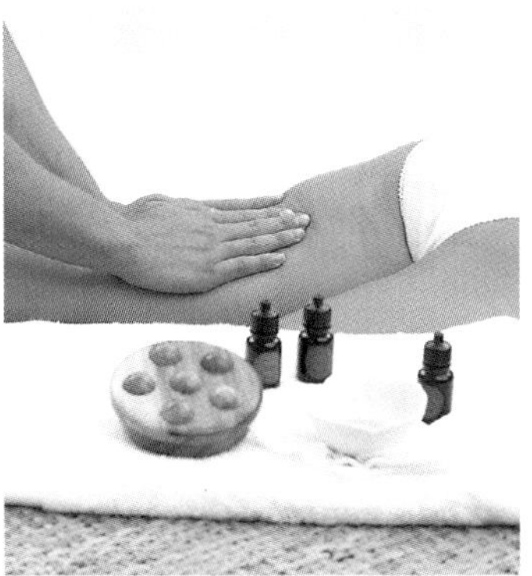

△ **1** Soothe, warm, and relax the thigh muscles with upward-flowing effleurage strokes such as integration and fanning motions. Repeat several times, always returning the stroke to the back of the knee by gliding your hands around and down the sides of the leg.

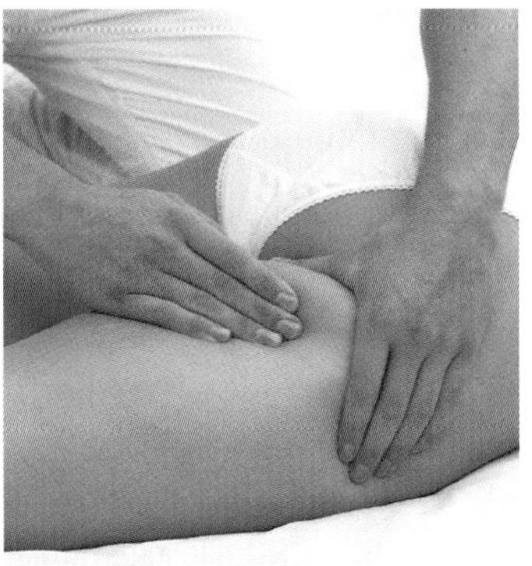

△ **2** The lifting, squeezing, and wringing action of kneading strokes enliven the thigh and buttock muscles and help the exchange of tissue fluids. Knead thoroughly over the whole area, following up with effleurage strokes to boost the circulation.

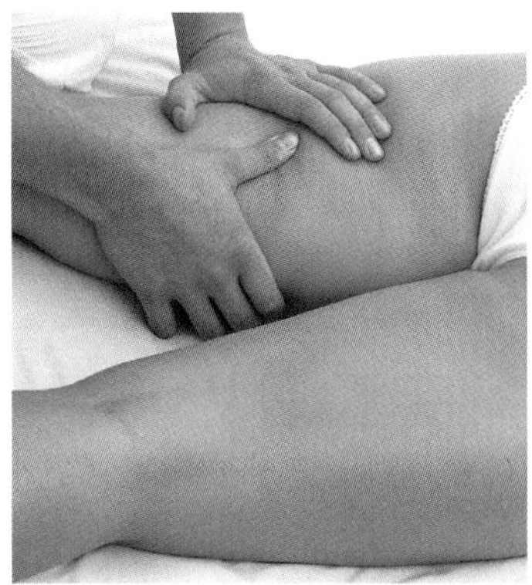

△ **3** Deep friction strokes help to break up toxic deposits. Sink and rotate your thumb pad on one area at a time, using your other hand to push the tissue towards the stroke. Follow these strokes with fanning motions to aid the elimination process.

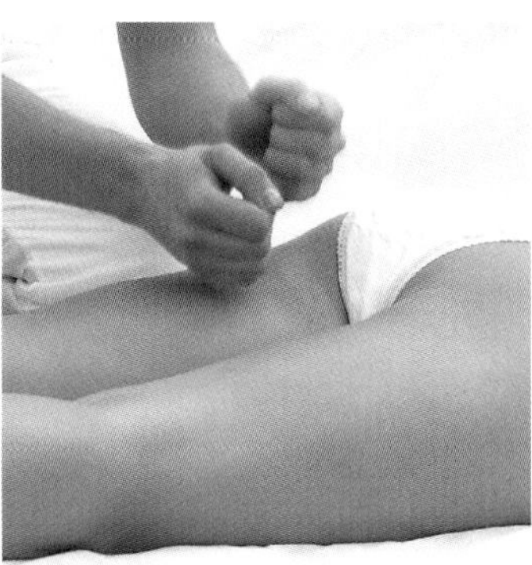

△ **4** Pummelling, hacking, and cupping strokes are ideally suited to cellulite conditions. Briskly strike the thigh and buttocks, one hand following the other in rapid succession, flicking off the skin at the moment of contact.

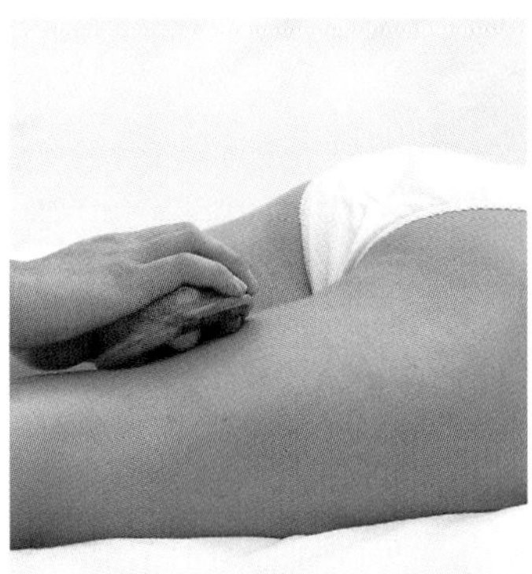

△ **5** Soothe the thighs and buttocks with effleurage strokes. If you have a mechanical roller, use it to add to the benefits of your cellulite massage by moving it in circular motions over the flesh. This is particularly effective when the skin is oiled.

Massage during pregnancy

Pregnancy is a time of great physical and emotional change for a woman, and it is important that, however busy, she finds the time to take good care of herself and her body. Massage is a soothing and beneficial therapy during this prenatal period, but because of complications and conditions that can occur, it is important to check first on its advisability with a family doctor or obstetrician.

Massage over the abdomen during the first three months of pregnancy should be avoided, and also in cases of toxemia, high blood pressure, severe water retention, and swelling of the hands, feet, and face. However, when a pregnancy is going smoothly, massage with the appropriate essential oils can help reduce feelings of nausea, minimize stretch marks, combat fluid retention, and alleviate the stress and strain on muscles and joints that result from carrying the extra weight.

staying comfortable

As the abdomen swells during pregnancy, it becomes more difficult to lie down comfortably. Use pillows to support the body, so lying on the side is comfortable while you massage.

▽ Place one pillow under the head, one alongside the body, to lean into, and one between the knees. This position enables you to make a gentle and relaxing contact hold, placing one hand over the abdomen and the other on the nape of the neck, holding for several moments.

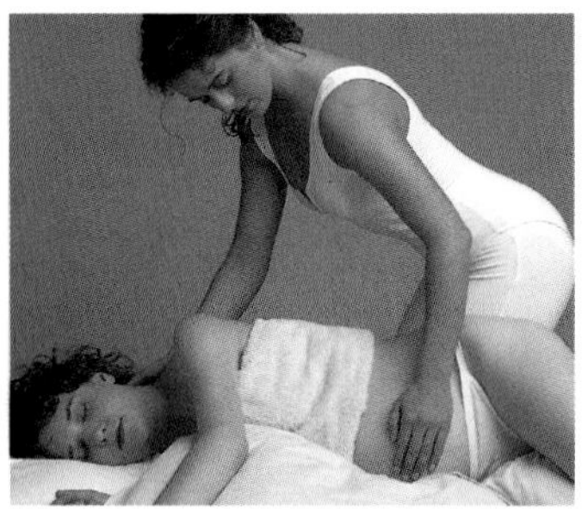

relaxing the shoulders

Loosening the shoulder joints takes the strain out of the upper back and chest, enabling the whole posture to carry the additional weight of the pregnancy.

▽ Encourage your partner to let go of the full weight of the arm and to allow you to control this passive movement. Place your right hand on the back of the shoulder to support it and, ensuring that the elbow remains flexed, begin to lift the arm by clasping the underside of the wrist and forearm with your left hand. Using your own forearm as a support, circle the arm forwards and back over the head. Do this three times with the movement coming from the shoulder joint. When you are ready to massage the other side of the body, rearrange the pillows and repeat this joint release movement on the right shoulder.

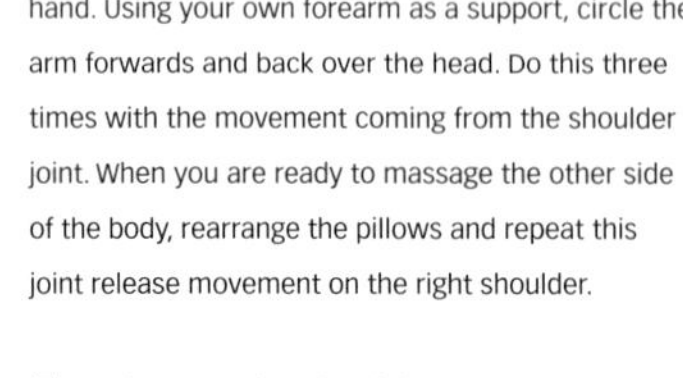

▽ **Gently massaging the abdomen in the morning and evening with a suitable oil blend can help to prevent stretch marks.**

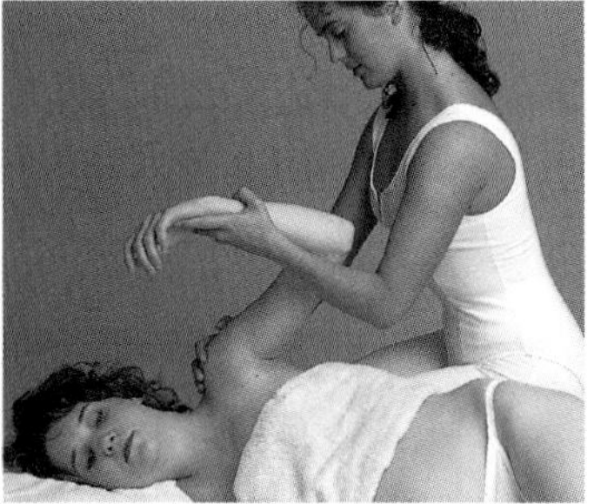

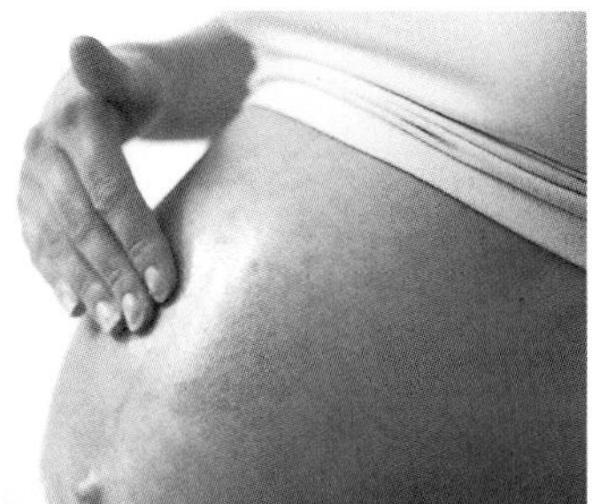

useful essential oils

The majority of essential oils are safe to use during pregnancy provided common sense is applied and the suggested guidelines given below are followed. Those to avoid are fennel, peppermint, and rosemary. A number of other oils stimulate bleeding, although no evidence has been found to suggest they endanger the foetus. However, they should be avoided during the first three months of pregnancy and after that used only in moderation if no alternative is available. These oils, which should be used with care and awareness, are as follows: chamomile, clary sage, cypress, jasmine, juniper, lavender, marjoram, nutmeg, peppermint, rose, and rosemary.

During the stages of pregnancy, some women can have a variety of uncomfortable symptoms, which may be eased by the following essential oils:

- for nausea: ginger, lemon, nutmeg, rosewood, sandalwood.
- to minimize stretch marks: mandarin and neroli or geranium and frankincense in a vegetable oil carrier enriched with carrot and wheatgerm oil.
- to combat fluid retention: choose from geranium, lemon, mandarin, neroli, and orange.

In the last few weeks of pregnancy geranium can be used to tone the whole reproductive system and assist the body in preparing for labour. During labour a variety of oils can be used for massaging the lower back. They include geranium, lemon, and neroli.

easing lower-back strain

Pregnancy can put a great deal of strain on the curvature of the lower spine and the surrounding muscles, sometimes leading to chronic back pain. While your partner lies sideways, focus your strokes on the lower back and buttocks, enabling the area to release its tension.

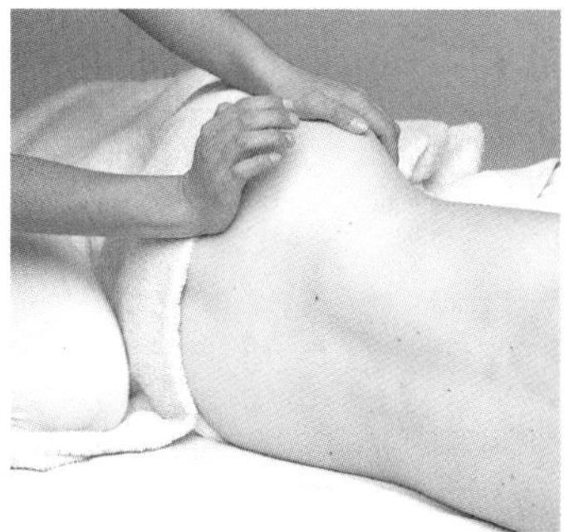

△ **1** Spread the oil over the lower back and buttocks, warming and soothing the muscles with soft effleurage strokes. Then begin to work deeper into the gluteal muscles of the buttocks, rotating the heel of your hand in one area at a time while supporting the hip with your other hand.

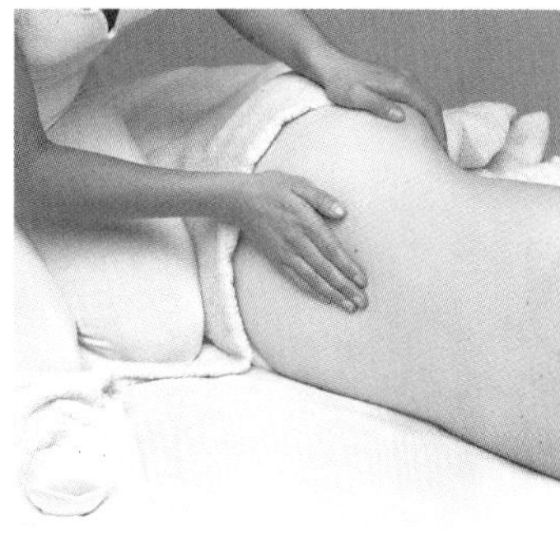

△ **2** It is common to see a pregnant woman instinctively placing a hand over the base of the spine to soothe away discomfort and pain. Bring relief to the muscles surrounding and covering the pelvic girdle and lower back with flowing, circular motions from the surface of your hand.

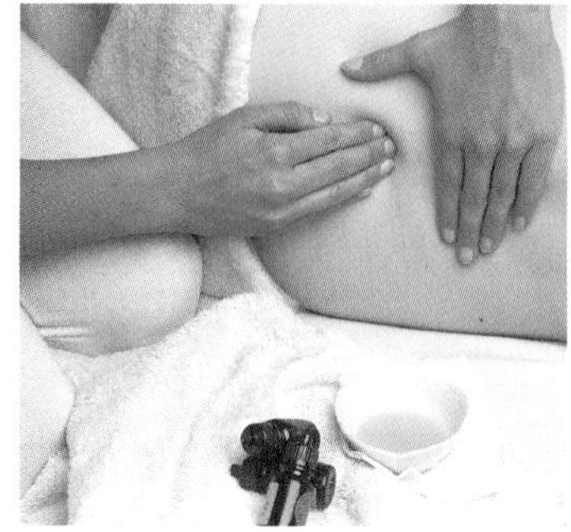

△ **3** Tiny, circular friction movements with your fingertips will deepen the remedial effects of your strokes on the lower back. Ease away tension in the muscle that covers the sacrum, the flat triangular bone at the base of the spine. Push the tissue towards the stroke with your other hand.

helping circulation

Smooth, flowing, and soft effleurage movements, stroking up over the feet, ankles, and legs, will help to boost circulation and to reduce the likelihood of puffy ankles and varicose veins, both common conditions during pregnancy.

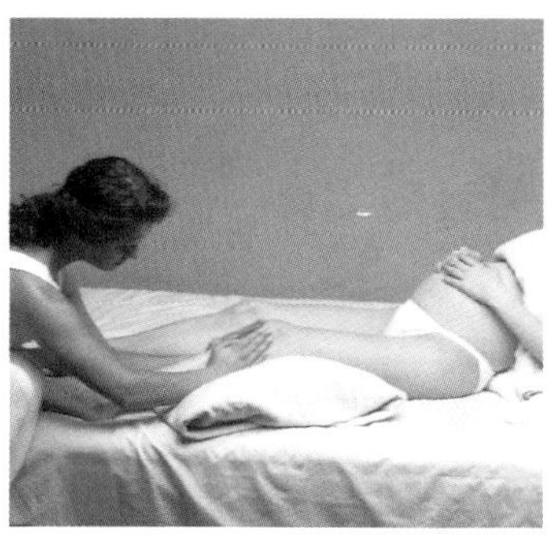

△ So that your partner can sit comfortably during a leg massage, the best position is usually to lean back on a mound of cushions or pillows, with a rolled-up towel to support the neck. It may also be helpful to place a pillow under the knees to take the strain off the thighs, buttocks, and lower back.

soft circles on the abdomen

After the first three months of a healthy pregnancy, you can gently massage the abdomen with the same soft circular motions that you would normally apply to the abdomen in a whole body massage.

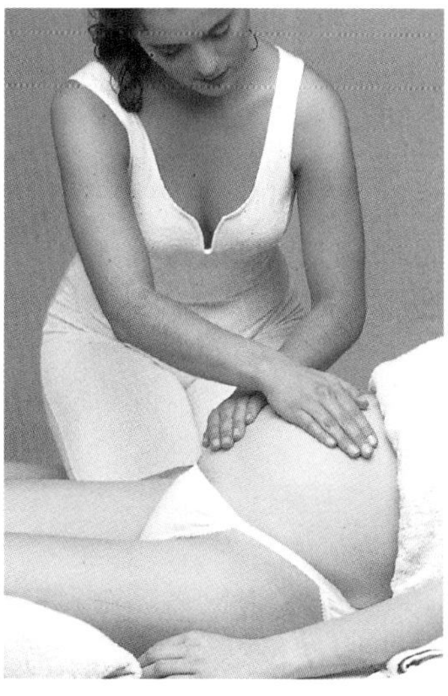

△ The warmth of your touch and the soporific motions will be very relaxing to both the mother and baby.

spine and shoulders

The best position for this massage is leaning into the support of a pillow while sitting astride a chair. This will allow the shoulders to fall forward so that the upper back becomes more open and available to touch.

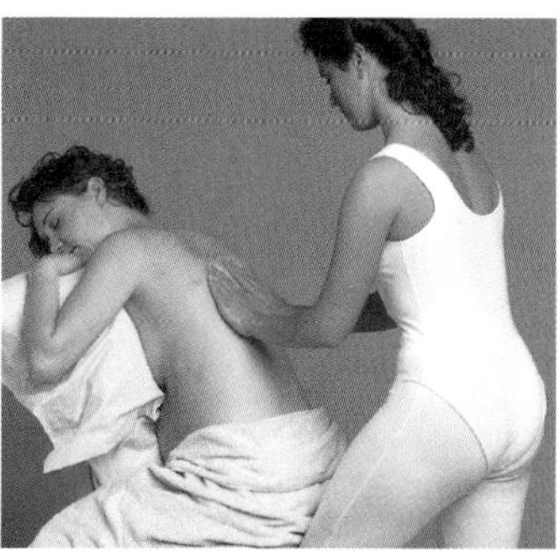

△ Begin with several effleurage integration strokes. Start at a point mid-back, and stroke your hands up each side of the spine before fanning out to encompass the shape of the upper back. When the muscles are relaxed, follow up with kneading on the shoulders and upper arms. Add some gentle friction with thumbs or fingers on tight spots beside the spine and shoulder blades. Complete with several more effleurage strokes.

Baby and child massage

It is never too soon to enjoy massage. In many parts of the world, it is customary for babies and children to be massaged by their mothers and carers. Touch is a natural expression of love, communicating warmth and security. In babies, massage helps strengthen the growing bond between mother and baby. Babies also enjoy it and usually sleep better afterwards. Children too are generally receptive to being massaged. The important thing to remember when working with babies or children is that their bodies are still developing, so they must be treated very gently.

massage for babies

When giving baby massage, focus on the chest and back, using light, smooth strokes. Do NOT massage the head, as this is too malleable. The best time to massage your baby is at the end of the day, before feeding and bathing. Although it may be the last thing you feel like doing, once you start you'll find it relaxes you both. If at any point you sense your baby is not enjoying the massage, then stop. The massage should only go on if you are both enjoying it.

preparation for massage

Make sure the room is warm, as babies feel the cold, and their body temperatures can drop quickly. Have a soft cloth or towel for your baby to lie on and, if you are using oil, warm it up before applying. In India, a blend of coconut and sesame oil is often used in baby massage, although almond, apricot or grapeseed oils are also suitable. Ideally the oil should be cold-pressed and organic.

▽ **All babies thrive on being cuddled and touched. Skin-to-skin contact is essential to the nurturing of an infant and an important part of the bonding process.**

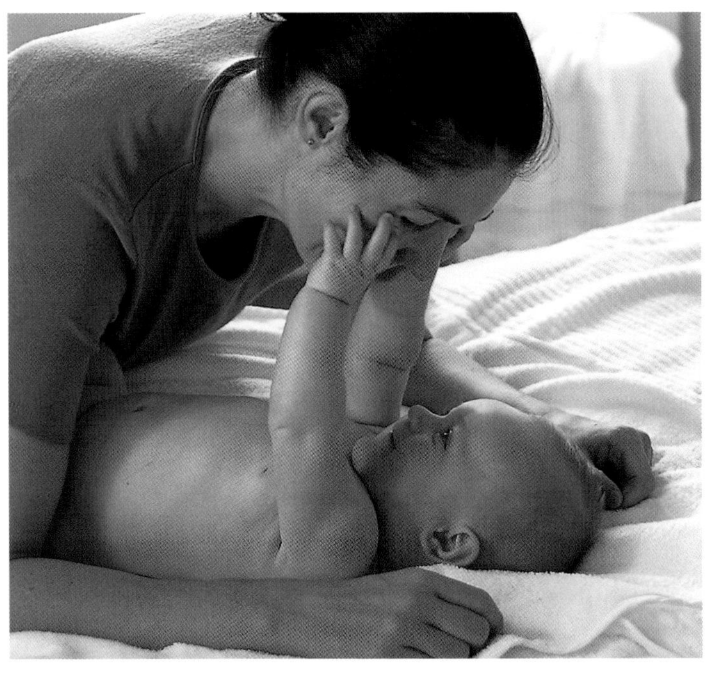

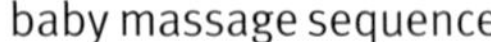

baby massage sequence

Begin the massage by playing and interacting with your baby. It is important to establish whether they are in the right mood.

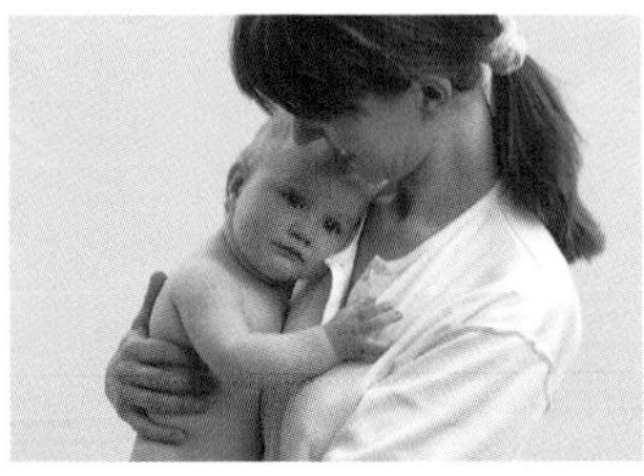

△ **1** Hold your baby close to you, so that the warmth of your body, the beat of your heart, and the rhythm of your breathing will comfort and soothe.

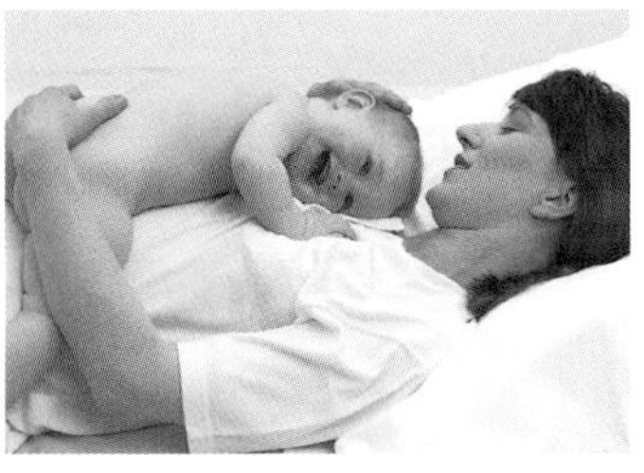

△ **2** Babies love to lie against the softness of your body. Place a soothing hand over the base of the spine, while gently stroking the head.

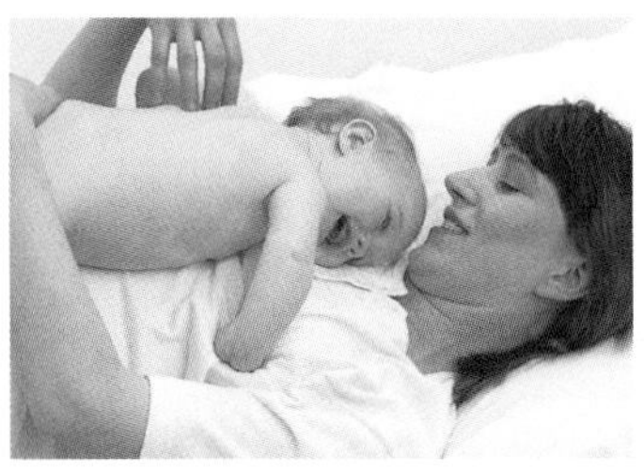

△ **3** Wriggling your fingertips softly up and down your baby's back will usually cause giggles of pleasure as the feather-like touches tickle and stimulate the soft skin.

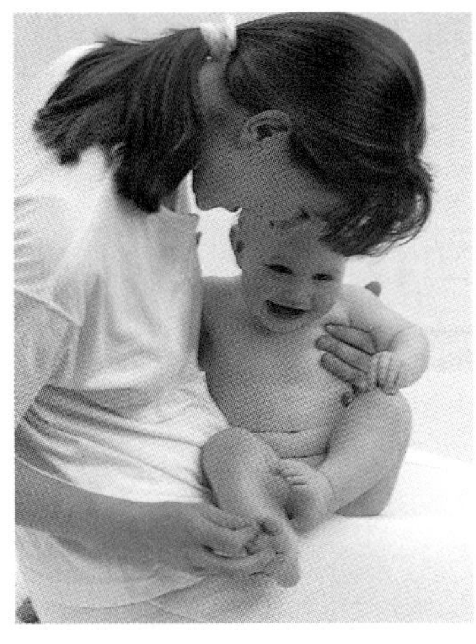

△ **4** Babies never seem to lose interest in their fingers and toes; use this fascination and wiggle and rotate the joints one by one.

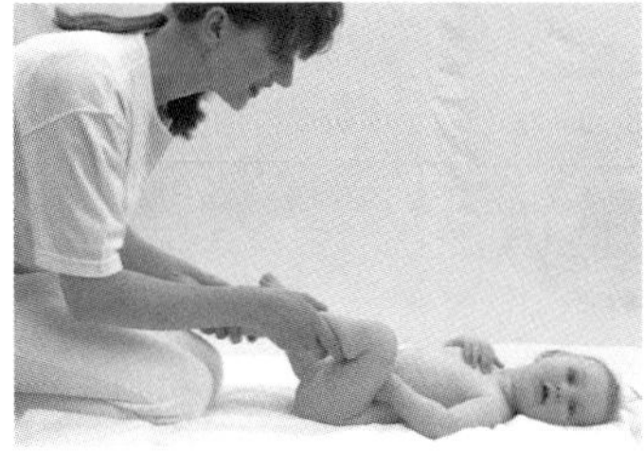

△ **5** Babies love a game of passive movements, where you move and gently flex the joints of the arms and legs. Bend one knee towards the body and then straighten out the leg. Carry out the same action on the other leg. Repeat several times.

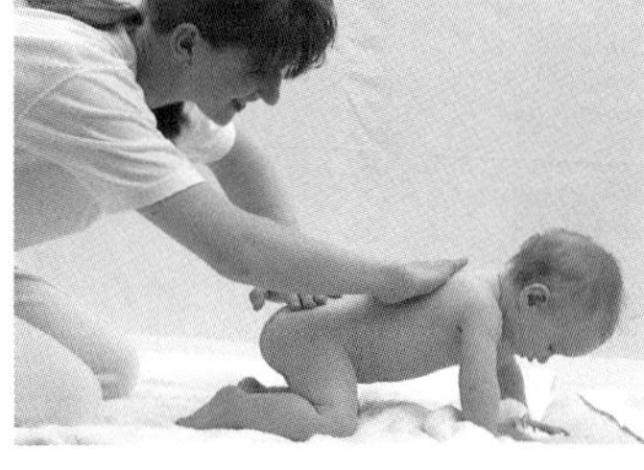

△ **6** If the baby can keep still for long enough, you can rub nourishing oil into the skin as you massage. Pour a little oil into your hands and rub it in gently, using circular movements on the baby's chest. Soft effleurage strokes on the back, such as a criss-cross motion and circles, will soothe and calm to complete the massage.

massage for children

When your massage partner is a younger child, you will probably need to find a higher chair, such as a kitchen stool, for them to sit on. You can also use cushions to raise the seat. Make sure the child's legs are not left dangling, by using cushions under their feet. Be flexible and creative in your approach, giving appropriate treatment when called for: you can offer a back or shoulder rub for instance if the child complains of a headache. A treatment that lasts between 5–10 minutes is usually sufficient. Be sensitive to how the child reacts, and don't try to persuade them to continue if they get restless or ill at ease.

When massaging teenagers, remember that they don't always welcome physical contact, and keep the massage as relaxed and informal as you can. Don't over-prepare the situation; take the opportunity when it comes to suggest a massage as part of your usual interaction with each other.

At the end of a massage with a young person, stand behind them and rest both your hands on their shoulders, with your fingers pointing forwards. Ask them to take a deep breath in and out. On the second out breath, gently press down with your hands and then let go. This helps to "ground" their energy and to release any remaining tension.

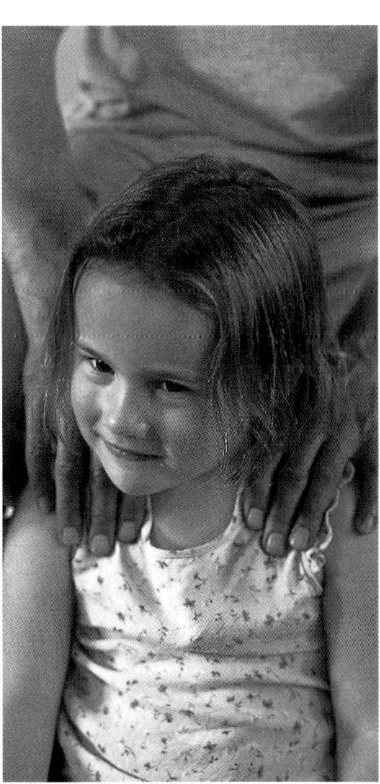

△ **You can do head massage on children from when they are aged about three years old. It is best to keep treatments light, short and sweet at this tender age.**

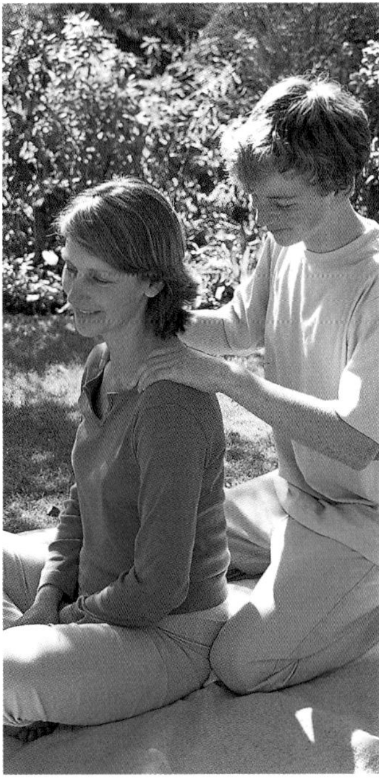

△ **Children learn by experience, and by receiving massage they can soon learn how to become proficient masseurs themselves, as happens in many parts of the world.**

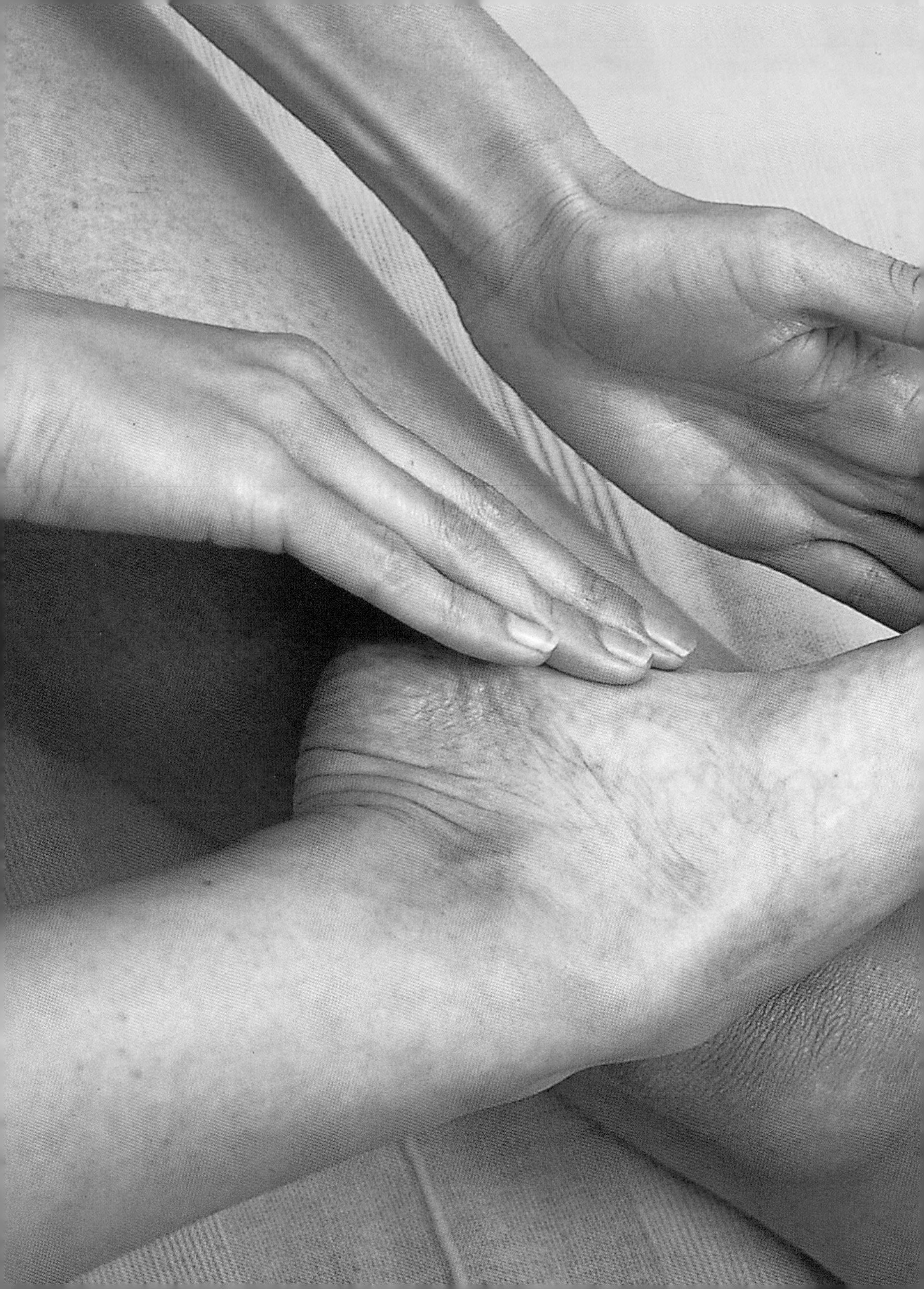

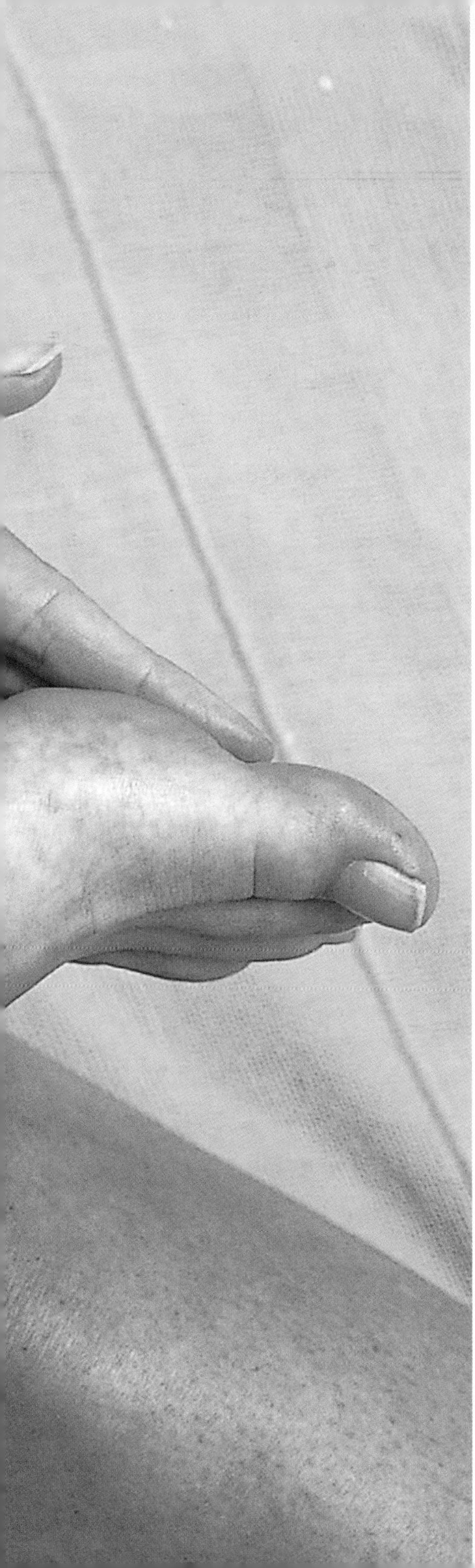

Part Four
Foot Massage

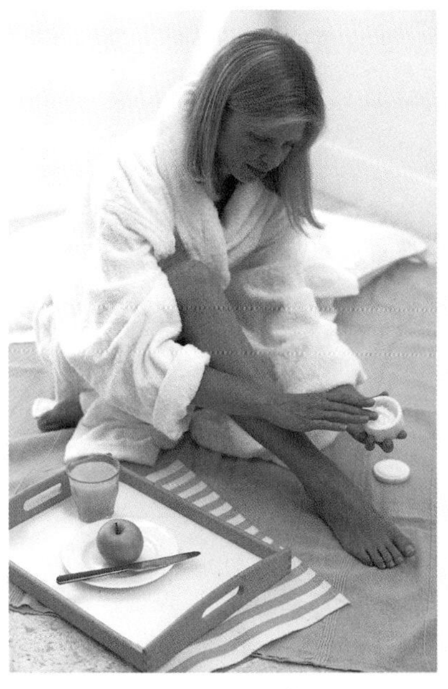

Introduction

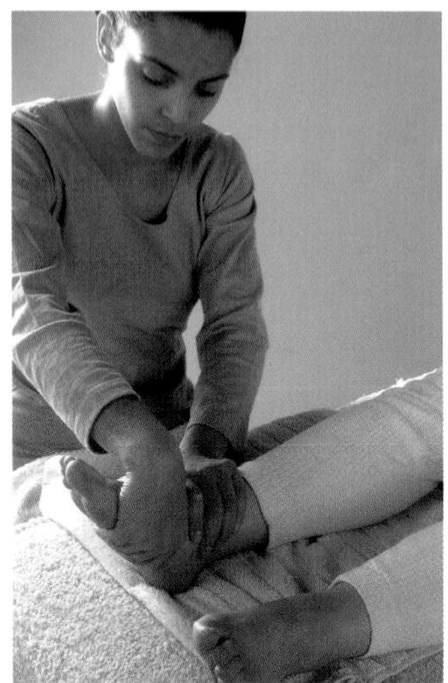

◁ **Foot massage techniques are broadly similar to those used on other areas of the body, with some minor adaptations.**

There are many different ways of working on the feet. It is worth spending the time to learn and assimilate fully the basic techniques of one method before going on to the next. That way, you will become adept at giving treatments.

therapeutic massage

Massage developed from our natural instinct to use touch to relieve pain: for example, we automatically rub an aching area, stroke a painful limb or hold an injured hand. Massage is highly relaxing to receive, making it an effective antidote to stress-related problems. For this reason, it has become very popular in recent years.

There are more than three thousand massage movements in common use, but you do not need to know more than three or four of them in order to give an effective foot treatment. The basic techniques are very easy to learn, and can be used at home to promote general well-being.

▷ **Essential oils can be added to foot creams for a healing and nourishing treat. Rose cream, for example, makes a superb moisturizer.**

Most massage practised in the West is Swedish massage. This was developed in the late 18th century by the Swedish gymnast, Per Henrik Ling. The therapy aims to bring about therapeutic results by manipulating the body's soft tissues: the muscles, skin, tendons and ligaments. A Swedish massage therapist will usually treat the whole body, but a treatment focusing on the feet and legs is also highly effective.

A variety of techniques are used, including stroking, kneading and fast rhythmic movements. These are delivered in a continuous flowing sequence. Oil is usually smoothed into the skin before and during the massage, to prevent pulling.

aromatherapy massage

In aromatherapy massage, oils extracted from plants are diluted in a carrier oil or cream, and then worked into the skin using Swedish massage techniques. The oils have delightful fragrances, which heighten the pleasure of the massage. They also have healing properties. Different oils can be used

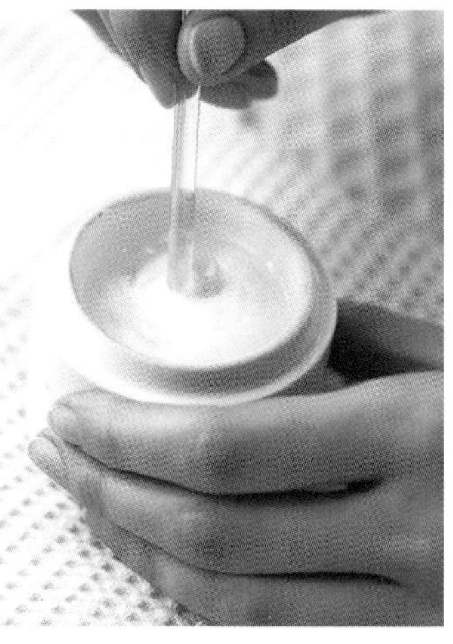

the birth of aromatherapy

Essential oils were originally used in cosmetics. In the early 20th century, a French chemist called Rene Maurice Gattefosse discovered by accident that the oils also had healing properties. While working in his laboratory he burned his hand. To ease the pain he plunged his hand into a bowl of cool lavender oil. He was impressed by the effect that it had in relieving pain, reducing redness and speeding up the skin's healing process. He went on to investigate the therapeutic properties of the oils, coining the term "aromatherapy" in 1928.

The use of essential oils combined with massage was developed by Margurite Maury, who worked with Gattefosse. She brought the idea of the everyday use of essential oils, to enhance health and well-being, to the wider world.

▽ **All kinds of plants yield essential oils with a wide range of healing properties. Roses are good for skin complaints.**

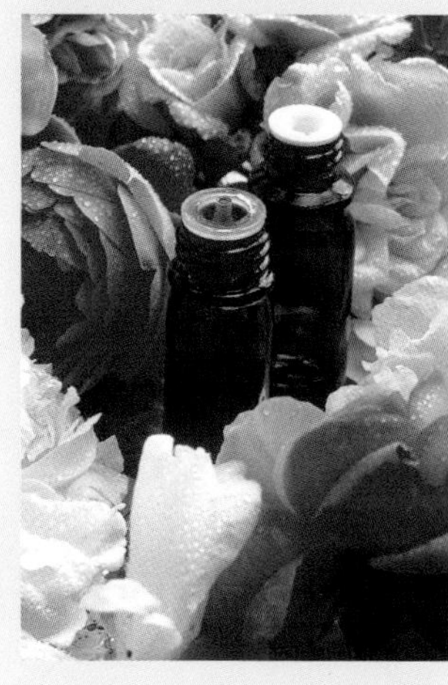

to induce feelings of calm, to boost energy or to treat minor ailments and relieve pain.

Aromatherapy foot massage is a highly enjoyable and easy way of using the therapy for self-help. You can also add the oils to baths and foot baths, incorporate them into nourishing creams for the feet and legs, or add them to compresses to help soothe away troublesome aches and pains. This book includes many suggestions for using essential oils, as well as recipes for luxurious or therapeutic aromatherapy home treatments.

reflexology

The therapy known as reflexology is a form of natural healing that focuses on the feet. It is based on the belief that there are specific reflex points on the feet which correspond to all the organs, systems and structures of the body. In reflexology, the points are stimulated by means of gentle finger-pressure. This helps to promote self-healing and good health in all kinds of ways.

Reflexology is a holistic therapy: it works on the whole person – the mind, body and spirit – rather than focusing on a specific condition or on a set of symptoms. Although reflexologists can detect specific problems, their main aim is to bring the whole body back to a natural state of balance and well-being. Over time, this can help to eliminate problems caused by specific disease.

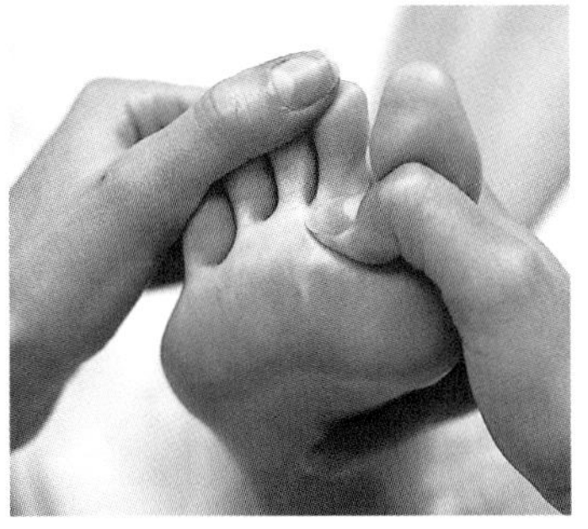

◁ In both reflexology and acupressure, specific points on the foot are said to correspond to other parts of the body. Pressing these points stimulates healing, and can be used to treat anything from a sore throat to digestive problems and backache.

acupressure

Like reflexology, acupressure is used to stimulate the body's own natural self-curative powers. Acupressure is similar to acupuncture in that they both use key energy points on the body – including many on the feet and legs – in order to bring about healing. However, while acupuncturists use special needles to stimulate the energy points, acupressure involves the use of finger or thumb pressure to work the points. Sometimes, the heels of the feet can be used for stimulation instead, or as well as, the fingers.

Acupressure can help to reduce tension, increase the circulation, and encourage the body and mind to relax. It helps to strengthen our resistance to disease, by relieving built-up stress and tension. One great advantage of the therapy is that it can be used as a quick fix, which can be done anywhere and at any time.

lymphatic drainage

One of gentlest forms of massage, lymphatic drainage massage works on the lymph system. Since lymph vessels are close to the surface, there is no need for heavy pressure. The body's lymphatic system is a secondary circulation system that supports the work of the blood circulation. The lymphatic system has no heart to help pump the fluid around the vessels, and therefore it must rely on the activity of the muscles to aid movement.

Lymphatic massage involves using sweeping, squeezing movements along the skin. The action is always directed towards the nearest lymph node: the main nodes used when treating the foot are located in the hollow behind the knee. Lymphatic drainage massage is hugely beneficial in helping to eliminate waste and strengthen the body's immune system.

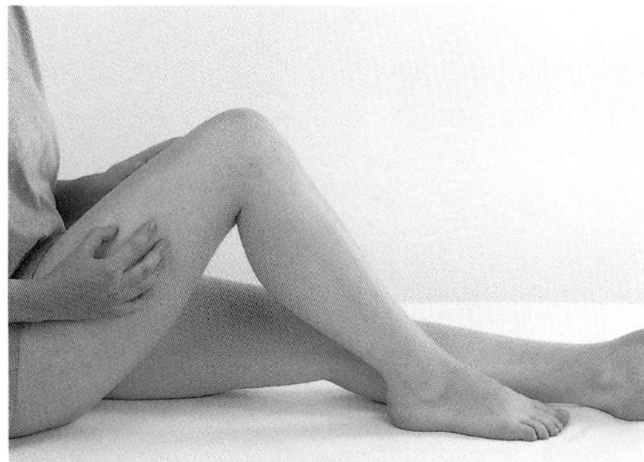

△ **1** To improve lymphatic drainage to the feet and legs, try a daily skin "brush", using your fingertips. Begin by working on the thigh. This clears the lymphatic channels ready to receive the lymph flood from the lower legs. Briskly brush all over the thigh from knee to top, three or four times.

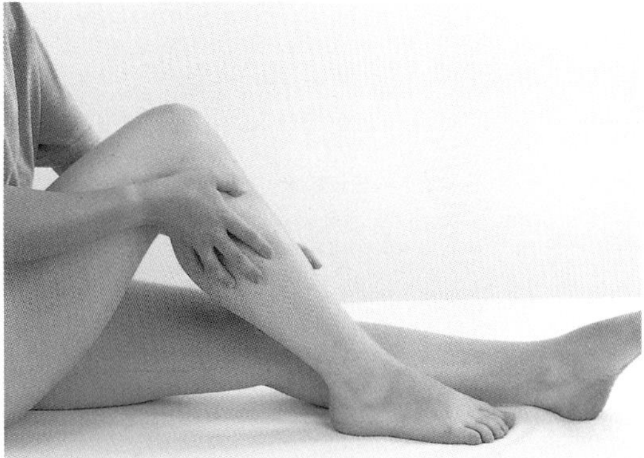

△ **2** Work on the lower leg in a similar way. Brush either side of the leg from ankle to knee, then treat the back of the leg. Follow this by brushing along the top of the foot, continuing up the front of the leg to the knee. Brush over each area twice more, making three times in total. Repeat on the other leg.

Caring for our feet

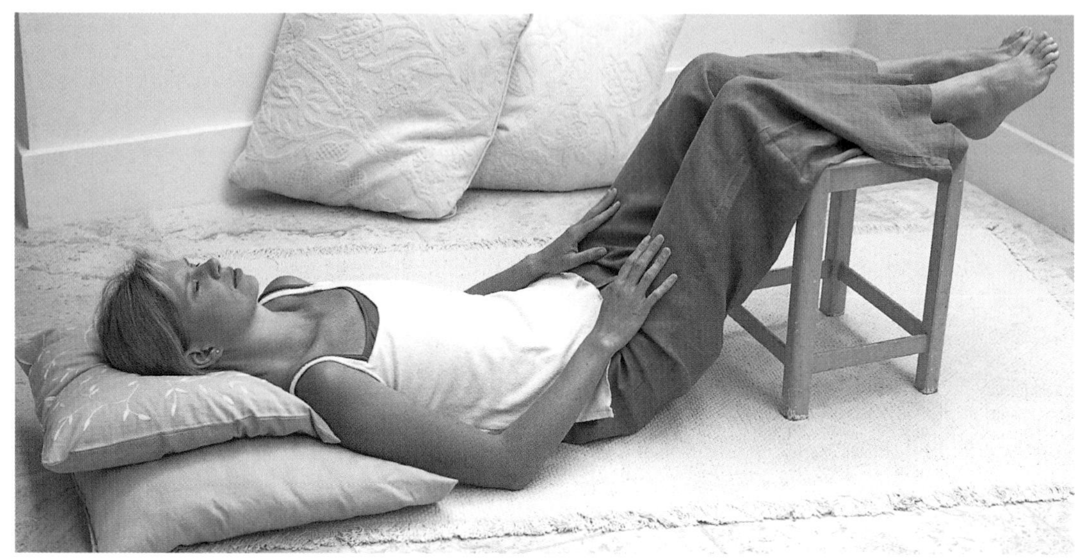

Our feet are an amazing construction. Twenty-six ingeniously shaped bones are bound together with bands of ligaments to form the basic structure of each foot. This structure is very strong – strong enough to bear the weight of our entire body – yet it is also remarkably supple. The foot is capable of making many intricate movements. Its dexterity is made possible through the actions of numerous small joints, as well as the 30 tiny muscles in the foot and by the leg muscles.

There are about 7200 nerve endings in each foot, making it highly sensitive to touch. The nerve supply comes from the sciatic nerve passing from the spinal nerve through the buttock and branching down the back and side of each leg to the foot.

helping the circulation

The foot is richly supplied with blood vessels. However, since it is at the end of the body and does not have its own pump, it depends on muscular activity of the foot and leg to keep a good return flow of blood to the heart. You can help the circulation in your feet by taking regular exercise – such as a daily walk – and by keeping your feet and toes moving whenever you are sitting down or standing up for long periods.

It is also beneficial to put your feet higher than your heart as often as possible – at least once a day. This will encourage any pooled blood to drain back down the legs. Regular massage will also keep the circulation of blood and lymph functioning well. This helps to remove any toxins from the feet, and also brings nutrients to them.

It is particularly important to put your feet up when you are pregnant, since you are particularly susceptible to varicose veins at this time.

pamper and protect

Our feet take a lot of punishment, and most of us take them for granted. Having a regular foot-care session can help to keep your feet healthy and prevent any problems

△ **Take time every so often to rest your feet above heart level. This helps to relax the muscles here and can be very soothing. It also lets blood drain away, which can help to prevent varicose veins and swollen ankles. Keeping fresh blood circulating will also help to nourish the skin.**

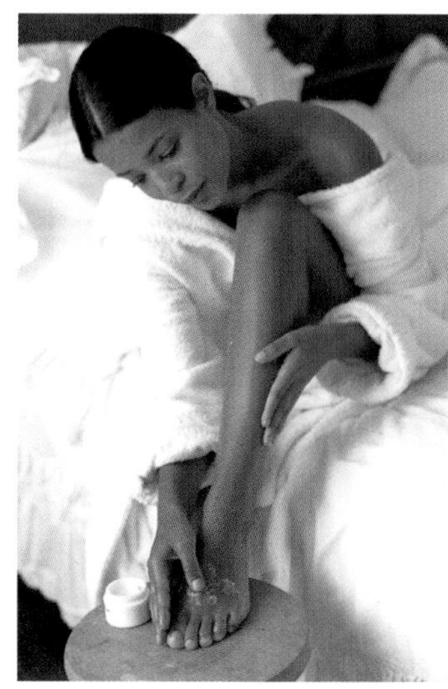

▷ **Pamper your feet on a regular basis; they take a great deal of punishment and richly deserve as much time and attention as you can manage.**

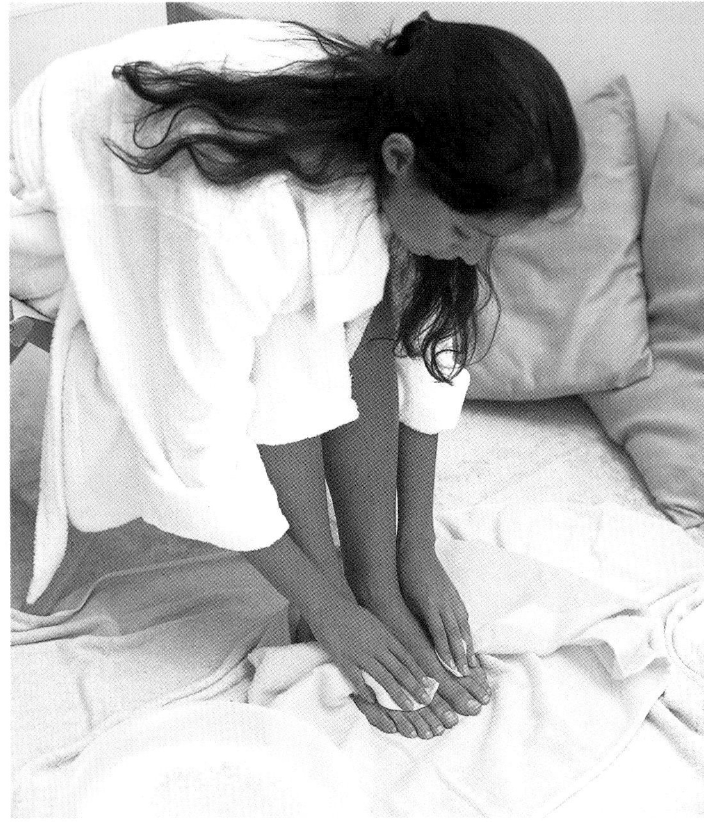

△ **Drying your feet thoroughly is an important part of good foot care and foot health. Special attention should be paid to drying the areas between the toes – allowing moisture to build up here can lead to problems such as athlete's foot.**

from arising. For a simple pamper, try soaking the feet for ten or fifteen minutes in warm water. Remove any hard skin with a pumice stone, then cut your toe nails. Always cut straight across rather than trying to shape the nail. This will help to prevent ingrowing toenails, which can be very painful. Moisturizing your feet daily will help to keep the skin soft and supple.

It is a good idea to visit a chiropodist for a professional pedicure at least twice a year. You should also act quickly if you notice flaking skin between the toes (athlete's foot), or a dark mark on the sole (a verucca) to prevent these problems from spreading. Seek medical advice if you develop any unusual symptoms on the feet.

the right shoe

You should avoid wearing high-heeled shoes since these distort the natural shape of the feet. The ideal shoe is not flat, but has a low heel.

Wearing badly fitting shoes puts unnecessary pressure on the feet, and it may lead to aching, blisters or bunions which are unsightly and can be painful. The idea that new shoes should hurt is a myth. Correctly fitting shoes should be comfortable from the first time of wear; they should not need to be "worn in".

Always try to buy new shoes in the afternoon. Our feet tend to swell slightly as the day progresses, and whenever they become hot. Shoes that you buy in the morning may feel tighter later in the day, and may restrict the blood and lymph flow to our feet and legs.

It is quite common for one foot to be slightly larger than the other. It is therefore important to try both shoes of the pair before making a purchase. Always buy the size that fits your larger foot, and buy foot pads or insoles, if necessary, to create a more comfortable fit for the smaller foot.

foot health

Do not massage anyone's feet if they have athlete's foot (tinea pedis) or a verucca, since they are both contagious. For self-massage of these problem areas, add 3 drops of essential oil of thyme to 5ml (1 tsp) of carrier oil. Vitamin E oil is therapeutic for these ailments.

▽ **The healthy foot is one that displays no signs of infection, skin breaks or ingrowing toe nails. Ideally the inner arch will be raised slightly off the ground as this is used as a shock absorber while walking and running.**

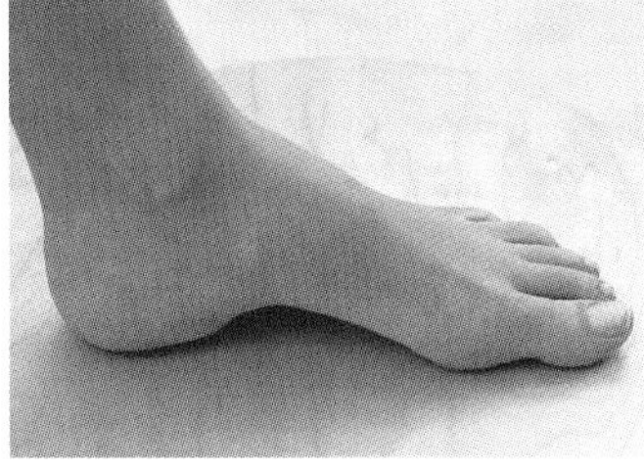

shoe-related allergies

Many chemicals are used in the adhesive, dye, rubber, tannins or metal commonly found in footwear. A small number of people suffer from allergic reactions to their shoes. It would be almost impossible to produce a shoe that is allergen-free because different people are allergic to different substances.

If you experience redness, itching or soreness in the feet, consult a doctor. He or she will be able to refer you to a dermatologist (skin specialist) if an allergy is suspected.

The dermatologist will usually perform a skin test to identify the substance or substances causing the allergy. You can then seek out footwear that is free of this particular chemical. If staff at the store cannot help, it is usually possible to check this information with the manufacturer.

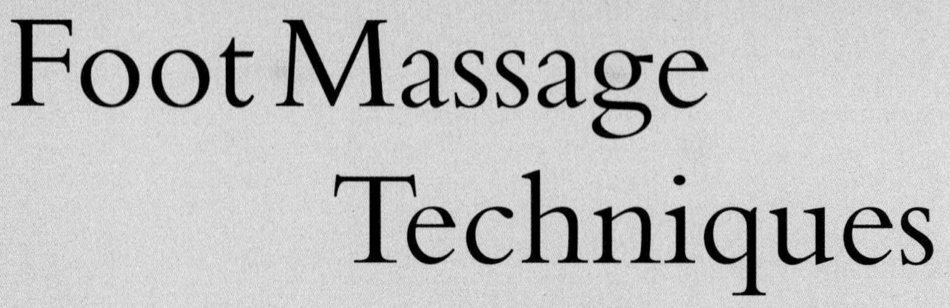

Foot Massage Techniques

Anyone can learn to give pleasurable foot treatments to themselves and others. This chapter covers the basic techniques of massage, aromatherapy and reflexology, and offers some classic types of routine. There is also advice on how to prepare for a treatment – from warming up the hands to creating a healing atmosphere at home.

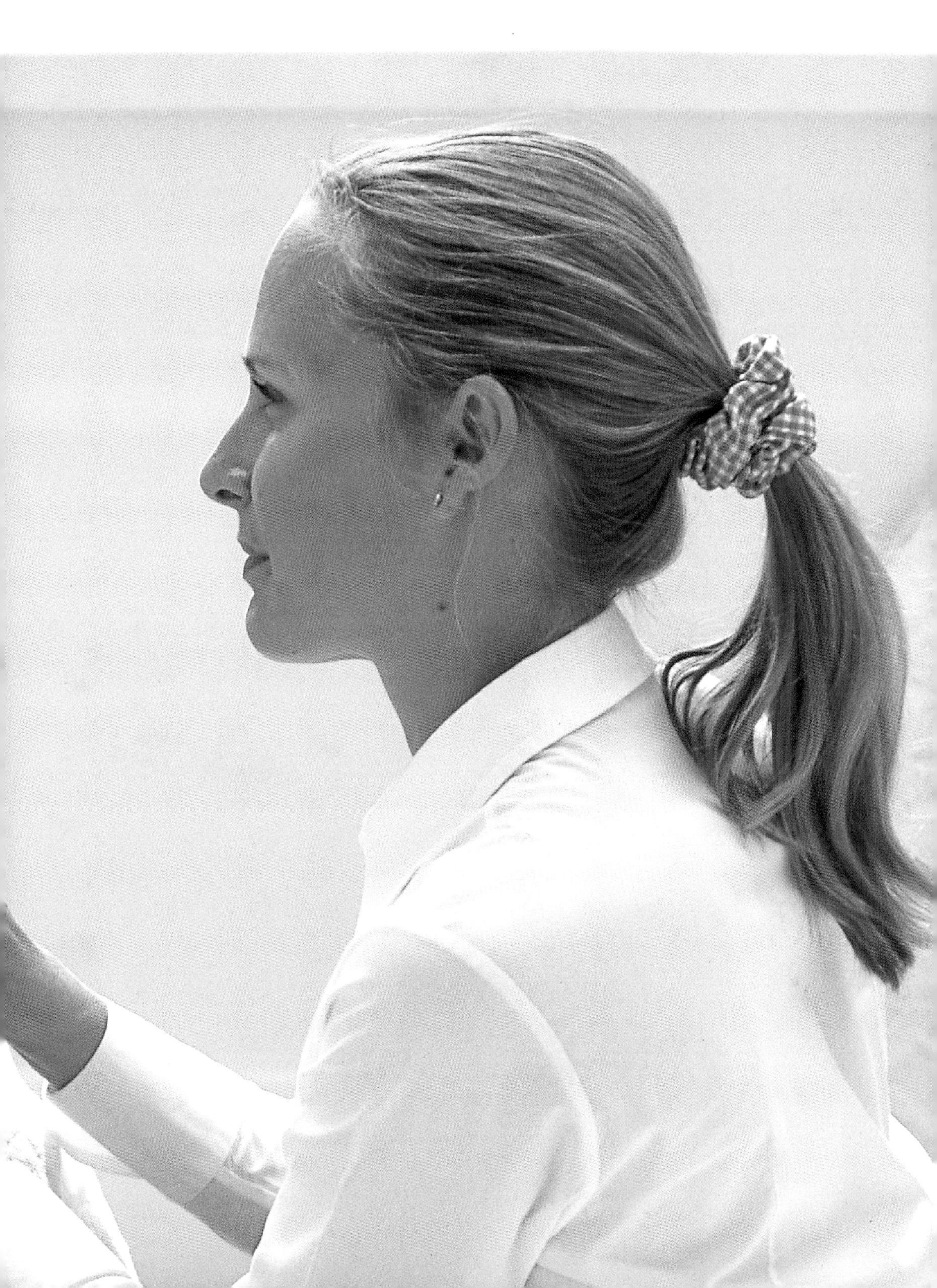

Foot massage strokes

You can give an excellent massage using just a few simple actions. Each movement can be performed twice or more, and your favourite few movements could be done three, even four times.

When you are learning new massage techniques, it is a good idea to try them out on yourself first. Practise until you become familiar with the different actions involved, and see how the movement feels when you vary the pressure. Always pay full attention to what you are doing. You will find that, if your attention wanders, your touch is unlikely to feel good. Feel your way into your hands and focus on the sensations here.

It is often helpful to massage without talking, except for when you are asking for or giving feedback. It is also much easier to concentrate on exactly what you are doing if you are quiet, and this will also help both you and the recipient to relax.

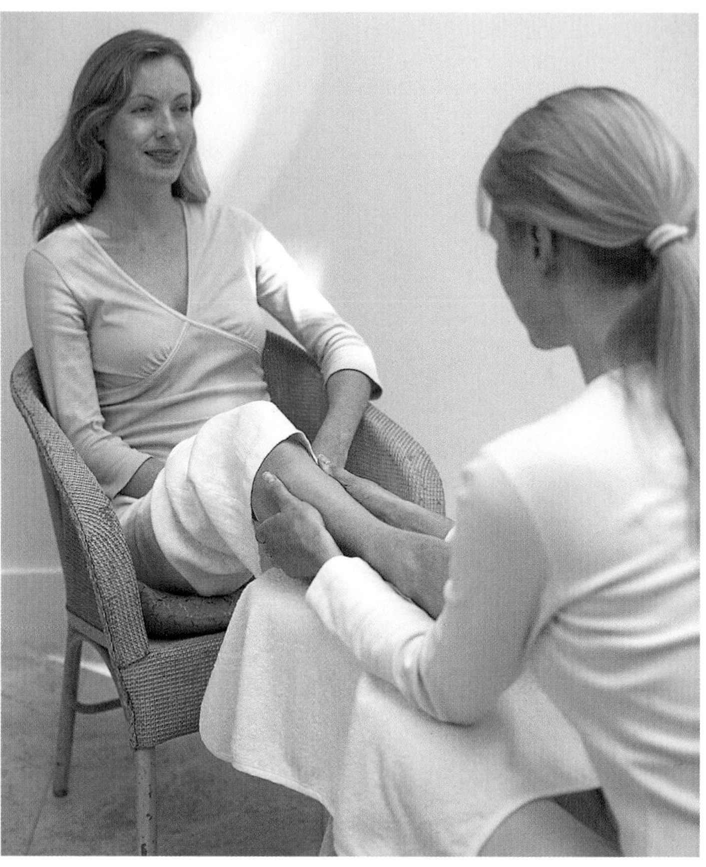

▷ If you are massaging someone else, make sure that he or she is comfortable, and that you are too. You will find it easier to concentrate if you maintain a good posture. Keep your back straight and your head balanced throughout the massage; imagine your head is connected to the ceiling and being pulled upwards. This posture will help you to use your body weight, giving depth to your movements.

getting feedback

People like different pressure. When you work on yourself, you get instant feedback about whether you are working at the correct level of firmness. When you work on other people, you have to monitor their reactions. Ask for feedback, but don't assume that you are getting it right just because the person doesn't tell you otherwise. Be aware of the person's general posture – if he or she is tense, you may be pressing too hard.

Always keep the pressure lighter on the top of the foot. The bones are closer to the surface than those on the sole, so it is easier to cause bruising and pain in this area.

massage aids

There are many aids now available for massage in general, and some can be suitable for use on the feet. Most masseurs say that it is better to use your hands if you are treating another person. However, some gadgets may help with self-treatment.

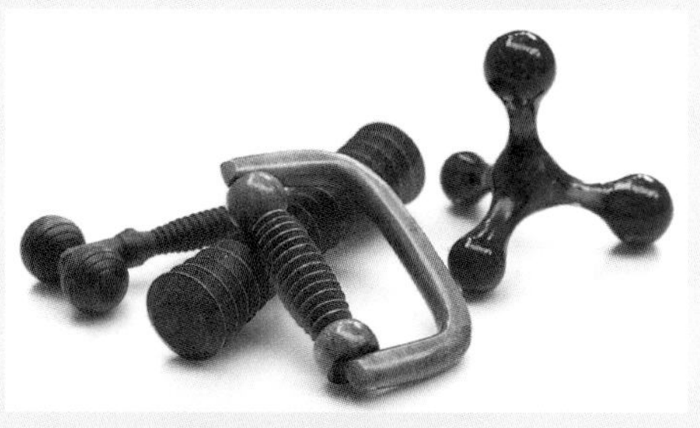

△ You may need to experiment with a few different massage aids to see what suits you best.

basic strokes

Always pay equal attention to both feet when you are massaging. You should start on the right foot, then move on to the left. The right side of the body is said to relate to your physical self; treating this one first will begin to relax muscle tension throughout the body, and will also boost the circulation and elimination processes. Treating the left foot will work on a physical level, too, but it will also help to release built-up tension in the sensitive emotional inner being.

▽ **Thumb circling**

Place the thumbs on the foot, one slightly higher than the other. Then, use the pad of alternate thumbs to massage the area all over, making small rotational movements. This movement is used for fleshy areas. It is good for the circulation and for warming the muscles of smaller areas.

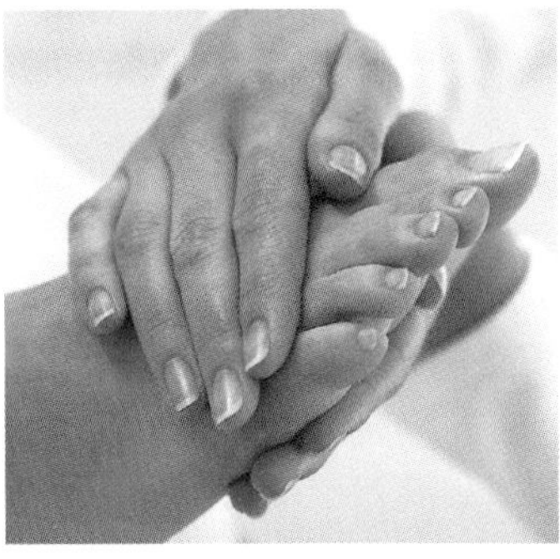

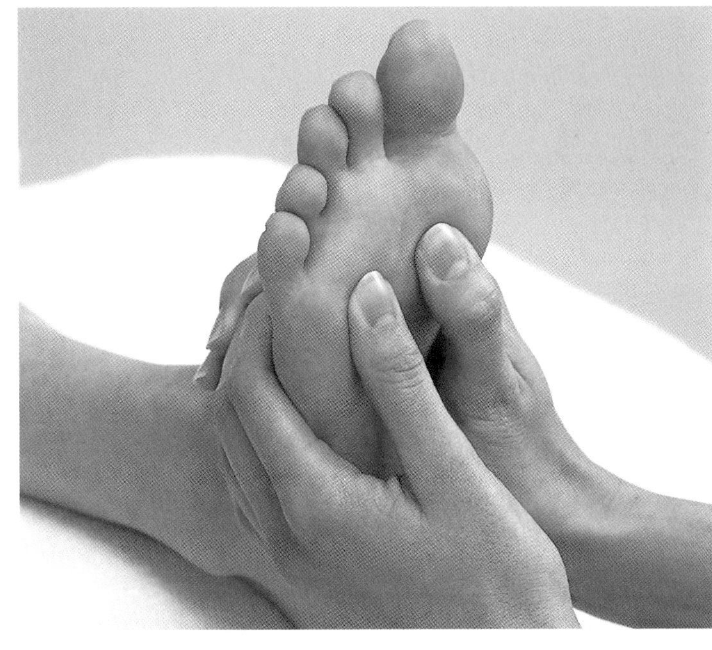

△ **Effleurage (stroking)**

Place your hands across the foot at the base of the toes. One hand should be on top and one below so the foot is sandwiched in-between them (sandwich hold). Slide your hands down the foot from the toes to the heel, then up from the heel to the toes. Repeat this movement twice more, or until the person feels relaxed. Use light pressure to start with, increasing it as you go. You usually start and finish a routine with effleurage, and it is also a good linking technique.

▷ **Knuckling (kneading)**

Make your hand into a fist. Press into the sole of the foot, using the flat part of the fingers from the knuckle to middle joint. Turn the fist as you press, so that you make a slight rotational movement. Cover the whole area from heel to toe. This movement is good for warming up the muscles, opening up the foot and releasing tension.

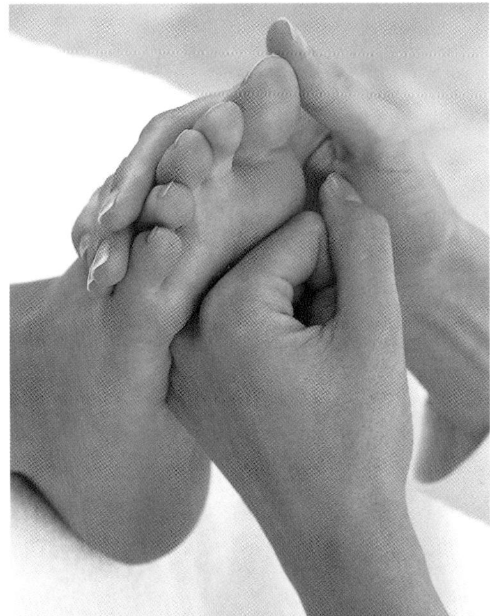

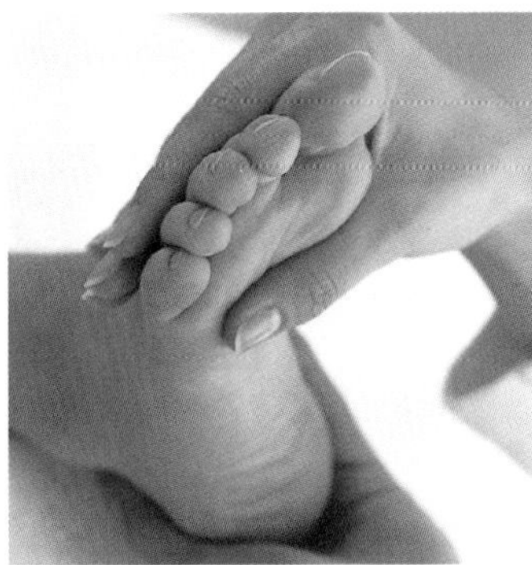

△ **Foot rotation**

Wrap your fingers around the top of the foot near the toes, and use your other hand to cup the heel. Slowly rotate the foot clockwise, then anticlockwise. Repeat, so you have rotated the foot in each direction twice. This movement loosens the ankle joint. It is important that you do not push the ankle further than its limits. Take particular care if treating someone with arthritis, diabetes or a foot disorder.

Spreading

▽ **1** To spread the top of the foot: place the thumbs and the heels of your hands on top of the foot, letting your fingers curl round to hold the sole. Pull the thumbs across the top of the foot towards the edges, keeping your fingers in position. Then return your thumbs to the starting position.

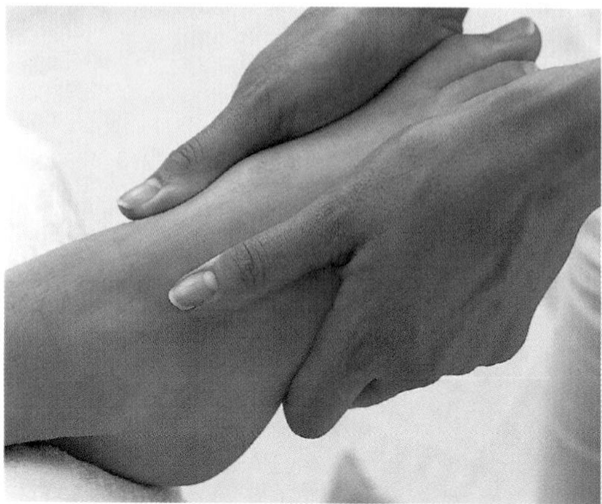

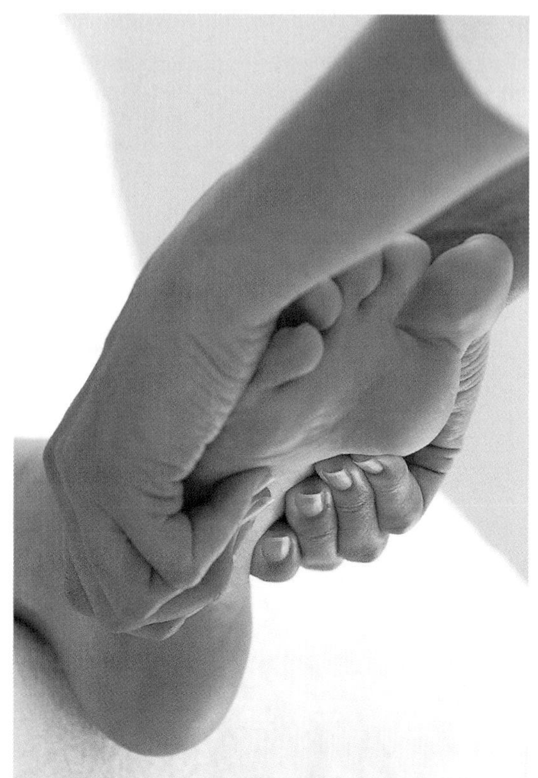

▷ **2** To spread the sole of the foot: keep your hands in the same position as before but reverse the action, so that you pull your fingers to the edges of the sole, leaving the thumbs in position. Start near the toes and work down the foot to the heel. This action works in a similar way to knuckling. It stretches the muscles and brings oxygen and nutrients to the area by improving blood flow.

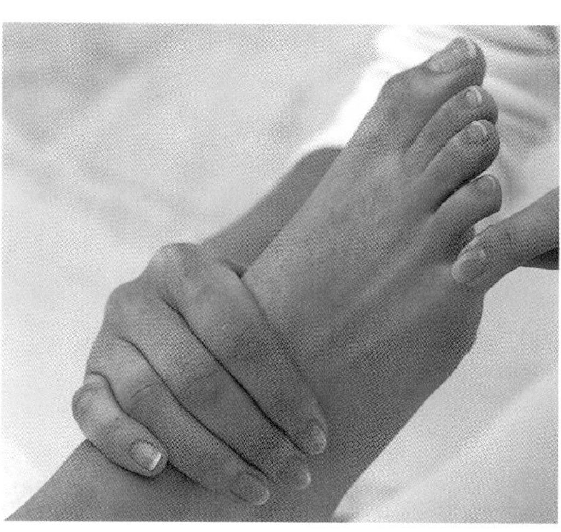

△ **Toe rotation**

Support the foot by placing your fingers across the top of it and curling your thumb underneath. Use your thumb and forefinger to grasp the base of the big toe. Gently rotate the toe in a clockwise direction, then anticlockwise. Work each toe in turn, ending with the little toe. This action helps to mobilize the joints and also improves the supply of nutrients and oxygen to the toes. Work gently, and take extra care if treating someone with arthritis.

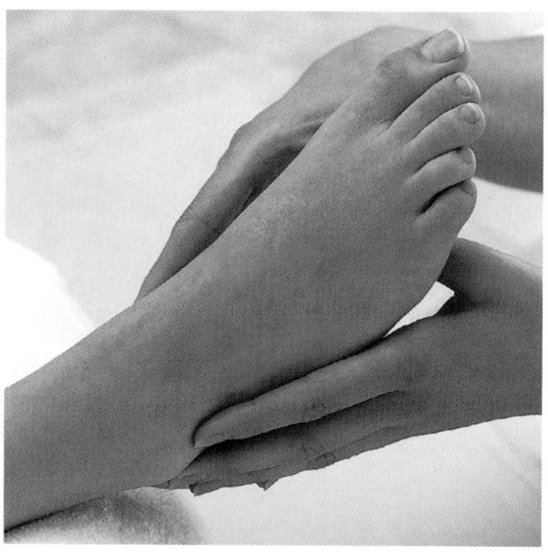

△ **Circling the ankle**

Circle around the inside and outside of the ankle bone at the same time, using the pads of your fingers. You can work quite strongly, provided that the person has no problems in this area. Work in a clockwise direction, then in an anticlockwise one. This movement helps to relax the ankles and improve mobility.

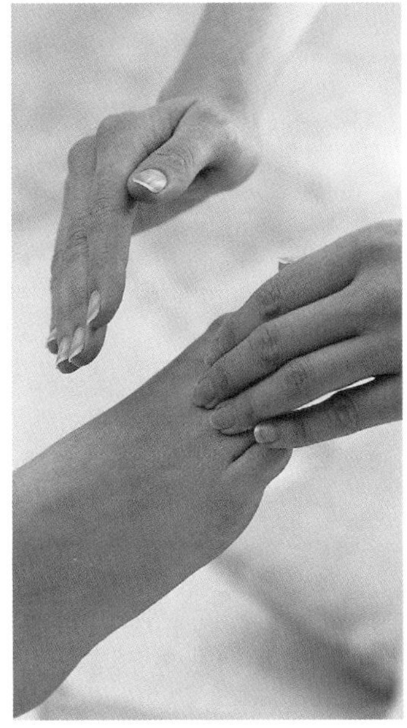

△ **Percussion (tapping)**

1 Use the tips of your fingers to tap all over the top of the foot. Work using alternate fingers. Do not tap too hard: the action should be pleasurable, and not a shock to the system. You can also use this movement on the sole of the foot.

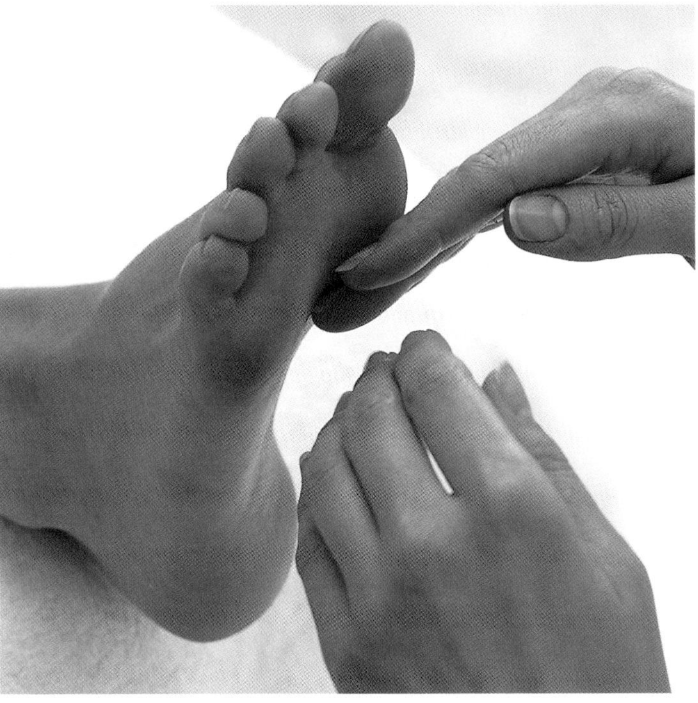

△ **2** To perform percussion on the sole: use the back of the hands to strike the sole lightly all over. This action is stimulating; it helps wake up the foot and increases the circulation. It is a good movement to do if the foot is cold. Be gentle if the person has arthritis, diabetes or a foot disorder.

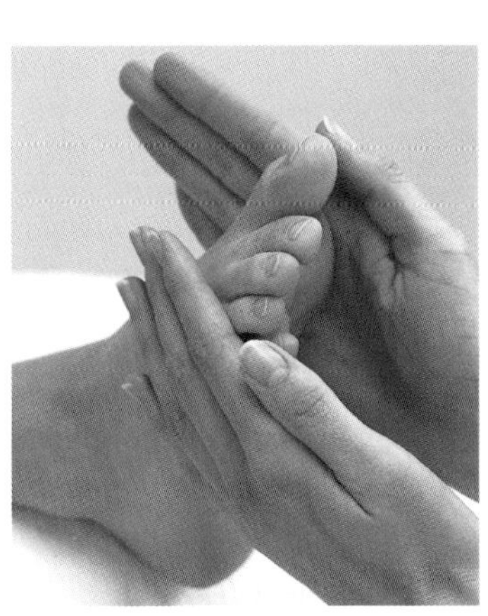

△ **Push-pull**

Place one hand on the outside of the foot and the other on the inside, so that the foot is gently wedged in-between them. Using the heel of the hands, pull one side towards you and push the other side away. Repeat, but this time reverse the action. Do this push-pull action twice more. This is a general movement which helps to open and relax the foot.

baby massage

Foot massage is a wonderful way to soothe and give pleasure to your baby. Always work very gently, massaging one foot at a time. As with adults, do the right foot first, then go on to the left. Try the following routine, or make up your own variation.

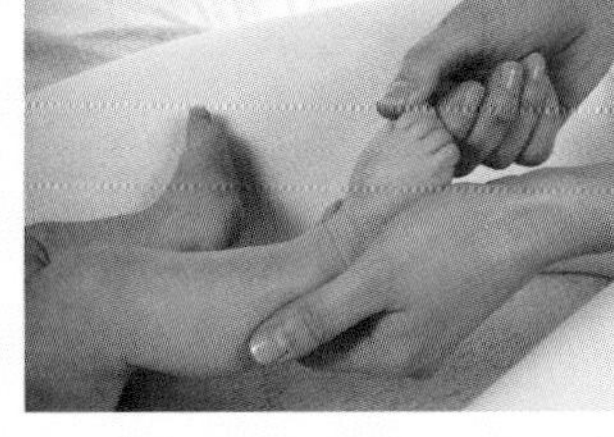

△ **Babies love to be touched – in fact, they cannot thrive without it.**

- Cup your left hand around the baby's right ankle, holding the foot in a confident way. Use the tips of your fingers to stroke the sole from heel to toe. Then stroke the top of the foot from toes to ankle. Do as many strokes as are needed to cover the area.
- Use two fingers to stroke the inner side of the foot, working from the big toe to the heel.
- Use two fingers to stroke down the outside edge of the foot in the same way.
- Use your right thumb to stroke across the sole, just below the ball. Start from the big toe side and stroke to the outer edge. Do this three times.
- To finish, gently hold the base of the big toe between your thumb and first finger. Gently stroke down to the tip of the toe. Repeat on the rest of the toes, ending with the little one. Then do the whole routine on the left foot.

Using oils

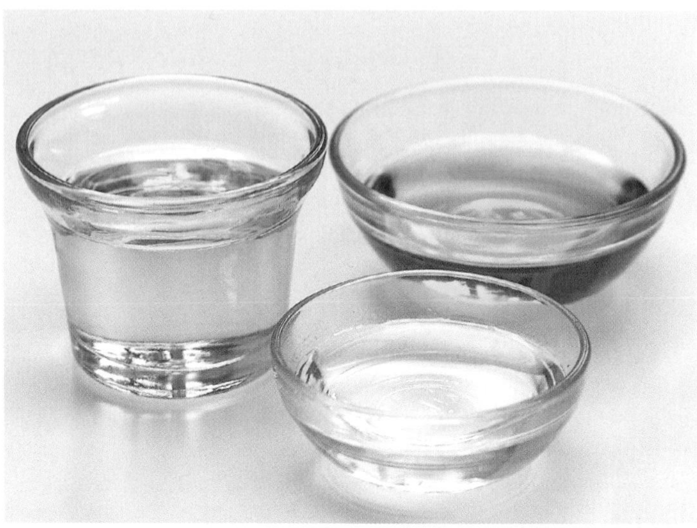

Using oils and creams to massage helps to keep skin soft, supple and moisturized, and prevents the build-up of hard skin. On a practical level, oil or cream helps to give "slip" so that your hands glide over the feet rather than dragging and stretching the skin. Oils and creams also give you the chance to incorporate essential oils, with their varied healing qualities, into the treatment - simply by adding some drops of essential oil to the cream or to an oil such as almond, grapeseed or olive. These three oils are popular choices for using on their own; they are known as "carrier" oils if drops of essential plant extract is added to them.

If your skin is dry, dehydrated or mature, it is best to use a massage cream instead of a carrier oil. The creams are heavier, take longer to be absorbed and leave a protective film on the skin, which helps to trap moisture, preventing further dehydration. It is rather like covering food with cling film in order to prevent it from drying out. Massage base creams are available from most drugstores and natural health stores, or you can make your own using one of the recipes in this book.

△ Many oils can be used as carriers, as long as they give good slip. Almond oil (front) is gentle and is suitable for most skin types, including very dry or dehydrated skin. Grapeseed (left) has almost no smell, so it is ideal for blending with essential oils. Olive oil (back right) is easy to get hold of, but it does have a strong smell that is difficult to disguise.

getting ready

Begin by pouring a little oil, just a drop or two, into the palm of one hand. If using cream, just one or two small blobs are sufficient. Rub your palms together, then move your hands, one over the other, in a hand-washing motion. This distributes the oil all over the back of your hands, your fingers and cuticles, which has the extra benefit of making them soft and supple. Add a little more massage medium into one palm, then gently bring your palms together, so you evenly cover both hands. The medium should not run all over the area but be just enough to give slip and shine. You are now ready to massage.

While working, observe the skin for changes in texture (from slippery to dry) and a gradual reduction in shine. At this point, add more massage oil or cream in the same way as described above.

If you are using a blend of different oils, it is worth making up enough to last for a few treatments and storing it in a clean, screwtop container. For an average-sized person, you will use about 10 ml/2 tsp of oil or cream for each massage involving the feet, and a little more when you are also massaging the lower legs.

using essential oils

Essential oils are made from natural plant ingredients and are a gentle and effective way to boost general health and treat minor ailments at home. However, it is very important to treat these oils with respect, as you would with any chemical or drug.

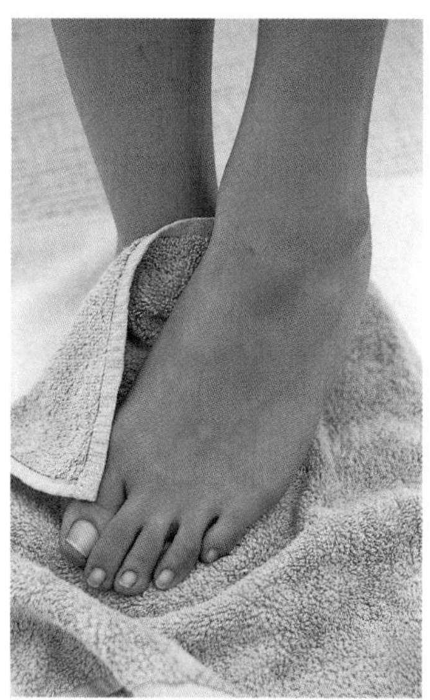

△ Massage oil into the skin until it is well absorbed. Give the feet a quick wipe at the end of an oil-based treatment to ensure that there is no slippery residue left. You can use the sole of one foot to rub the towel over the top of the other, so that you do not have to bend down.

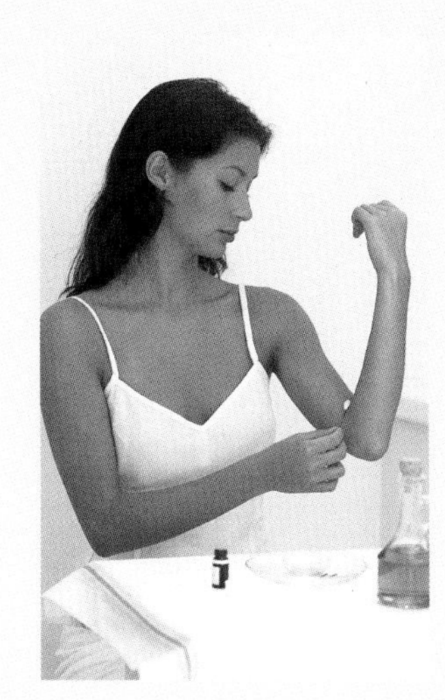

oil blends

Essential oils must always be well-diluted in a carrier oil or massage cream before being applied to the skin. As a general rule, blend one or two drops essential oil to 5ml (1 tsp) carrier. If making a larger quantity, keep the ratio of essential oil to carrier constant.

◁ **It is a good idea to patch test essential oils before using them. Add 2 drops of essential oil to 2 drops of carrier oil. Massage into a patch of the delicate skin on the inside of your arm and leave for six hours; if no reaction occurs it is probably (but not certainly) safe to use. If a reaction occurs, apply lots of carrier oil to the area to help neutralize the effects. Do not rub the area.**

Use less essential oil (1 drop per 10ml carrier) if:

- your skin is sensitive
- you are allergy prone
- you are on high-dose medication
- you are pregnant
- you are treating a child.

If blending in a bottle, shake well to mix. If blending in a dish or a pot of cream, stir well using a clean spoon handle. Do not be tempted to add more than the suggested amount of oil when following a recipe. When adding oil to an aqueous cream, you should put the essential oil into a spoon of carrier oil or vodka first, and then blend this mixture with the cream.

Never use an oil unless you know it to be safe, and avoid using any oil with women who are pregnant, children, the very old and the sick unless you have specifically checked its suitability. The most direct and effective method is to add a few drops of oil to a carrier oil, and then gently smooth it in. Breathe deeply as you massage for maximum therapeutic effect.

Nobody knows exactly how the therapy works, but it is thought that the scents stimulate nerve endings in the nostrils. Messages are then sent to the areas of the brain that are concerned with moods and emotions, and may trigger a reaction here. Pleasant smells are also thought to have an effect on the hypothalamus, a mysterious organ deep within the brain which regulates our sleep, body temperature, metabolism and the libido.

The oils used in aromatherapy massage can also have a direct effect on the nerve endings in the areas of the skin where they are applied. Lavender and tea tree, for example, have been known as healing plants for centuries. These and other oils with antifungal, antiseptic and anaesthetic ingredients have an instant first-aid effect when they are rubbed into the skin.

The massage routines in this book recommend good oils to use, or you can experiment with your favourite aromas. If you prefer not to use oil when you massage (or if you are giving a reflexology treatment, in which your hands need to be dry), you can burn the oils in a vaporizer instead – although the effect will not be as strong.

baths and compresses

A warm bath or footbath allows you to absorb the oils through your skin as you lie back and relax. Soak for at least ten minutes breathing deeply all the while. The oils do not disperse well in water so you will need to dilute them in a base oil or in full-fat milk. Add to the filled bath (not to running water) and swirl the water with your hand.

If you are having a footbath, keep a boiled kettle close at hand so you can top up the water in the bowl as it cools. Footbaths are a good way of relieving aching or swollen feet; they are also a good way to soften the feet before a pampering session.

For bruising, pain or arthritic joints, try an aromatherapy compress. Use a warm compress for general pain, aching or arthritic joints, and a cold compress if the area is inflamed, swollen or hot.

To make a compress, fill a bowl with hot or very cold water, then dilute your chosen essential oils in a carrier. A good blend to try is 4 drops geranium, 3 of bergamot and 3 of clary sage with 10ml (2 tsp) grapeseed oil. Add the blended oils to the water and swish around. Soak a small towel or facecloth in the water, wring it and hold on the affected area. Replace the cloth often so that the temperature remains constant.

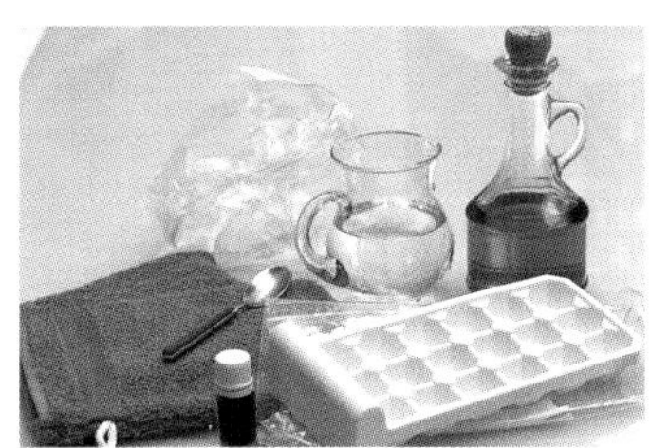

△ **For a cold compress, use chilled water, or freeze an essential oil and water mix in an ice cube tray to make aromatic ice-packs. You can also place a sealed bag of crushed ice or a bag of frozen vegetables over the compress to help keep the area cold. Never apply ice directly to skin.**

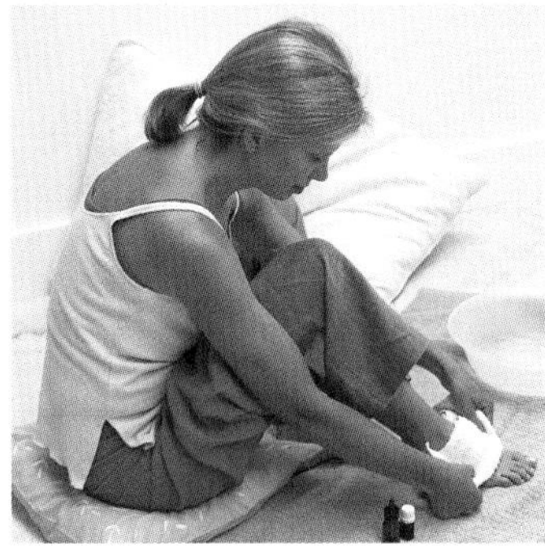

△ **A warm aromatic compress effectively soothes an aching ankle. Secure the compress in place with a bandage or a thin, clean scarf, and then rest with your feet above the level of your heart for 15 minutes.**

Reflexology and acupressure

The therapy of reflexology is based on the idea that health-giving energy flows around the body. When this energy flows freely, physical and mental well-being is maintained. If the energy flow is blocked or stagnant, we can become unwell or unhappy.

Reflexologists believe that gentle pressure applied to points on the feet – known as reflexes – can be used to stimulate energy flow and release any blockages. The feet contain a "map" of the entire body: every organ and body structure relates to a precise point on the top, side or sole of the foot. For example, the brain is connected to the top of the big toe, while the bladder point is at the base of the heel.

When an area of the body is out of balance, the related reflex will be tender to the touch. Sometimes small granules may be felt around the reflex. These granules are thought to be accumulated waste which has solidified in the form of calcium crystals or uric acid. A reflexologist will gently work a tender point, which helps to break down waste deposits and restore energy flow through the zone. The massage-like action also has the effect of stimulating the circulation of blood and lymph to the area, and it feels highly relaxing.

The hands also contain a map of the body. However, they are not as responsive as the feet so they are usually used only for self-help.

mapping the feet

Reflexology is a holistic therapy that aims to bring the whole body back to balance. For this reason, a full treatment always encompasses work on both feet. The majority of reflexes are on the sole of the foot, but some are on the top or along the side. In general the right foot relates to the right-hand side of the body, while the left relates to the left-hand side. Some organs are sited on only one side of the body, and therefore the related reflexes appear on only one foot.

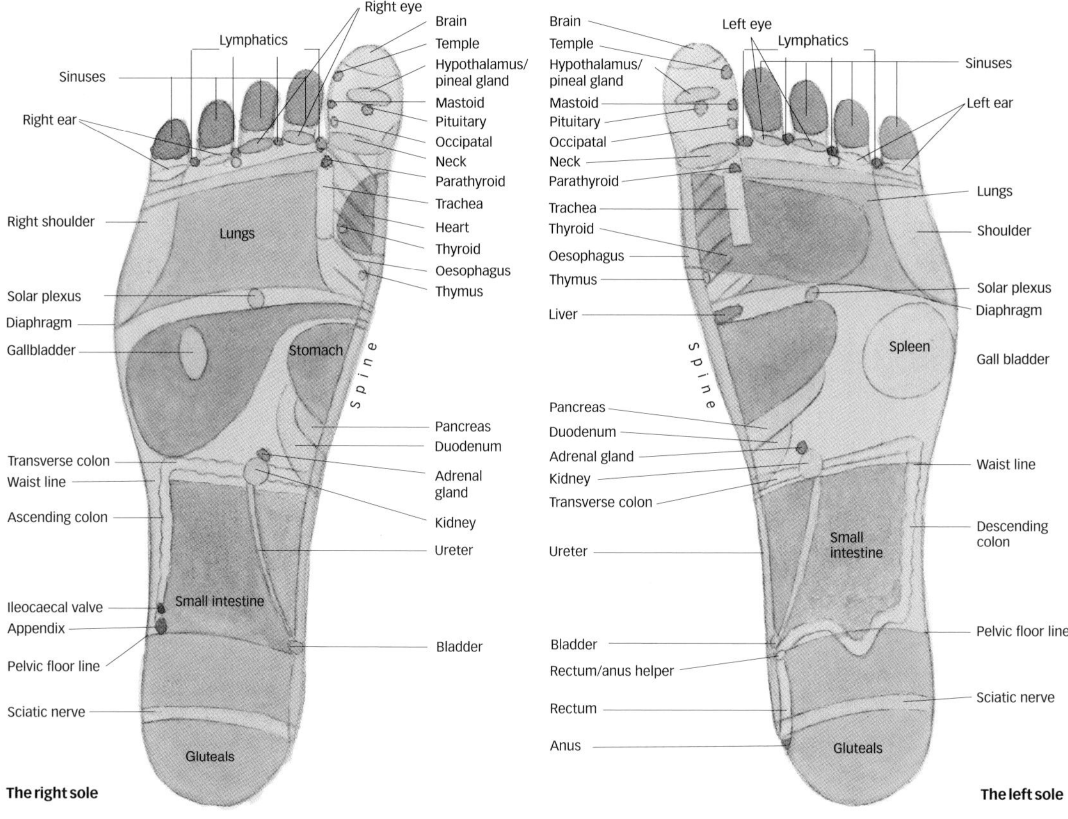

The right sole **The left sole**

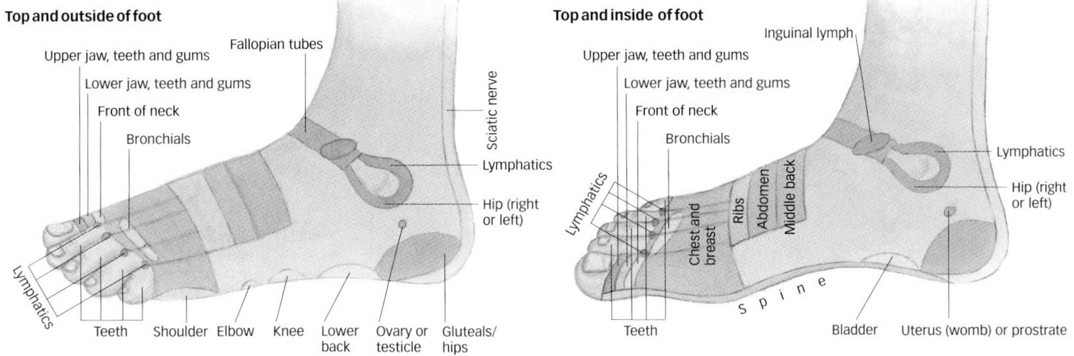

acupressure

Like reflexology, acupressure aims to restore our natural ability for self-healing by encouraging energy flow around the body.

In acupressure, energy is said to flow through invisible channels, called meridians. Most of these are named after the organs of the body – Liver, Heart and Kidney are all important meridians. In Chinese medicine, our organs represent aspects of our emotional well-being as well as physical health: the kidneys are associated with grief, while the heart is connected to joy.

As in reflexology, gentle pressure is used to stimulate the energy points, and points in one area of the body are used to promote healing elsewhere. However, while reflexology concentrates on the feet, acupressure involves points all over the body.

Stomach 45 is on the outside of the base of the nail of the second toe. Press if you have indigestion, or are recovering from a late night.

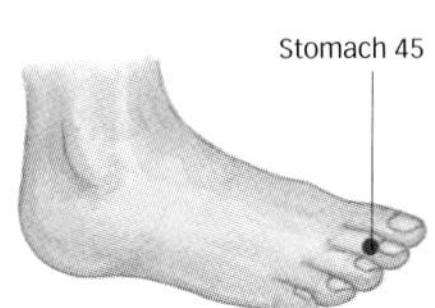

Liver 3 – known as Bigger Rushing – is a useful point to press if you are feeling stressed. It is in the groove between the big toe and second toe, where the bones meet.

Liver 2 is in the webbing between the big toe and the second toe. It is another good stress-relieving point, and it can help to ease constipation.

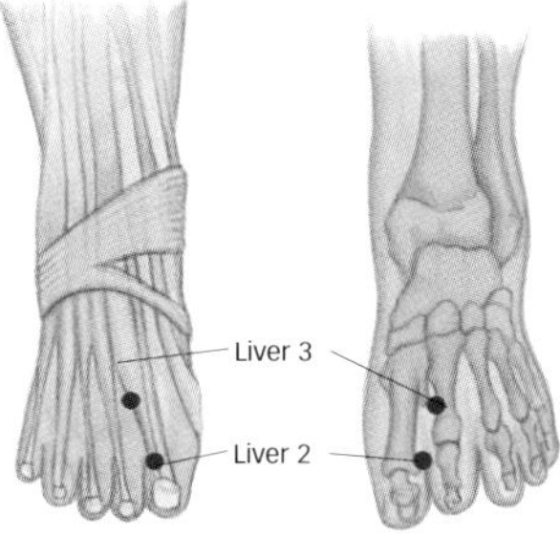

useful acupressure points for self-help

To stimulate an acupressure point, place the tip of your thumb over it. Press gently for a minute or two, making a small rotational movement as you do so. You may notice some tenderness or tingling in the area; ease the pressure if you feel any discomfort. Do not use these points if you are pregnant or seriously ill, unless otherwise recommended by a professional acupuncturist.

Bladder 62 is known as Calm Sleep. It is a very soothing point, and can help to ease insomnia. It is in the first indentation directly below the outer anklebone – about one-third of the distance from the outer anklebone to the bottom of the heel.

Gallbladder 41, which is called Above Tears, is on top of the foot. It is 2.5cm (1in) above the webbing of the fourth and fifth toes, in the groove between the bones. It is good for migraines and headaches that affect one side only.

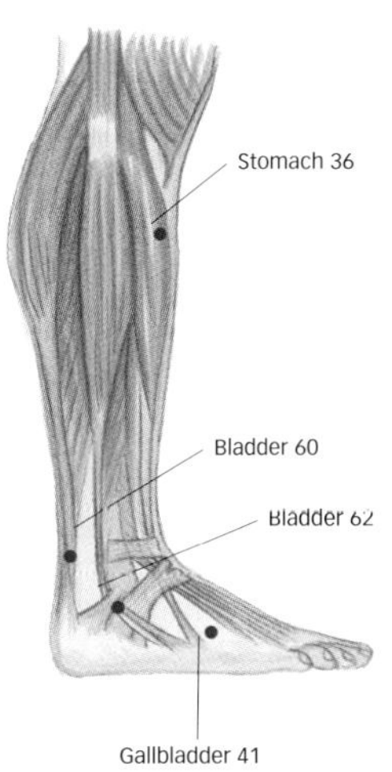

Try pressing **Stomach 36** if you need a quick energy boost. It is called the Three Mile Point – supposedly because it was used by the Chinese army when they needed to push themselves a few miles further. You will find it four finger-widths below the kneecap, and one finger-width from the outer edge of the shinbone. To check you are on the right spot, move your foot up and down – you should feel the muscle flexing beneath your fingertip.

Bladder 60, also known as High Mountains, is midway between the back edge of the outer ankle bone and the achilles tendon. This is a good general relaxation point.

Spleen 6 is a good first-aid point to press if you are feeling faint. It can also help relieve period pain and aids the digestion. The point is four finger-widths above the inner anklebone, close to the back of the shinbone. **Spleen 4** is found in the upper arch of the foot, one thumb-width from the ball – a helpful point if you are fighting off a cold.

Kidney 6 is also known as the Illuminated Sea. It is good for insomnia and can also ease the symptoms of menopause. The point **Kidney 3**, or the Bigger Stream, is helpful if you are feeling depleted and drained.

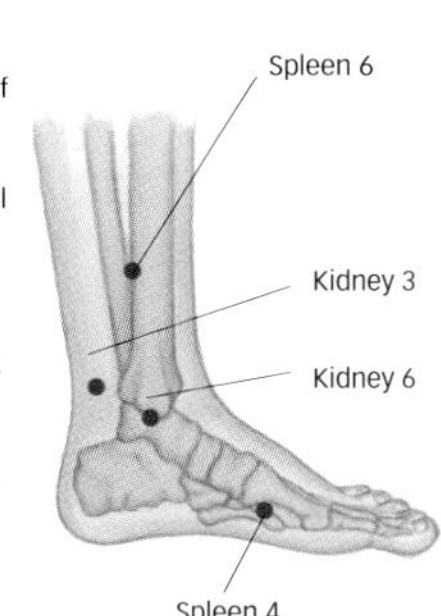

Reflexology techniques

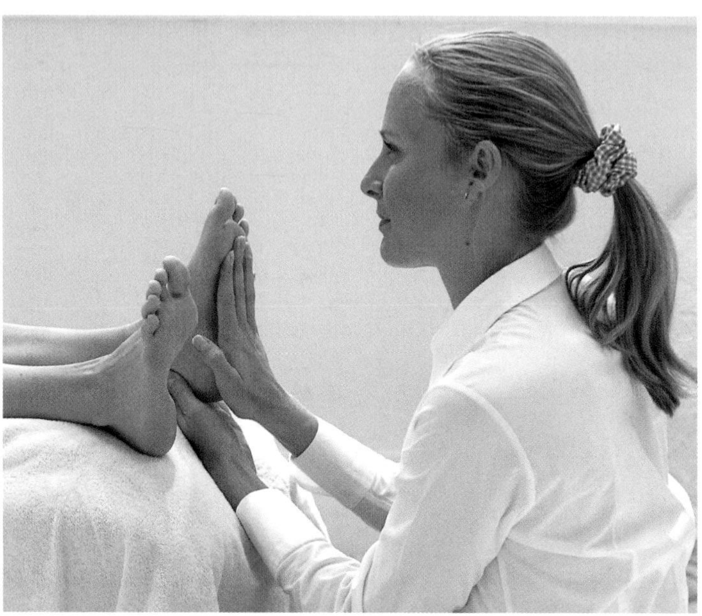

◁ Establish a connection with the person you are treating before starting a reflexology treatment, and always ask the recipient how he or she is feeling. Placing your hands on the soles of the feet before you begin is a reassuring and centring experience for both giver and receiver.

Reflexology is a method of self-healing that can easily be done at home. The basic movements are simple to learn. Once you have become familiar with them, you can use reflexology to treat minor ailments as well as to boost the general well-being of yourself and your family and friends.

When doing reflexology, wear comfortable clothing that does not restrict your movements: in particular, do not wear a tight top. Maintain good posture throughout; try to keep your back straight and your shoulders relaxed. Remember to breathe naturally and deeply – many people tend to hold their breath when they are concentrating.

What every reflexologist needs is a good touch. To a certain extent, this comes with practice. However, it is always very important to check the responses of the recipient, and to ask him or her for feedback. Practise the hand exercises given in this book regularly: this will help you to develop suppleness in your wrist and fingers.

Have a glass of water after giving a treatment. If you are treating another person, offer him or her a drink as well.

giving a treatment

Always start a reflexology treatment by giving the feet a gentle massage. This helps you to connect with the person you are treating, and it will help you to connect with your own body when self-treating. Massaging also gets the fingers mobile, and it encourages both you and the recipient to relax. The simple self-massage and relaxing massage treatments on the previous pages are good routines to do at this point. A short massage should also be given after the reflexology treatment.

You can either give the full reflexology routine – described on the following pages – or you can focus on a particular area of the body, or on a symptom. If doing a full treatment, remember to work gently, and do not repeat the routine more than once a week. If you are working on specific points rather than doing the full routine, then two or three treatments a week should be sufficient. Do not treat anyone with a major illness or severe problem, or a woman in the first three months of pregnancy.

getting the pressure right

Reflexology should neither hurt nor tickle – aim for firm, pleasurable pressure. The pressure will need to be varied depending on the size of the person's foot, his or her general health and individual tolerance level. In general, the pressure applied to bony areas such as the top of the foot should always be lighter than that applied to fleshy areas, such as the heel or ball. The pressure used when treating a child or an elderly person should always be significantly lighter.

Start off using a light pressure, then gradually increase to tolerance level. Do not overtreat particular points – keep to the number of times suggested.

hand preserver

This great lotion can be used every day to keep your hands soft.

ingredients

- 15ml/1 tbsp avocado oil
- 15ml/1 tbsp almond oil
- 15ml/1 tbsp petroleum jelly or glycerine
- 1ml/⅕ tsp vitamin E oil
- 10 drops essential oil. Use any one or a combination of these: rose, sandalwood, geranium, lavender, neroli.

Combine the ingredients in a small bowl. Transfer to a 50ml (2fl oz) screwtop jar.

basic techniques

Anyone giving a reflexology treatment needs soft skin, so moisturize daily. Always check that your nails are clean and short before treating. This is even more important for reflexology than for massage since you press into the skin.

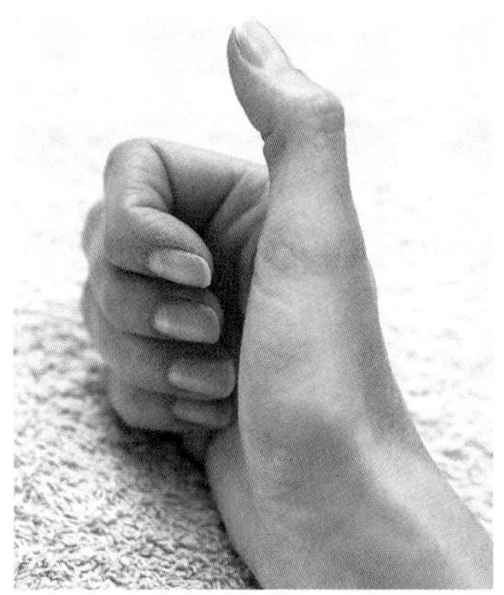
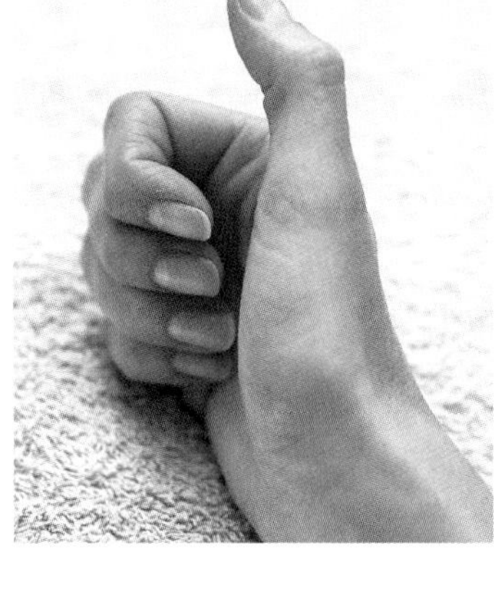

△ **Thumb walking or crawling**
Hold your thumb straight up in front of you, then bend it from the first joint and straighten it again – this is the basic technique used in thumb walking. Place the thumb on the skin, and use alternate bending and straightening movements to "walk" across the area. This has been likened to the crawling movement of a caterpillar.

▷ **Rotation on a point**
This movement is used for sensitive reflexes. Place the pad of your thumb on to the reflex point, then use your other hand to bring the foot slowly into the thumb. Rotate the foot in a circular movement around the thumb.

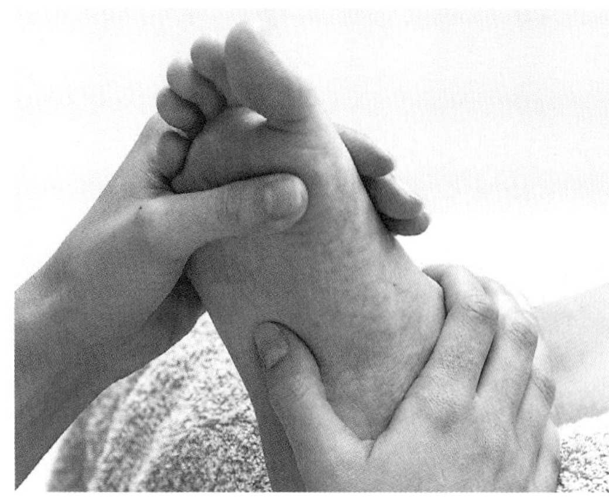

▷ **Pinpoint, or hooking**
This is used for small reflexes or those that are difficult to locate. Place your thumb on the point, and apply pressure. Now, keeping the pressure steady, move the thumb on to the uppermost tip in a "hooking" action. Move the thumb back to the original position.

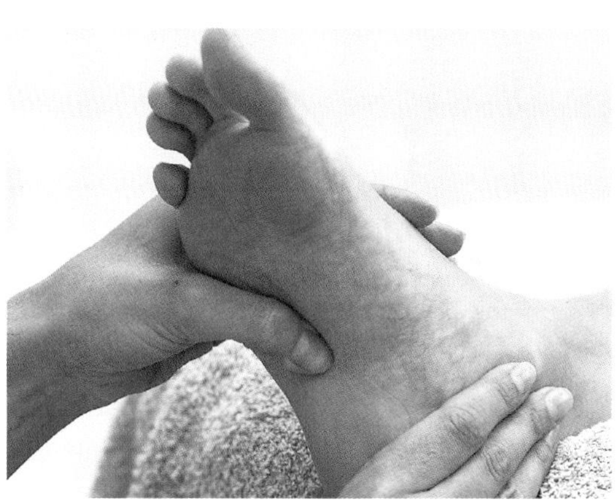

△ **Finger walking or crawling**
This technique is the same as the thumb-walking technique described above, but you use the index (first) finger instead. The action is used on the top of the foot and other areas where the flesh is thinner and less pressure is required. You can use another finger if you find that easier.

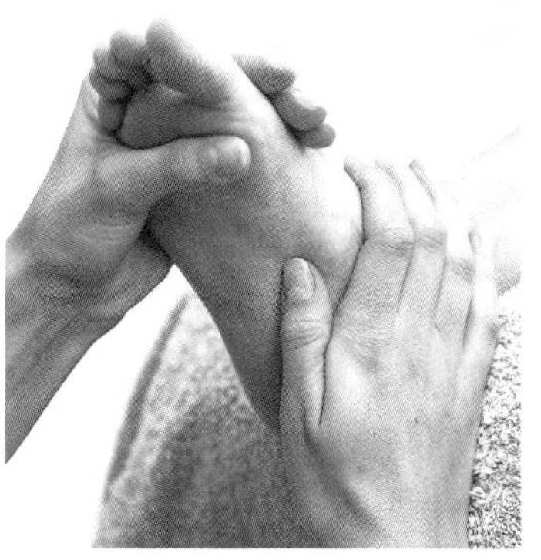

△ **Holding and supporting**
One hand is used to support while the other works the reflex. Always support the foot while you are working. Position your working hand close to the holding hand: this allows you to support and control the movement of the foot. It also gives the recipient a feeling of security.

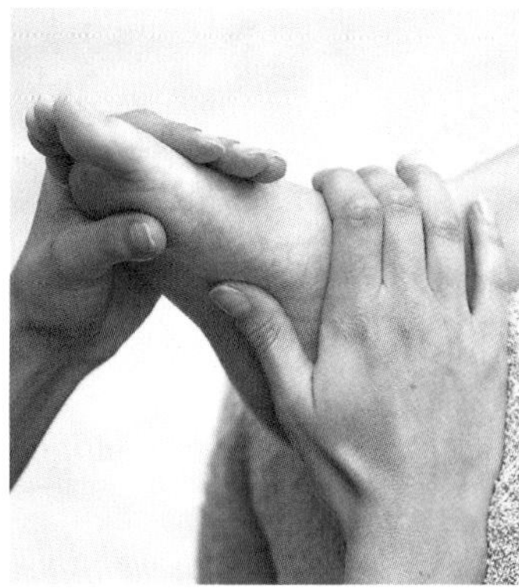

△ **Pressure circles on a point**
Hold the foot comfortably with one hand and place the flat pad of the working thumb on the reflex. Press into the area and then slowly circle your thumb gently on the point. This movement is usually used for very sensitive areas.

A complete reflexology treatment

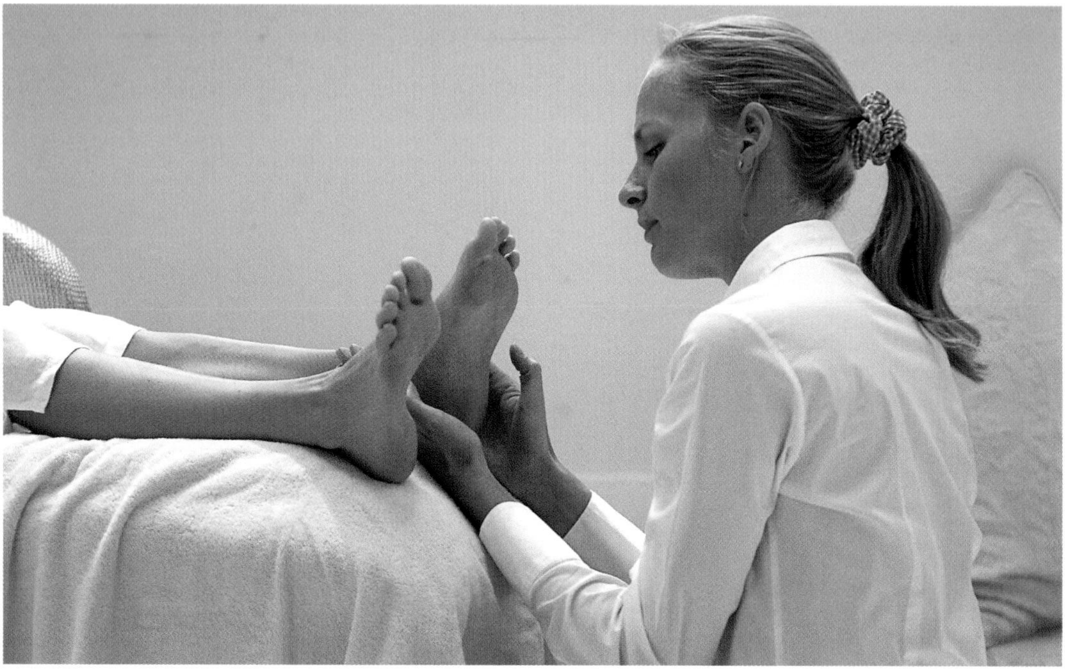

A full reflexology routine treats the whole body, and can be a great way to enhance general well-being, and boost energy. Reflexology treatments work best if the recipient is mentally and physically relaxed, and if he or she is breathing well. For this reason, the first movements in the routine work on the diaphragm and solar plexus reflexes. These points are powerful relaxants which encourage natural, deep breathing. The third movement in the routine treats the head and brain. Stimulating this reflex helps to clear the mind, and also prepares the brain to receive and send messages to and from the rest of the body.

Although each reflex point relates to a specific organ or part of the body, it will also have an effect on other areas. For this reason, it is important that you work round the foot in the exact order given. Be sure to treat all the reflex points on both feet. Ideally, you should perform reflexology on the right foot first (unlike massage, where it is not so important which foot is attended to first).

Reflexology can be very powerful, so it is important that you do not repeat a movement more than the amount of times specified here. You should also not give more than one treatment to the same person – or to yourself – in a week.

△ This is a long routine so make sure that both you and the person you are treating are comfortable. In particular, it is important that the feet are at the right height so that you do not have to bend to reach them. The recipient can lie on a couch, or sit in a chair with the feet propped up on a footstool, with you sitting or kneeling directly in front.

in the hands

The hands, as well as the feet, contain a stylized "map" of the body. Reflexologists tend to treat the feet because they are more sensitive, but the hands can be easier to use for self-treatment. A person's hands may also be used for treatment if they are very frail or have a foot problem.

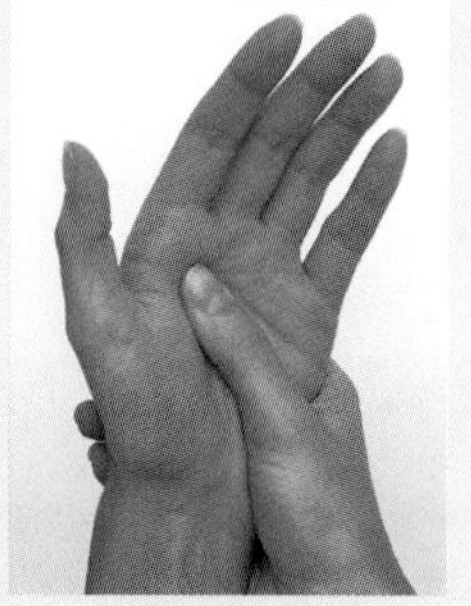

▷ The point being pressed here is connected to the solar plexus. It is an excellent reflex to stimulate if you are feeling anxious or stressed. Breathe deeply as you work it.

holistic reflexology routine

Before starting the treatment, give the person a short foot massage. This helps to release tension in the foot, and allows the person to get used to your touch. You may use a massage oil or cream, but you should blot this off with a towel to prevent your hands from slipping when you are working on the reflexes. At the end of the treatment, massage the feet again. This time, you can leave the oil or cream to sink in. Here the right foot is treated first, then the left.

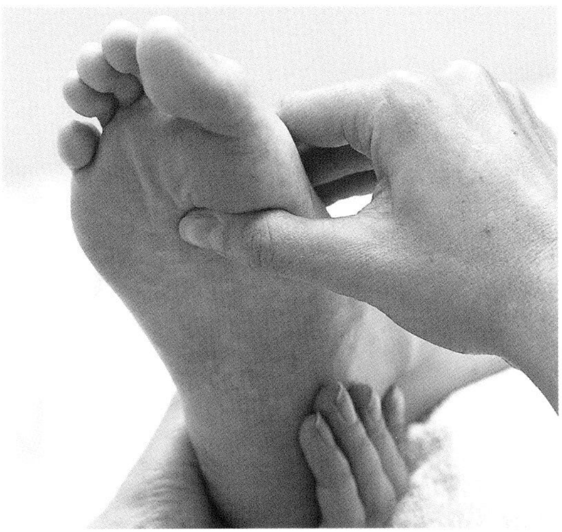

△ 1 **Diaphragm (sole)**
Cup the right heel in your left hand. Place your right thumb on the edge of the foot, so that it is on the big toe side just below the ball. It should be pointing across the foot, towards the inside edge. Now walk the thumb across the sole in a crawling motion, remaining just below the ball. Repeat the movement once more.

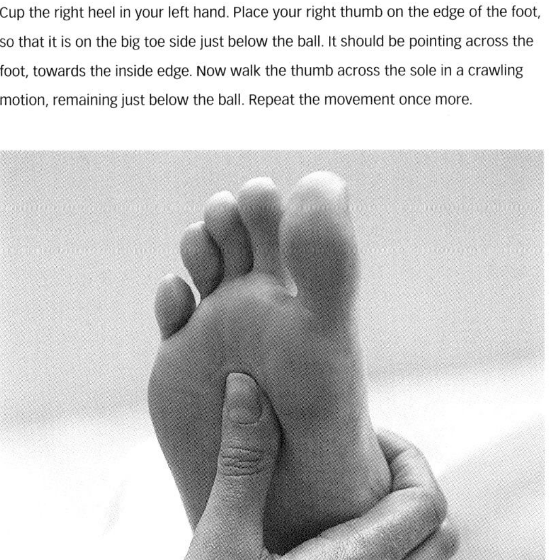

△ 2 **Solar plexus (sole)**
Repeat the action described in step 1, but this time stop when you reach the point directly below toes two and three. Turn the tip of your thumb so that it points towards the toes and press three times on the solar plexus reflex. Then continue the crawl to the outer edge of the foot. Do this movement twice.

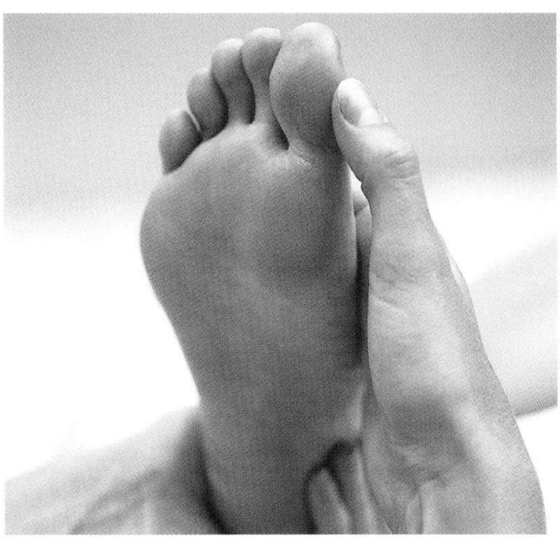

△ 3 **Head and brain (big toe)**
Continue cupping the heel. Use the right thumb to crawl up the outside of the big toe, going over the top and down the inner edge, in a large horseshoe shape. Then crawl up the back of the big toe from the base to the top. Do as many crawls as necessary to cover the entire surface area.

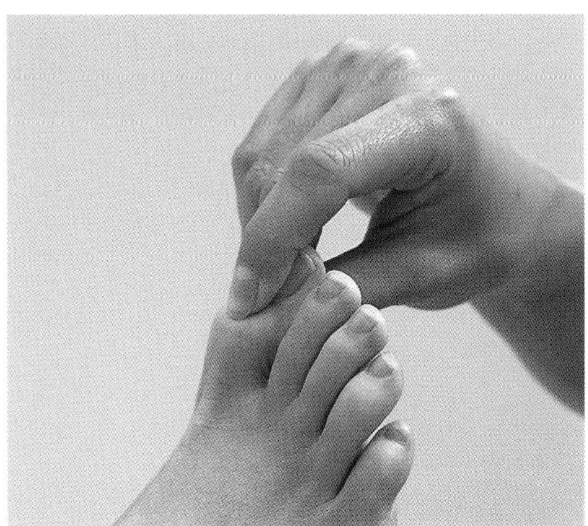

△ 4 **Face (front of big toe)**
Continuing to cup the heel, use the right index finger to crawl down the front of the big toe (finger walking). Use your thumb to keep the toe steady as you do this. Crawl from the top of the toe to the base, and do as many crawls as necessary to cover the entire surface area.

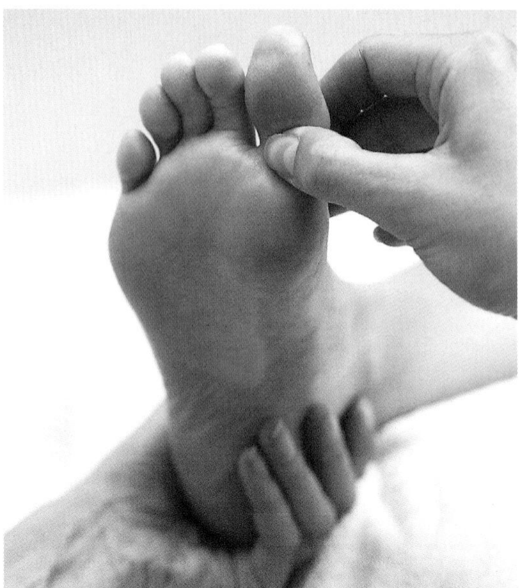

△ **5 Front and back of neck (base of big toe)**

Place your index finger on the base of the big toe, at the edge of the foot. Finger-walk around the front of the big toe, until you reach the join between the big and second toes. Now use your thumb to crawl around the back of the toe, again starting from the edge of the foot and stopping at the join between the toes.

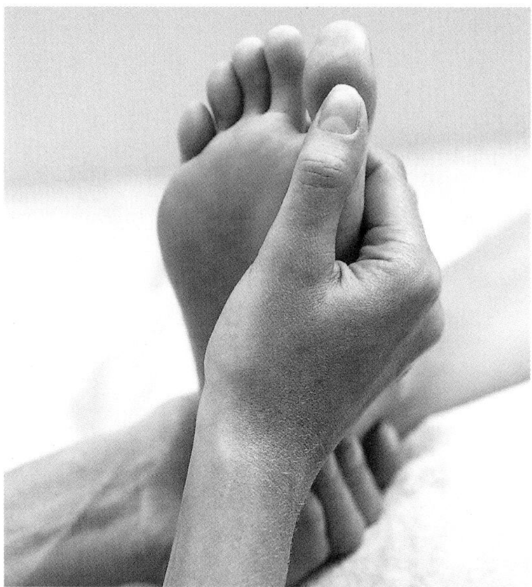

△ **6 Pituitary (back of big toe)**

Continue cupping the heel. Place your right thumb in the centre of the widest point on the big toe and press deeply on the reflex here three times. **Do not work this point on a woman who is pregnant.**

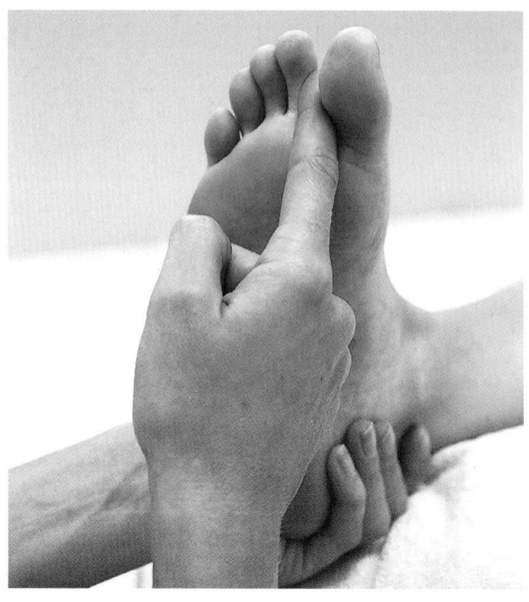

△ **7 Cranial nerves (four small toes)**

Place your right index finger in-between the big and second toes, angling it towards the second toe. Finger-walk up the second toe and down the other side, making a horseshoe shape. Finger-walk over the next three toes in the same way. Now repeat the whole movement.

treating between meals

You should not give reflexology to someone who has eaten a heavy meal within the last two or three hours. On the other hand, a person should not have reflexology treatment on an empty stomach, as their energy levels will be depleted and they will not respond to the treatment as well as they should. If the person that you are treating has not eaten for several hours, or if he or she is hungry, offer a small snack such as juice and biscuits before starting the routine.

▽ **A glass of orange juice and a couple of biscuits will help to boost the person's energy before a reflexology treatment.**

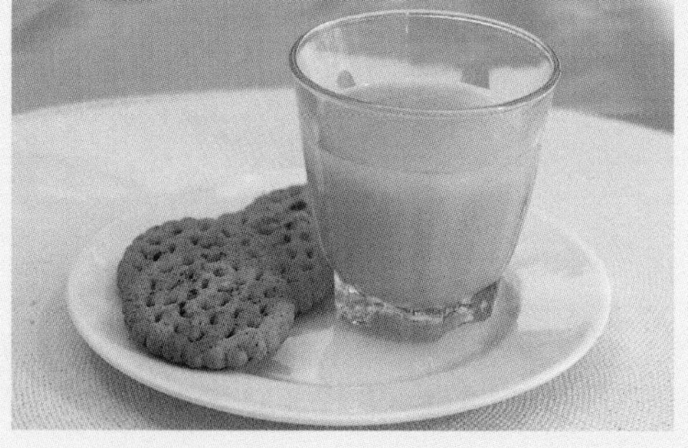

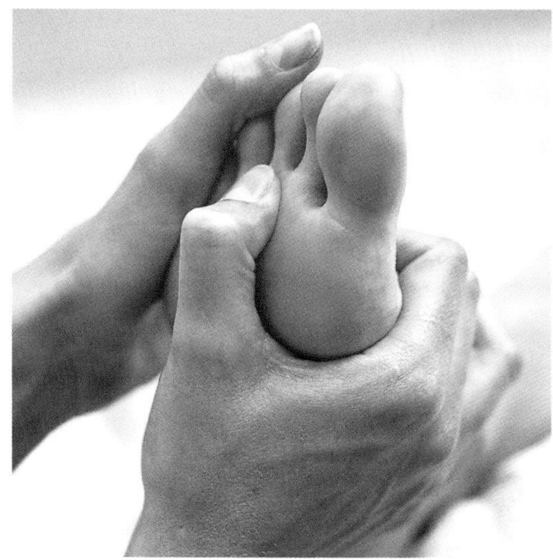

△ **8 Sinuses, teeth and gums (back and front of four small toes)**

Support the toes with your left hand. Thumb-walk up the back of each toe: start at the base and crawl up the centre-line to the top. Repeat the movement, but pause when you reach the fleshy bulb of each toe, press in and slide the thumb up to the top. Now, use your index finger to walk down the front of each toe – start at the top and support the base of the toe. Do as many crawls as needed to cover the area.

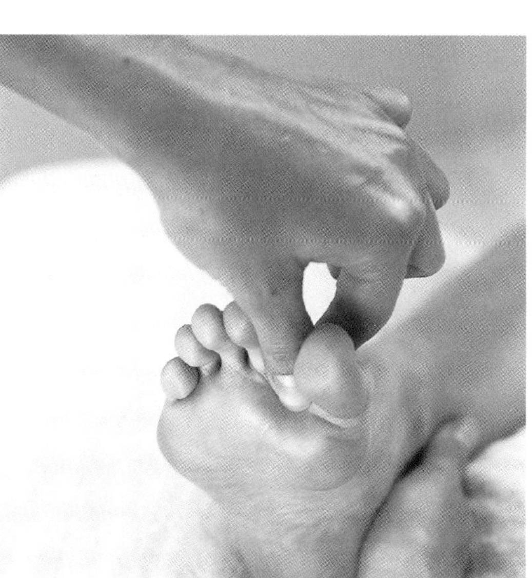

△ **9 Lymphatic glands (webbing between toes)**

Support the foot by cupping the heel. Use your index finger and thumb to pinch and release the webbing between the big and second toes. Repeat on the webbing of the other toes in turn, working gently. Now place your index finger between the big toe and second toe. Slide the finger down the groove on the top of the foot, by a distance of about half its length. Draw back along the same groove.

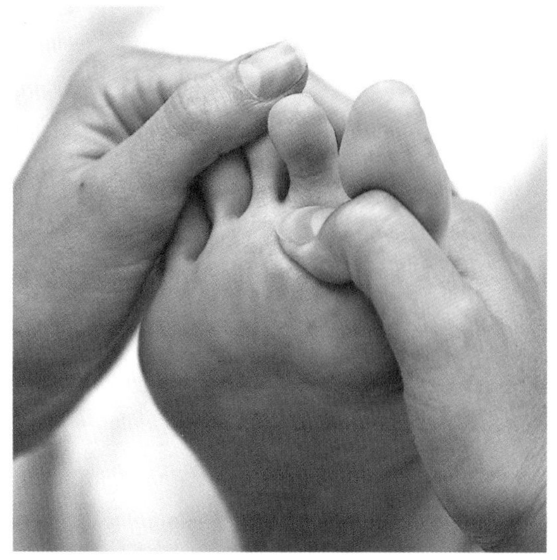

△ **10 Eyes and ears (under the toes on the sole)**

Use your left hand to hold the tops of the toes and bend them back slightly; this exposes the ridge on the sole underneath the toes. Starting on the inner edge of the foot, use the right thumb to crawl along the ridge to the outer edge. Exert a good downward pressure as you thumb-walk. The eye reflex is located under toes two and three, while the ear reflex is under toes four and five.

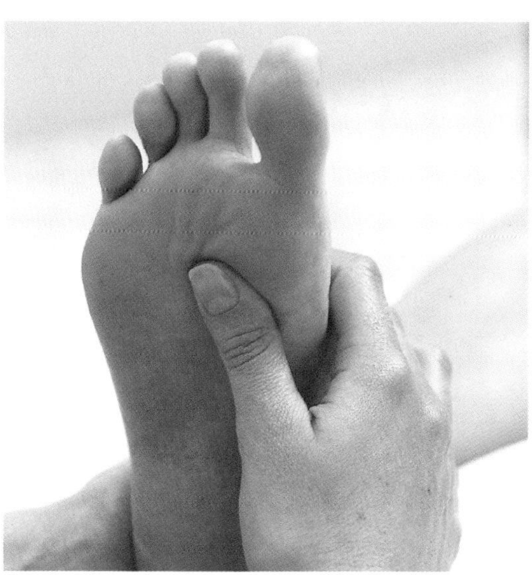

△ **11 Thyroid, parathyroid, thymus (sole)**

Cup the heel in your left hand again. Use the thumb of the right hand to crawl along the diaphragm line, which runs across the foot at the base of the ball: start at the inner edge of the foot and thumb-walk until you are directly in line with the point between the big and second toe. Turn the thumb to point upwards, and thumb-walk up until you reach the base of the toes.

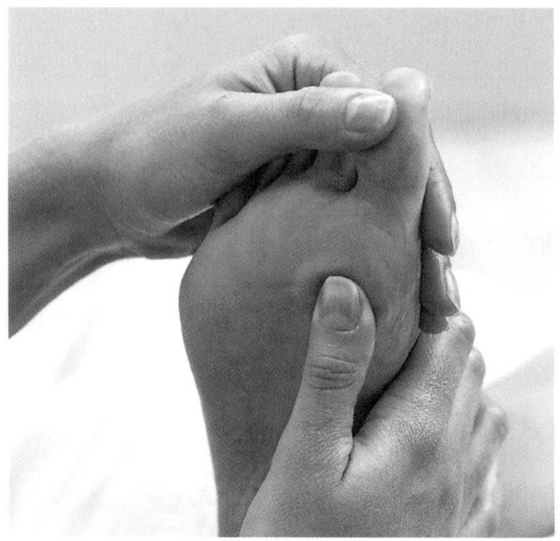

△ **12 Oesophagus, chest, lungs, heart, shoulder (sole)**
Now gently grasp the top of the toes. Place your right thumb on the diaphragm line at the edge of the foot; this thumb should be pointing up, towards the big toe. Using your thumb, make crawling movements up the ball of the foot to the base of the big toe. Do as many crawls as necessary to cover the area. Now, work in the same way to cover the area of the ball of the foot from toe two to toe four. Finally, cover the area under the little toe.

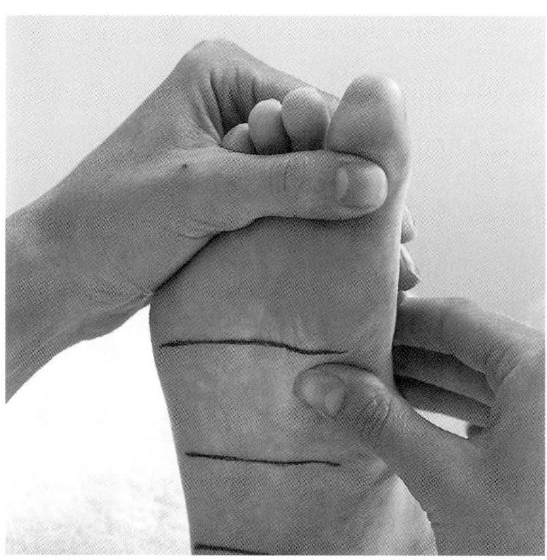

△ **13 Upper abdominal area (sole)**
The upper abdomen reflex is located between the diaphragm line and the waist line, which is in the arch of the foot (marked above). Use the right thumb to crawl across the foot from the inner edge to the outer edge. Repeat the movement as many times as you need to in order to cover the entire area twice. The reflexes for the liver, gall bladder and duodenum reflex are in this area on the right foot; the stomach, pancreas and spleen reflexes are on the left foot.

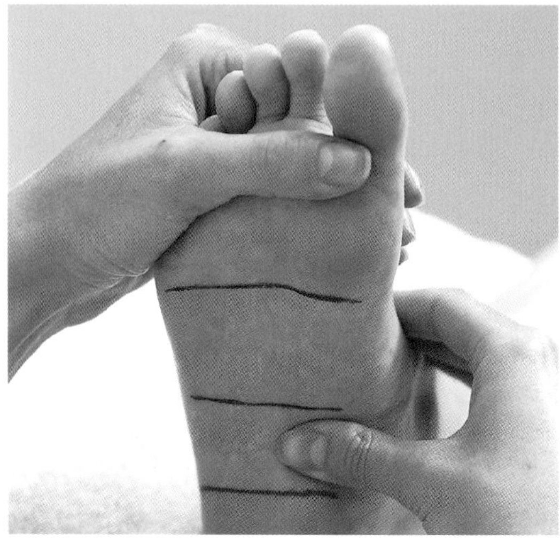

△ **14 Lower abdominal area (sole)**
Here you work in the same way as for Step 13, but you cover the area between the arch (waist line) and the edge of the heel pad (the pelvic floor line). Again, crawl with the right thumb across the foot as many times as necessary to treat the area. Do the movement twice. The reflex for the small intestine is in this area.

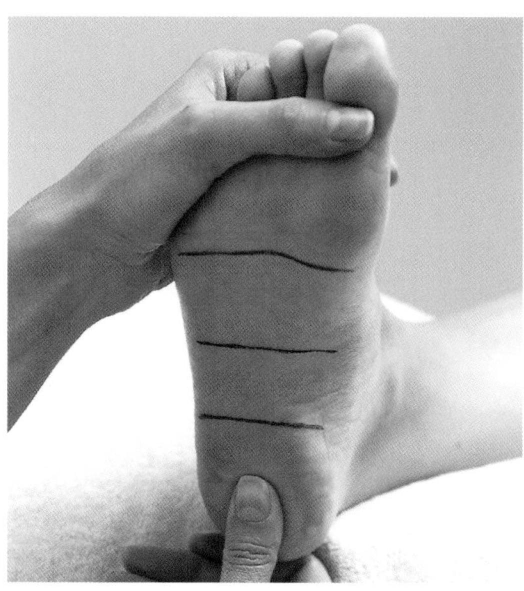

△ **15 Lower back pelvic and sciatic (sole)**
Continue to support the foot at the toes. Start at the back of the foot, and use the right thumb to crawl up through the heel pad, stopping when you reach the soft flesh. Use as many crawls as needed to cover the entire pad, always working in the same direction. Now, place the thumb on the inner edge of the heel, so that it points across to the outer edge. Crawl across the heel as many times as necessary to cover the entire area.

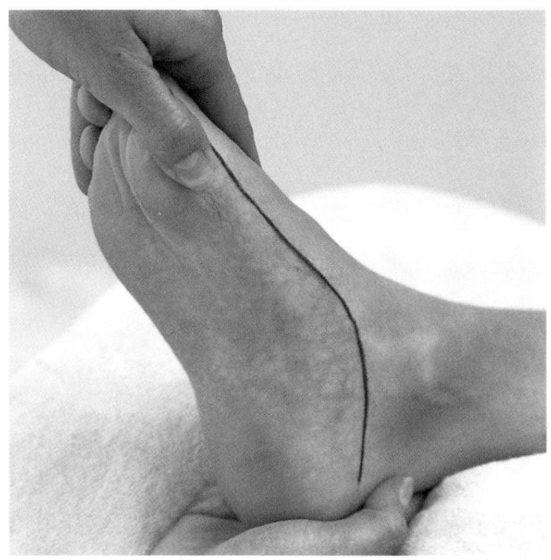

△ **16 Spine (inner edge of the foot)**

Cup the heel with your right hand. Crawl the left thumb down the inner edge of the foot. Start from the first joint of the big toe and work to the heel, following the bone (as marked above). Change hands and crawl back upwards, this time pressing upwards into the bone as you crawl. Do the movement twice in both directions. Most conditions benefit from work to the spine, because nerves run from here to all areas of the body.

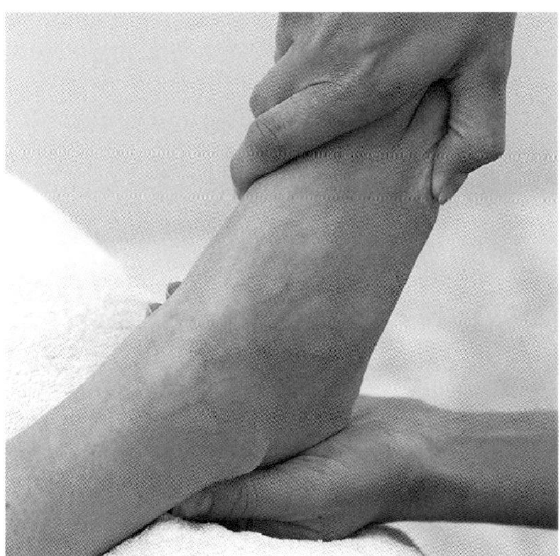

△ **17 Shoulder, hip and knee (outside edge of the foot)**

Now cup the heel firmly but gently in your left hand. Thumb-walk right down the length of the outside edge of the foot, from the base of the little toe to the heel. Then work back up to the toe along the same line. Do this movement twice in both directions. It is important to work this area of the foot thoroughly as you are treating three very different parts of the body.

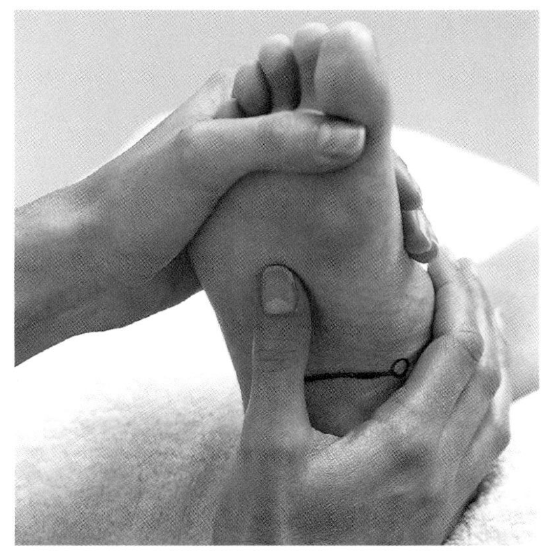

△ **18 Kidney (sole)**

Support the foot by gently holding the base of the toes. Put your right thumb on the waist area, which crosses the centre of the arch; the tip should be pointing towards the join between toes two and three. Make one tiny crawl up the foot; this is the kidney reflex. Press twice, rotating the thumb as you do so (pressure circling). Release the pressure for a second, then make two further pressure circles on the same point.

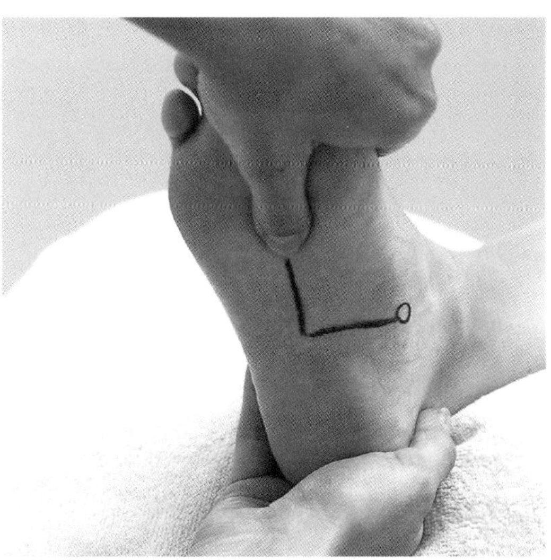

△ **19 Ureter and bladder (sole)**

Now use the right hand to cup the heel. Turn the left thumb to point towards the heel and crawl down the ureter reflex to the line where the heel pad and the soft flesh of the foot meet (as marked). Now, turn the thumb again and crawl up on to the inner side of the foot. You will reach a soft, fleshy mound, which is the bladder reflex (circled). Press on this point three times.

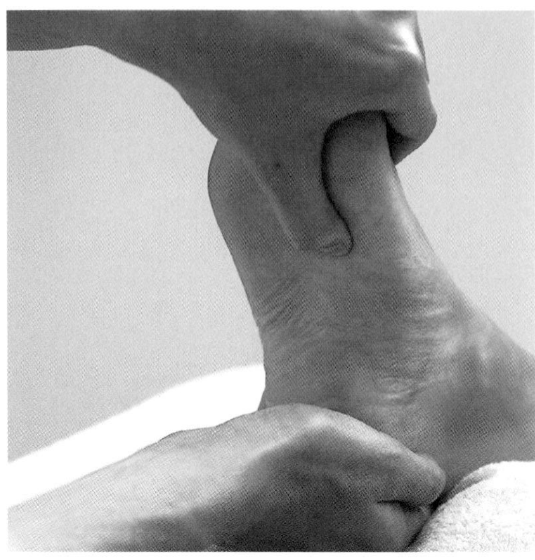

△ **20 Adrenal gland (sole)**

Continuing to cup the heel with the right hand, place your left thumb on the kidney reflex again. Move the thumb across the foot so that it is directly below the second toe. Turn the thumb around so that it is pointing towards the heel, then hook into the flesh and pull back towards the toes. Do three distinct hook-in and back movements on this point.

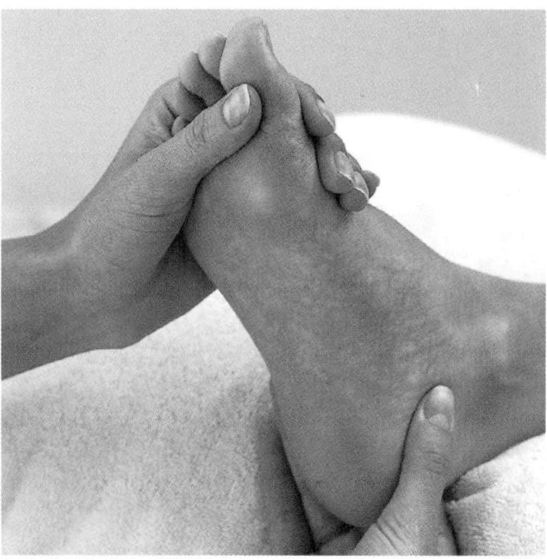

△ **21 Uterus (female) or prostate (male) (inner side)**

Hold the toes with your one hand (whichever feels easiest to you). With the other hand, place the thumb midway along an imaginary line running between the ankle bone on the inside of the foot and the back corner of the heel. Press this point three times. As you press, rotate the thumb slightly (pressure circling) so that you are covering an area the size of a large coin. **Gently stroke rather than press the area if you are treating a woman who is pregnant or has an IUD fitted.**

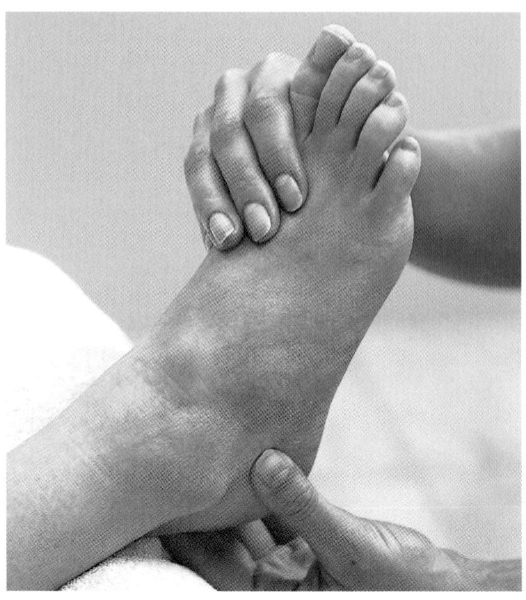

△ **22 Ovaries (female) or testes (male) (outer edge of foot)**

Find the same midpoint on the outer side of the foot. Press in the same way. (You may find it easier to swap your hands over.) **Stroke rather than press this area if you are treating a woman who is pregnant.**

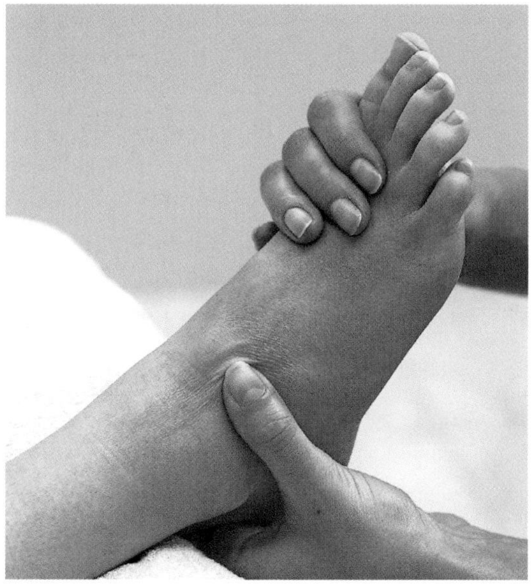

△ **23 Fallopian tube (female), vas deferens (male) (top of foot)**

Continuing to hold the toes with one hand, use the thumb of the other hand to crawl across the top of the foot on the crease line between the leg and foot. Work from the outside ankle area to the inner ankle area. Repeat.

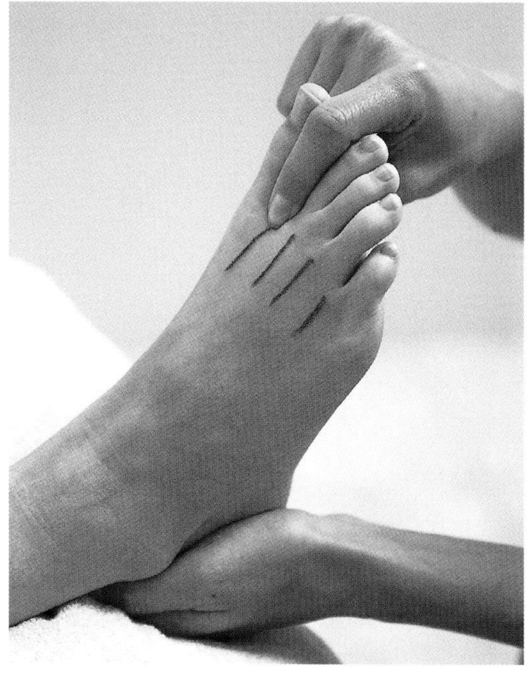

△ **24 Breast area (top of foot, at base of toes)**

Cupping the heel in your left hand, use the index finger of the right hand to crawl down the top of the foot from the base of the toes to a point corresponding with the diaphragm line (the base of the ball). Now, crawl backwards over the same area. Do as many crawls as needed to cover the breast reflex, which starts between the big and second toes and ends between the fourth and little toes. Repeat steps 1-24 on the left foot, then bring both feet together to finish.

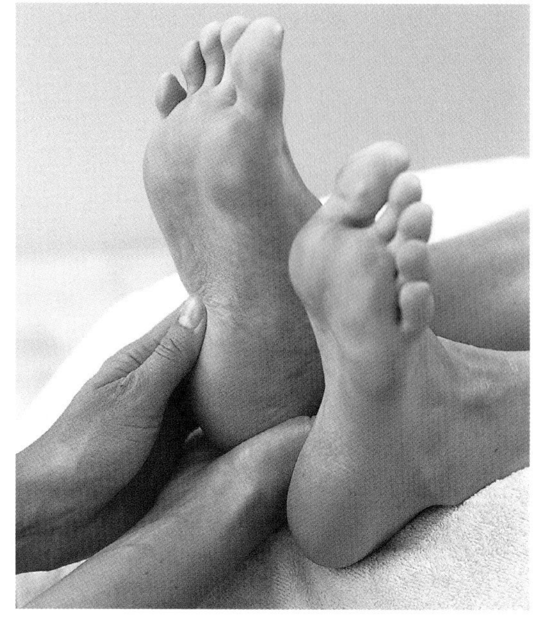

△ **25 Colon/large intestine (soles of both feet)**

Start at the edge of the right heel, in line with the join between toes four and five. Thumb walk up the right sole to the middle of the foot. Now thumb-walk across both feet until you are in line with toes four and five on the left foot. Crawl down to the left heel pad, then a little way across the foot until the thumb is in line with toes three and four. Turn the thumb to point towards the heel and make three deep pressure circles here. Crawl to the inside of the left foot, make two pressure circles, then crawl down about two-thirds of the heel – to the anus reflex. Make three deep pressure circles. Repeat the movement three times.

treating with care

Being able to offer friends and family a reflexology treatment is very satisfying. However, it is important to be sure that you are treating people safely and responsibly. Always ask if someone has any major illnesses. If so, it is probably wisest to offer a gentle massage rather than reflexology. Similarly, if the person is experiencing any severe or unusual symptoms, advise him or her to get a diagnosis and treatment from a doctor before giving reflexology. People with conditions such as arthritis can benefit from reflexology, but they should ideally check with their doctor before receiving treatment, and you should always work very gently.

If treating a woman, check whether there is any chance that she is pregnant. Do not treat a pregnant woman in the first three months, or if she has experienced any problems. Some points must not be pressed at all during pregnancy.

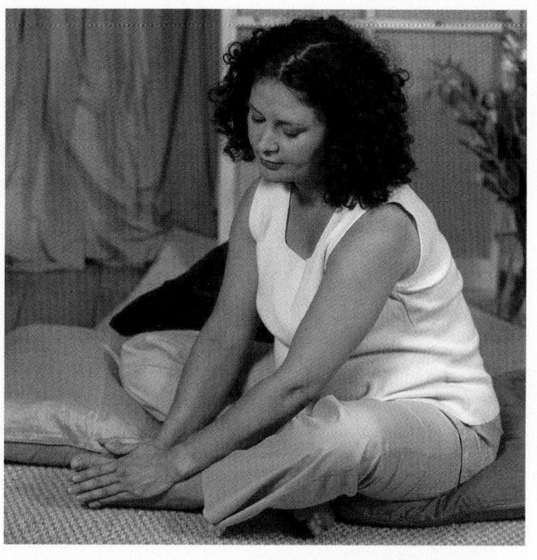

▷ **Reflexology can help to alleviate some of the common symptoms of pregnancy. However, you should not treat if the pregnancy is unstable.**

Setting the scene

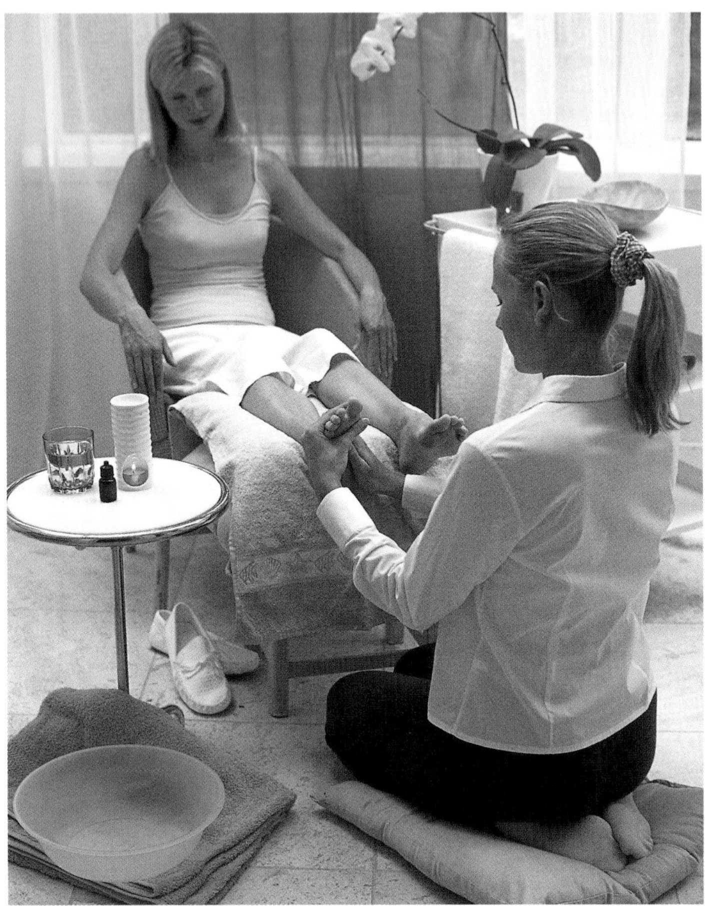

fragrant room spray

Try this sweet-smelling spray.

ingredients

- 5ml/1 tsp vodka
- 20ml/4 tsp rosewater
- 3 drops of your favourite oil

Blend the ingredients in a 30ml (1fl oz) bottle. Shake well, then spray into the air. Don't spray on to furniture or fabrics.

◁ Keep your massage space clean and attractive. Using matching towels will help to create a luxurious and professional atmosphere. Be sure to get everything ready before you start massaging, so that you do not have to stop halfway through the treatment.

Always try to create a relaxing atmosphere in the room where you are treating, whether it is yours or someone else's. Ideally, the area should be warm, inviting and quiet. A few simple preparations will help to give any room a suitably supportive atmosphere for relaxing massage or reflexology work.

First of all, make sure that you are somewhere private, and that you won't be disturbed during the treatment or immediately afterwards. Turn off any phones, including mobiles, close the door and shut the windows if there is noise outside. Ignore the doorbell if it rings while you are treating, or make a previous arrangement with another family member to deal with any callers. Make sure that nobody else will come into the room while you are treating; interruptions will break your concentration as well as the relaxing flow of the massage.

clear away clutter

Tidy and clean the room, and clear away any clutter. You want as few distractions as possible when you are massaging.

Decide where you are going to massage. The floor is a good option because there is usually plenty of room to move about. It can be hard on your knees, so make sure that you have a few floor cushions to hand. The person you are massaging should sit in a comfortable arm chair with their legs supported on a small table or stool. You want to be able to reach their feet without bending or twisting in any way.

Have any massage oils and equipment that you will be using to hand. You'll want two or more towels; at least one to place under the foot being worked and another to keep the resting foot warm.

Sitting or lying down for any length of time can cause some loss of body heat, so make sure the room is warm. On cool days and evenings, you may like to offer the person a light blanket to keep him or her feeling warm and secure.

creating atmosphere

Where possible, have soft lighting. Turn off bright lights that are positioned directly overhead or in direct line with eye contact – either yours or the person you are treating. A couple of lamps will usually give

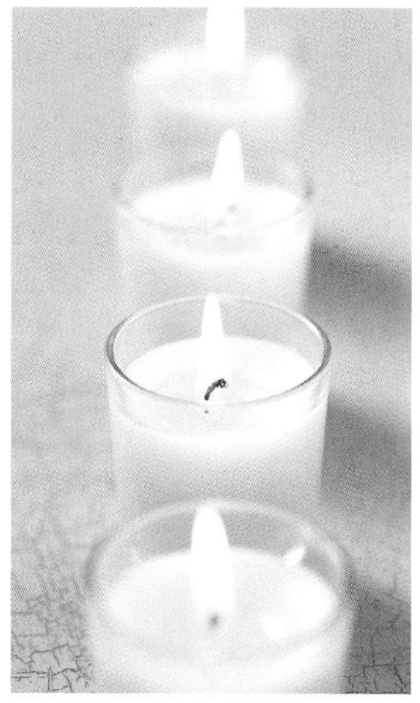

△ **A few candles will help to create soft relaxing lighting in the room. Scented candles will often help to lift the mood, too.**

enough light, and you may also like to light a few candles in the room. A flickering candle helps to create an atmosphere that is calm and cosy.

Flowers always look attractive. If you have dried or fake flowers, try adding a drop of essential oil to three or four cotton buds and place them in the arrangement. Rose, jasmine, neroli, violet and ylang-ylang are good oils to try: they give appealing, slightly heady, floral aromas.

Other ways to introduce pleasant smells into the area are by using scented candles or by burning an essential oil in a vaporizer. You could also use an essential oil room spray half an hour before treatment. However, don't use a strong scent, since some people may find it off-putting.

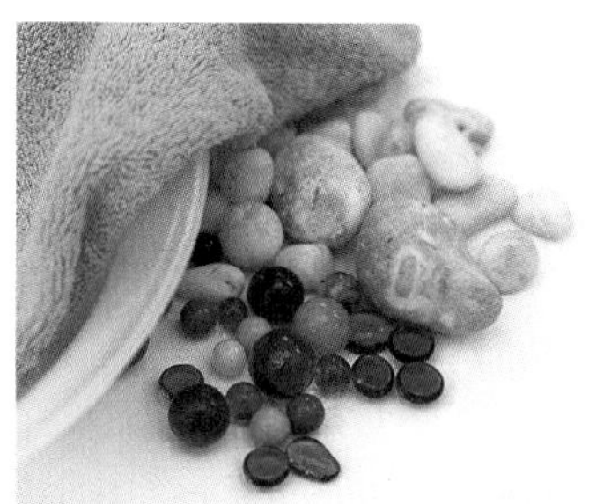

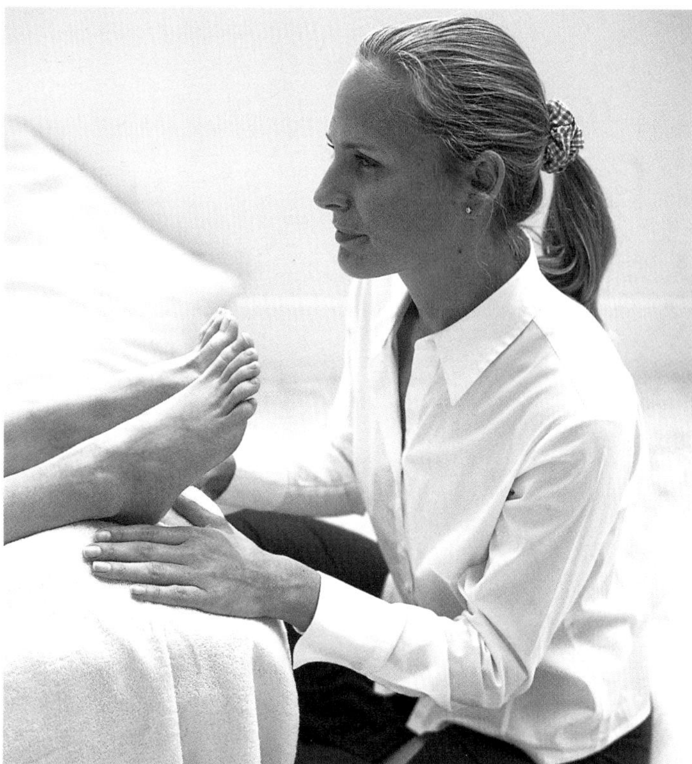

Most people like music, but tastes vary, so choose soft instrumental music that is relaxing to mind and body, and keep the volume low so that it is not intrusive. Always ask if silence is preferred.

preparing yourself

Once the room is ready, prepare yourself. Wash your hands and check your nails are well trimmed. There should be no danger of them catching the recipient's skin.

Spend a few moments centring yourself before you start the massage. Sit comfortably with both feet flat on the floor. Relax your shoulders and face, then breathe slowly and deeply for a few moments. Posture and breathing are vital for an effective massage treatment. To warm up your body carry out some stretching sequences combined with

◁ **Suggest that the receiver has a footbath before you treat them, particularly if he or she has come at the end of the day. Place a layer of marbles or pebbles in the footbowl. The receiver can roll their feet backwards and forwards over them for a relaxing mini-massage.**

△ **Always make sure that you can reach the person's feet easily. You should be able to keep your back straight as you work.**

deep breathing exercises. Relax and warm your hands with a quick self-massage to ensure they are supple and soft.

When all is ready and you are about to start, see if you can feel the healing energy of your hands. Bring the hands together in a prayer-like position, but pull them apart just before they touch. Do this two or three times before you start. You may feel a slightly pulling or tingling sensation as you do so – this is the energy of your hands.

post-massage

After the massage or treatment, let the person relax for a few minutes. You may decide to leave the room for this, or simply to sit quietly beside him or her.

Drink a glass of water, and offer one to the receiver as well. Suggest that he or she spends the next hour or two quietly, in order to appreciate fully the relaxing effects of the foot treatment.

The Foot Massages

Your feet can transport you into realms of pleasure. They are one of the most sensual and sensitive parts of your body, and a loving touch applied here can be wonderfully relaxing, energizing or stimulating. Here are some fabulous foot treatments that will soothe your spirits, and restore your soul.

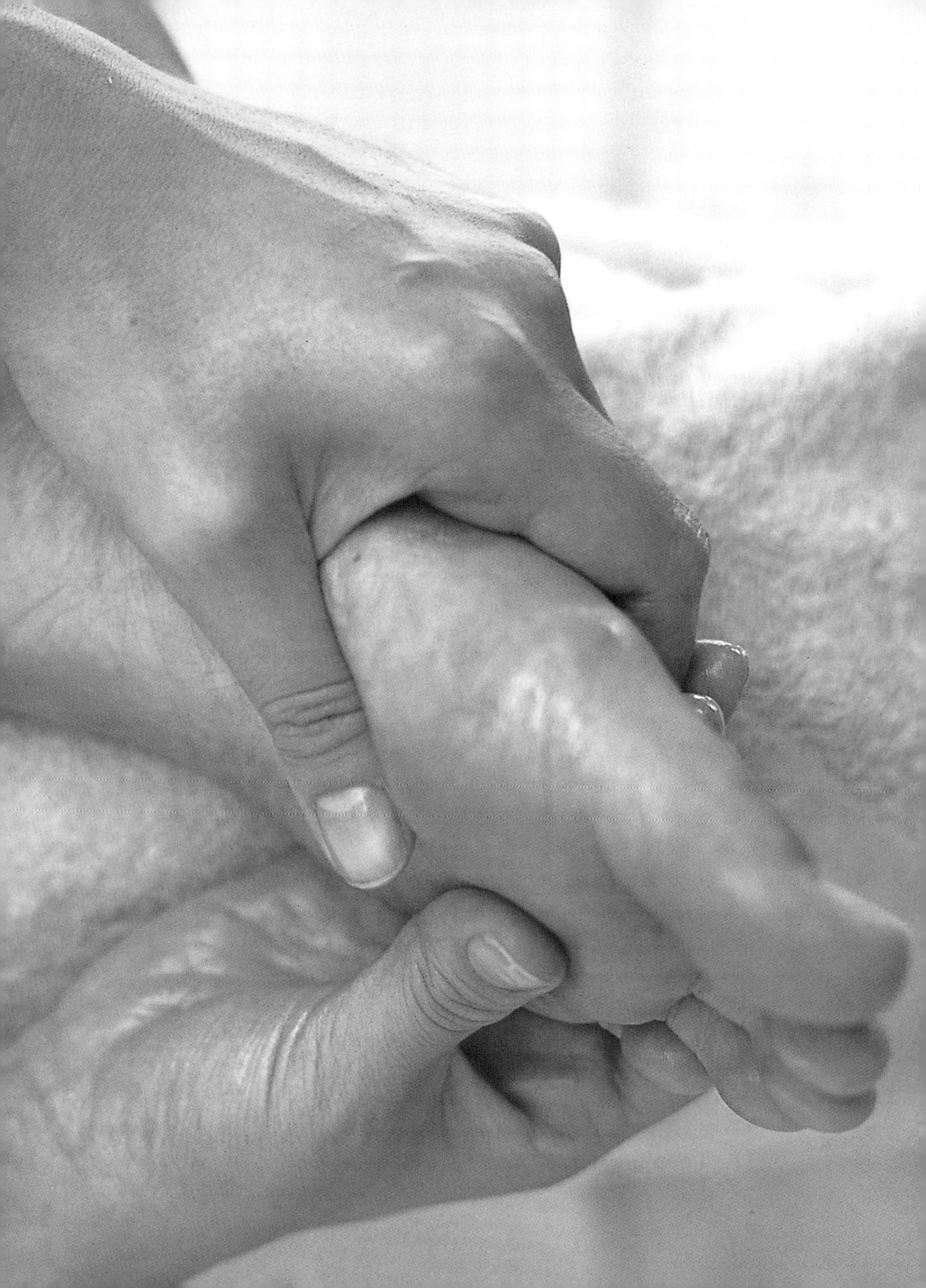

Simple self-massage

All that is needed for a simple self-massage treatment is an understanding of a few basic strokes. After that, it is a matter of practice so that you become comfortable with the different techniques involved.

Self-treatment is a great way of learning massage, because you have your own physical responses to guide you. It is important to get yourself into a relaxed position: you should not need to twist your back or the knee in order to reach the foot. If you are comfortable, you will find it much easier to detect the subtle differences between different strokes and types of pressure, and your reactions to them. You will instantly know when you have got the technique right, and when your touch is sufficiently sensitive and pleasing.

Once you have mastered the basic routine described here, you will be able to adapt the techniques to suit your particular needs and your different moods. You'll also find it much easier to learn the other treatments in this book.

easy self-treatment

This is a quick, simple and effective massage that helps to soothe the tired muscles. It can be used at any time as a treatment to relax and refresh the feet, as a quick pick-me-up or as a way to boost your vitality and energy. You can use a cream or massage oil if you like. This basic massage is best done while sitting on the floor, with the resting leg stretched out in front of you.

△ **3** Place your foot on the floor, beside the knee. Hold the foot so that your fingers curl round the sole and your thumbs and heels are on top. Spread the top of the foot by sliding the thumbs apart, applying firm pressure and keeping your fingers in place.

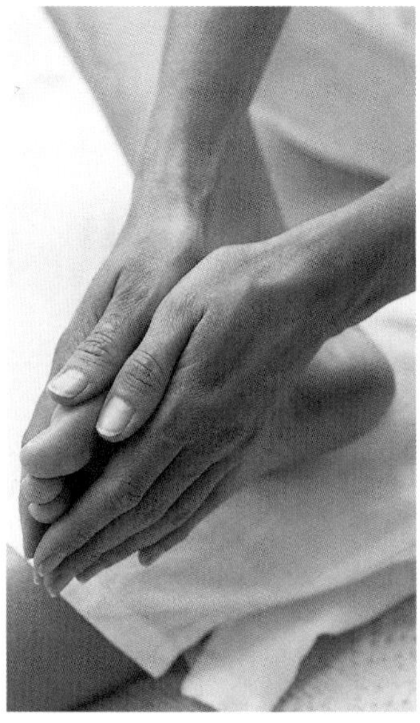

△ **1** Bring your right foot to rest on your left knee; make sure that you are sitting in a comfortable position. Start with gentle stroking. Grasp the foot between your hands, in a sandwich hold, then slide them up the foot, from your heel to the toes.

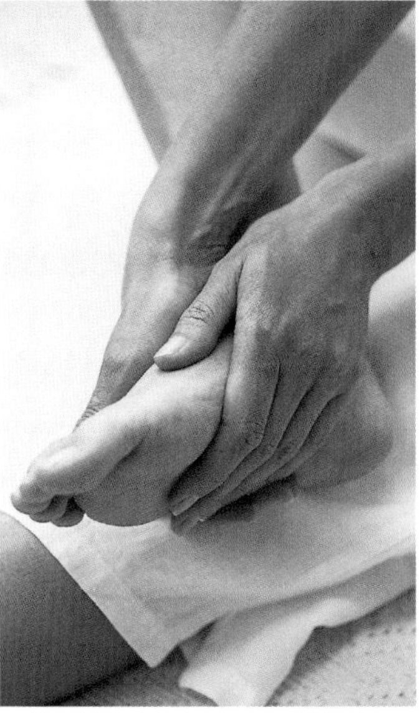

△ **2** Keeping the foot in the same position as before, slide your hands in the opposite direction – down the foot from the toes to your heel. Keep the pressure steady and firm. Now repeat these up-and-down sliding movements two more times.

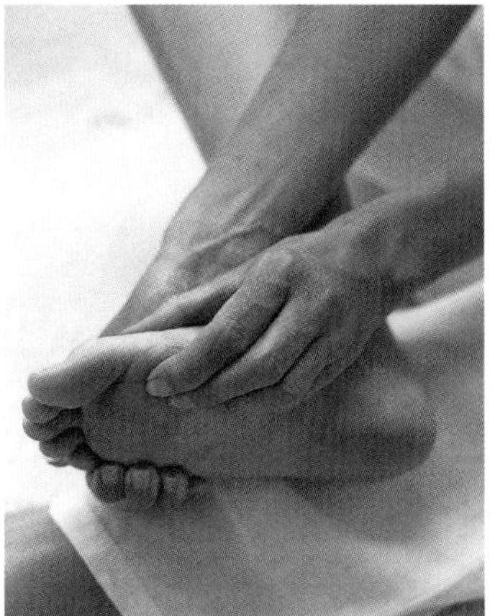

△ **4** Now lift up your foot and place it on your knee again. Place your hands in the same position as in step 3. Now, pull the fingers slowly outwards so that you stretch and spread the sole of the foot. Apply firm pressure as you do so.

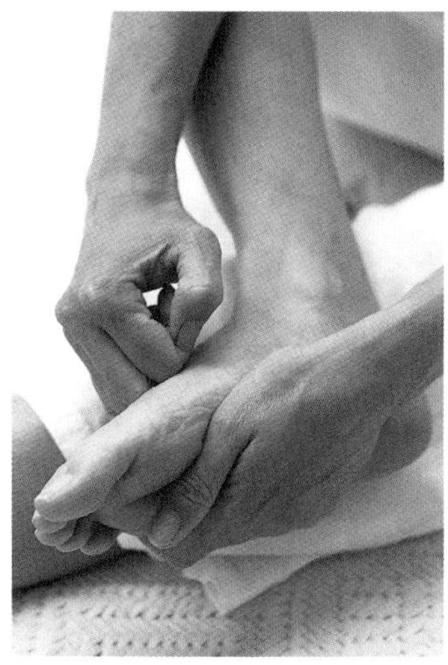

△ **5** Support the sole of the foot with your left hand. Make a fist with your right hand. Use your knuckles to apply light pressure to the top of the foot, making circular movements. Now support the top of the foot with your right hand. Use the knuckles of the left hand to work the sole, applying deeper pressure.

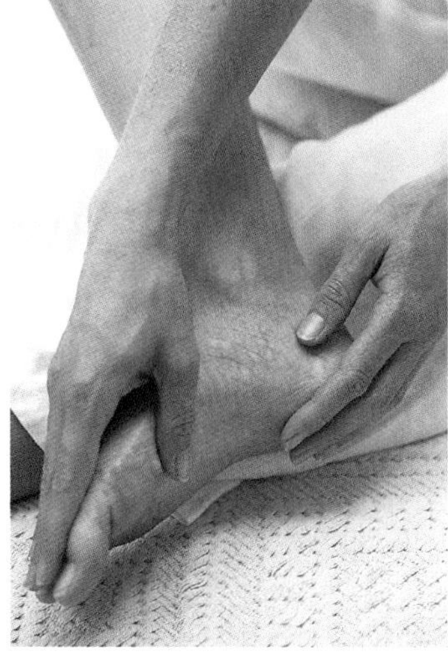

△ **7** Continue to support the heel of your foot with your left hand. Place the right hand over the top of the foot, placing your thumb on the sole. Now, gently stretch and push the foot downwards. Again, stretch only as far as feels comfortable. Do steps 6 and 7 once more.

different strokes

When giving yourself a foot massage, take the opportunity to experiment. Try out different strokes, levels of pressure and combinations of the two. People vary considerably in what strokes they like best, and in particular how much pressure they enjoy. What you like can also change depending on your mood and the part of the foot being worked.

As a general rule:

Fast strokes are stimulating and energizing.

Slow rhythmic strokes have a hypnotic, relaxing effect.

Deep pressure can be used to release muscular tension, relieve stress or to enhance vitality.

Gentle pressure is soothing and has a calming effect on both the mind and the body.

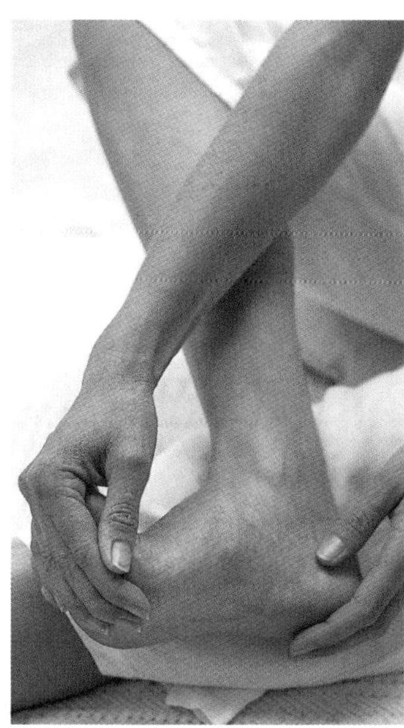

△ **6** Hold the heel of your foot with your left hand, then grasp the ball with your right. Pull the ball of your foot gently upwards so that you stretch the sole. Make sure that you stretch the foot only as far as feels comfortable.

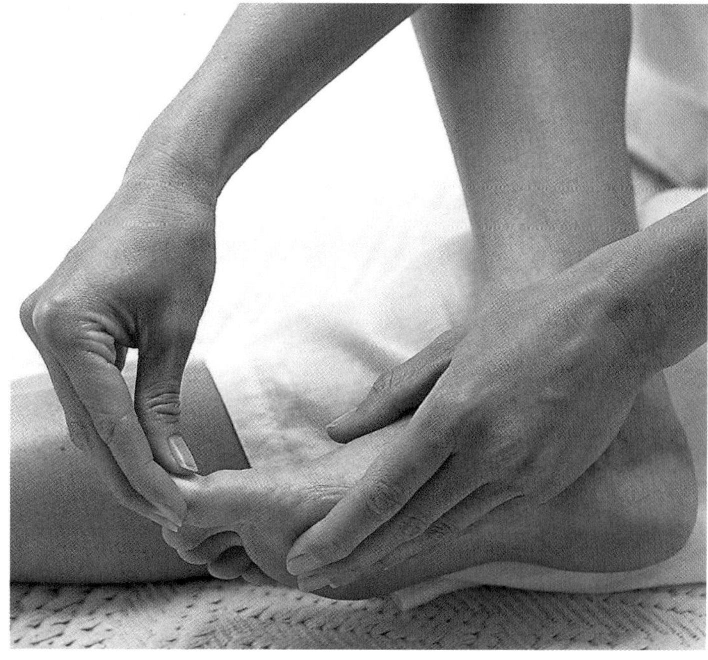

△ **8** Support the foot near the arch with your left hand. With your right hand, hold the big toe near the main joint. Gently rotate the toe first in a clockwise direction, then in an anticlockwise direction. Repeat the action on each toe, finishing on the little one. Now, repeat steps 1 to 8 on your left foot.

Soothing relaxer

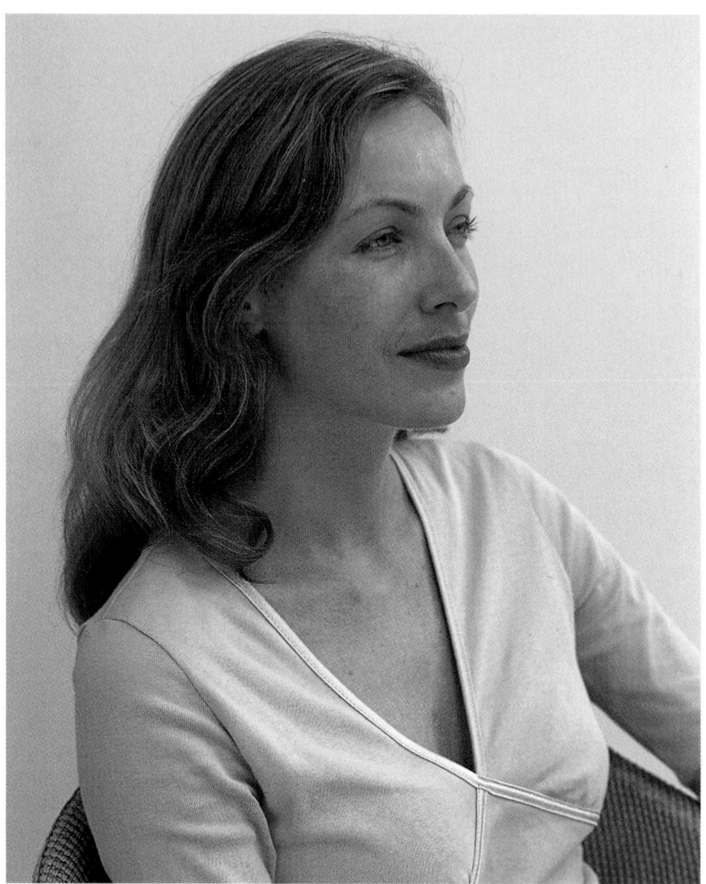

Self-treatment is wonderfully soothing. However, nothing you do to yourself can quite match the sensation of leaning back and letting someone else do the work, as in this routine. There is something utterly relaxing about having your feet massaged; tension seems to drain out of the whole body almost as though a tap had been opened. Perhaps because the feet are so far away from your head, it feels easy to let your mind release worries and anxieties, too.

teach a friend

A relaxing foot massage is a wonderful gift to be able to offer others. It's also worth persuading a friend to learn this short routine, so that you can benefit from it.

△ **This treatment should leave you thoroughly relaxed. Take some time to sit quietly after the routine. If you are giving it to someone else, leave them alone for five or ten minutes so that they appreciate the full effects.**

Anyone can do it even if they have never learned massage techniques before.

There is no need to make any special arrangements in order to do this massage. It can be done anywhere, and works well if the person is sitting on the sofa watching TV or if you are in the garden on a warm, sunny afternoon. You can use it to give a friend a pick-me-up after a late night, and it can also be done in the morning to set someone up for a long, stressful day.

calming massage routine

If you like, you can incorporate this massage into a longer pamper treatment for the feet. You may also like to use some favourite aromatherapy oils to heighten the effects. Neroli and sandalwood or rose and bergamot would be excellent soothing blends to use. Take some time to relax afterwards, too – perhaps with a cup of herbal tea.

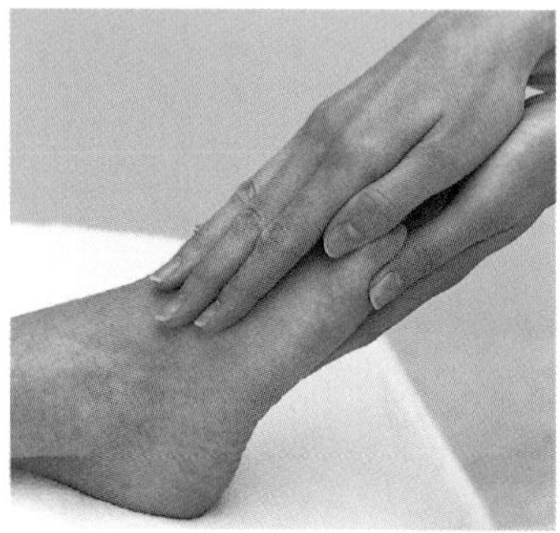

△ **1** Start with the right foot. Hold the foot between your hands – place one hand lengthways over the top of the foot, with the other underneath it. Slide the hands up the foot to the toes, then back down again. Repeat the action at least three times, increasing the pressure as you go.

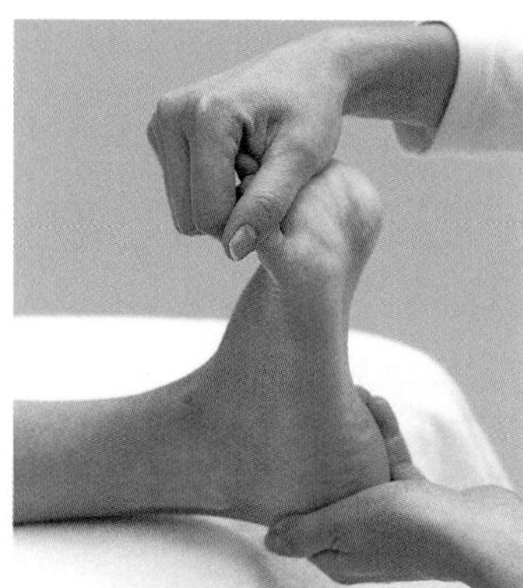

△ **2** Support the heel of the foot in your left hand. Gently grasp the toes with the other hand and then slowly push the top of the foot towards the leg. This gives the sole a good stretch, which helps to release tension. Do not push further than feels comfortable.

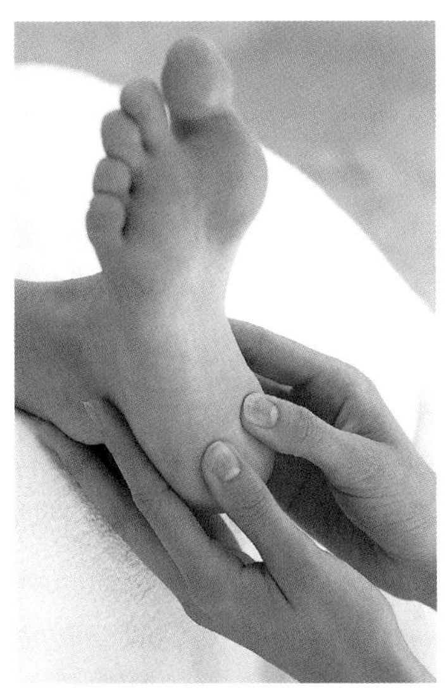

△ **3** Place both of your thumbs on the heel of the foot, with one thumb positioned slightly higher than the other. Now start to massage, by making tiny circles with the thumb, using alternate thumbs. Work your way right up the foot, to the top of the sole, and remember to use much lighter pressure on the arch than on the heel and ball.

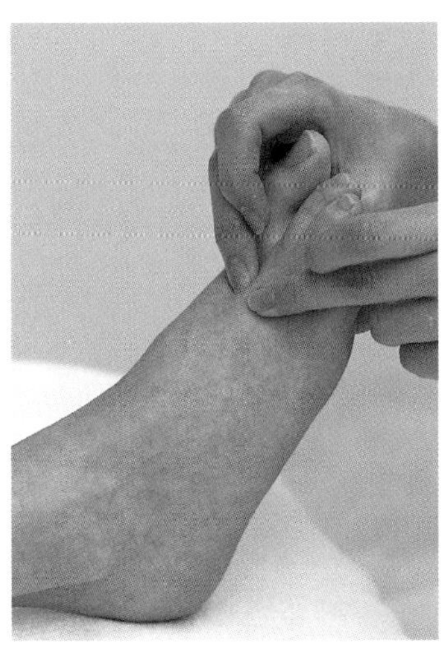

△ **4** Massage the top of the foot, using your two middle fingers to make tiny circular movements. Start in the groove between the big and second toe, and work down the entire foot to the ankle. Repeat the movement, this time starting in the groove between the second and third toes. Work across the foot in this way until you reach the little toe.

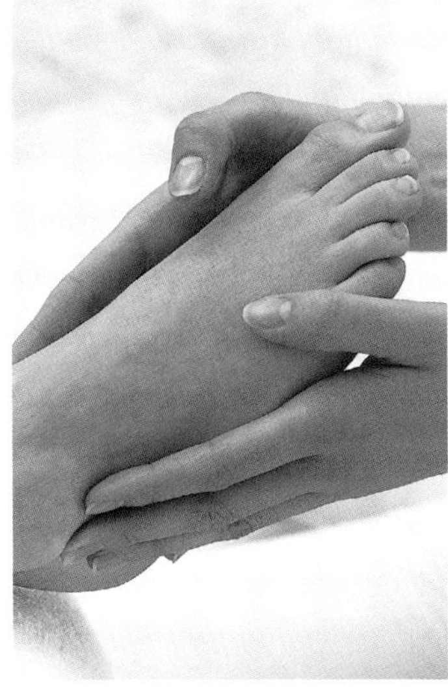

△ **5** Place both of your hands on either side of the foot, in such a way that your fingertips are positioned next to the ankle bones. Now, using firm (but pleasurable) pressure, massage in a clockwise direction around both ankle bones at the same time. Repeat the movement, but this time working in an anticlockwise direction.

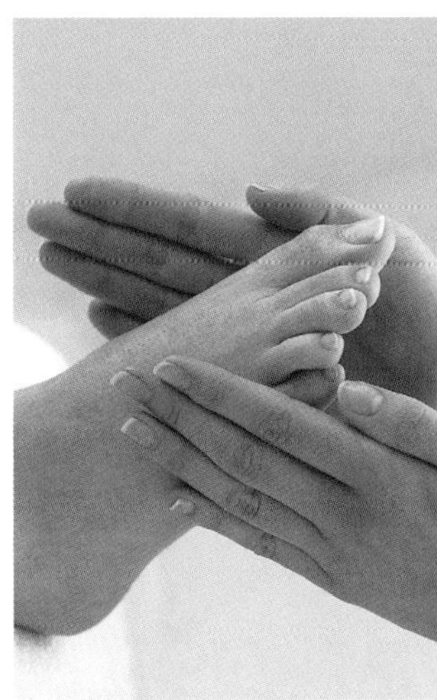

△ **6** Place your hands either side of the foot, so that it is wedged in-between them in a sandwich hold. Using a gentle push-pull action, pull one side of the foot towards you and push the other side away at the same time. Repeat, but this time reverse the action so that you push the first side away, and pull the other towards you. Do the movements twice more.

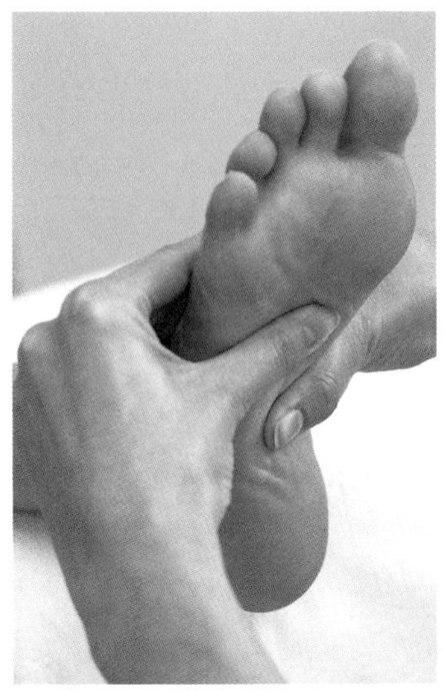

△ **7** Now place your thumbs on the sole so that they point in opposite directions. Wrap your fingers around the top of the foot to keep it steady. Slide the thumbs up the sole, making a criss-cross movement – so that first the left thumb slides above the right, then the right one slides above the left. Start at the toes and work down the foot; then work back up to the toes.

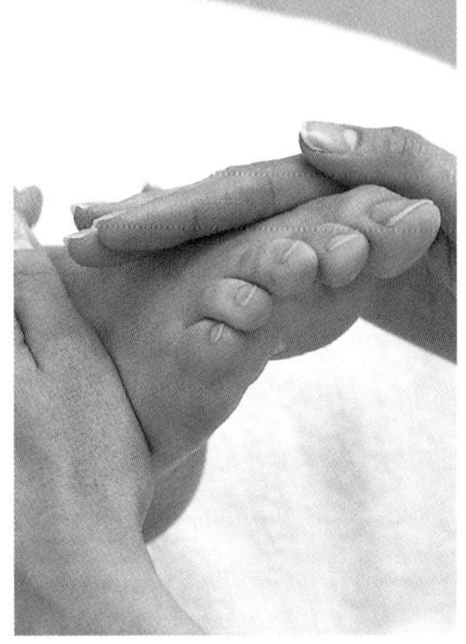

△ **8** Finish the massage by making feather-light strokes on the top and sole of the foot, using alternate hands. Cover the whole area two or three times, or longer if you feel that the person is really benefiting from this relaxing action. Now repeat the whole sequence on the left foot.

Start the day massage

The ancient Greeks believed that a daily massage was one of the best ways of keeping the body healthy. Few of us have time for a full treatment, but a quick self-massage for the feet is a great way to start the day. This routine is designed to be relaxing yet invigorating – a real wake-up call.

▽ It's worth getting up 15 minutes early so that you can enjoy a relaxing start to the day. A foot massage doesn't take long, but it can make all the difference to the way you feel.

wake-up routine

Ideally you will be relaxed before starting this sequence. However, don't worry if you wake up feeling anxious; you will find it almost impossible to remain so once the massage is underway. Start with the right foot, then repeat on the left.

▷ **1** To start, get into a comfortable position in a peaceful spot. Have a glass of juice and some fruit on hand to enjoy after the massage. Choose a favourite cream or essential oil blend to apply to the feet – they should have reasonable slip but should not be dripping.

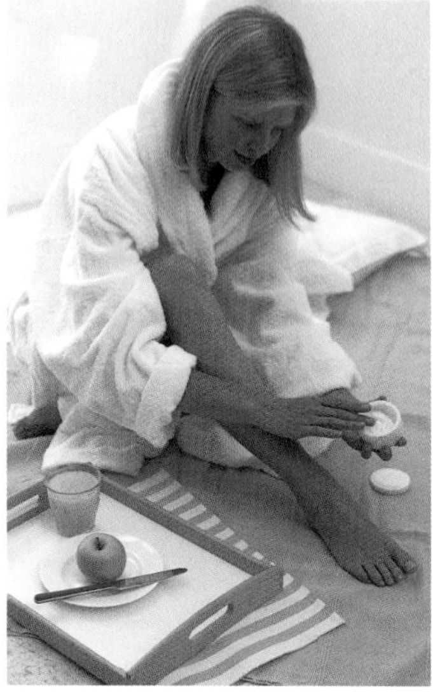

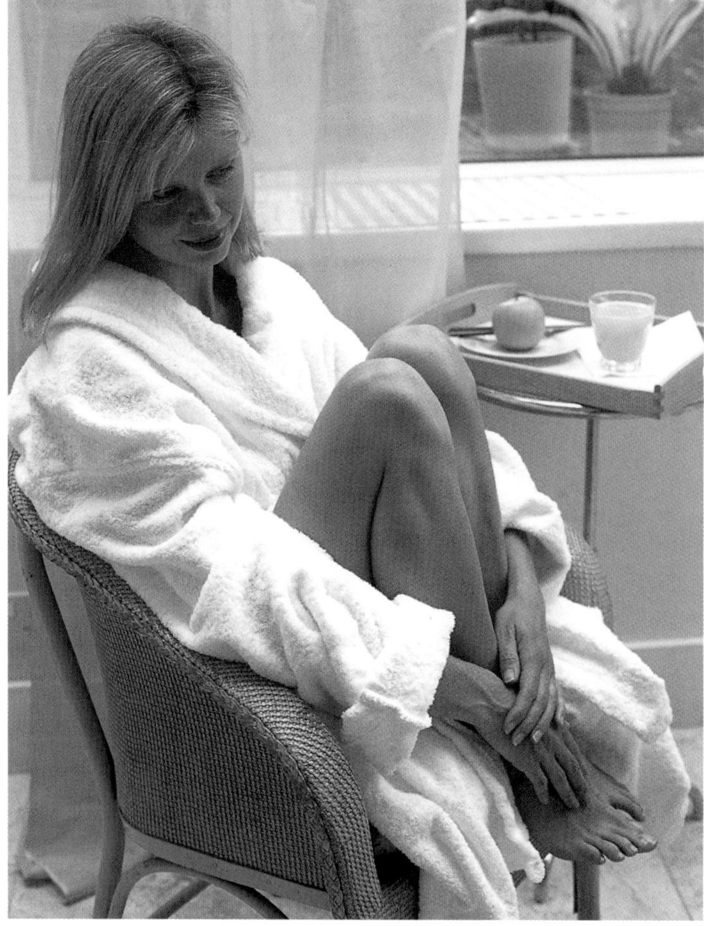

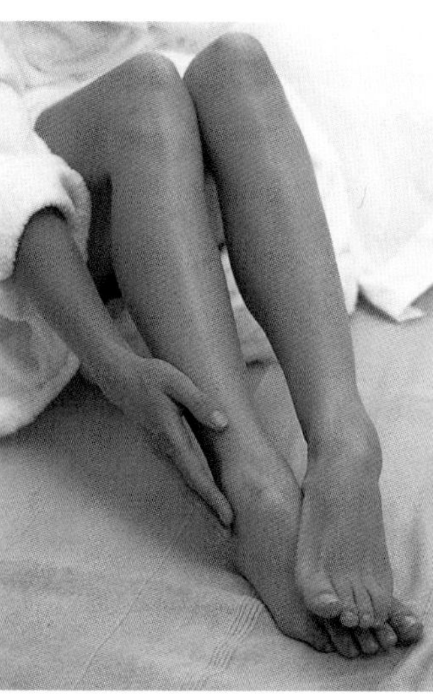

△ **2** Use your fingers to rub the cream or oil liberally over the top of the right foot. Then place your left foot on top, and use the sole to massage from the toes to ankle. Apply heavier pressure on the toes than to the top of the foot, which is more delicate. Take particular care around the ankle area.

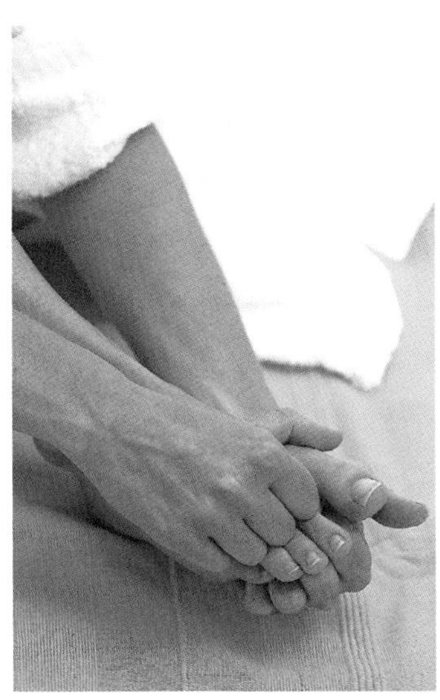

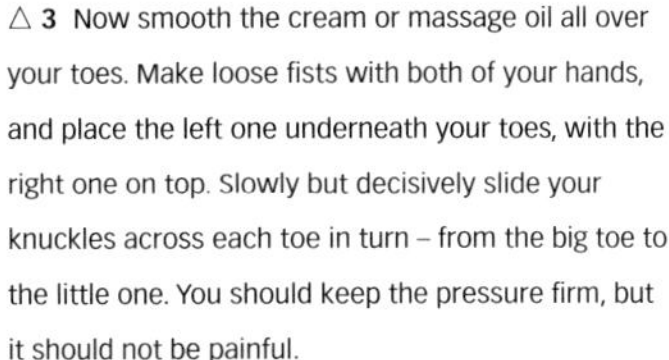

△ **3** Now smooth the cream or massage oil all over your toes. Make loose fists with both of your hands, and place the left one underneath your toes, with the right one on top. Slowly but decisively slide your knuckles across each toe in turn – from the big toe to the little one. You should keep the pressure firm, but it should not be painful.

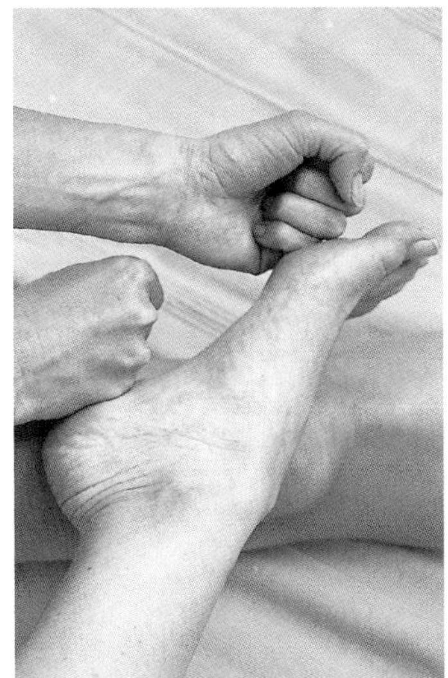

△ **5** Rest the heel of the right foot on your left knee and apply the cream or oil to the sole. Make fists of both hands. Use the outside edge of alternate fists to strike the sole of the foot, starting at the toes and working towards the heel area. Hit the foot harder on the ball and heel than the arch, which should be struck only lightly,

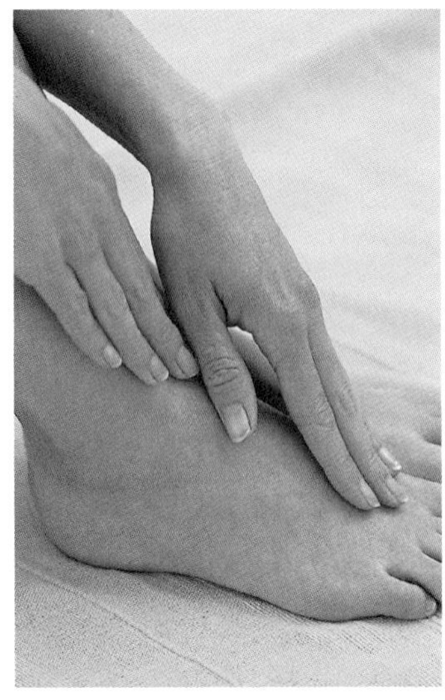

△ **6** Add more oil or cream to your hands, then rub the palms together to spread it evenly. Use alternate hands to stroke the top of the foot, starting from the toes and working down to the ankle. Begin with a feather-light touch to encourage relaxation, and then increase the pressure to a strong energizing level. Keep it pleasurable at all times.

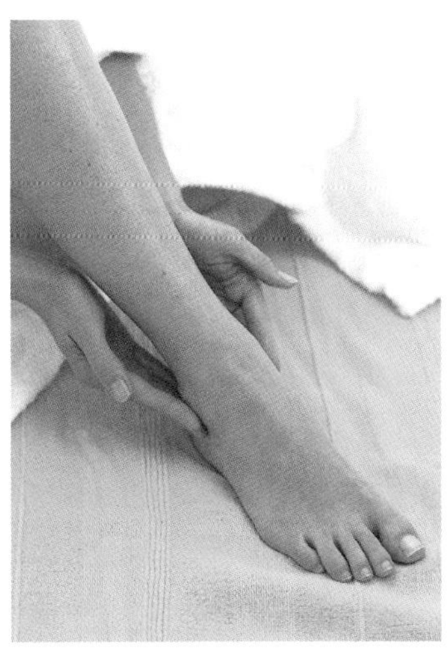

△ **4** With plenty of cream or oil on your hands, massage around both sides of the ankle at the same time. Work in a clockwise direction, making three distinct rotations. Repeat, this time working in an anticlockwise direction. If you are still feeling sleepy or if your ankles feel tight or tense, repeat the movement in both directions.

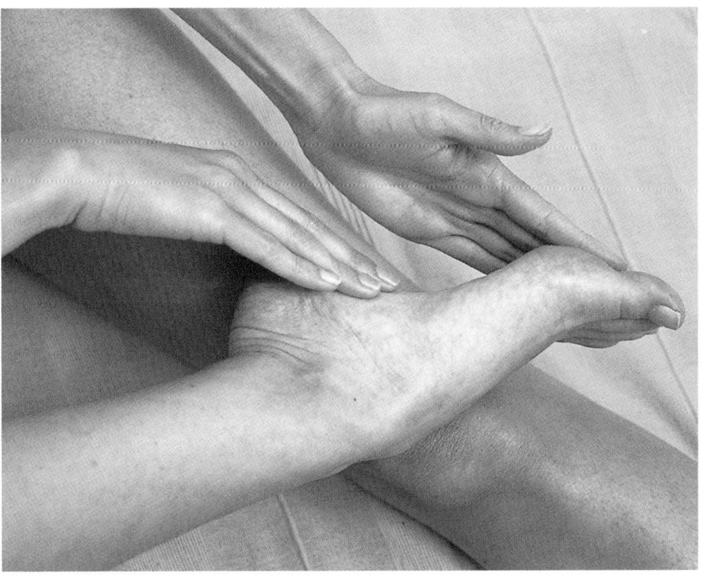

△ **7** Now rest the heel on your left knee, exposing the sole. Add a little more oil or cream to your hands and rub the palms together to spread it evenly through them. Use alternate hands to make long sweeping strokes down your foot from the toes to the heel. Again, start with light touch to aid relaxation, then gradually increase the pressure. Now repeat the sequence on the left foot.

Recharge your batteries

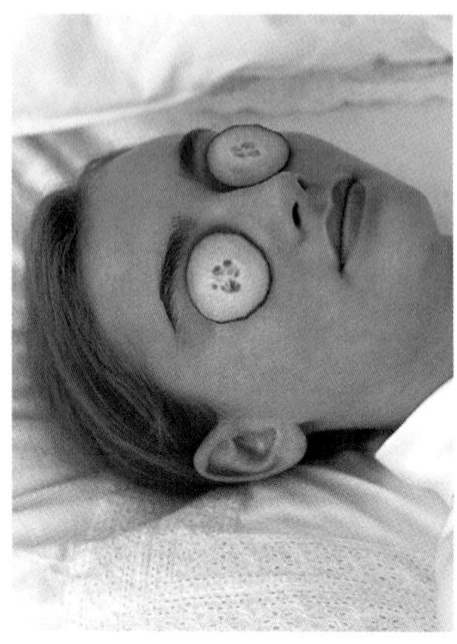

◁ Slices of cucumber or potato placed over the eyes while your feet are being massaged will enhance the general revitalizing effect.

Most of us don't have enough time in our lives to relax and recharge. Ideally, we should stop and rest whenever we feel tired or low in energy, but we often need to keep going because of work, home or social commitments.

This treatment is designed to soothe and revitalize at the same time, so it should leave the recipient feeling refreshed and energized. It is an excellent treatment to do if someone is going out in the evening after a hard day at work, or in the middle of a busy or stressful week.

The routine can easily be adapted for self-treatment – and used as an instant pick-me-up wherever you happen to be. It is great for days when you can't stop – but feel you can't go on.

the power of silence

Try to work in silence except when you need to ask for and receive feedback – a few minutes of calm can help to increase the restorative effect of this massage. The person you are treating may like to cover his or her eyes with slices of cucumber or raw potato; these will have a restorative effect, and closing the eyes will also reduce any temptation to chat.

Give the recipient a glass of water to sip before and after the massage – dehydration can increase feelings of fatigue. It is also good to eat a small snack – a piece of fresh fruit would be ideal – to boost energy levels. If possible, he or she should take a short walk in the fresh air after doing the routine.

revitalizing routine

Make sure the recipient is sitting comfortably. Suggest that he or she takes a few moments to relax the shoulders and face muscles, and to take a few deep breaths before you start.

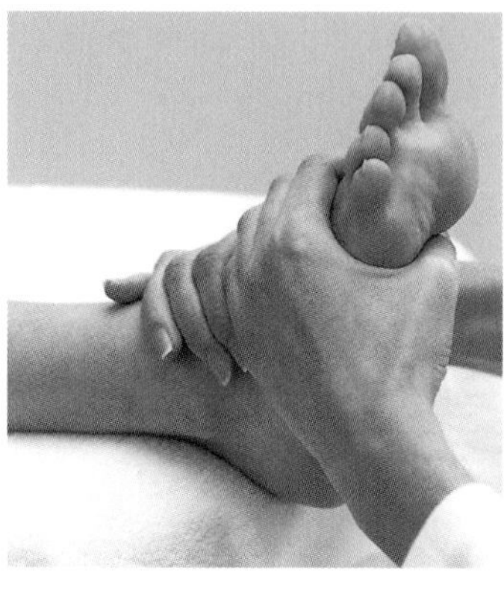

△ **1** Stroke the sole and top of the right foot, using alternate hands. Cover the foot three times or more. Now place your thumbs on the sole and the fingers on the top, one hand slightly above the other. Move the hands in opposite directions, in a gentle twisting action – as if wringing out a wet cloth. Start near the ankle and work up to the toes, then work back down the foot. Repeat the action once more.

tonic massage cream

This thick cream works well with the revitalizing routine, and it is suitable for any skin type. Made in the following quantity, it will last for about 12 treatments. You can substitute other essential oils for the peppermint and petitgrain if you like. Try cypress and lemon to aid detoxing, rose and mandarin for total indulgence, or rosemary and geranium for an uplifting effect.

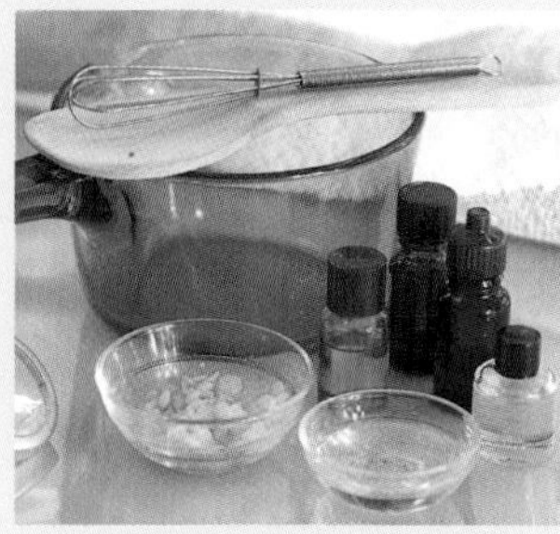

△ **You can make a superb massage cream using just a few natural ingredients.**

ingredients

- 20ml/4 tsp almond oil
- 40ml/8 tsp avocado oil
- 20ml/4 tsp rosewater
- 5ml/1 tsp lecithin granules
- 10g/¼fl oz beeswax
- 8 drops each petitgrain and peppermint essential oils

Put the almond oil, avocado oil and beeswax into a ceramic or stainless steel jug. Stand in a saucepan that is half-filled with water. Heat on a low temperature, stirring occasionally until the wax melts. Remove the jug from the water. Add the lecithin and beat the mixture vigorously, then stir in the rosewater. Allow the mixture to cool (but not to become completely cold). Now mix in the essential oils. Scrape the cream into a clean, screwtop jar.

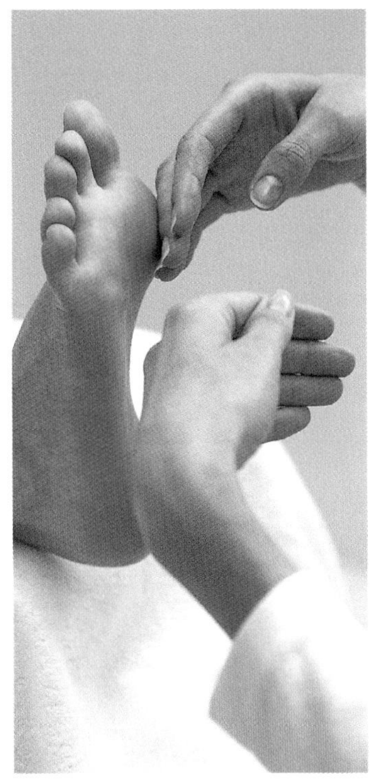

△ **2** Briskly but lightly, use your palms to slap all over the top of the foot, working from the ankle to the toes. Then use the back of your hands to slap all over the sole – the pressure can be heavier here. Do this a few times. It helps to increase the circulation, removing toxins and bringing nutrients and oxygen to the area.

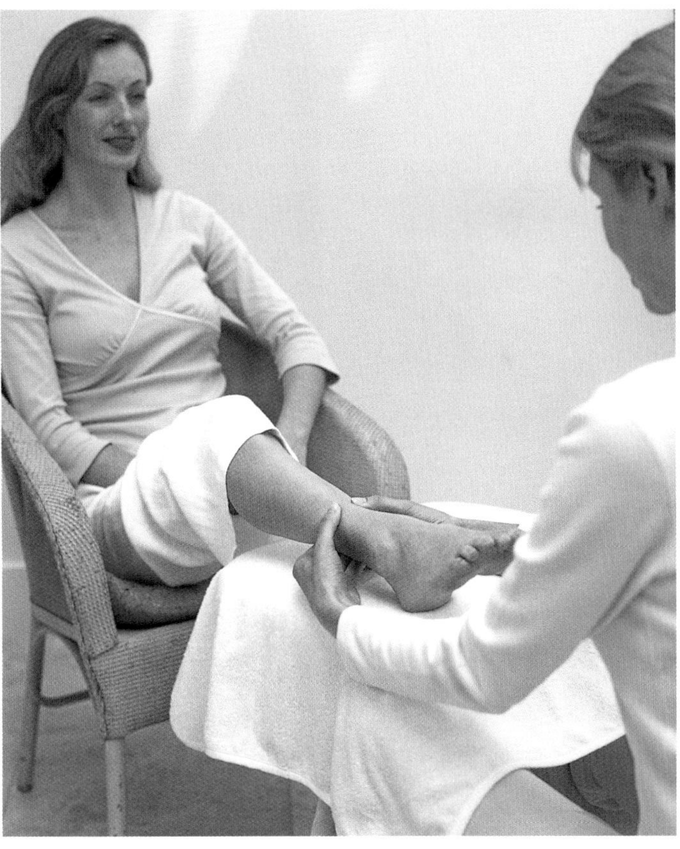

△ **4** Place your thumbs either side of the shinbone. Use the tips to massage, making little circles. Work up the leg from the ankle to the knee. Slide the hands back down to the ankle, without applying any pressure. Repeat.

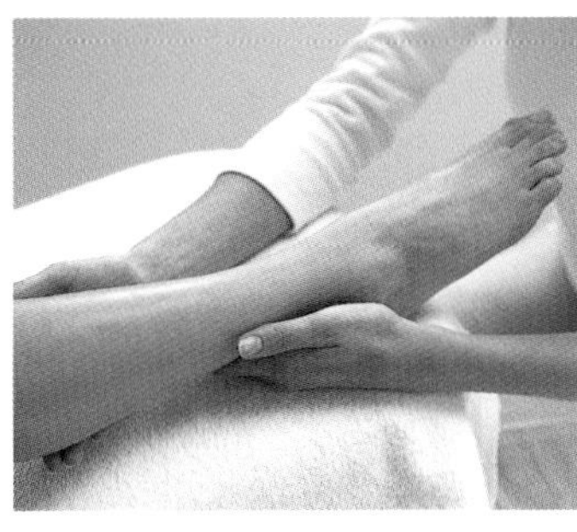

△ **3** Hold the foot behind the ankle to keep it steady. Cup the other hand around the calf muscle, then squeeze and release. Start from just above the ankle and work up the leg to just below the knee, squeezing every part of the muscle. Now slide your hand back to the ankle and work up the leg in the same way twice more. Tension often collects in the calves, and this is a good way to release it.

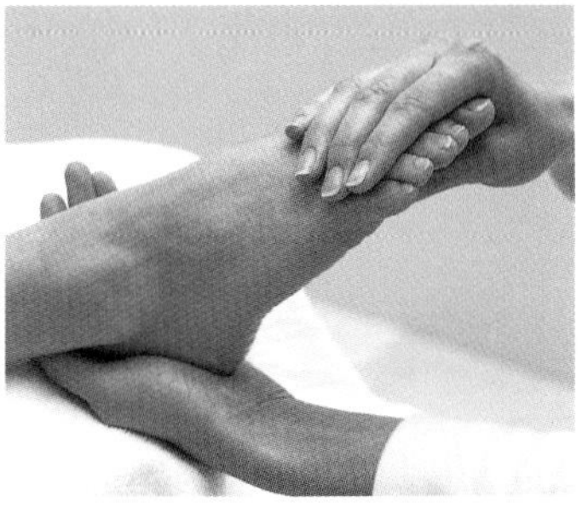

△ **5** Cup a hand around the heel to support the foot, while resting your other hand against the base of the toes. Gently push the foot away from you three times – remember that you should never push it further than it will go naturally. Now do a forward stretch (shown): place the hand on top of the foot near the toes and pull them gently towards you. Do this pulling movement three times.

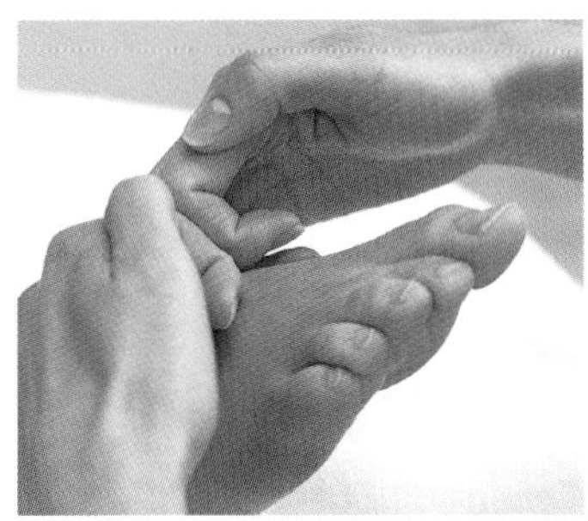

△ **6** Curl your fingers to make very loose fists with your hands. Rest the flat area between the top two joints of each fist on top of the foot, and use to massage, making small circular movements. Start near the toes and work down the foot to the ankle, then work back up again. Repeat. End the routine by stroking the sole and top of the foot, as in Step 1. Repeat the whole sequence on the left foot.

And so to sleep

When you sleep well, you wake up feeling refreshed and ready for the activities of the day. Sleep is also essential for good health: while we rest, the cells in our body repair and regenerate, our detoxifying organs do their work unimpeded, and our blood pressure drops. All this helps to combat stress and improves our ability to fight off illness.

Regular sleep is a key element of a healthy lifestyle, along with exercise, a good diet, and drinking plenty of water. Exercising helps tire you out, so it can aid sleep, as can certain foods such as starchy carbohydrates.

getting into a routine

Your sleep is likely to be better if you have a regular routine before bedtime. Having a warm bath and a warm, milky drink each night will help you to relax. If you do these things each evening, you will start to associate them with bedtime, and this will get you in the right frame of mind for sleep.

A foot massage is another great way of relaxing. It is particularly good if your mind is buzzing with thought, because it redirects your attention from the head to the feet – the grounded part of your body.

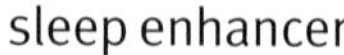

sleep enhancer

This is a very simple self-treatment routine that you can do before bedtime. You use the feet to massage each other, so that there is no need for you to bend down. An oil-based spray is used, so that you can massage without pulling the skin. You can do the routine sitting on your bed, but put a towel down to protect the cover.

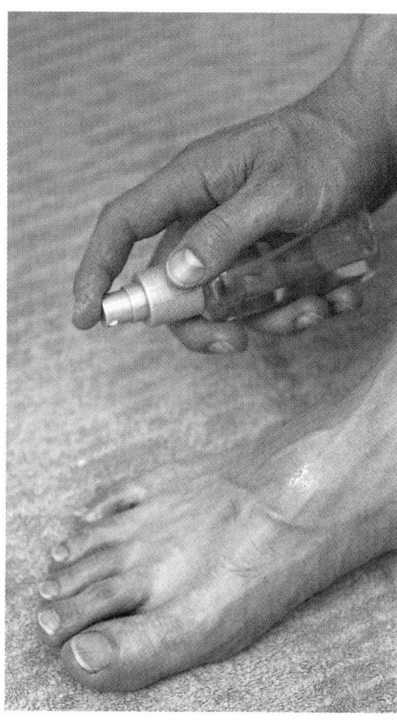

△ **1** Place a large towel underneath your feet. Spray a large, clean tissue with the sleep-time oil spray (see box, right), then spray the top of your right foot. Drop the tissue on top of the foot, and use the sole of the left foot to wipe it all over the top of the right one. Discard the tissue. Repeat on the left foot, so that the top and sole of both feet are lightly perfumed.

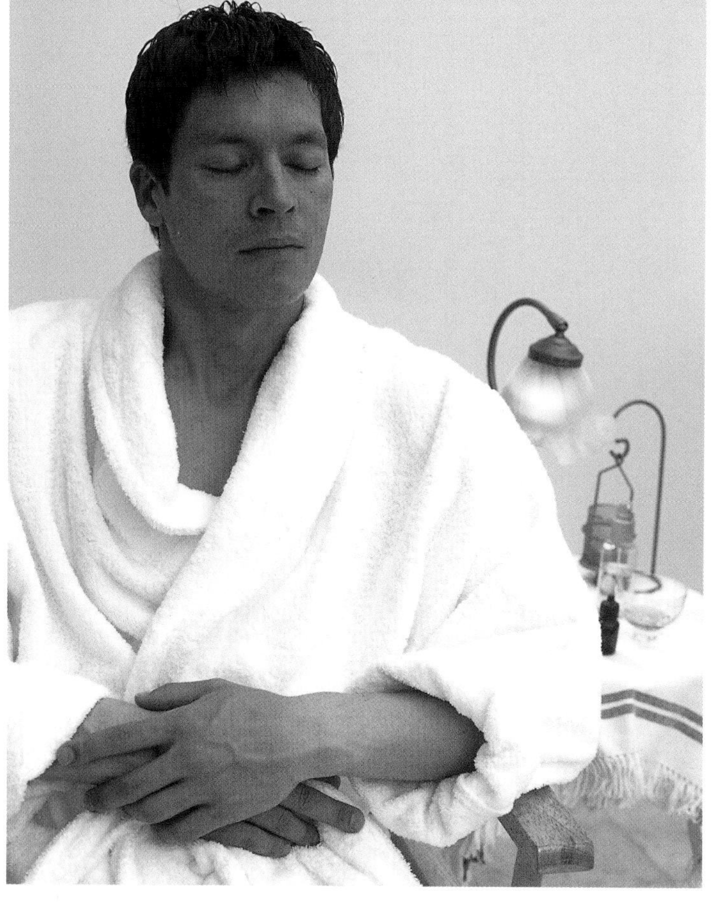

◁ **It is good to get ready for bed before doing this treatment. Ideally you should do it in the bedroom, either sitting in a comfortable chair or lying down in bed, in which case you can go straight to sleep afterwards. If you find yourself getting sleepy, do not feel you have to finish the routine but simply let yourself drift off.**

sleep-time oil spray

This oil spray uses chamomile and lavender oils, which are prized for their relaxing and sedative properties. Neroli and marjoram can also be used, if you prefer their aromas. You can adapt the spray for other occasions by changing the oils: a combination of bergamot, clary sage, geranium and lemon, for example, will make a cleansing spray that is great after a workout and shower.

ingredients

- 25ml/5 tsp grapeseed oil
- 25ml/5 tsp almond oil
- 20ml/4 tsp jojoba oil
- 10ml/2 tsp rosewater
- 10ml/2 tsp glycerine
- 20 drops each lavender and chamomile essential oils.

Mix the first five ingredients together, then stir in the essential oils, mixing well. Transfer to a clean 100 ml/3 ½ fl oz spray bottle. Shake before use.

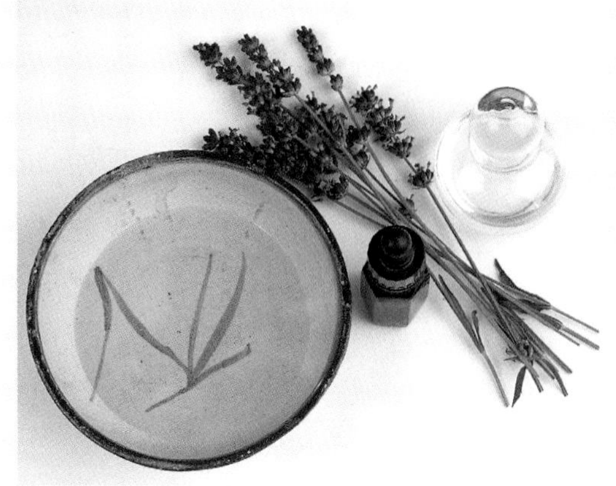

△ **Essential oil distilled from lavender is well known for having a calming effect and for promoting deep, peaceful sleep**

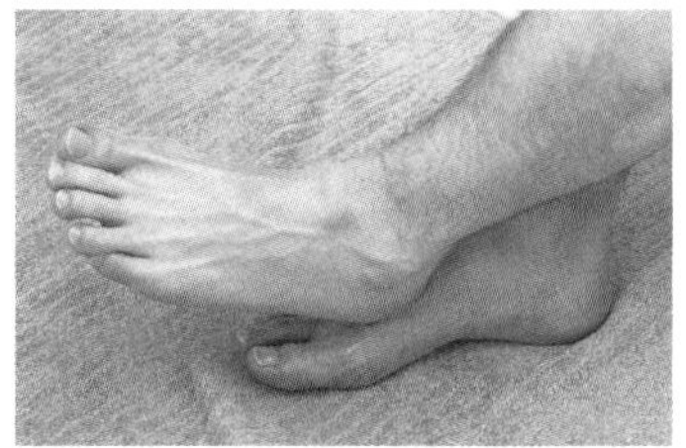

△ **2** Bend your right knee so that the right foot lies flat on the floor or bed. Use the heel pad of the left foot to massage the right toes. Work up and down each toe in turn.

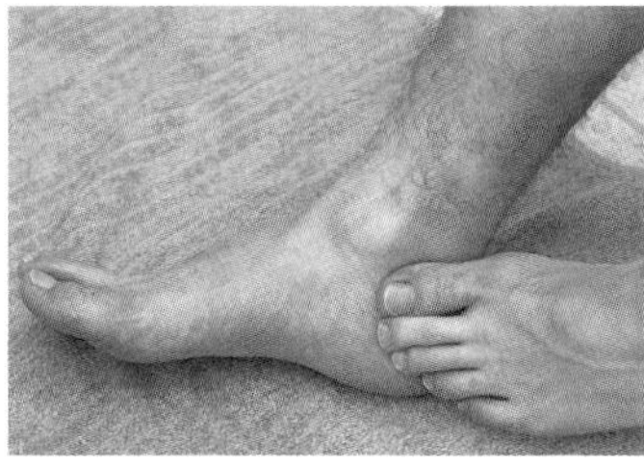

△ **3** Slide the left heel up to the right inner ankle. Use the left heel to massage all around and on top of the ankle bone. Then massage all over the same area with the toes of the left foot. Try to establish a soothing rhythm to the movements. The beauty of these kinds of self-massage techniques is that they can be done anywhere and at any time. So, you can easily try this kind of movement as you sit and watch television or sit on an aeroplane, for example.

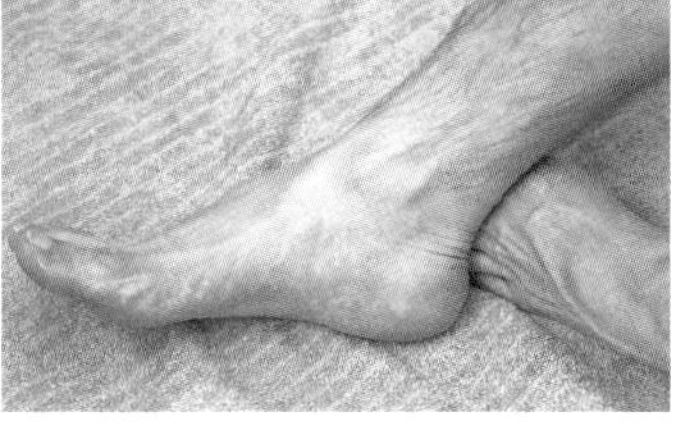

△ **4** Push the left foot around to the back of the right heel, as shown. Now use the toes and the top of the left foot to massage all round the right outer ankle – a quick and easy self-massage technique.

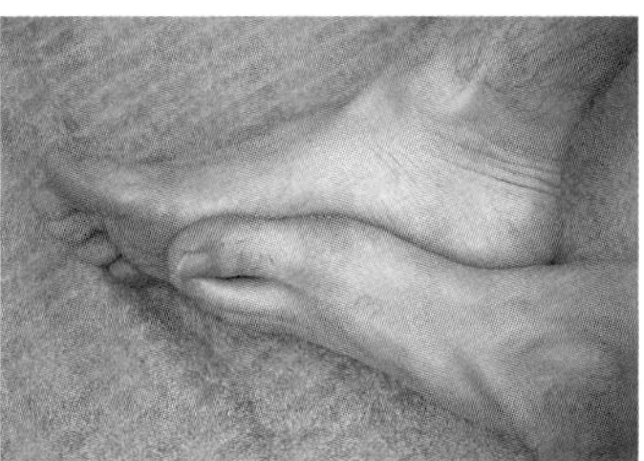

△ **5** Turn the right foot so that it is resting on its outer edge. Use the sole of the left foot to massage up and down the sole of the right. Now repeat steps 2-5 on the left foot. To end, rub the soles of the feet on a towel to ensure they are free from any residue of oil. If you are sitting up, close your eyes, lean back into the chair and relax for ten minutes. If you are in bed, then simply switch off the light and get into your normal sleeping position.

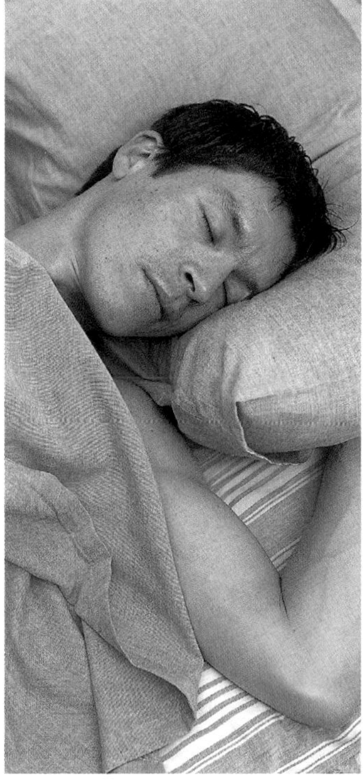

△ **How much sleep you need depends on how old you are and also on your individual constitution. Babies sleep up to 16 hours a day, while older people may need only six hours a night. Most adults need between seven and ten hours a night.**

Foot pamper session

Most of us neglect our feet – particularly in the winter months when they are not on show. Setting aside time for a regular treatment will help you to care for your feet and keep them healthy all year round.

This is a great routine to do at the weekend, or whenever you have some time to yourself. You'll need at least an hour to do it properly – or you can really indulge yourself and take two hours over it.

Think of a pamper session as a time to relax; working on the feet is a great way of taking your mind off day-to-day worries and allowing yourself to focus on feeling good. It is also great to share a pamper session with a friend – set aside an afternoon so that you can really indulge yourselves. You may like to give each other a foot massage at the same time, using one of the relaxing treatments in this book.

Doing a full pamper session once a month will greatly improve your feet's appearance, and will also soften the skin and help the circulation. It is also an excellent way of pepping up your feet at the start of the summer or before going on holiday. You can also shorten the routine and use it as a basis for a mini-pamper session. You may like to do this each week, to keep your feet looking and feeling good in-between full pamper sessions.

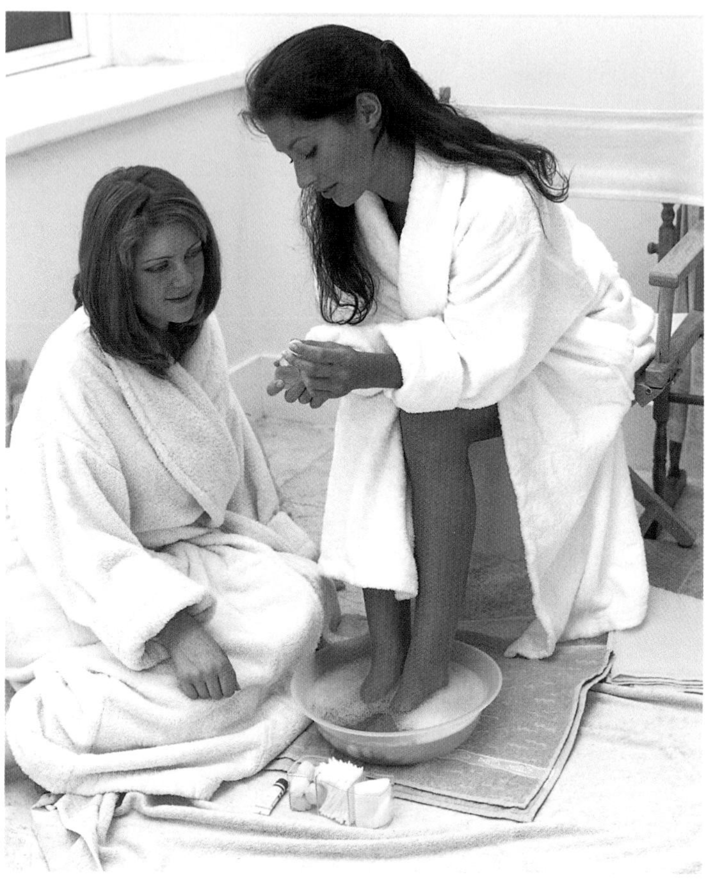

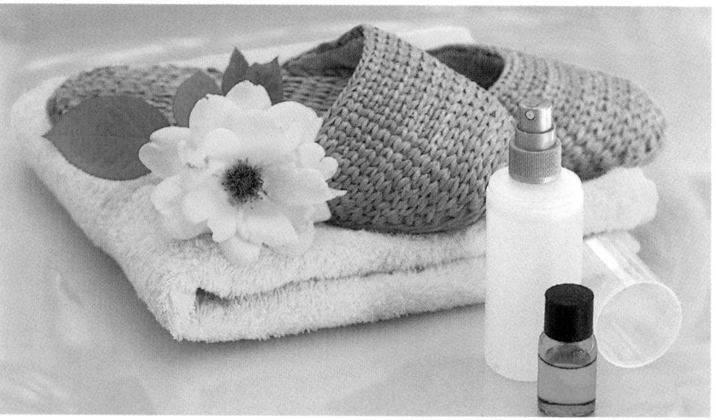

△ Instead of meeting a friend in a bar or restaurant, suggest that you spend an afternoon or evening enjoying a pamper session. It is a good way of spending some relaxed time together, and you could give each other a foot massage at the same time.

◁ Once you start the foot treatment, you won't want to stop, so get everything ready beforehand: lotions, oils, sprays and thick, fluffy towels. Make sure you have a pair of comfortable slippers to slip your feet into after the treatment.

foot care routine

This routine uses the luxury foot scrub described overleaf. If you don't have time to make it, buy one that includes essential oils so that you can benefit from their soothing properties. You'll also need foaming bath or foot gel, a large foot bowl, one large towel and two smaller ones, two plastic bags to slip your feet into, a pumice stone and other items for the pedicure.

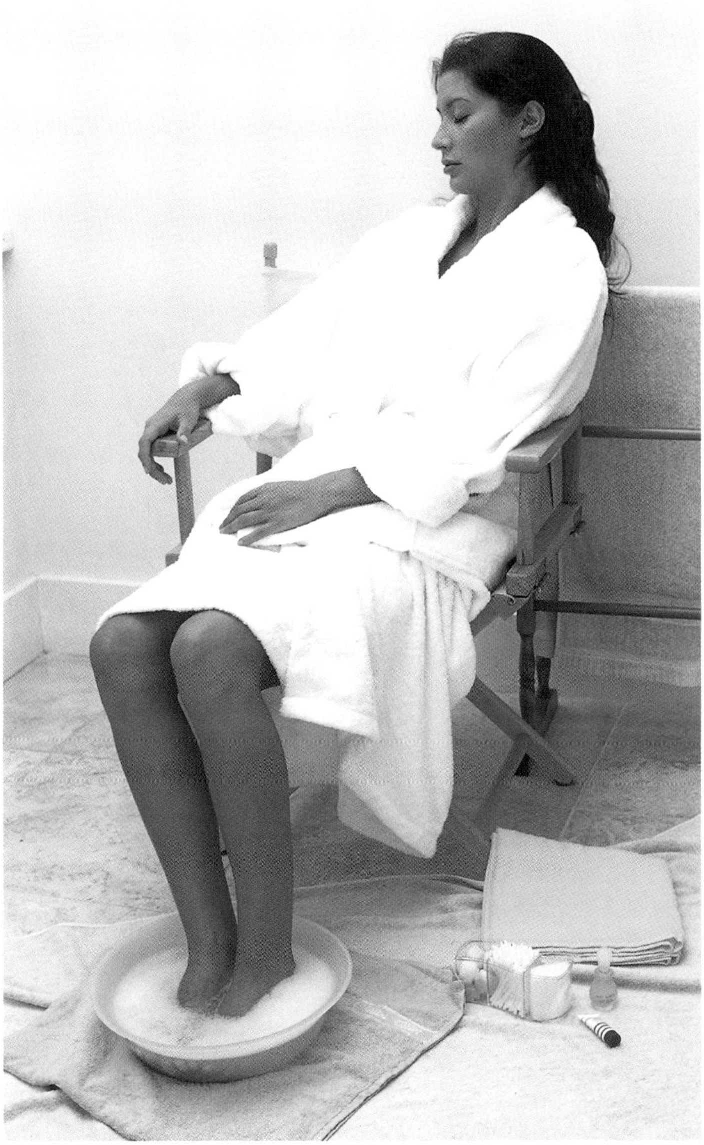

△ **1** Half fill a large bowl with warm water. Place the bowl on a large towel on the floor. Add a little foaming gel, and perhaps a couple of drops of essential oil which have been diluted in a carrier oil or in full-fat milk. Swish the water around with your hand to create plenty of bubbles and to release the aroma of the essential oil. Put both feet into the water, then sit back and relax as you soak them for a good five minutes. Remove your feet from the bowl and rub on the floor towel to remove most of the water.

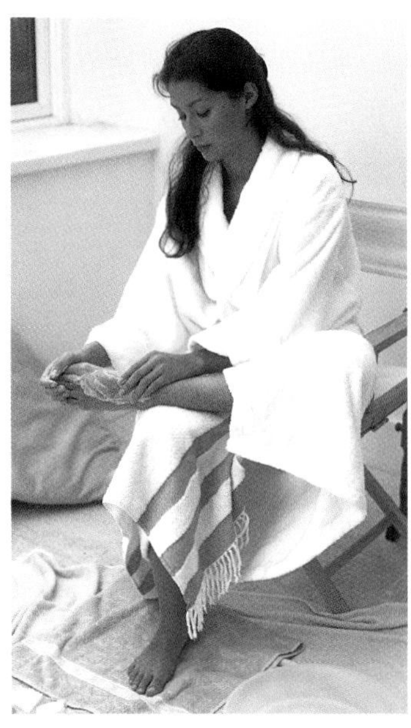

△ **2** Put a towel on one knee and rest the foot of your other leg on top. Massage the foot scrub all over the sole and toes: pay extra attention to any rough skin. Place the foot in a plastic bag and secure.

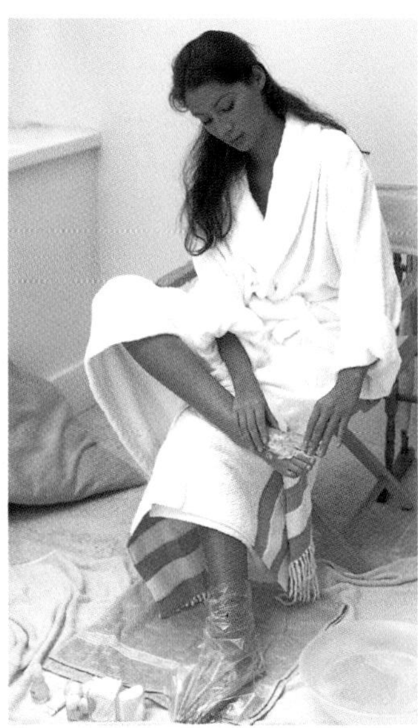

△ **3** Repeat on the other foot. Relax for ten minutes, then remove the bags from your feet, sliding the bags down so that they remove most of the scrub. Dip your feet back into the water. This will now be cool, and will stimulate the circulation.

grooming the feet

A pedicure will keep your feet looking great, and will also help to keep them healthy. You need a few special items in order to give yourself a pedicure. Once bought, they will last for ages, so it is worth the investment. Leave out the polish if you prefer to keep your nails natural.

what you need

- Nail polish remover – choose one with a conditioner.
- Cotton wool – to separate the toes while applying polish.
- Nail brush or orange stick (with the tip covered with cotton wool) – for cleaning under the nail.
- Hoof stick or cotton wool buds – to push back cuticles.
- Toe nail clippers – these are easier to use than scissors.
- Emery board – toe nails are harder than finger nails, so you'll need a strong one.
- Cuticle remover – to soften and loosen the cuticle.
- A base coat – to create an even surface.
- Polish colour of your choice.
- Clear top coat – to help seal the polish and prevent chipping.

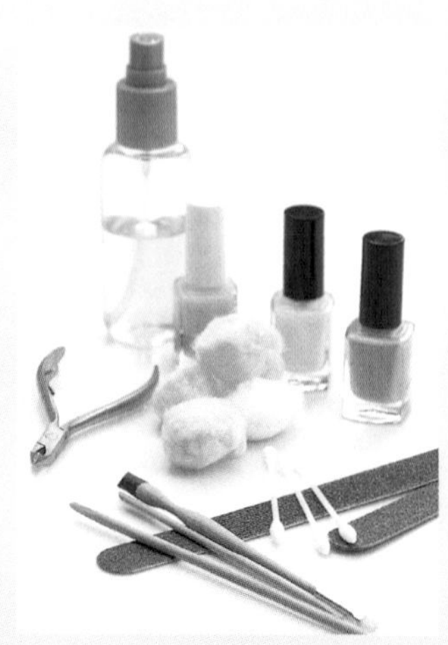

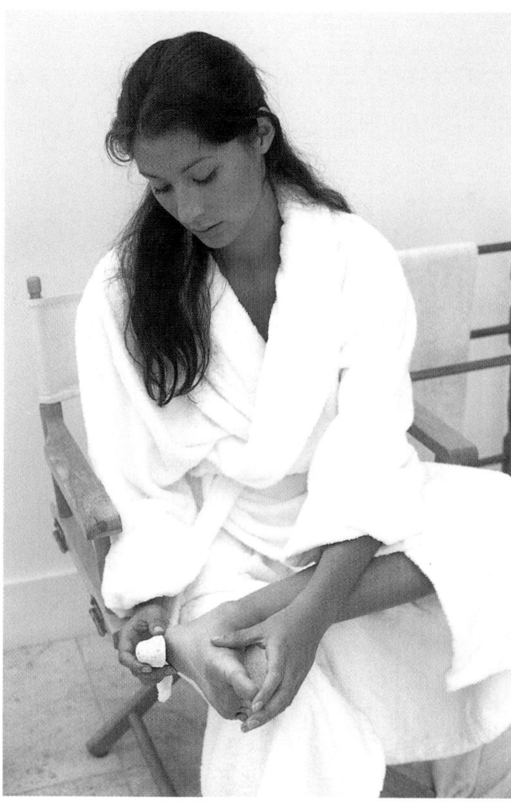

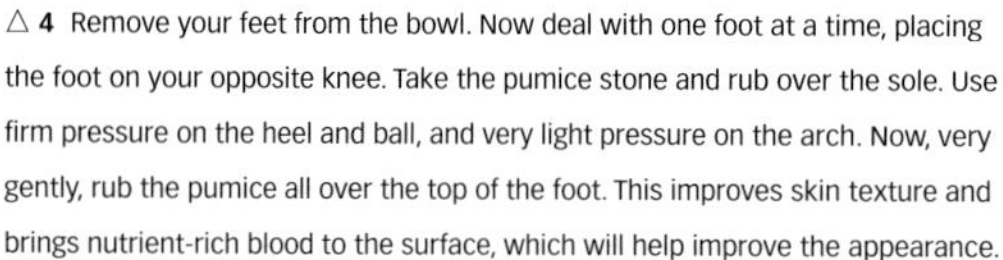

△ **4** Remove your feet from the bowl. Now deal with one foot at a time, placing the foot on your opposite knee. Take the pumice stone and rub over the sole. Use firm pressure on the heel and ball, and very light pressure on the arch. Now, very gently, rub the pumice all over the top of the foot. This improves skin texture and brings nutrient-rich blood to the surface, which will help improve the appearance.

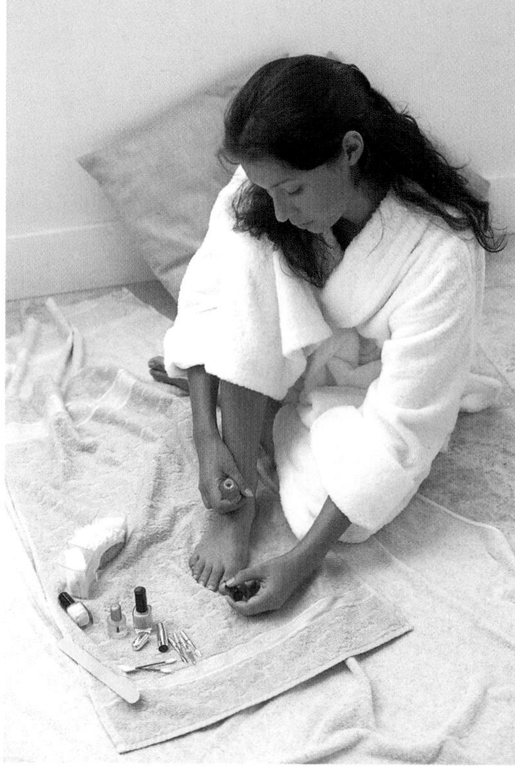

△ **5** Trim the nails straight across, then smooth the edges with an emery board. Use a cotton-wool bud to apply cuticle remover, wait a few minutes, then gently push the cuticle back with a hoof stick. Soak the feet again, then carefully clean under the nail. Dry the feet, then apply base coat, polish and top coat; use cotton wool to separate the toes and allow each layer to dry before applying the next.

luxury foot scrub

This grainy scrub is an excellent cleanser and exfoliator for the feet.The oils and glycerine have a nourishing, moisturizing effect, while the Fullers earth and salt help to soften and deep-cleanse. The essential oils are added for an aromatic, feel-good factor. Choose whichever oils you like best, or use the blends suggested.

This scrub can be used whenever you feel that your feet need a bit of a boost. It should be applied after a warm bath or shower when the feet are damp but not sopping wet. For the best results, though, use it as part of the full pamper session, as described on these pages.

ingredients

- 5ml/1 tsp almond oil
- 5ml/1 tsp jojoba oil
- 5ml/1 tsp glycerine
- 5g/1 tsp each Fullers earth and rock salt
- 10ml/2 tsp foaming foot or bath wash
- 2 drops mandarin and 1 drop geranium essential oils – you could also use lavender and lemon here.

In a small, clean bottle, mix together the foaming wash, essential oil and glycerine. Shake and set aside while you prepare the other ingredients. Put the Fullers earth and rock salt into a medium-sized dish and mix together well. Add the almond and jojoba oils, and mix well. Add the glycerine mixture to the bowl, and mix all the ingredients together with a metal spoon. You should now have a paste with a runny consistency, which can easily be applied to the feet.

▽ Always soak your feet before applying the foot scrub. You can use a foot spa if you have one. This will give a strong massage at the same time as you soak. However, be aware that foot spas are not advised if you have high blood pressure.

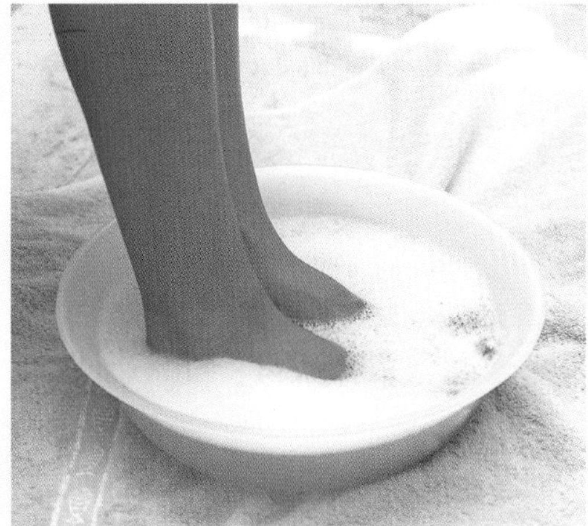

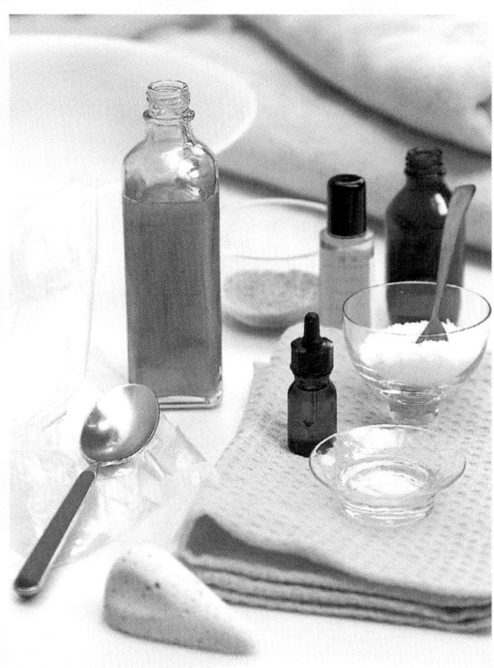

△ To make the luxury foot scrub, you'll need a mixing bowl that is large enough to hold all the ingredients, a metal spoon and a small clean bottle. Other equipment used in the pamper routine includes a pumice stone, a couple of freezer-type bags to put on your feet and three towels, one large one to protect the floor and two smaller ones for resting and rubbing the feet.

▽ A mini pamper session can be achieved by soaking the feet in warm suds for ten minutes. Use a loofah or nail brush to scrub and deep cleanse, then pumice all over the soles of the feet. Pat them dry, then give a quick massage using a blend of neroli and lemon essential oils well diluted in almond oil.

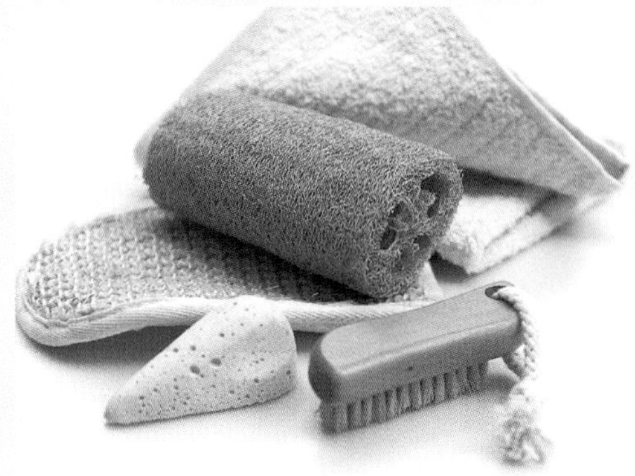

Detox treatment

Fast foods, sugary or salty snacks, alcohol, coffee and tea all contain toxins, which can build up in the body and cause us to feel lethargic and unhealthy. Even if you have a healthy lifestyle, you are still exposed to poisonous substances in the atmosphere. The air that we breathe contains chemicals, gases and dust particles, and it can pollute our land, water and food.

The body is a highly efficient machine, and it is constantly working to remove toxins from the circulation. However, an unhealthy diet, stress or late nights all put the body under pressure, and can affect how well its elimination systems work. Regular exercise supported by a healthy diet and a weekly detox massage regime will help improve your circulation, eliminate waste from the muscles and keep the detoxifying organs in good working order.

It is also important that you drink plenty of water. We lose fluid daily through the natural elimination processes of urination, defecation and sweat. This fluid needs to be replaced. To maintain good health and an efficient detox system we should drink at least three large glasses of water each day.

the role of the feet

The feet are the most distant part of the body – that is, they are furthest away from the heart, the main circulation organ. Toxins and wastes therefore tend to collect in the feet, particularly around the joints. Regular foot massage helps to break down and eliminate these toxins, and also to mobilize the joints. At the same time, it improves the circulation. This has a knock-on effect throughout the body, aiding the natural purification processes.

cleansing routine

It takes only a few minutes to do this simple routine, but it can have a highly beneficial effect on your general well-being. Use gentle strokes at first, to help relax the foot, then increase the pressure as you go on. If you like, use a massage cream or an oil of your choice.

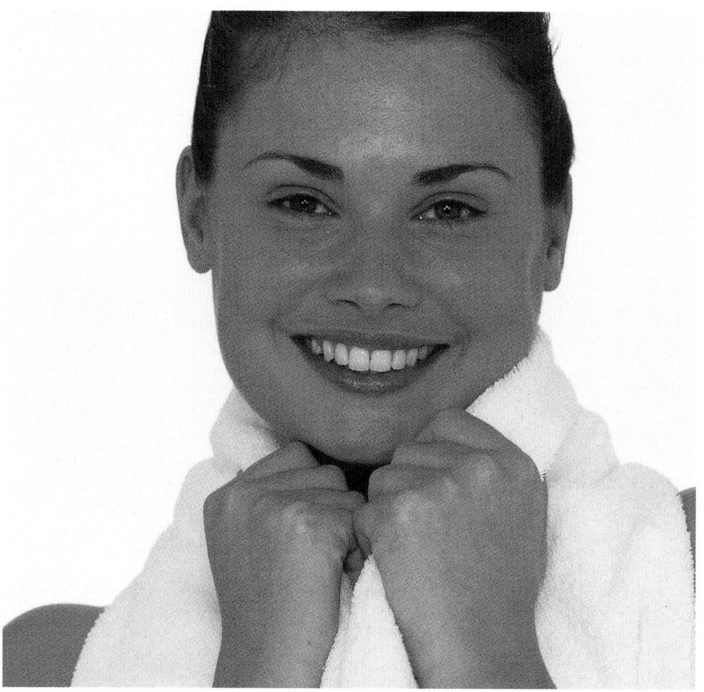

△ You can include the foot detox routine in a fuller programme of cleansing and relaxing. Dedicate some time – perhaps a full day – to enhancing your well-being. Enjoy some brisk exercise, such as running or fast walking, as well as some gentle stretches. Drink plenty of water and eat small, healthy meals consisting of whole grains, fresh vegetables and fruit.

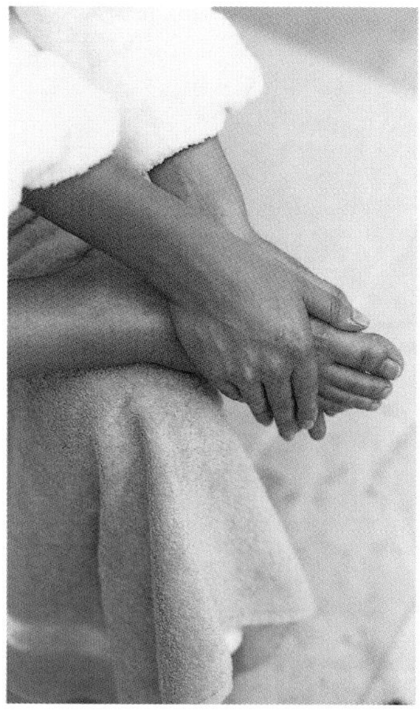

△ **1** Bring your right foot to rest on your left knee. Place your right hand across the top of the toes and your left hand underneath them, with the fingers of both hands pointing towards the outside edge. Gripping the foot between the hands, in a sandwich-like hold, slide both hands down to the heel then back to the toes. Do the movement three times in each direction. Repeat on the left foot.

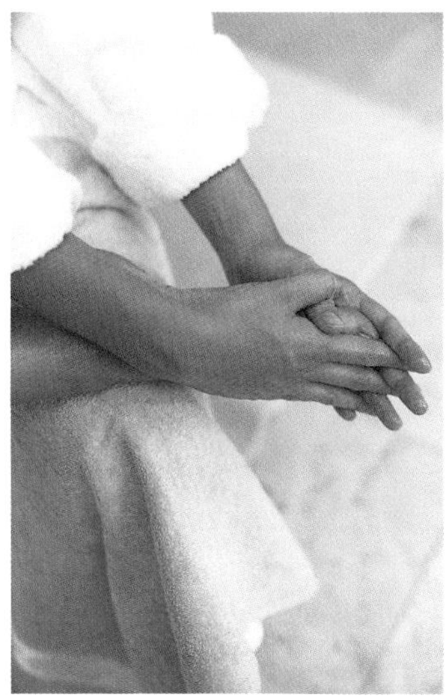

△ 2 Put your left hand on the right sole, fingers towards the toes. Place your right hand on the top of the foot in a similar position. Link the fingers of both hands across the tops of the toes. Now gently pull the hands apart, sliding one down the sole and the other down the top. Do this three times. Then, repeat the movements on the left foot.

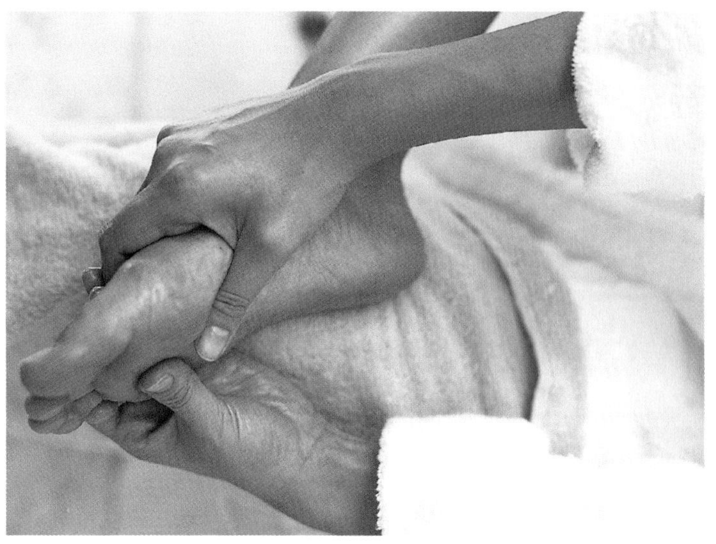

△ 4 Place the thumbs of each hand across the sole of the right foot, so that they point towards opposite sides of the foot. Start off as close to the toes as you can. Using a strong pressure, slide your thumbs backwards and forwards across the sole, pulling out to the edge of the foot each time. In this way, work down the foot to the heel, then back up to the toes. Do this three times; this movement helps to improve circulation and eliminate waste. Repeat the whole movement on your left foot.

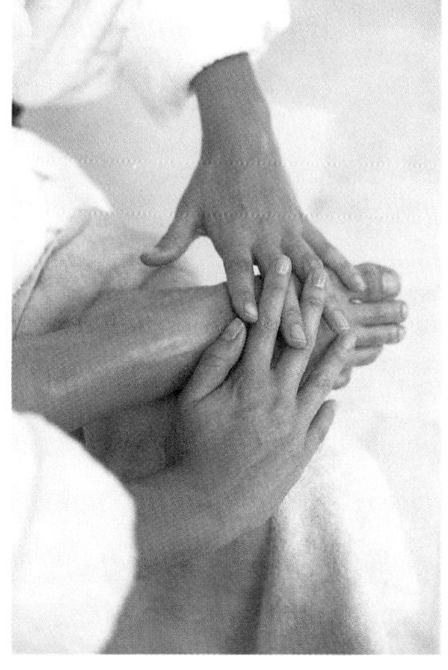

△ 3 Link your fingers together over the top of the right foot. Keep pressing down into the foot at the same time as you pull your fingers apart and draw them towards the edges of the foot. Work in this way from toes to ankle, then work back to the toes; this helps to eliminate waste. Repeat on the left foot.

what is detoxing?

Toxins can build up in the body, causing us to feel tired and drained. Detoxing is a way of cleansing the body of these impurities by helping the body's natural elimination processes. Most people benefit from the occasional detox – having a healthy day once a month can be a great way to keep energy levels up. It will also benefit your skin, hair, nails and general well-being.

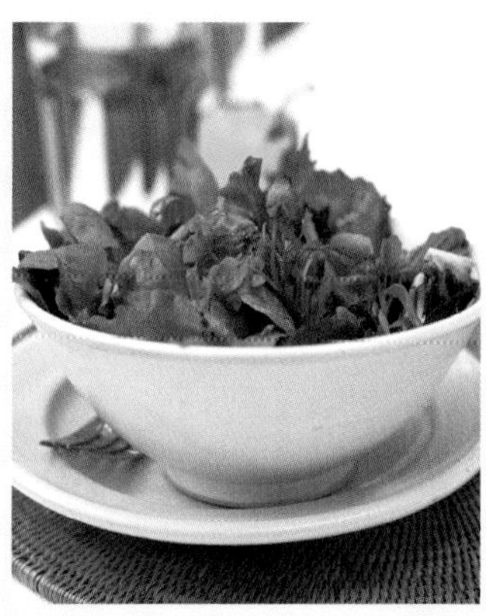

△ Raw, fresh foods play a vital role in any body-cleansing programme.

how to detox

There are different approaches to detoxing. The most extreme one is fasting – abstaining from all foods and drinking only water, herbal tea and juices over a short period.

Fasting tends to slow the digestive system, so it can be counter-productive and is not recommended for most people. Your body is more likely to benefit from a gentle programme that does not place it under pressure. A detox is best done over a day or two. During this time eat little and often, having only fibre-rich, healthy foods such as raw or lightly cooked fruits, vegetables and grains. Do several sessions of gentle exercise and get lots of rest. Drink plenty of water to help flush toxins away. You can also drink fresh juices, and herbal teas. Massage speeds the detox process, and brings a pleasurable, relaxing element to the day.

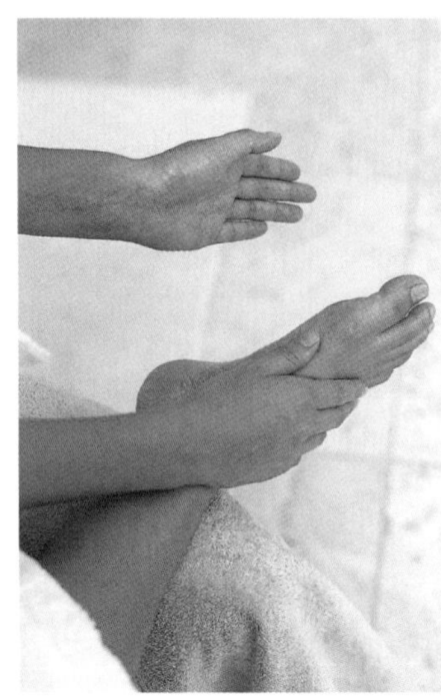

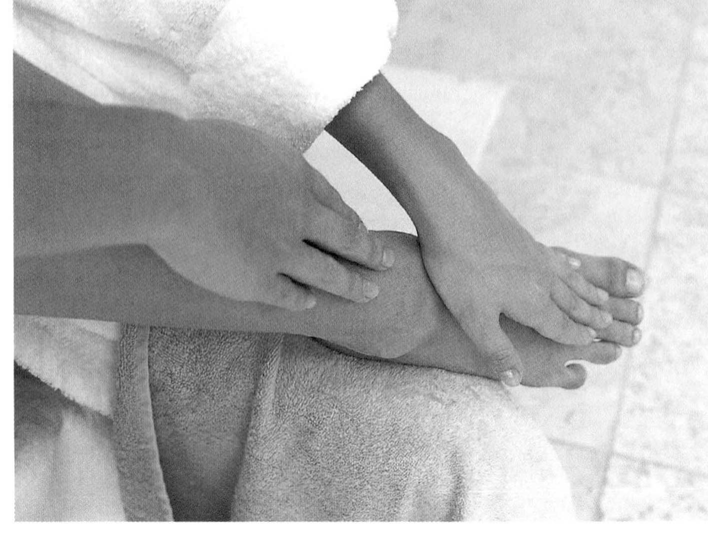

△ **5** Put the right hand on the top of the right foot, fingers pointing towards the toes. Put the left hand in a similar position on the sole. Using alternate hands slap the foot all over, moving up and down between the heel and toe to boost the circulation. Pressure should be harder on areas where the skin is thick. Slap all over four times, then repeat on the left foot.

△ **7** With alternate hands, make light strokes from toes to ankle. Do ten strokes with each hand, using the whole palm. Now stroke five times with each hand, making the pressure as firm as is bearable. Finally, start with the fingers interlaced between the toes. Do five medium-pressure strokes with each hand. Repeat on the left.

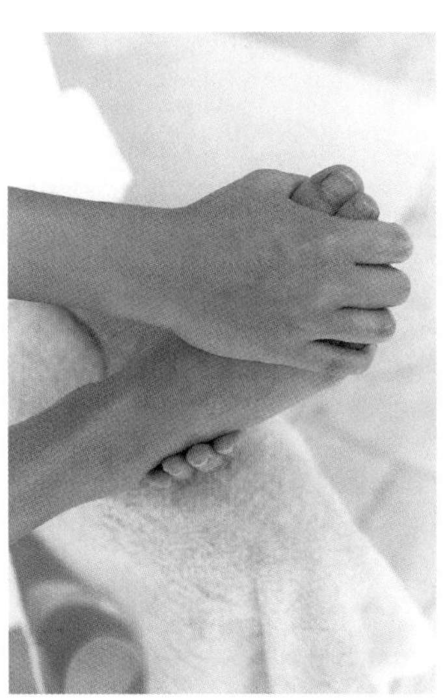

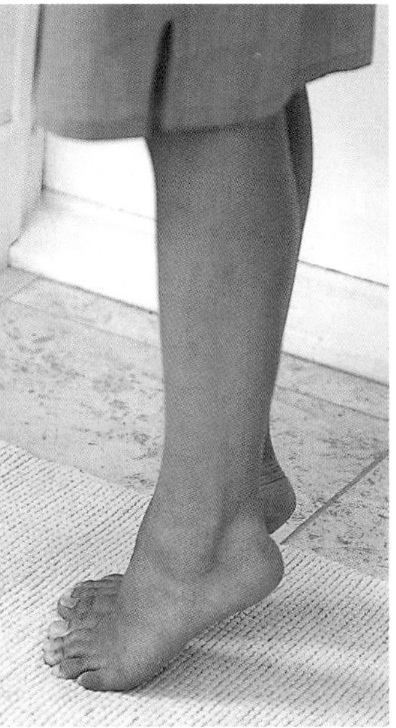

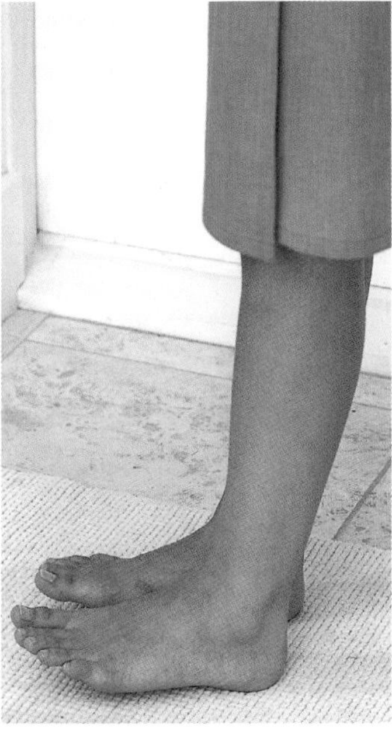

△ **6** Hold the toes of the right foot in your right hand and cup the heel in your left hand. Circle the foot, rotating it from the ankle three times clockwise, then three times anticlockwise. This action helps to mobilize the joints. Rest then repeat. Do not force the ankle beyond its limits. Repeat on the left.

△ **8** Stand up straight. Keep breathing as you lift both heels off the ground and hold them there for a slow count of ten. Return the heels to the floor and count to five. Do this muscle stretch three or four times, depending on your fitness level. You can rest your hands on a chair back if you feel unsteady.

△ **9** This movement stretches the tendons as well as the muscles. Standing upright, firmly press your heels into the floor as you lift the forefoot and toes off the ground. Hold to a count of five, return feet to start point. Rest to a count of five. Do the movement three times. Again, use a chair if you find this difficult.

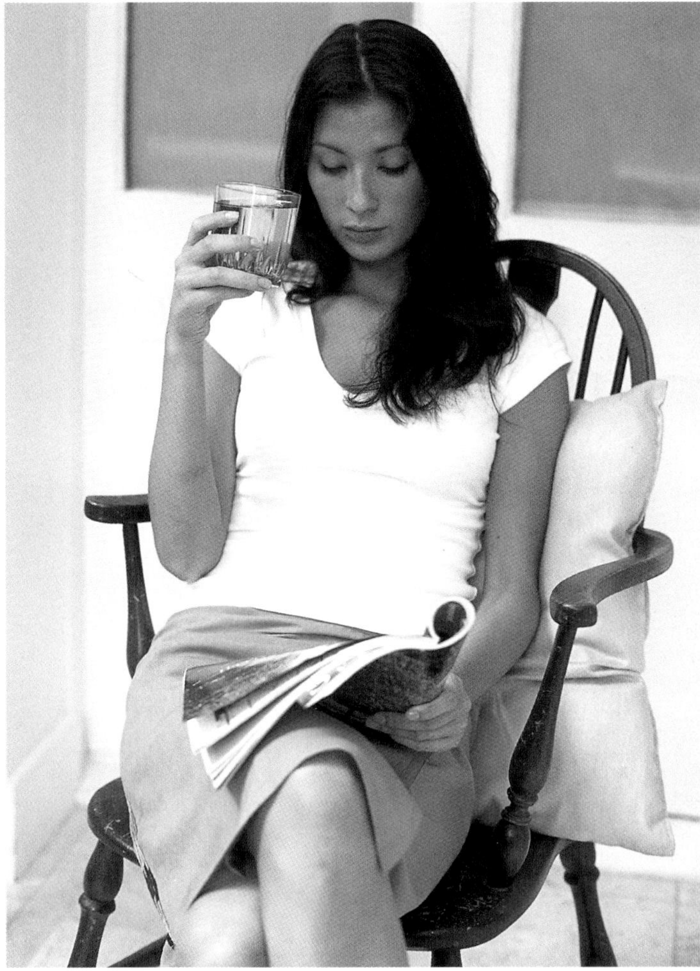

◁ **10** When the massage is over, sit down quietly. Enjoy some peaceful time on your own or read a magazine or book. Spend at least 20 minutes relaxing. During this time, drink a large glass of water or fruit juice. This will help the elimination processes started by the massage routine.

after the routine

If possible, you should try not to do too much after doing the detox routine. If you have time, it is a good idea to combine this treatment with other health-enhancing activities. For example, you may like to do some gentle exercise – such as swimming, walking, yoga or Pilates. You could also go for a sauna; impurities are passed out of the body in sweat.

Make sure that you drink plenty of water. If you like, add a slice of lemon to zing up the taste; lemon has cleansing properties so this will aid the detoxifying process. Try not to eat any sugary, salty or processed foods, at least for the rest of the day. The best foods to help the body get rid of wastes are those that contain plenty of fibre. Eat fresh fruit and vegetables, in the form of juices, soups and salads, together with whole grains such as wholemeal bread, wholewheat pasta or wholegrain rice.

For the best results, you should do this detox routine every week or so. Combined with regular exercise, a healthy diet and drinking plenty of water, it will help to keep your system working well, and prevent the build-up of toxins in the body.

vitamin-packed juicing

Drinking freshly made juices is an easy way to up your nutrient intake and boost your energy levels without placing the digestion under any strain. Here are some good juices to try when you are detoxing, or at any time.

- Apple, orange and carrot: packed with vitamin C and energizing fruit sugars to give you a lift.
- Papaya, melon and grapes: papaya is soothing on the stomach, and this juice can also help the liver and kidneys.
- Carrot, beetroot and celery: a good juice to kickstart the system in the morning. Try using 100g (3½ oz) beetroot to three carrots and two celery sticks.
- Cabbage, fennel and apple: a cleansing juice with antibacterial properties. Use ½ a small red cabbage, ½ a fennel bulb, 2 apples and a spoonful of lime juice.

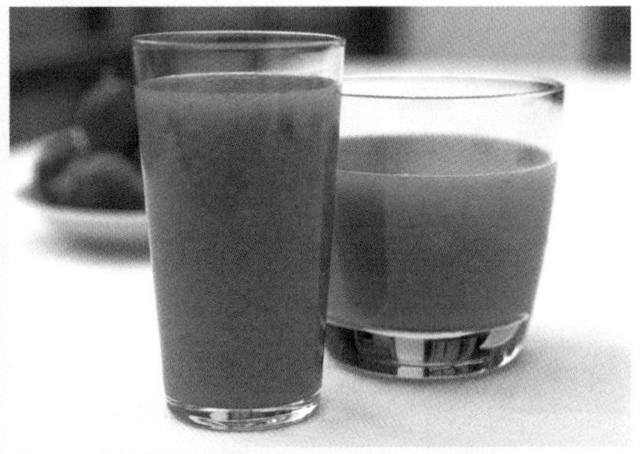

△ **Fruits and vegetables are packed with vitamins and nutrients. Use the freshest produce, and buy organic whenever you can.**

De-stress and unwind

The modern world presents us with more opportunities and choices than we have ever had before. With these new opportunities come new challenges, responsibilities and the need to make an ever-increasing number of decisions. Our everyday life now involves a multiplicity of claims on our time, involvement, commitment and energy.

It is not surprising, then, that we all feel overwhelmed occasionally. Stress has become one of the biggest health problems in the western world, and most of us are affected by it at some point in our lives. Sometimes, a little stress can be helpful; it may galvanize us into action, for example, or motivate us to finish a necessary task. All too often, though, it is counterproductive, and leaves us feeling exhausted, anxious and less effective than we might otherwise be.

the need for rest

The best antidote to stress is rest. However, when you are feeling tense, it can be hard to relax. The solution is to slow yourself down so that your mind becomes quieter and the tension drains out of your body.

There are many ways to do this, but giving yourself a foot massage is probably the quickest. Not only does it require you to focus on what you are doing, which always helps to clear the mind, but you are working on one of the body's most sensitive areas. It is almost impossible not to relax when your feet are being stroked and pummelled.

Do this routine in a quiet place where you won't be disturbed; close the door and switch off the phone. After the treatment, give yourself a few minutes simply to sit and listen to the sound of your breathing.

essential oils for de-stressing

Using an essential oil that has soothing and uplifting properties will heighten the relaxing effects of this routine. Add a few drops of your chosen oil to a carrier and massage into the feet at the start of the routine, or heat in a burner. Good stress-relieving oils include geranium, lavender, bergamot, jasmine, chamomile, neroli and rose. Choose one with an aroma that really appeals to you.

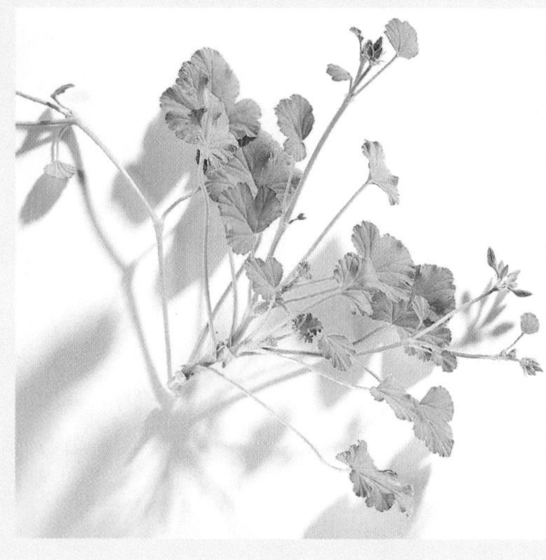

▷ **Geranium is a sweet-smelling oil that has a soothing effect on the nervous system. It can also be helpful for PMT. Use it on its own or combine with rose or lavender.**

releasing tension routine

This de-stressing routine has been designed to help you to let go of strain and tension. Try to relax your whole body as you do it; this will enhance the effects. The routine could be practised each day – perhaps after work – but a one-off at any time will bring rewards.

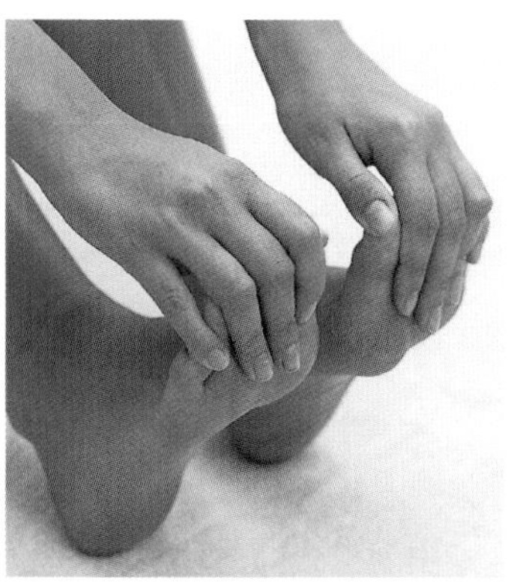

△ **1** Stretch both feet out in front of you, toes pointing upwards. Bend forwards and bring your fingers to rest on the ball of the foot, then pull your feet gently back towards you.

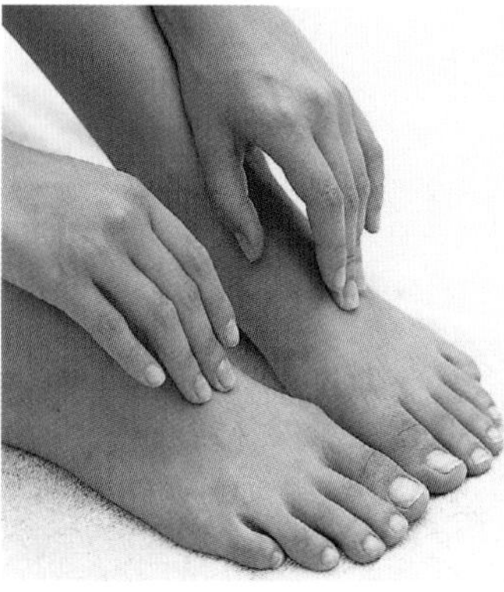

△ **2** Massage the grooves that start between the toes and run up the foot: use the two middle fingers of each hand to make small circles. Start between the two biggest toes, then do the others in turn. Repeat.

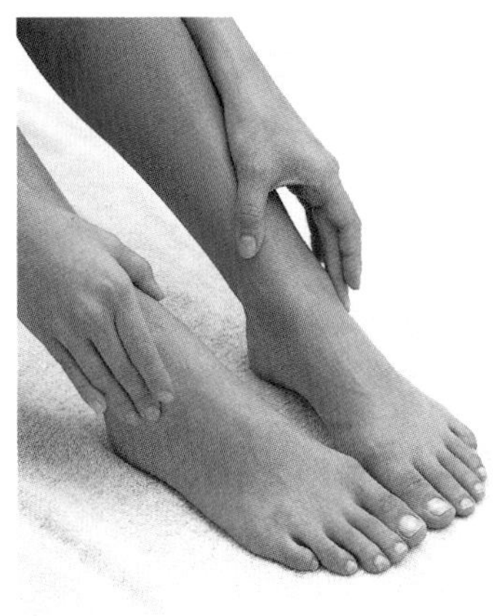

△ **3** Massage around both outer ankle bones at the same time, using the two middle fingers of each hand. Massage first in a clockwise direction, then in an anticlockwise direction. If an area feels tender or tight, repeat the movement in both directions. Do the same on the inner ankles.

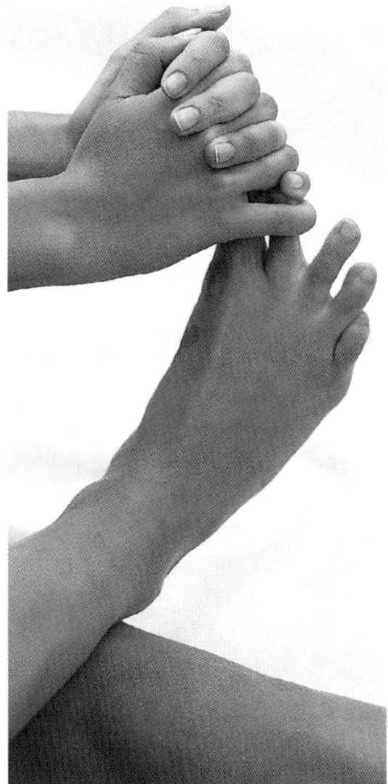

△ **4** Place one hand on the sole and the other on the top of the right foot. Cup your hands together, interlocking your fingers. Slide the hands over the tips of your toes, pulling and separating each one as you go. Repeat on the left foot.

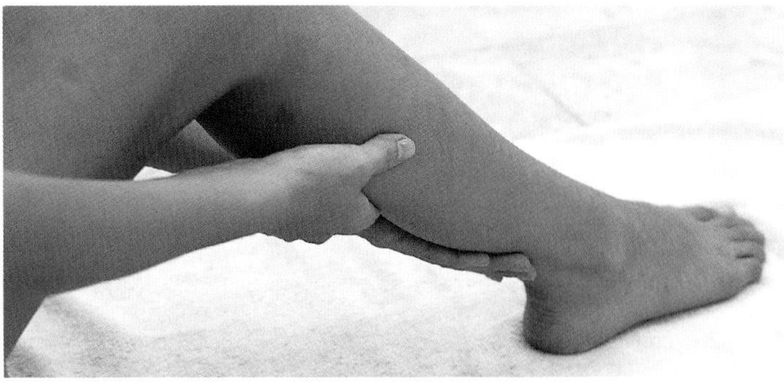

△ **5** The next step is to massage the Achilles tendon and muscles of the lower leg. This helps to relieve tension in the feet and legs; it works best if you oil your hands first. Begin the massage on the right leg. Use alternate palms to work up from the back of the heel to behind the knee. Massage the area twice. Repeat on the left leg.

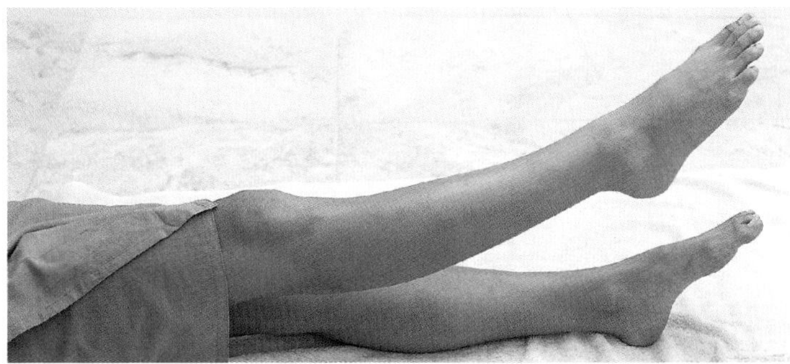

△ **6** Lie on the floor or sit on a chair. Stretch both feet out in front of you. Make scissor movements by crossing the right foot over the left, then the left over the right. Keep your feet and toes pointing straight up towards the ceiling. Work each leg ten times. Rest for a few moments, then repeat the exercise.

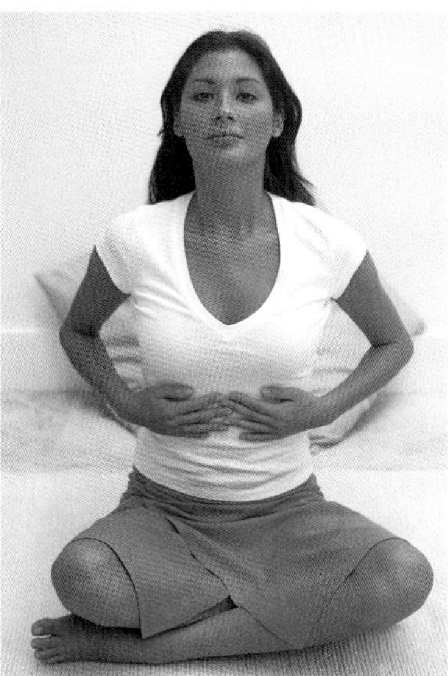

◁ **7** Sit in a comfortable position, eyes closed, fingers resting on your solar plexus. Allow your breathing to follow its own rhythm. Quietly repeat to yourself a meaningful two-syllable word, such as re-lax or hea-vy. This helps to soothe your mind while simultaneously encouraging your body to unwind and de-stress. Don't worry if you feel a little awkward or find this difficult at first. With practice, your voice will become calm and low, and your breathing deep and slow.

Sports routine

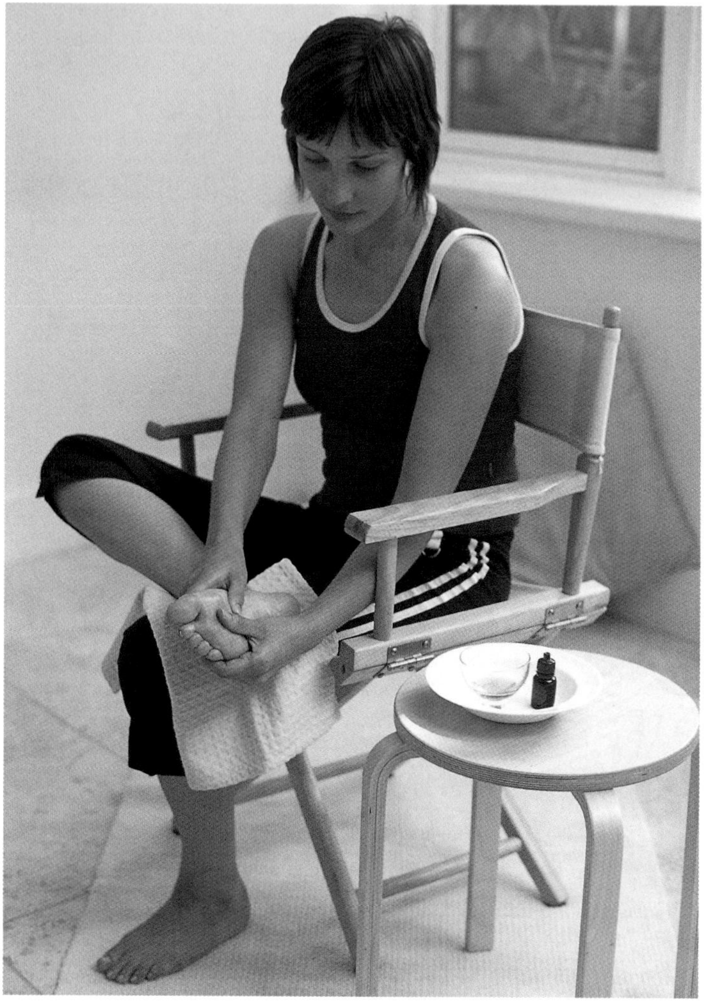

◁ **If you wish to use oil for this routine, add a few drops to your palm. Rub the hands together to distribute the oil, then briskly rub all over the right foot and lower leg – you should add enough oil to create a light sheen but not so much that the skin becomes greasy. Oil the left side when you are ready to massage it. Afterwards, wipe off any excess with a towel before putting your shoes back on.**

It is essential to warm up properly before doing any type of sport. Warming up helps to prevent cramp and reduces the possibility of aches and pains – you are much more likely to get injured if your muscles are cold.

Cool-down exercises after a work-out are also important. They give the body a chance to come back to a balanced state after its exertions. Warm-ups and cool-downs also help you to manage the transition between normal life and exercise and back again.

Massage is a valuable addition to your usual warm-up and cool-down routines. It is a good way of connecting with your body, and becoming aware of any held tension or awkwardness that you may be experiencing. It is also good to pay some attention to the feet, which bear the brunt of much of the exercise that we do.

soothing foot powder

This is a great powder to use before or after doing sports. It will help to keep the feet dry and fresh. Tea tree is a vital component because of its antiseptic qualities, but you could use rosemary or sandalwood instead of the lemon – choose whichever has the most appealing aroma.

ingredients

- 150g/5oz rice flour
- 150g/5oz orris root powder
- 150g/5oz bicarbonate of soda
- 1 tsp boric acid powder
- 6 drops each lemon and tea tree

Mix together the rice flour, orris root powder and bicarbonate of soda. Add the boric acid powder and mix well. Drop in the essential oils, and stir well until they are thoroughly absorbed. Now transfer your powder to a clean, plastic shaker.

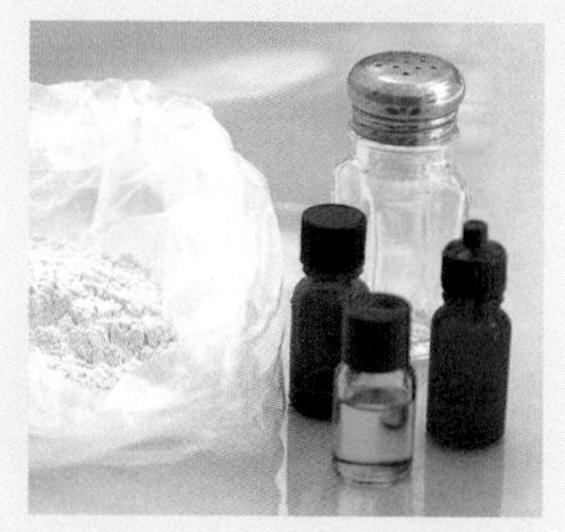

before a work-out

This short routine is easy to do in the gym or at home. Start on the right foot, and then do the left. For the first two moves, sit down and bring the foot you are working on to rest on your knee.

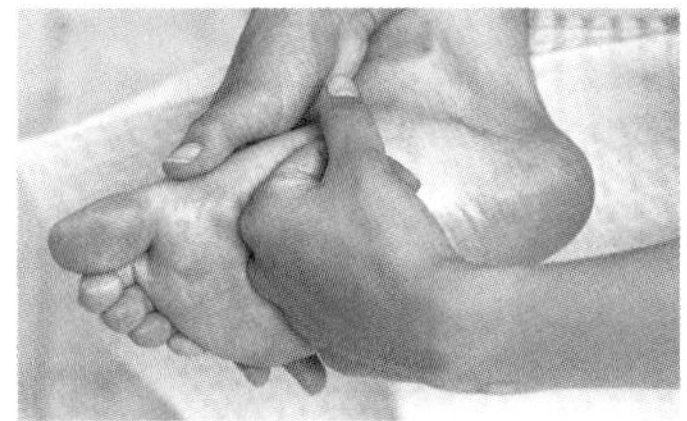

△ **1** Hold the top of your foot in your right hand and make the left hand into a loose fist. Use the flat area between the knuckle and first joint to knead the sole. Work all over the foot, starting at the heel. Use firmer pressure for the heel and ball, and light pressure on the arch. Massage the sole area three times.

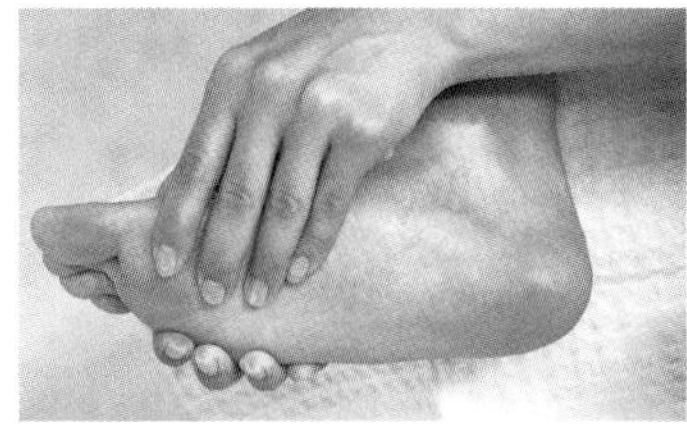

△ **2** Place the thumbs on top of your foot, near the toes, and let the fingers of both your hands curl round the foot to meet in the middle of the sole. Keep your thumbs in position and press the fingers in deeply, then pull them out to the edges to spread the sole. Slide the fingers back to the middle and work in this manner down the foot towards the heel. Repeat.

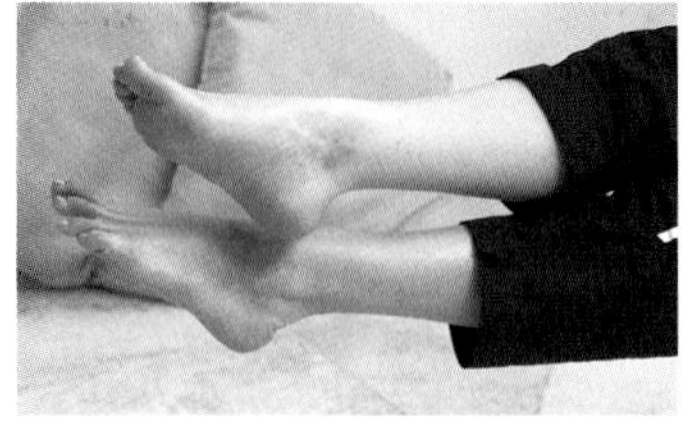

△ **3** Sit down on the floor or on a very stable chair with your legs stretched out in front of you. If on the floor, raise your feet up. Now cross them alternately and rapidly, one over the other in a scissor-like action. Keep the feet straight and the toes pointing upwards. Do the movement at least ten times with each leg.

after a work-out

After exercise or a sporting activity, have a warm shower to help relax your muscles. If you are at home, it is a nice idea to soak your feet in a large foot bowl half-filled with warm water. Add 10ml/2 tsp of almond oil blended with two drops each of rosemary and tea tree. Dry your feet thoroughly before the massage.

▷ **1** Start with the right foot. Use the thumb and index finger of your left hand to pull your big toe straight. Hold to the count of five. Gently rotate it in clockwise direction, then anticlockwise. Do the same to all the toes in turn, ending on the little one.

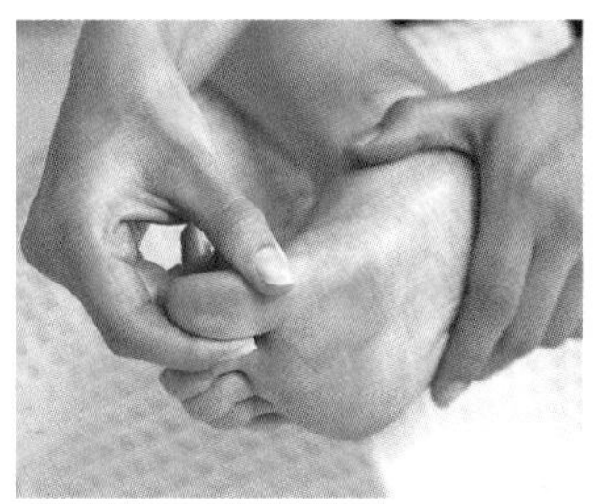

▷ **2** Using the back of the fingers, slap all over the foot. Start on the sole, then do the top of the foot. Repeat so that you cover the entire area twice. Make the slaps as heavy as is tolerable; they should be lighter on the top of the foot than on the sole. This is an excellent action for breaking down toxins.

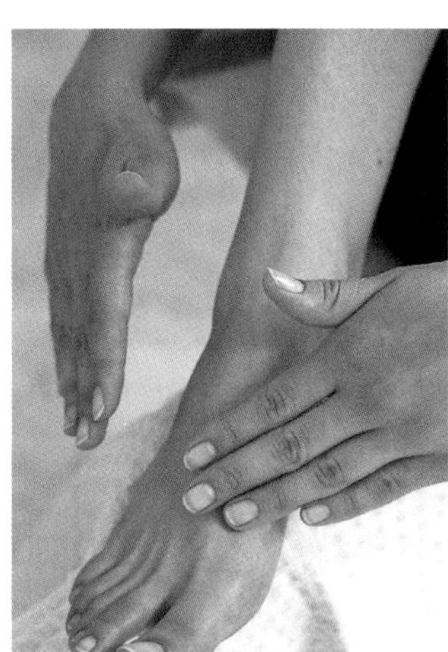

▷ **3** This movement is good for eliminating cramp in the calf. Put the first two fingers of the left hand on the Achilles tendon, then slide upwards to the base of the calf muscle. Press in and make deep circular movements on the spot. Continue to work in this way as you move up the leg, so that the entire muscle is treated. Slide your fingers back down to the Achilles tendon. Do the movement five times in total.

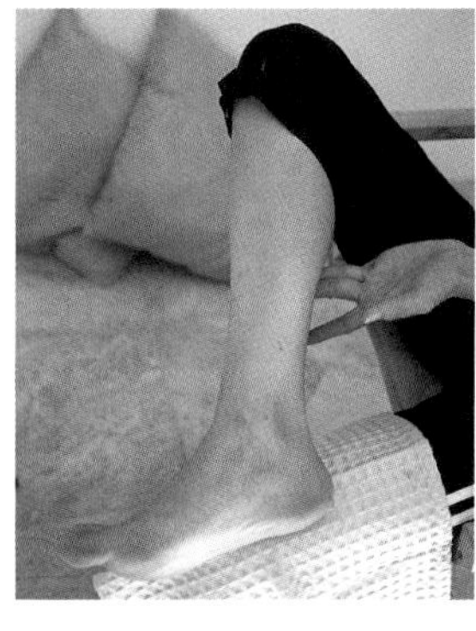

▷ **4** Finish off with some brisk stroking up the back of the leg, using both of your hands. Briskly stroke up the lower leg, from the ankle to the knee. Slide the hands down to the ankle and repeat twice more. Now repeat the whole sequence on the other leg.

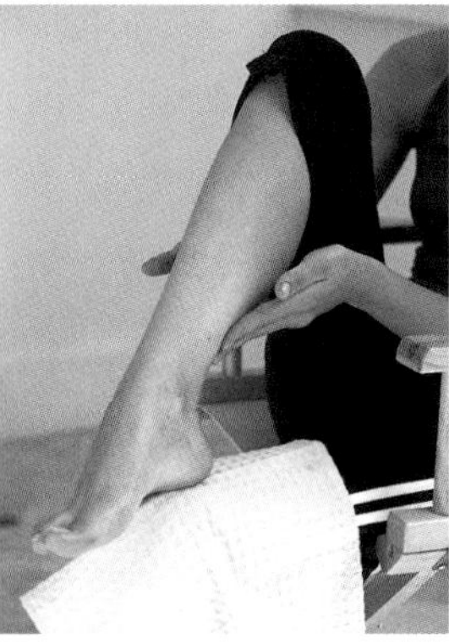

Take a break

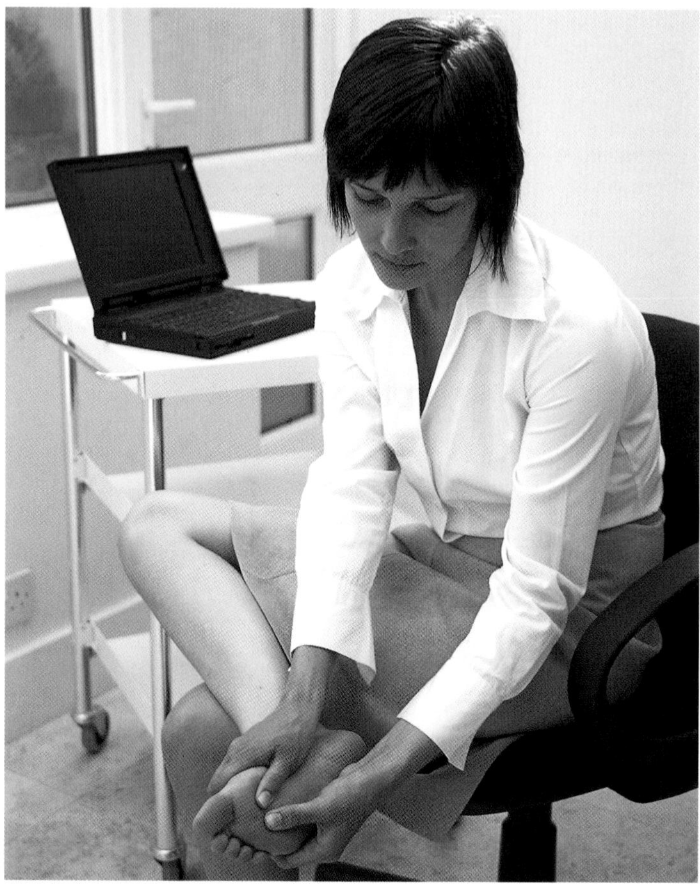

We often have to work or fulfil other obligations when we are feeling under par, because it just isn't possible to take a day out every time we feel a little unwell. Even on a good day, your energy will inevitably flag at various points.

Taking regular breaks from work is always beneficial – and, in the long run, will help you to work more efficiently. If possible, get some fresh air every day, perhaps taking a short walk during your lunch hour. Many office workers eat lunch at their desk, but it is important to get away and have a proper break. Make sure you have healthy food, such as fruit, to snack on at other times of day, too. This will stop you from relying on quick sugar fixes, such as chocolate and biscuits, to keep your energy up. You should also drink plenty of water – have a litre bottle to hand, and top up regularly.

Giving yourself a quick treatment can be a great way to revitalize body and mind. The treatments given here are easy to do in the office, or in a quiet area of any workplace.

◁ If you work in one place all day, such as an office, you may find that you feel low at certain times. If you also work on a computer, you are likely to develop tension in the shoulders and neck. Giving yourself a quick self-treatment will make you feel cared for, and will help to release tightness in the back of the body.

quick cure-all

The reflexology points that treat the spine also have an effect on the whole nervous system. Working these points may help to shift a headache, backache or shoulder tension, and it is a great way to give yourself a general boost.

Remove your shoe and bring one foot to rest on your left knee. Turn the foot to expose the inner edge. Starting at the base of the big toe, walk your thumb along the bone and down to the heel, using a caterpillar-like crawling motion. Now thumb-walk back towards the toes, but this time press up into the bone as you go. Repeat the movements on the other foot.

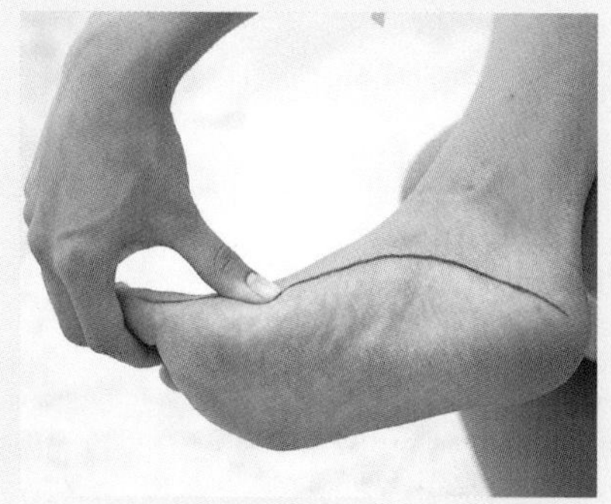

▷ The spine reflexes run along the inner edge of each foot. As you work the points, try to be aware of any areas of tenderness, and give them a gentle massage.

general pep-up

This easy revitalizing routine uses a combination of massage and reflexology. It's easy to do at your desk or in any quiet corner. Start with the right foot, then repeat on the left.

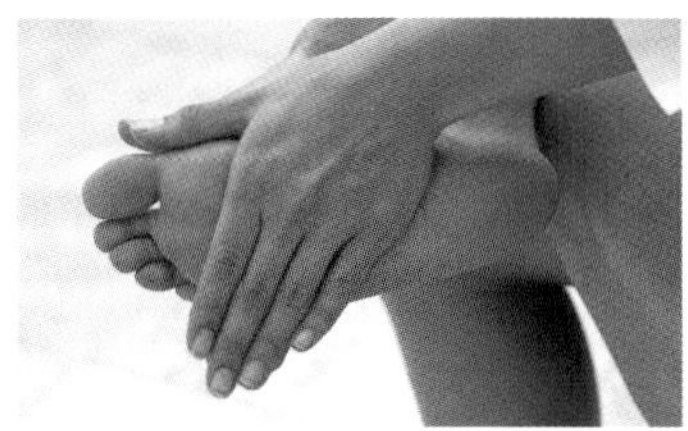

△ **1** Place your right hand over the top of the foot and your left hand on the base, in a sandwich hold. Gently slide your hands up from toe to heel and back again. Press the lower hand in so that the pressure is firmer on the sole. Do this three times, or more.

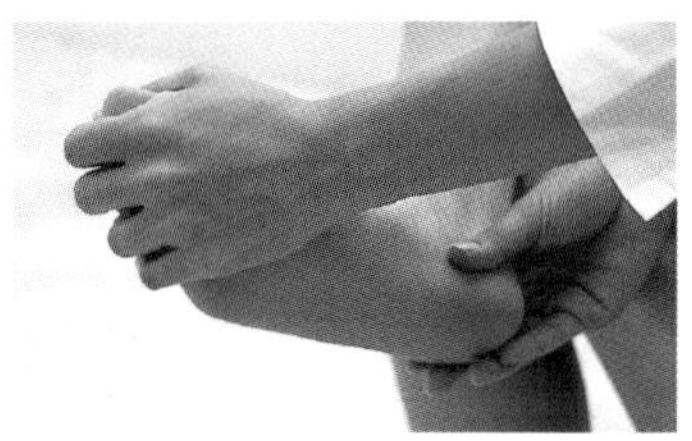

△ **2** Cup your heel in your right hand for support. Hold the top of your toes with your left hand and rotate the ankle gently. Do this first in a clockwise direction, then circle it anticlockwise. Repeat until you have done three circles in each direction.

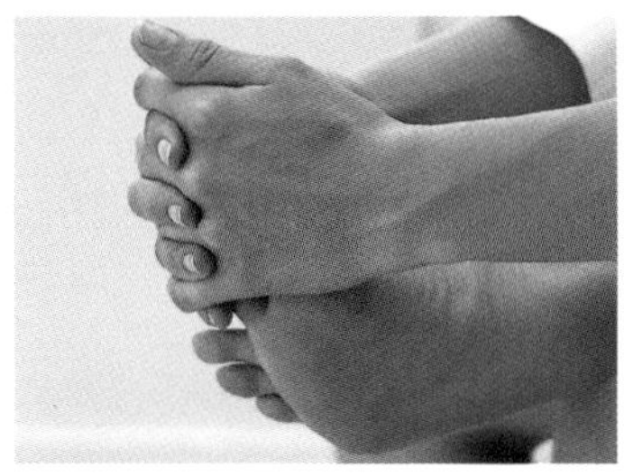

△ **3** Clasp your hands over the toes, so that they join directly over the little toe. Slowly pull along the top of the toes, allowing each one to open out as you go. This releases tension in the head area.

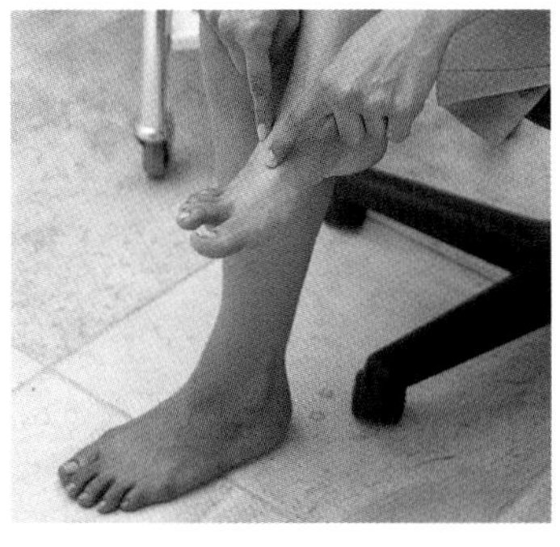

△ **4** Move your foot so that you can reach the top easily; you may like to rest it on a stool. Use both index fingers to make tiny circles all over the top of the foot. Work from the base of the toes up to the ankles. Vary the pressure depending on how you are feeling; light pressure is very relaxing, heavier pressure will have an energizing effect.

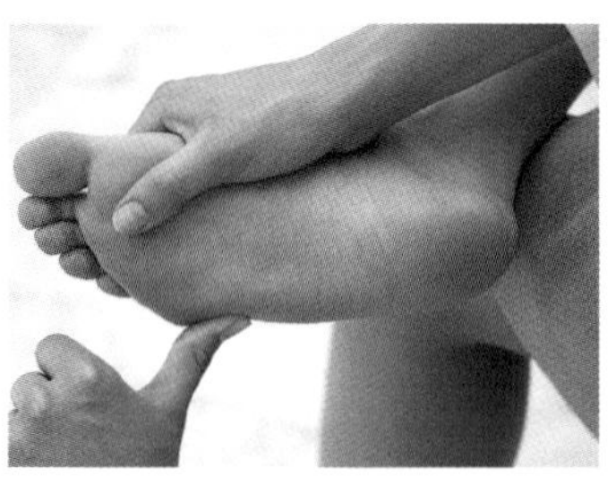

△ **5** Support the inner edge with your right hand, and use your left thumb to crawl down the outside edge. This works on the shoulder, hip and knee, relaxing the muscles in these areas.

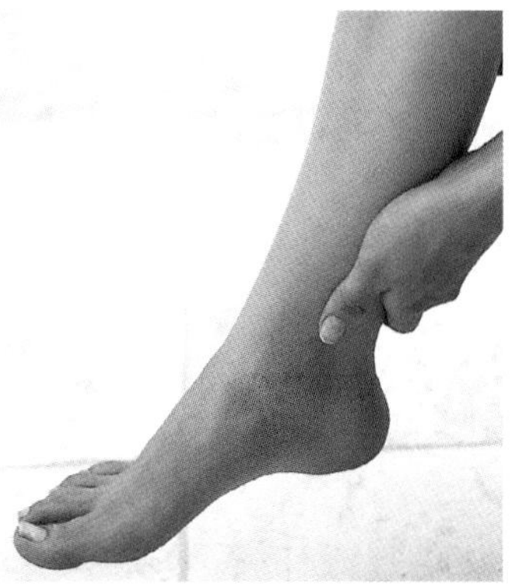

△ **6** Massage the back of the leg, using alternate palms to stroke briskly from the top of the ankle to just behind the knee. This is a good energizing movement to end the routine. Now repeat the whole sequence on the left foot and leg.

relieving headaches, sore throats and neck tension

Here is a excellent treatment for headaches or sore throats that are related to tiredness, stress and tension. This will also help if you have tension in the neck. Do it on both feet.

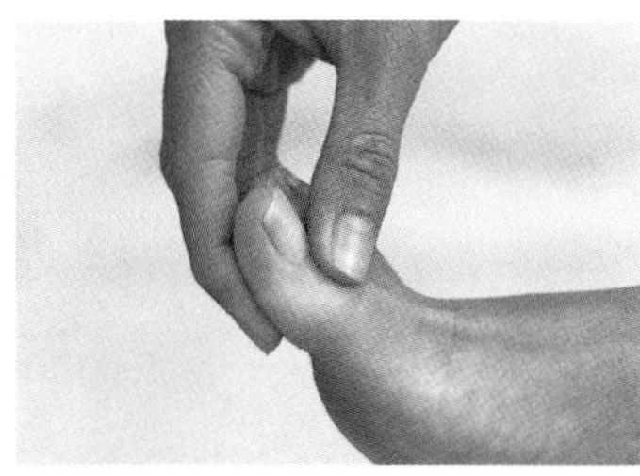

△ **1** Take off your shoes and raise up your right foot. Using your thumb and index finger, pinch your big toe all over. Do the sides, back and top. This action is good for the head and neck.

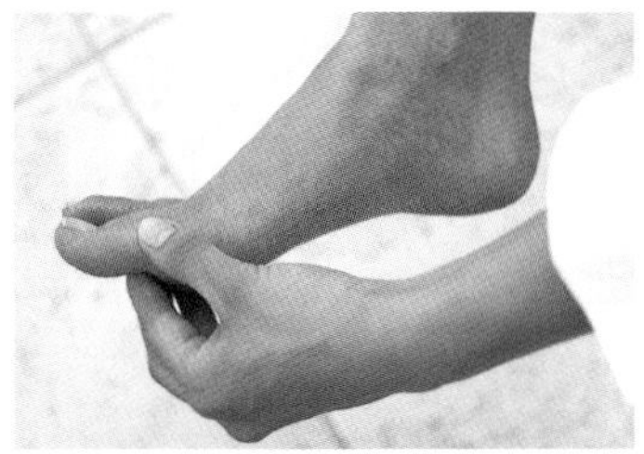

△ **2** Use your thumb to walk around the top of the big toe from the outside to the inside. This is a reflexology technique used to relax the throat area.

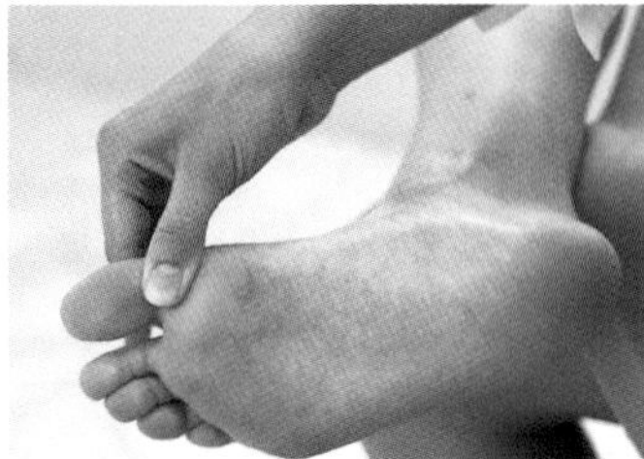

△ **3** Use your thumb to walk from the outside to the inside of the big toe, along the base. This helps relax the muscles at the back of the neck and base of the skull, which may be implicated in a tension headache.

Tonic for tired legs

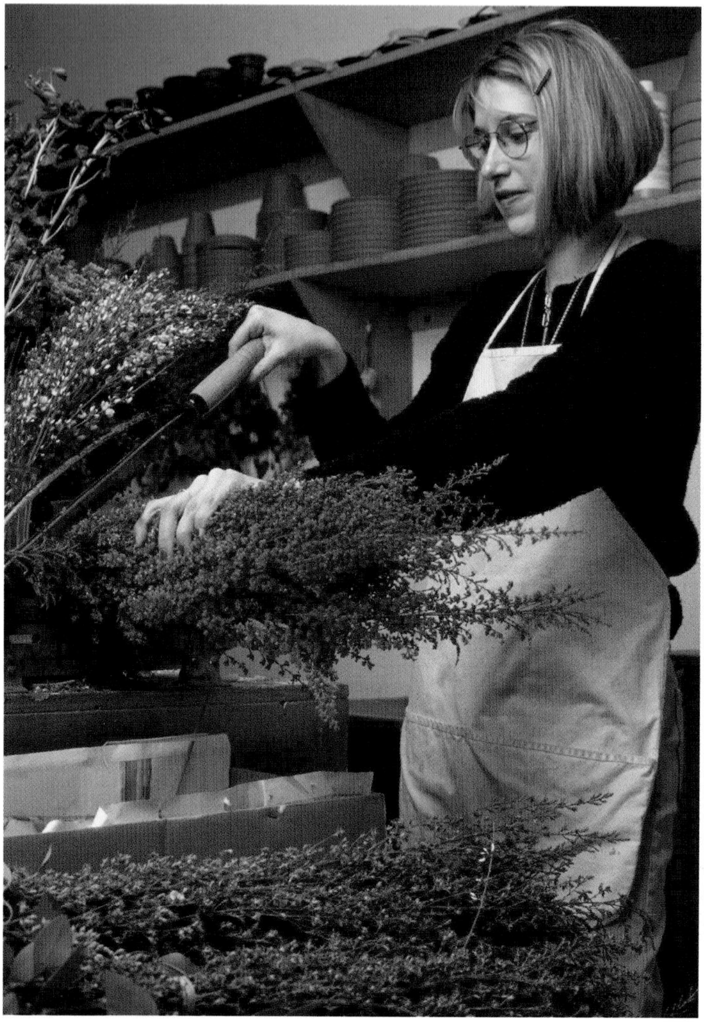

◁ **All kinds of occupations, particularly those in the service industry, require people to be on their feet for much of the day. Taking a quick break every so often to practise some simple exercises will relieve aching and heaviness, and may prevent long-term problems from developing.**

Standing on your feet all day long is not good for your circulation. The force of gravity means that fluid tends to pool in the ankle and feet area.

Muscles do not get a good supply of oxygen and nutrients unless they are moving. If you stand still for a long time, there will also be build-up of waste, which can make the muscle feel tired and achy. A sluggish circulation is the main cause of varicose veins. It also tends to make your skin very dry.

If you need to be standing for long periods, take regular breaks so that you can sit down. You should also keep your feet moving from time to time – walk on the spot, or go up on to the balls of your feet for a few seconds, then release.

quick rejuvenating routine

These simple foot-and-leg exercises will help to keep your circulation moving and should be done at regular intervals. They are particularly effective at the end of the day.

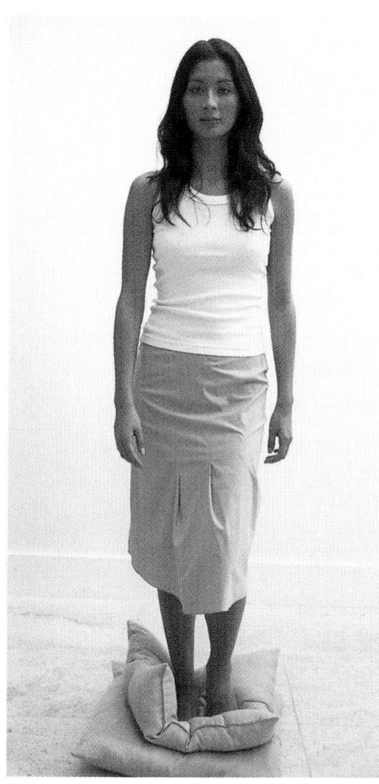

△ **1** Stand on a beanbag, or a couple of cushions if nothing else is available (the many tiny beans used in a bean bag have a pleasurable massaging effect). Try to balance for a few moments. Move your feet one at a time, in a walking motion. This gets all the leg muscles working, and kick-starts the circulation. Have a chair or wall nearby in case you feel unsteady.

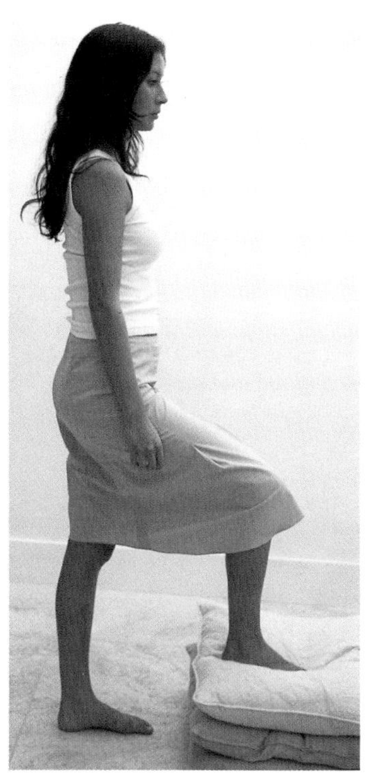

△ **2** You need a step for this exercise. The easiest place to do it is at the bottom of the stairs, or you could improvise with a stack of folded towels or cushions. Use alternate feet to step up. Do up to ten steps with each foot, depending on your fitness level. This also works the muscles, and helps to raise oxygen levels in the leg.

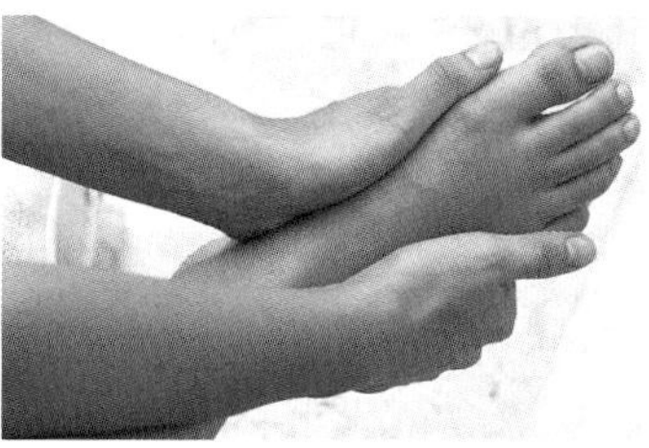

△ **3** Sit down, and rest the right foot on your knee. Place the thumbs on top of the foot, pointing towards the toes, and wrap the fingers round the sole. Draw the thumbs out to the edges of the foot. Return to the start position, and draw the fingers to the edges of the sole. Do this alternate spreading movement all along the foot, starting at the toes and ending at the ankle.

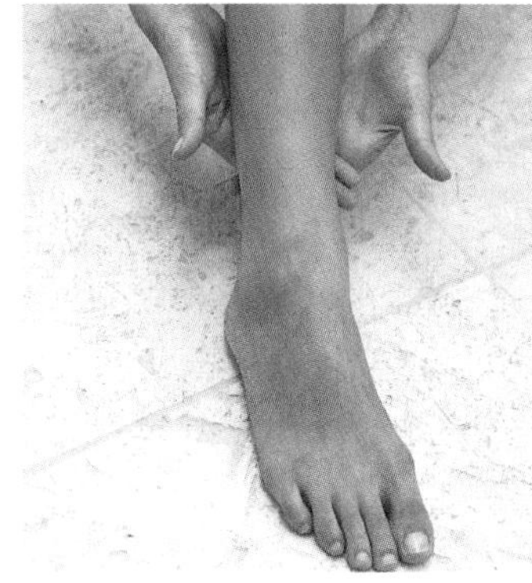

△ **4** Place your hands on the calf above the ankle area. Cross the back of one hand over the palm of the other, as shown, ready for the following step.

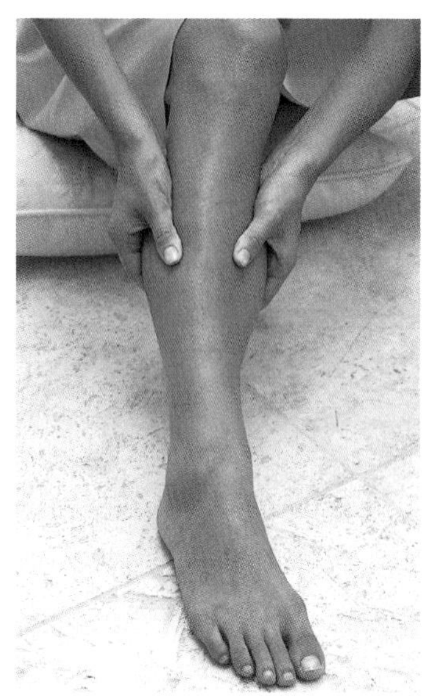

△ **5** Now grasp the sides of the calf muscle with your thumbs. Pull back the thumbs to squeeze the muscle between thumbs and fingers. Work up your entire calf muscle to just below the knee. Repeat.

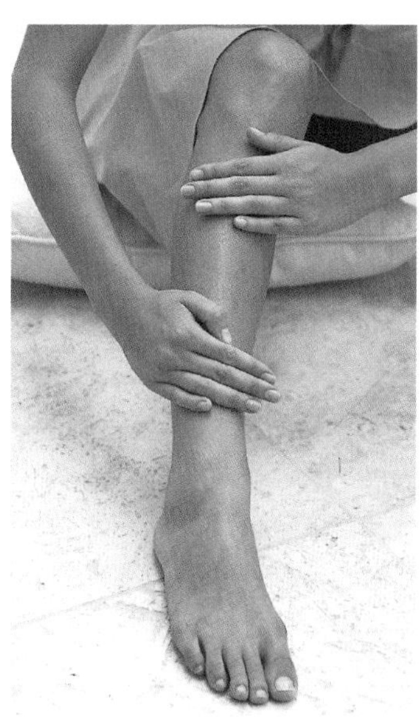

△ **6** Stroke up the front of the leg from ankle to knee, using alternate palms. Use soft pressure. If you wish, stroke a diluted essential oil into the leg in step 6 of the routine, shown here. Good oils to help the circulation and aid relaxation include a blend of geranium and rosemary. Repeat on the other leg.

at the end of the day...

It is an excellent idea to rest with your feet above hip level for at least 15 minutes at the end of the day. A good way of doing this is to use the following modified yoga pose. Find a place next to a wall and put a folded blanket, rug or mat on the floor. Sit on the mat with the side of one buttock against the wall. Lie down and at the same time bring your legs up against the wall, then move onto your back. The backs of your legs should be flat against the wall, your buttocks should touch the base of the wall, and your body should be straight. Stay like this for 15 minutes.

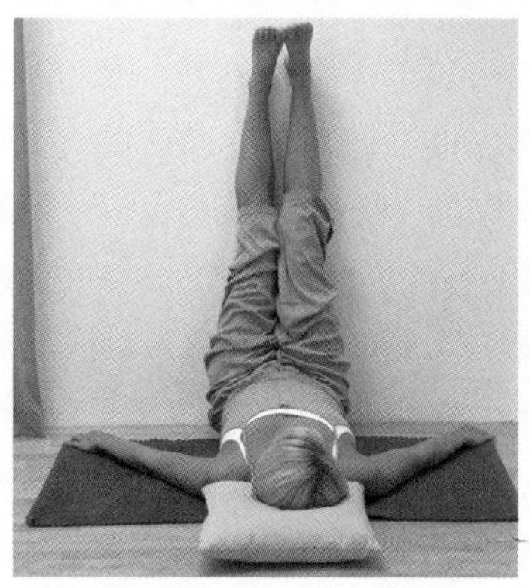

△ **As you rest in this circulation-restoring position, relax your arms and close your eyes.**

Travel tips

Travelling is hard on the body. Whether in a car, train or aeroplane, we tend to sit in cramped conditions and often need to maintain the same posture for many hours.

A few simple techniques can make travelling more pleasurable, and reduce any negative effects on the body. First of all, make sure that your clothes are comfortable and do not restrict your movements.

If you are travelling by car, stop the vehicle and get out at regular intervals. Walk around for a few minutes; stretch your arms above your head and out to the sides and drop your neck towards each shoulder in turn. Raise and drop the shoulders a few times to relieve tension here.

On a plane or train, get up and walk down the aisle from time to time. Every half an hour or so, do some foot and leg exercises to keep the circulation moving.

On aeroplanes, the air is dry and your feet and ankles can swell. If you are flying, it is important to wear comfortable shoes with laces so that they can expand with your feet. You should also wear loose socks – or compression socks as advised by the airline or your doctor. If you take your shoes off, put them back on a few hours before landing so that your feet have a chance to get used to them. Drink lots of water during the flight, and take no alcohol, since it has a dramatic dehydrating effect.

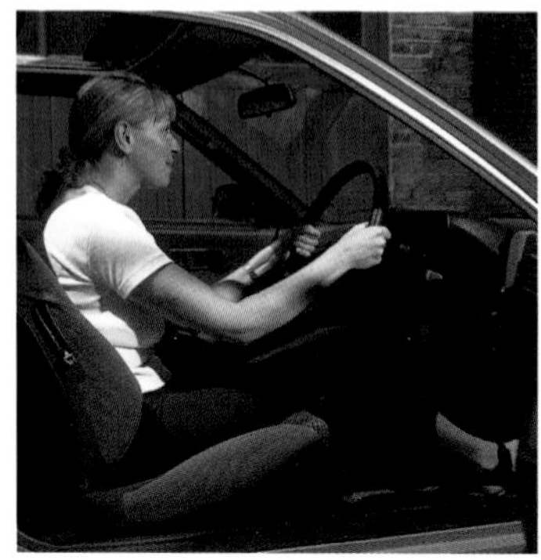

◁ Travelling often involves sitting in fixed positions in a cramped space for long periods of time. This is bad for all of the body, and it takes a heavy toll on the legs and feet. Make sure that you don't slump forwards, like this woman, but sit up straight. It may help to place a wedge-shaped cushion under the buttocks.

foot exercises in transit

Keeping the feet moving during a long air, bus or train journey minimizes swelling and helps to reduce the risk of deep-vein thrombosis (DVT), a potentially life-threatening condition. You should also do any exercises that are recommended by the airline. You will need an inflatable travel neck cushion to do the following routine.

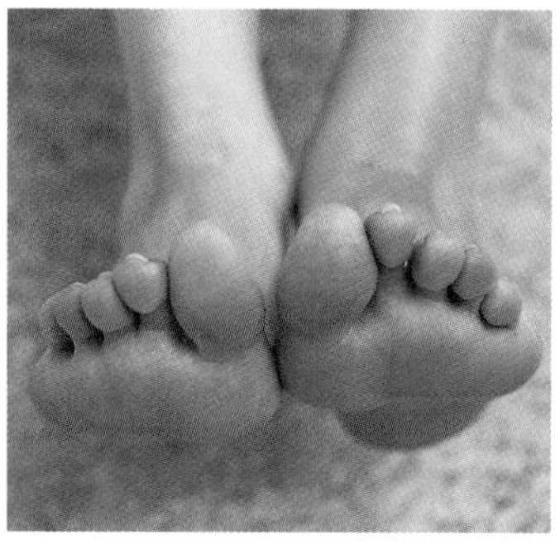

△ **1** Take off your shoes (and socks if you wish). Press the heels into the floor and lift your toes. Pull your toes towards your shins as far as you can; feel the stretch in the front of the lower leg. Then stretch them the opposite way, by pressing the toes into the floor.

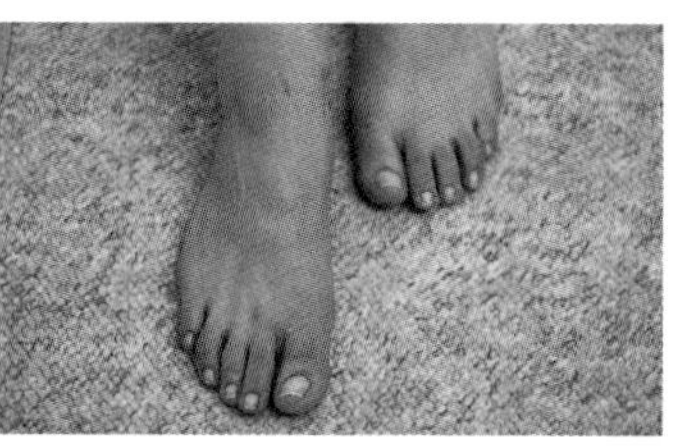

△ **2** Slide one foot forwards, then slide it back as you slide the other one forwards. Repeat this alternate action many times, starting off slowly and increasing the speed. If doing the exercise in bare feet, do not press too hard or you will get carpet burns.

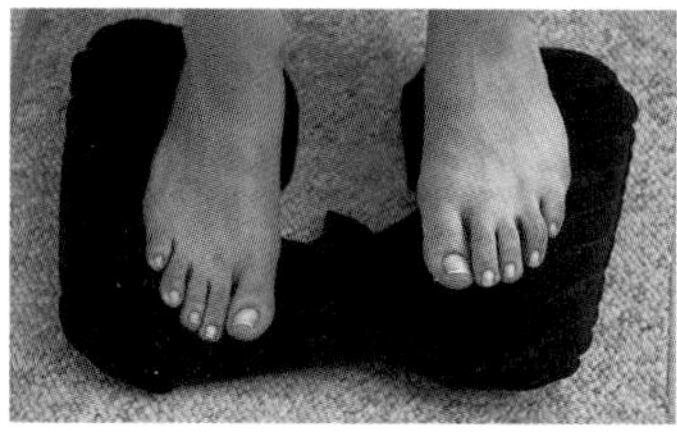

△ **3** Inflate a neck cushion to about three-quarters capacity. Place under the feet, then press alternate feet down as though you are walking. Push down hard enough to move the air from side to side.

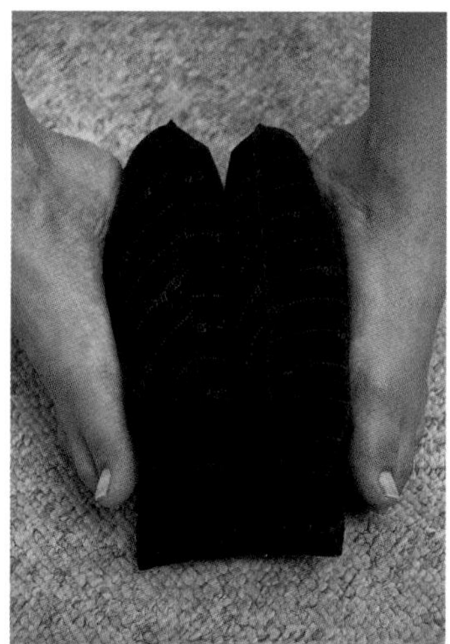

△ **4** Now fold the cushion in two and place it between the soles of your feet. Keeping the cushion in position, try to push your feet together. The partially inflated cushion provides resistance, giving a good workout for the thigh and buttock muscles. You will also feel the stretch in the abdomen. Relax, then push again a few times. Do the whole routine at regular intervals – twice an hour – during the flight.

jetlag routine

These steps will specifically help to relieve the symptoms of jetlag. They are an excellent way of keeping yourself going so that you can go to bed at the correct time.

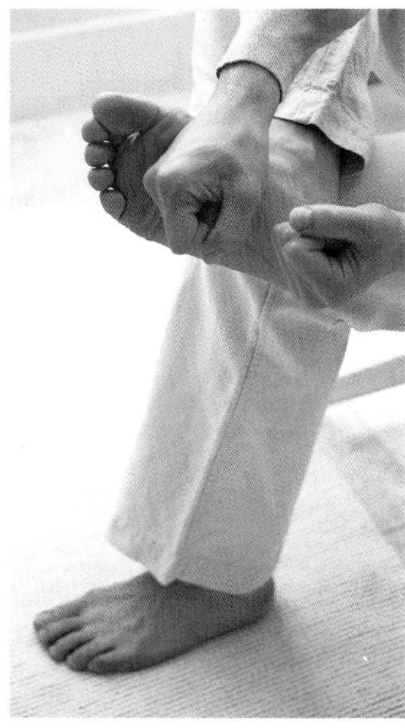

△ **1** Curl your hands into loose fists. Use the flat edge on the little finger side to strike the sole of the foot. Strike all over, working from toe to heel, then back to the heel.

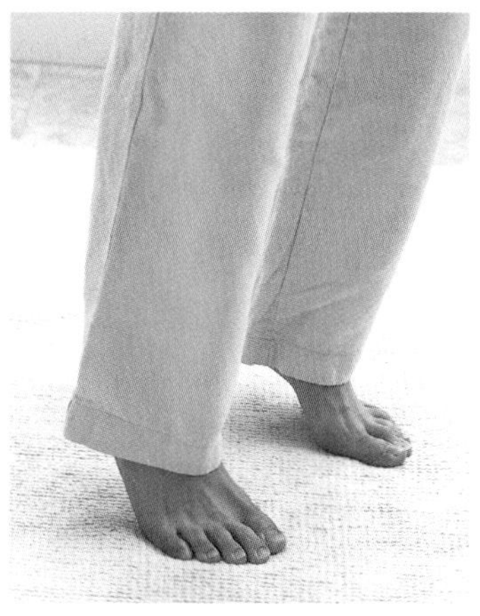

△ **2** Stand up. Stand on the balls of your feet to the count of ten – hold on to a chair or wall if you feel at all unsteady. Relax, then repeat.

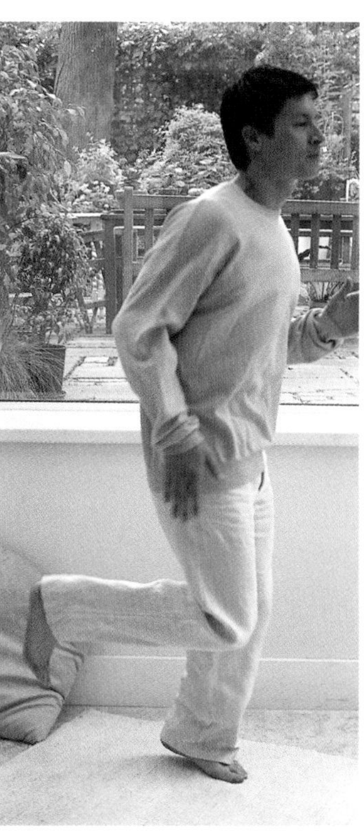

△ **3** Run on the spot to a count of 30. Relax for a count of 10, then run again. Do this about five times, depending on your fitness level.

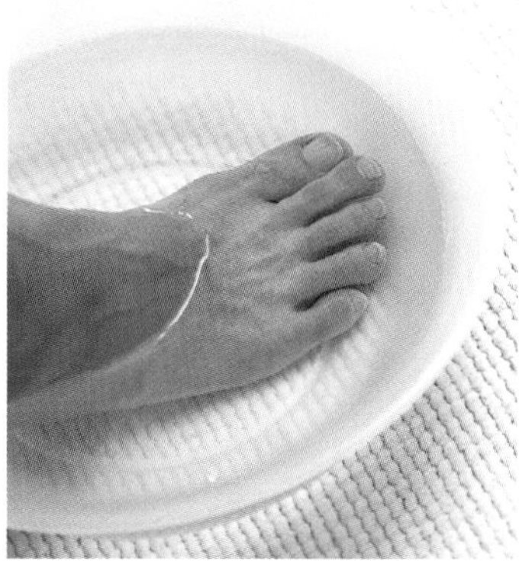

△ **4** Fill a large bowl with cool water (not too hot or cold), or run a very shallow, cool bath. Now place your feet in the bowl or bath. Lift up the toes, then the heels a few times. Rotate your right foot from the ankle, ten times clockwise, ten times anticlockwise. Do the same with the left foot. Repeat the rotation on both feet.

travel beads

Wearing an anklet or bracelet of wooden beads soaked in appropriate oils is a great way of staying fresh and relaxed in crowded places. It also helps to keep germs at bay, as you jostle with fellow travellers.

ingredients

- 5ml/1 tsp almond oil
- 1 drop lavender oil
- 1 drop tea tree or niaouli oil

Mix all the oils. Roll some unpainted, unvarnished wooden beads (you could just use a few) in the oils, leave for five or six hours, then thread onto a cord. Wear on the wrist or ankle (loosely) during a long journey.

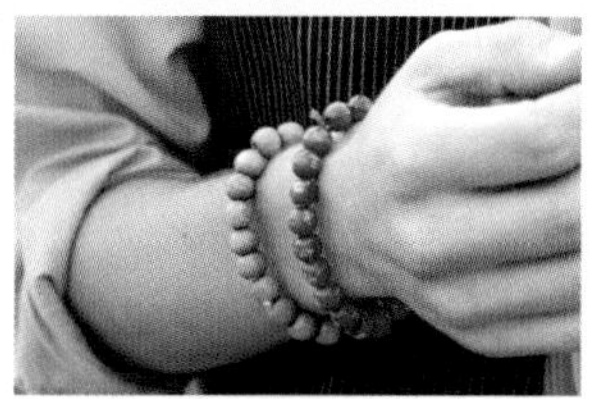

△ **A bracelet of wooden beads soaked in healing oil makes a natural travel talisman.**

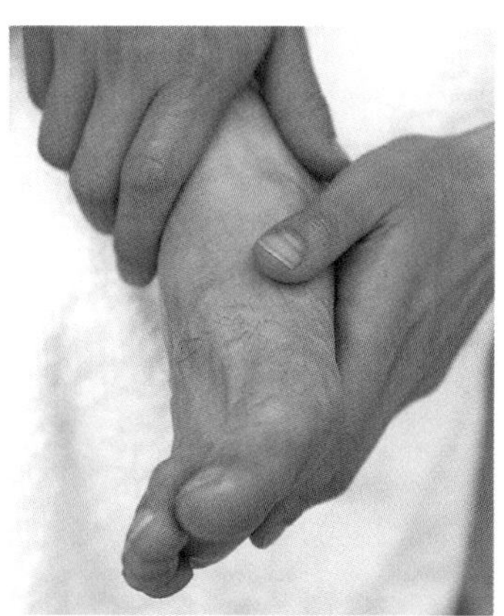

△ **5** Dry your feet. If you like, apply a tonic spray or some talcum powder, or stroke some revitalizing oil into your feet: rosemary is a good uplifting oil to use. Stroke the foot gently to warm up the muscles again.

Circulation booster for the later years

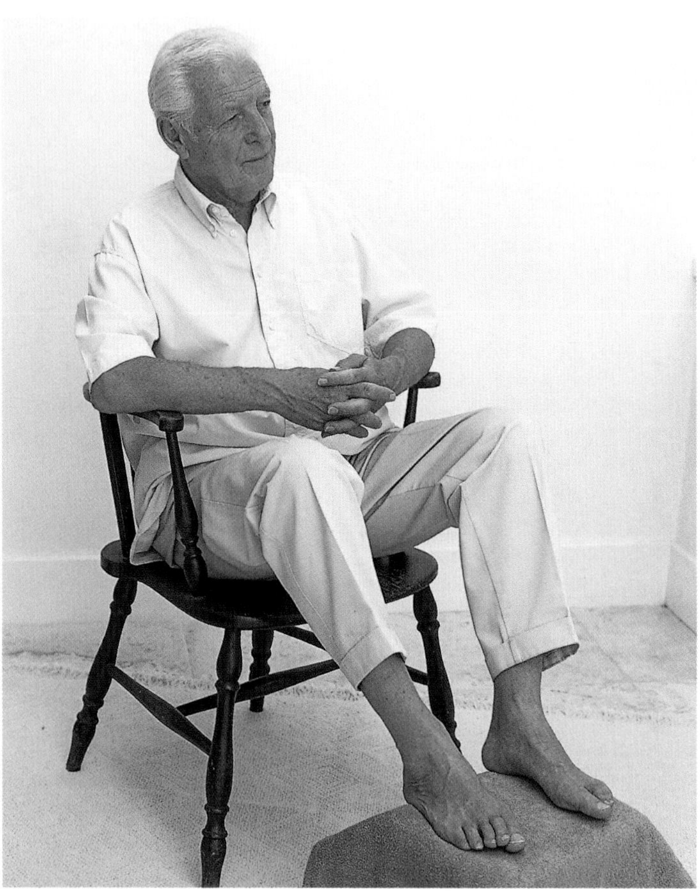

Everyone can benefit from foot massage. Older people, in particular, will benefit from the increase in blood flow that massage brings. We tend to become less active as we age, with the result that our circulation becomes less efficient. Self-treatment once a day will help to keep the feet healthy, bringing oxygen and nutrients to the area and boosting the circulation throughout the body. It will also help to keep the ankles and toes as mobile as possible.

The skin often becomes dehydrated when we are older; using a massage cream in this routine will help keep it moisturized.

△ **Self-massaging the feet once a day will help keep your circulation flowing. Always sit down to treat yourself. Rest your feet on a low stool so that you do not have to bend as far to reach them. Cover the stool with a towel to protect it from any foot spray or oil.**

safe for all

This treatment is very safe; it is fine to do if you have varicose veins, arthritis or other age-related complaints. The routine featured here is designed for self-treatment, but it can also be given by another person if you find that easier.

self-treatment routine

You need a towelling strap with loops for this routine, or you can improvise with a long folded towel, as shown. You also need some empty cotton reels threaded through some strong cord. At the start of the routine, it is good to use a light spray on the feet. You can make your own (plenty of light carrier oil, a little rosewater and glycerine and some of the essential oils listed below). Otherwise, use a ready-made spray.

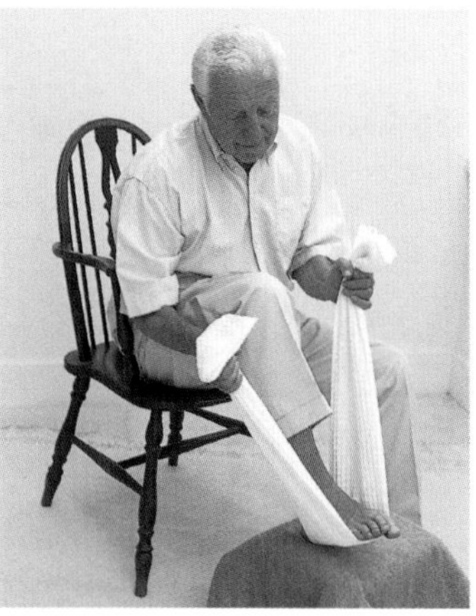

△ **1** Rest your feet on a footrest, covered with a towel. If using a spray, turn the right foot on to its edge to spray the sole, then straighten it up to spray the top. Drop a tissue on to the foot and rub with your left foot to blot excess spray. Now rub your soles over the towel on the footrest until they feel warm. Put the strap under your right foot and pull from side to side. Work all over the sole, from toe to heel, three times.

good oils for older skin

Try using one of these oils in a foot spray, or add a few drops to a carrier and smooth into the skin.

- Sandalwood, which is relaxing
- Cypress, which is stimulating
- Clary sage, which has pain-relieving properties

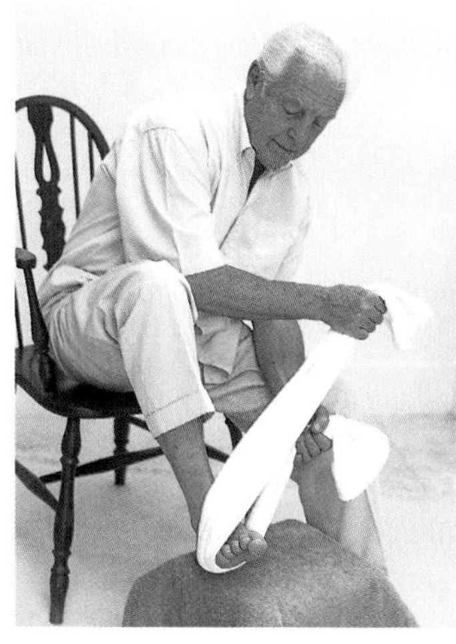

△ **2** Now turn the foot back on to its outside edge. Holding the strap out to one side, pull it back and forth so that you are gently rubbing the top of the foot as you did the sole. Again, work over the area three times, from toe to heel.

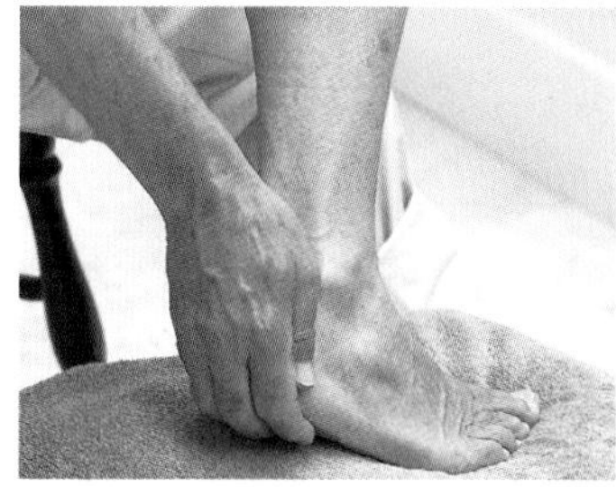

△ **3** Place the middle fingers of your right hand at the base of your heel. Draw them slowly up the back of the heel, using as firm a pressure as you can comfortably tolerate.

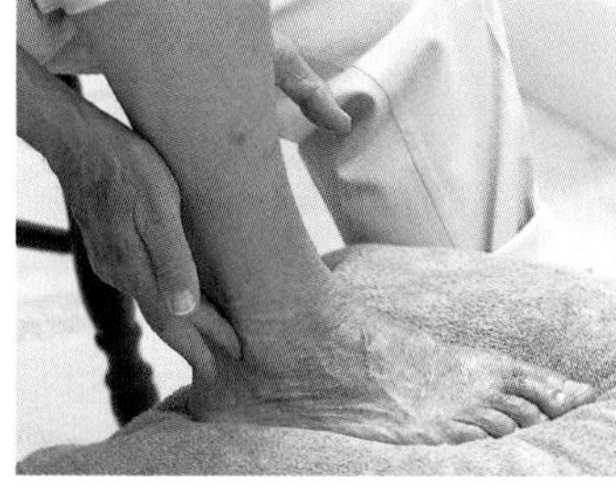

△ **4** Use the fingers of both hands to circle round the inner and outer ankle at the same time. Do steps 3 and 4 once again.

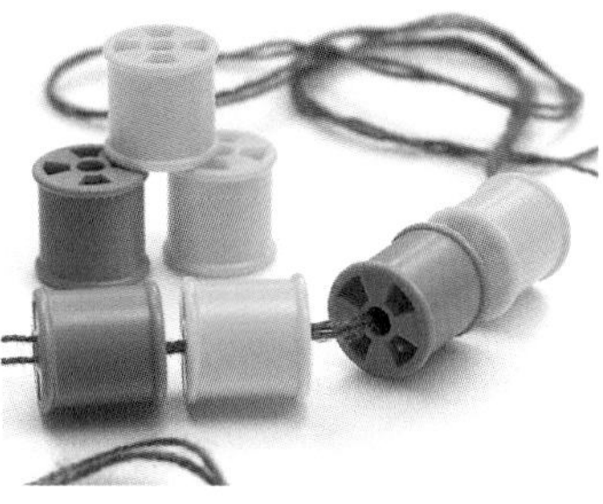

△ This routine involves using a home-made massage aid consisting of several cotton reels threaded on to a strong piece of cord or string. The string should be roughly the length of your leg. Devices such as these can be very helpful if you have difficulty bending down, or if it feels uncomfortable to rest your foot on your knee.

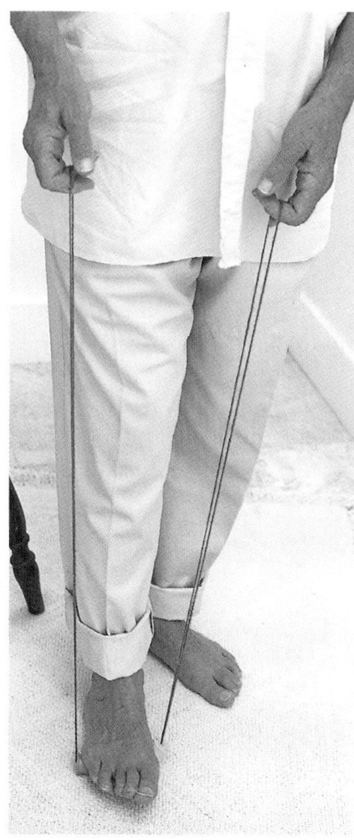

△ **5** Stand up (stay seated if you are unsteady). Place the threaded cotton reels under your right foot and hold the ends of the cord. Roll your foot backwards and forwards on the reels from heel to toe. Do five complete rolls in each direction.

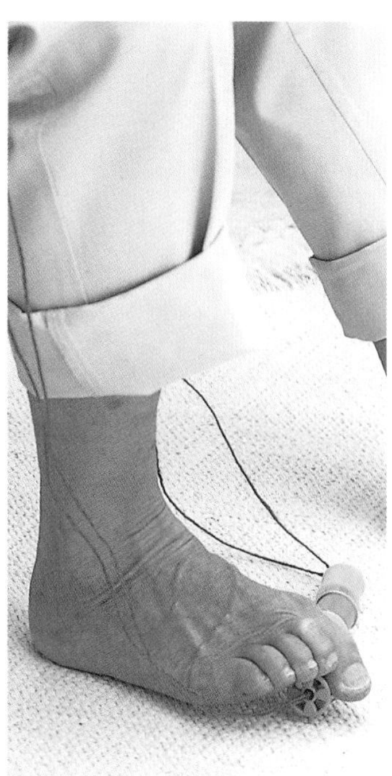

△ **6** Sit back down again, keeping the cotton reels under your right foot. Now try to pick up one or two of the reels with your toes. Practise this lifting exercise five times, making sure that you get all of your toes working.

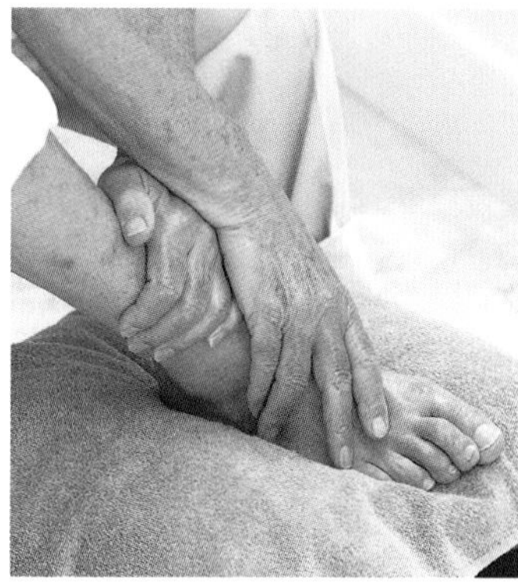

△ **7** Place a little nourishing oil in your hands and rub the palms together to distribute evenly. Using alternate hands, stroke over the top, then the sole, of the right foot. Continue stroking until there is no oil residue left on the top or bottom of your foot. Now repeat the whole routine on your left foot. Make sure there is no oil on the soles of your feet before you get up, so that you don't slip.

Getting closer

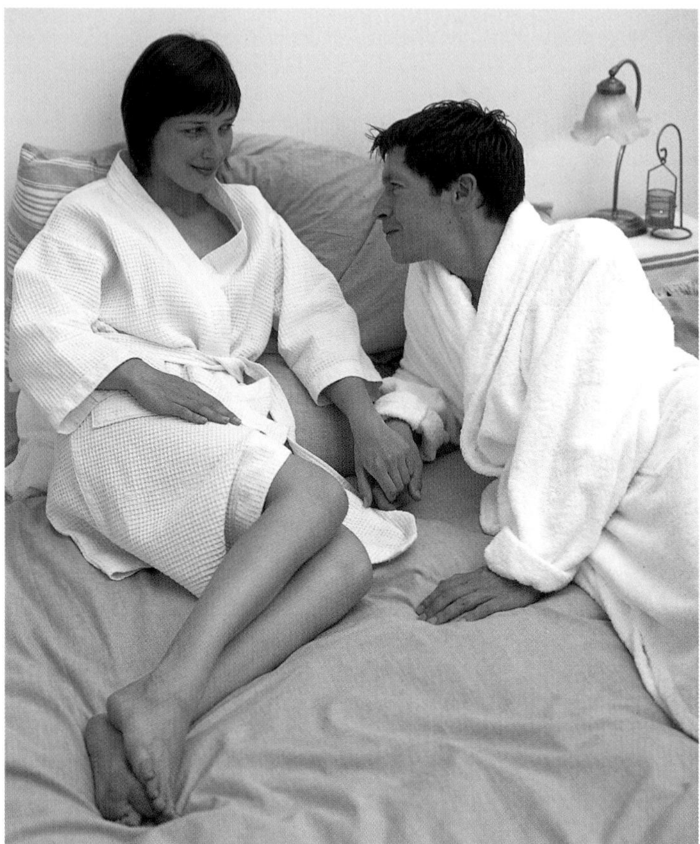

◁ This is a lovely massage to do in the bedroom, perhaps after a warm, relaxing bath or shower. Arrange plenty of cushions or pillows at the head of the bed, so that your partner can lean back and enjoy the massage.

aphrodisiac bath oil

The warm and spicy aroma of this sensual bath oil blend will linger seductively on the skin for some time after your bath – the perfect prelude to an intimate foot massage.

ingredients

- 100ml/3½fl oz almond oil
- 20ml/4 tsp wheatgerm oil
- 15 drops rose essential oil
- 10 drops sandalwood essential oil

Pour the almond and wheatgerm oils into a bottle with a screwtop or tight stopper, then add the essential oils. Shake well.

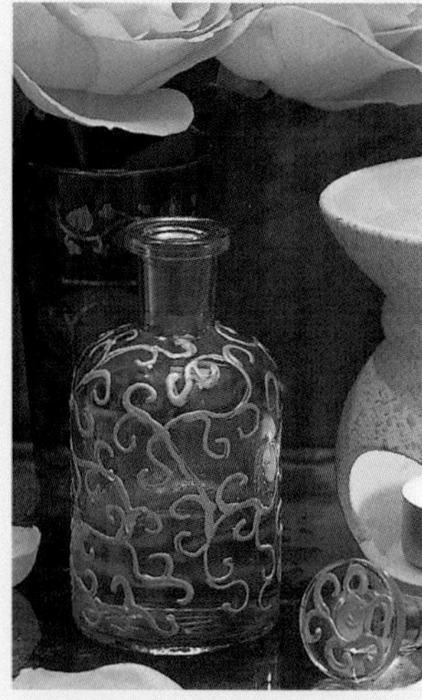

△ Storing oils in pretty bottles helps set the mood, but bottles like this are not ideal. Choose dark glass to keep the oils' aroma for as long as possible.

Sometimes, our days seem to be so filled with work and other commitments that it can be hard to make space for our most important relationship. Massage gives you an opportunity to spend some quiet time with your partner, without the TV, radio or other distractions.

A foot massage is a wonderful way of treating your partner, and for him or her to treat you. It allows you to touch each other in a loving, gentle way that is not necessarily always sexual. As well as soothing and calming the body, foot massage offers a quick route to reconnecting with each other, and re-establishing intimacy.

creating the right mood

When sharing massage with your partner, take a few moments to create an ambience of warmth and intimacy. Make sure that your bedroom is tidy, and that any clutter is cleared away. Have plenty of cushions on the bed so that you can lie back and relax. Use soft lighting – turn off overhead lights and use lamps or candles instead.

You might like to have music playing while you massage. Use the aroma of intoxicatingly-scented essential oils to add sensuality to the experience if you wish. Sandalwood is a warm, heady oil that is said to have genuine aphrodisiac qualities.

sensual foot massage

Try this routine with a relaxing or sensual essential oil, such as geranium or sandalwood, diluted in almond or another carrier oil. Place a towel over the bedcover to protect it from the oil.

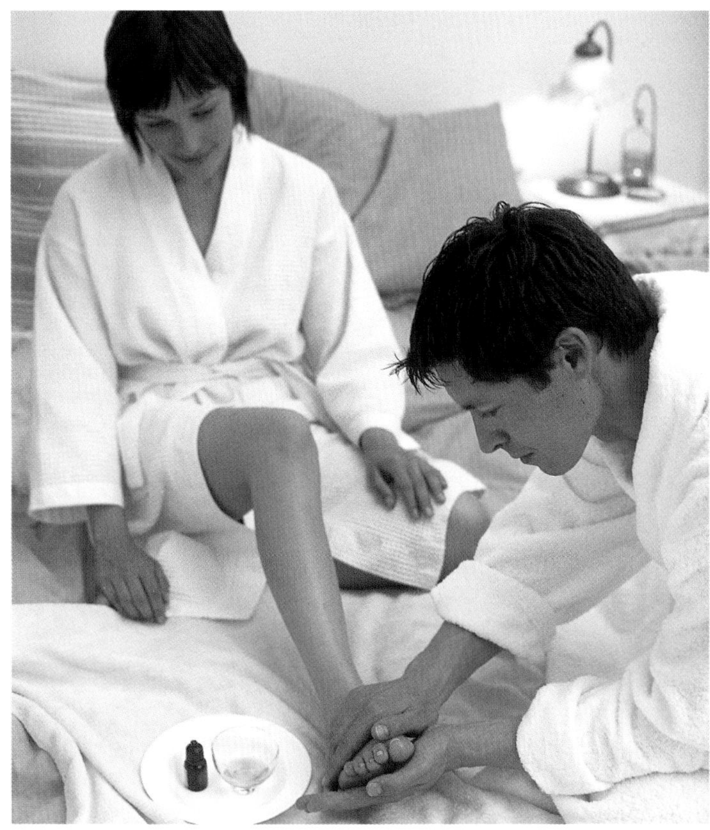

△ **1** Put three or four drops of massage oil in your hand, then lightly rub the palms together to spread it evenly. Take the right foot in a sandwich hold, with one hand across the top of the foot and the other across the sole. Hold for a minute or two, breathing quietly as you maintain contact.

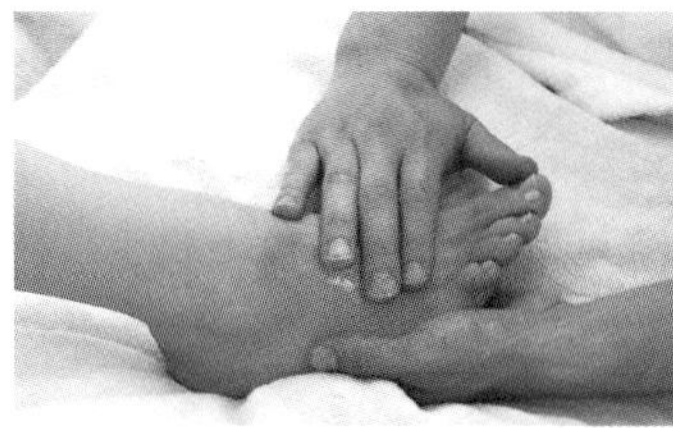

△ **2** Keeping the same hand position as Step 1, stroke the hands down the foot, towards the ankle, then slide back to the toes.The pressure should be firm, but pleasurable. Do this movement three times.

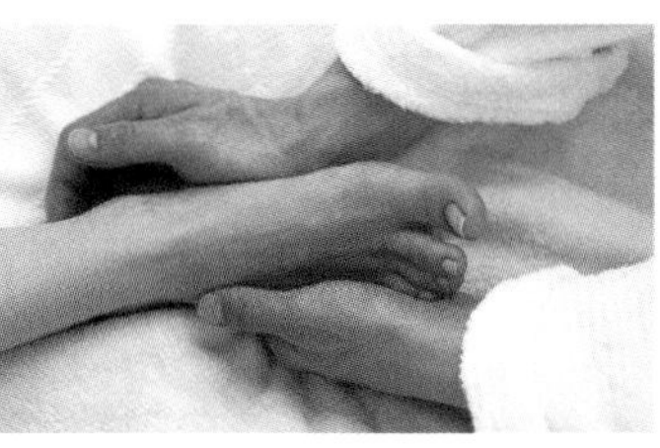

△ **3** Support the outside edge of the foot, so that the toes rest on the heel of your hand. Use the heel of the other hand to stroke down the inside edge of the foot from the big toe to the base of the heel. Work slowly and smoothly. Return the hand to the toe, and fan the inside edge in the same way twice more.

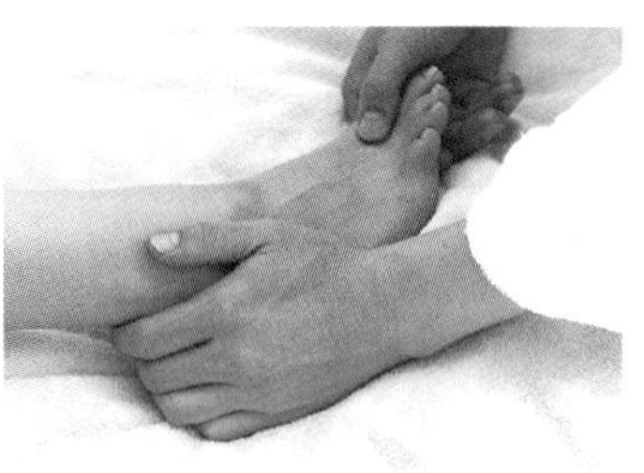

△ **4** Now support the inside edge of the foot, by holding your partner's toes quite firmly. Use the other hand to stroke down the outside edge of the foot, from the little toe to the base of the heel. Stroke back down to the little toe, working slowly and smoothly. Repeat this action two more times.

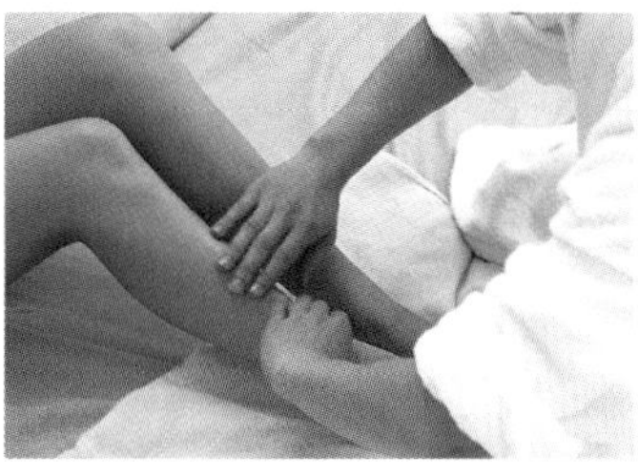

△ **5** Ask your partner to bend his or her knee, so that the foot rests flat on the bed. Apply a little more oil to your hands, then place both hands on the top of the foot – one slightly higher than the other. Stroke down the foot from the toes, and continue to stroke up the leg to the knee, using light pressure. Slide back down to the toes, using no pressure. Repeat twice more.

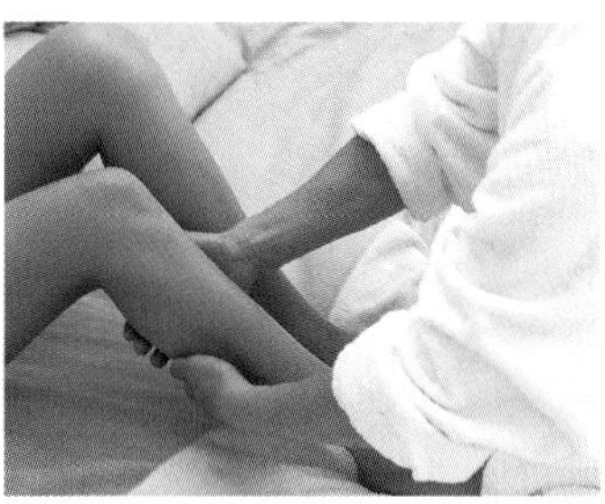

△ **6** Cup both hands around the heel, so that they point in opposite directions and one is higher than the other. Slide the hands up the lower leg to the knee: this helps release stored tension, so keep the pressure reasonably heavy. Slide down to the heel area, using no pressure, and repeat twice more. To finish, use alternate hands to stroke over the top and sole of the foot. Repeat the sequence on the left foot.

Therapeutic Foot Treatments

Most of us experience minor ailments from time to time, and many people suffer recurrent symptoms. In this section you will find some quick footwork that you can use to alleviate common and repetitive problems such as tension headaches, menstrual pain and insomnia.

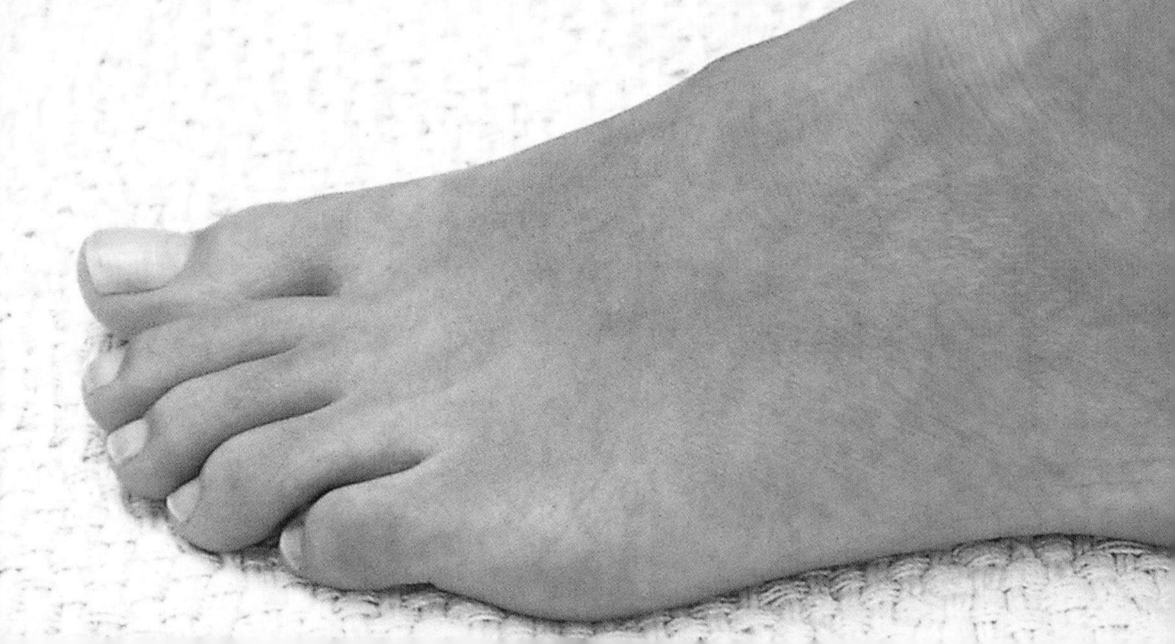

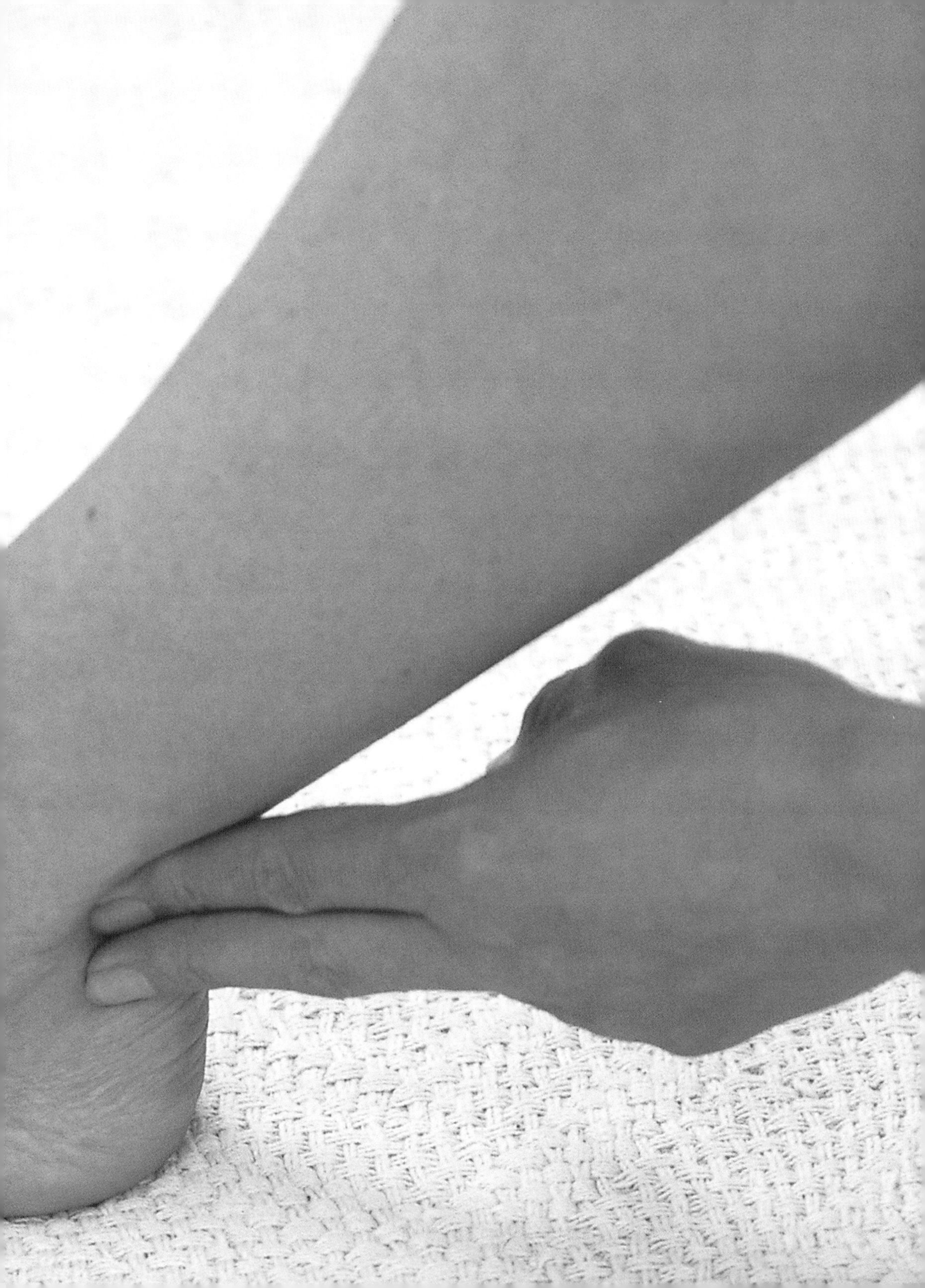

Arthritis

Arthritis is inflammation in the joints, which causes stiffness and pain. There are many kinds of arthritis: one of the most common forms is osteoarthritis, which is usually a result of wear and tear associated with age.

It is important for people with arthritis to take gentle exercise on a regular basis. This helps keep the joints mobile.

Massage can also be very helpful in encouraging mobility; the foot routine given here will help to loosen the ankle and toe joints. This treatment has a relaxing effect, and will improve the circulation of oxygen to the joints, which is also beneficial.

mobility-improving routine

Do this short routine as often as possible – a daily treatment gives maximum benefit. You can do it in the garden or anywhere both giver and recipient can sit down. When treating someone with arthritis, always work gently; in particular, do not force the joints past their limits.

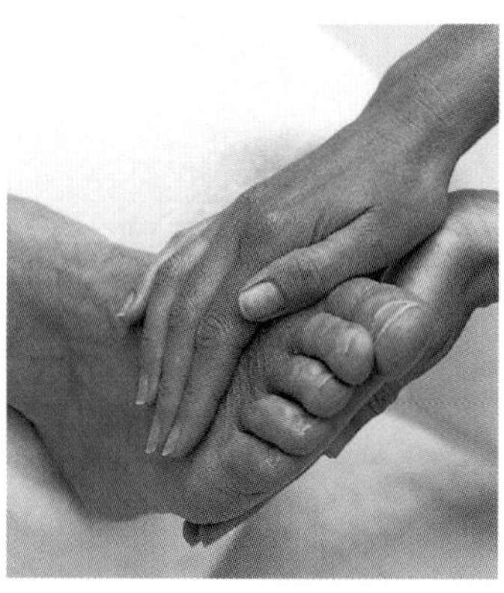

△ **1** Start with the receiver's right foot. Place one hand above and one hand below their foot, so that you are clasping it in a sandwich hold. Slide both hands down the foot from the toes to the heel, then slide them back. Press into the foot with the lower hand, so that you are applying firmer pressure here than on the more delicate top of the foot. Make sure that you ease the pressure when you are crossing the softer tissues of the arch.

If you like, use massage oil or cream in the routine. Try adding a few drops of lavender and camomile essential oils, which are anti-inflammatories. Marjoram and black pepper are also helpful oils to use, for arthritis, since they can reduce stiffness.

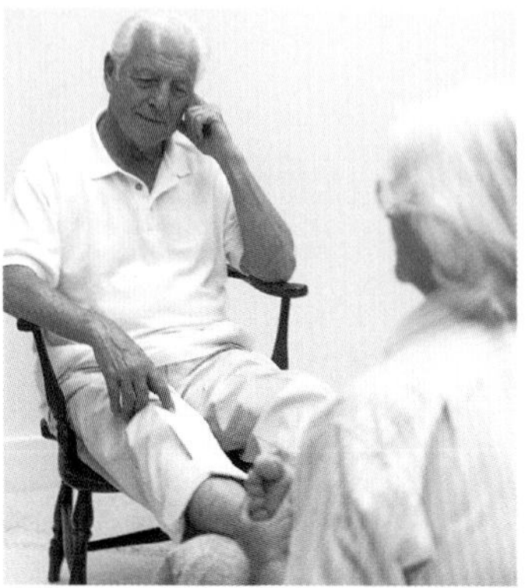

▷ **Mature skin can be very dry, so it is good to use a massage cream rather than oil when giving this treatment to an older person. Place a pillow on your lap, cover it with a towel and rest the person's feet on top. Apply some cream to your hands, then rub the palms together to distribute it. Stroke the medium all over the feet.**

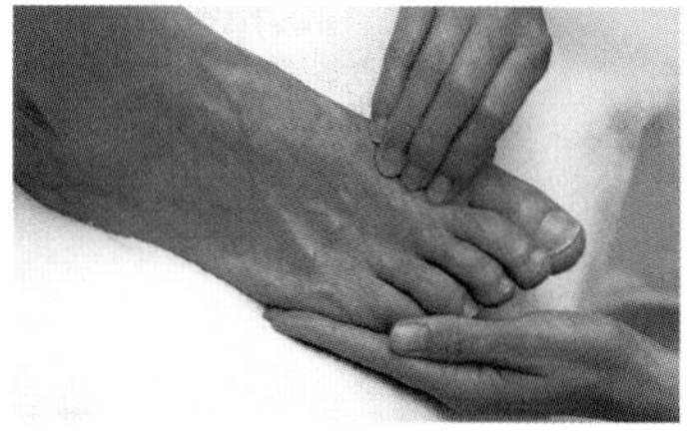

△ **2** Using the three middle fingers of your right hand, make small circular movements down the grooves between the long bones of the foot. Start in the groove between the big and second toes, then work down to the one between the two smallest toes. Use firm but not heavy pressure. Rest the inner side of the foot against your left hand to keep it steady.

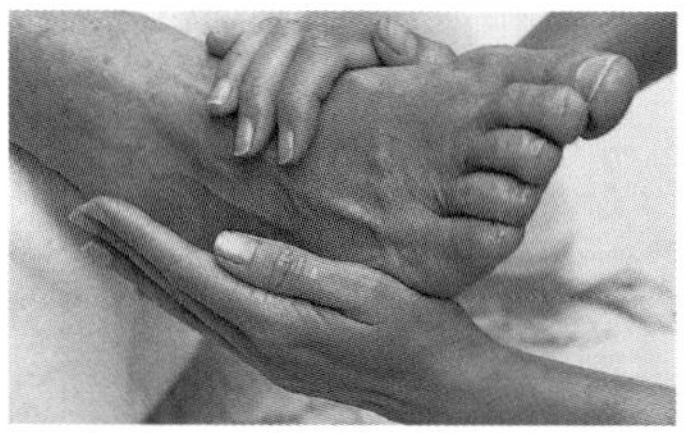

△ **3** Use the fleshy part at the base of the left thumb for this movement. Slide the pad down the outside of the foot, working from the base of the little toe to the heel. Use strong pressure, but keep it pleasurable. Steady the foot by wrapping the right hand around it, with the heel of the hand on the sole.

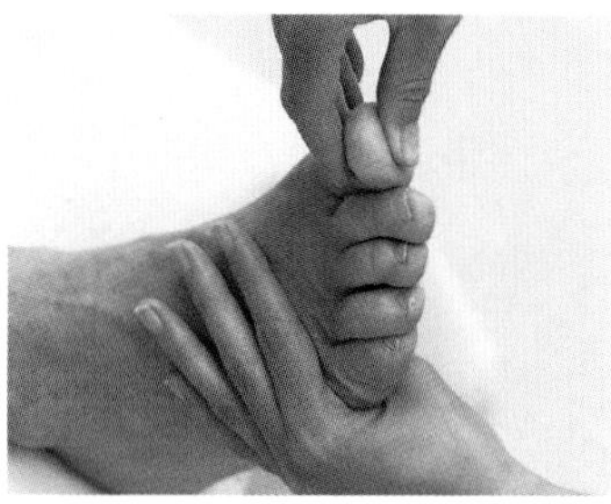

△ **4** Supporting the foot, hold the base of the big toe. Rotate it three times clockwise, and three times anticlockwise. Work gently. Repeat on all the toes.

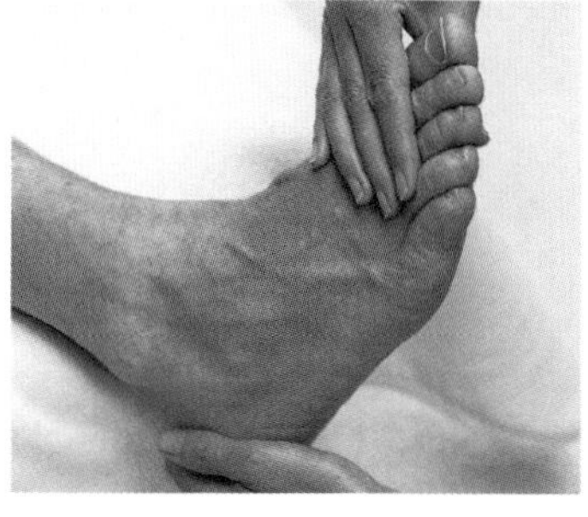

△ **5** Cup the heel for support and wrap the right hand around the foot, with your thumb on the ball. Slowly rotate the foot three times clockwise, and three times anticlockwise. Do not push the ankle beyond its limits. Repeat step 1, then repeat the routine on the left foot.

Muscle strain

It's easy to strain, or pull, a muscle. It happens when the muscle is put under excessive pressure - for example, if you lift a heavy object or make a quick, twisting movement. The muscle fibres may become overstretched, or even torn, and they can take several weeks to heal.

Muscle strain is more common where there is sudden movement or if the muscle is worked hard in a way that is unfamiliar. It is particularly likely to occur if you exercise without warming up the muscles properly, or if there is a burst of activity after a period of inactivity. For example, if you have taken no exercise for months and then do a long workout at the gym.

If you strain a muscle, you need to rest it to allow it to heal. Applying an ice pack or cold compress will help to reduce inflammation, while massage will keep the circulation going.

massaging a strained calf

This self-treatment helps to relieve pain and promote healing after a calf strain. Repeat several times a day, and combine with applying cold compression to the area.

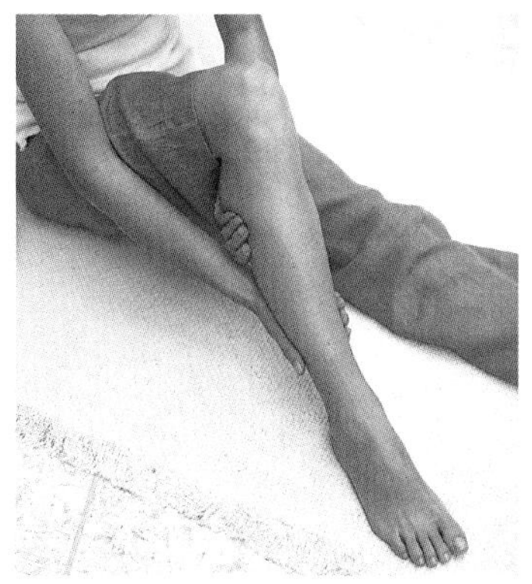

△ **1** Sit on the floor, or on a chair with your leg supported on a stool in front of you. Place your hands on the back of the lower leg, one above the other. Starting above the ankle, squeeze the calf muscle, then release. Work up the leg in the same way to just below the back of the knee. Slide your hands back down to the ankle, then repeat. Do this three times, making the pressure as hard as you can tolerate.

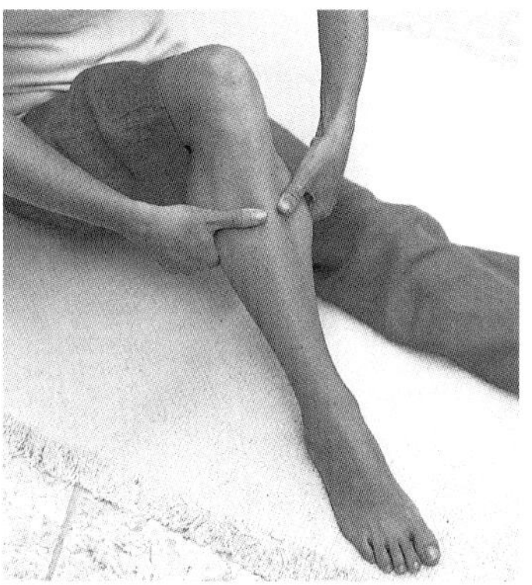

△ **2** Place your thumbs over the shinbone, curling your fingers around the back of the leg. Use your fingers to pull the muscle slowly out to each side, to give it a good stretch. Again, start just above the ankle and work up the leg to just below the back of the knee. Slide your hands back down to the ankle and repeat the action three or four times.

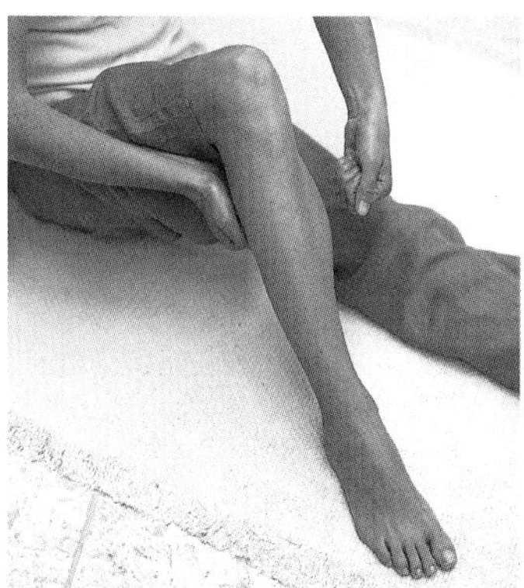

△ **3** Make your hands into fists. Push the calf muscle backwards and forwards from the sides, using alternate fists. Work from the top of the muscle to the bottom, then work back up again. Go up and down three more times (making eight times in total), increasing the speed as you progress. Keep the pressure comfortable at all times. Repeat on the other leg.

cold compress

ingredients

- 10ml/2 tsp grapeseed oil
- 4 drops geranium essential oil
- 3 drops each bergamot and clary sage oils

Fill a bowl with ice-cold water and mix in all the oils. Soak a cloth in the water, wring out and put on the affected area for 15 minutes.

treating a sprain

Sprained ankles are common in childhood. This soothing spray is a good one to have in your first aid kit.

ingredients

- 25ml alcohol or surgical spirit
- 5 drops geranium oil
- 5 drops chamomile oil

Put the alcohol or surgical spirit into a 30ml (1fl oz) spray bottle. Use a plastic one if you are likely to be carrying it around. Now drop in the essential oils, then close the lid and shake vigorously to mix. Spray the affected area, then apply an ice pack to the area; to improvise an ice pack, wrap some ice cubes or a pack of frozen vegetables in clean cloth. Use the spray and ice pack treatment twice a day.

Headache and migraine

Most of us suffer headaches at some time or other. The most common cause is tension. A tension headache often feels like a tight band around the head, and it can last for many hours. There can be many different triggers for this type of headache, including stress, noise, tension in the neck and prolonged watching of television. Dehydration is another common cause.

Migraines can be very debilitating. They often manifest as a throbbing ache at the front of the head, which may be accompanied by flickering light, numbness or vomiting. A migraine can be brought on by certain foods, such as chocolate or red wine, by stress or by other triggers.

relieving symptoms

The foot treatments featured here may help alleviate a headache or migraine. If you develop a headache, you should try drinking some water, in case you are dehydrated. Eating a healthy snack and getting some fresh air or gentle exercise may also help. Many sufferers of migraines find it helpful to lie down in a dark quiet room until the attack passes.

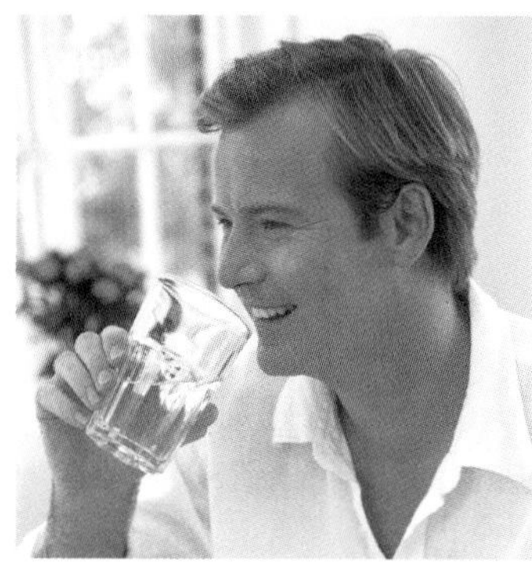

△ **Keep a check each day of how much water you are drinking. Many headaches are simply caused by dehydration, which is a common result of today's dry, centrally heated work and home environments.**

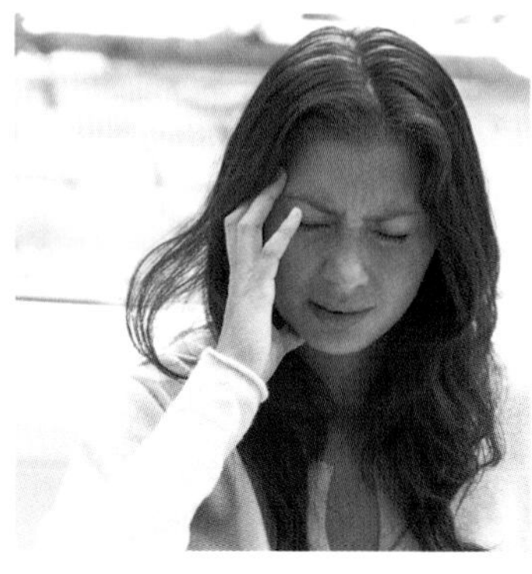

caution

You should see your doctor if you experience any unusual, very severe or persistent headaches.

◁ **If you suffer from recurrent headaches, you should try and identify possible triggers so that you can avoid them. It may help to discuss the problem with your doctor.**

reflexology routine

This routine is based on reflexology; you can use the techniques on yourself or on another person. Give a short foot massage before and after the treatment, to help with relaxation. Make sure that you treat both feet – the routine is shown here on the right foot. If you want to use oil, lavender and chamomile are good choices. Juniper may help an allergy-related headache.

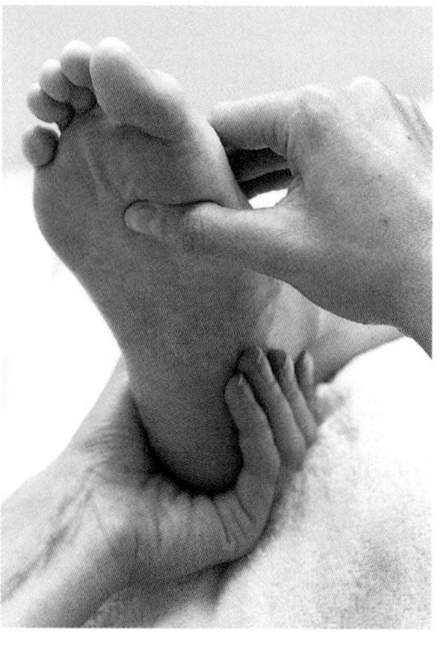

△ **1** Cup the heel with your left hand. Put your right thumb on the edge of the foot, just below the ball and in line with the big toe. It should point towards the inside edge. Thumb-walk across the sole, staying below the ball as you go, then repeat once more. This movement works on the diaphragm, which helps you to breathe deeply, sending oxygen and nutrients to all parts of the body.

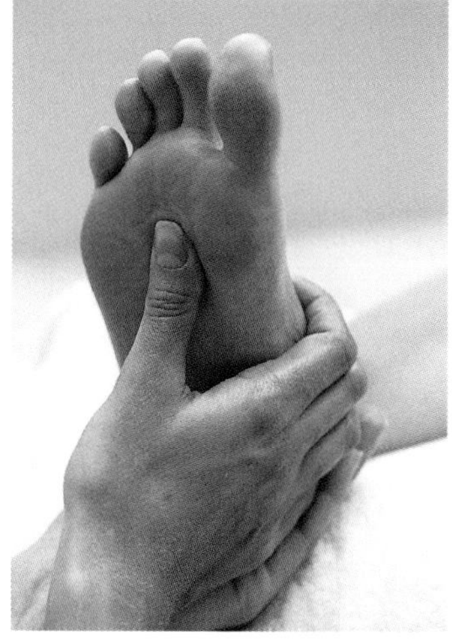

△ **2** Repeat the action described in step 1, but this time stop when you reach the point directly below toes two and three. Turn your thumb so it points up towards the toes, and give three distinct presses; this is the solar plexus point, which also helps with relaxation and breathing. Continue the crawl to the outer edge of the foot. Repeat the whole movement one more time.

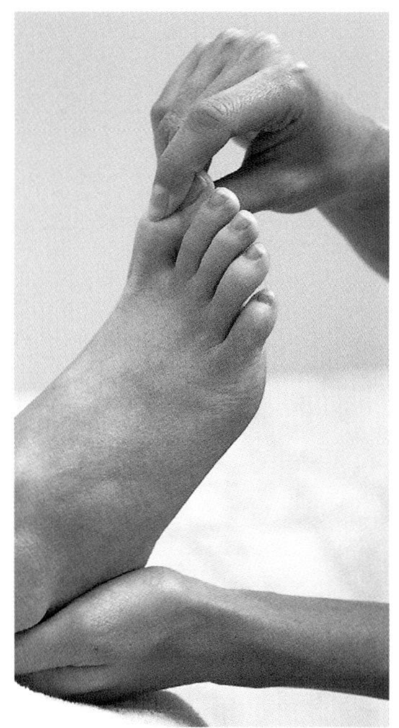

△ **3** Supporting the heel of the foot with one hand, use the index finger of your other hand to crawl down the front of the big toe, from the top to the base – use your thumb to keep it steady. Do as many crawls as necessary to cover the surface area. This action works on the front of the head.

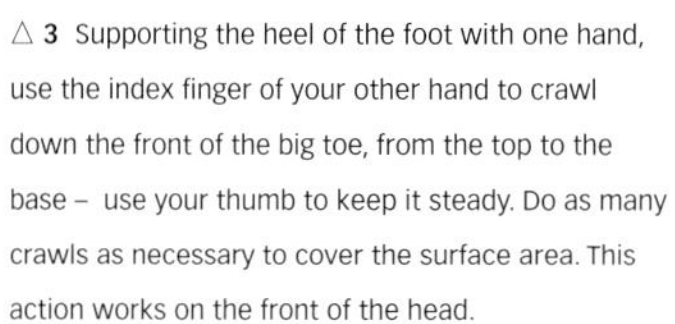

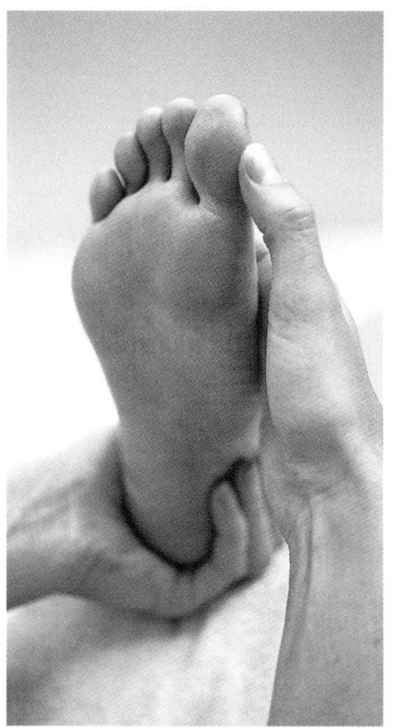

△ **4** Now, use the right thumb to crawl up the outside of the big toe, over the top and down the inner edge, making a horseshoe shape. Then crawl up the back of the big toe from the base to the top. Do as many crawls as it takes to cover the entire surface area. This helps to relax the head muscles and balance nerve functioning here.

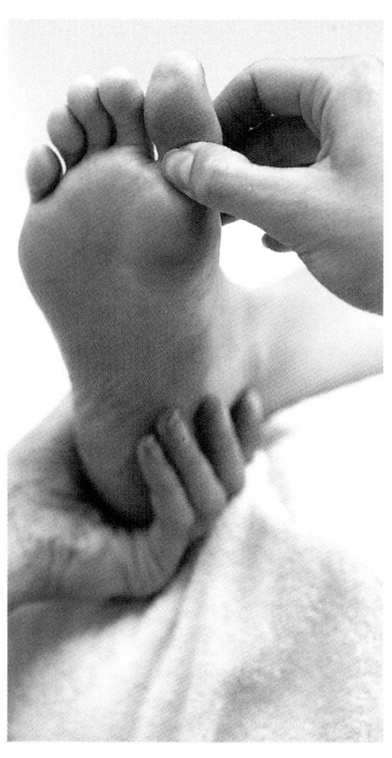

△ **5** Keeping the hold position, use your thumb to crawl around the base of the toe, from the outside of the foot to the webbing in-between the big toe and toe two. This works on the back of the neck, which may be a factor in a headache. Now repeat the whole sequence on the other foot.

quick acupressure routine

Although this is a short treatment, it is very soothing and can help to shift the discomfort of a headache surprisingly rapidly. Experiment with this and the reflexology routine to see which one works best for you.

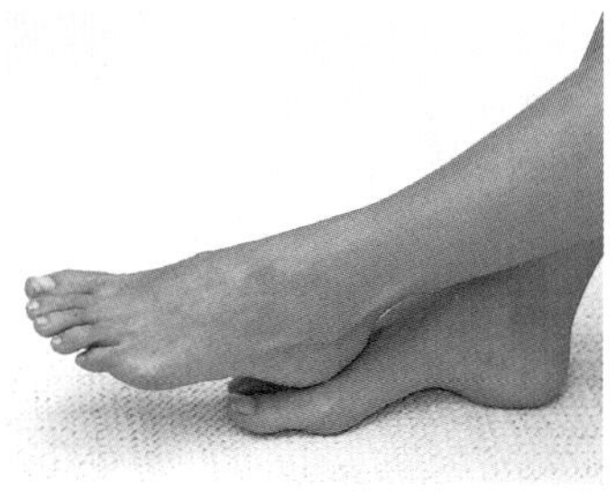

△ **1** Place your right foot flat on the floor. Use the outer edge of your left heel to rub the top of the right foot along the groove between the big and second toe. Rub back and forth from the base of the toes to halfway up the foot, to the count of 50. This soothing action at the Liver 3 point, helps to release tension. Change feet and do the other side.

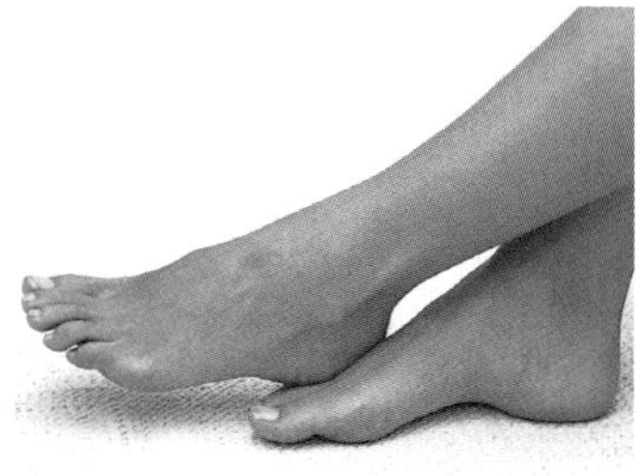

△ **2** Use the same action as described in Step 1, but this time rub the groove between the fourth and little toe. This activates Gallbladder 41, a point which is excellent for migraines, or one-sided headaches. Again, rub backwards and forwards to the count of 50, breathing deeply as you work. Then repeat on the other foot.

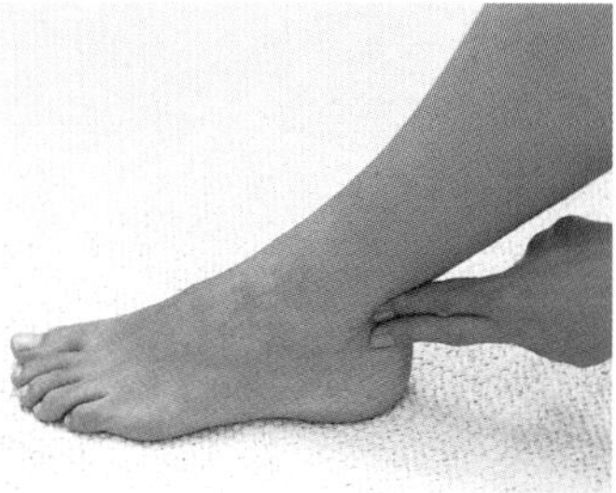

△ **3** Place your two middle fingers between the back edge of the heel and the Achilles tendon. Hold the pressure for the count of 30, release for a couple of seconds and then repeat. This point is Bladder 60, which may relieve headaches on the top or back of the head. It is also a good general relaxer. Now repeat on the other ankle.

Back and neck pain

Neck and back pain is part of everyday life for many people, and almost everyone experiences it at some point. Pain in this area of the body can be caused by certain disorders, but it also commonly occurs as a result of lifestyle factors – for example, office workers often spend long periods sitting in a slouched position, which puts pressure on the back.

Muscle strain can occur when people place excessive demands on the back – for example, if you spend hours digging the garden, make a sudden movement or do some unfamiliar exercises. Women often suffer back pain during menstruation or when they are pregnant.

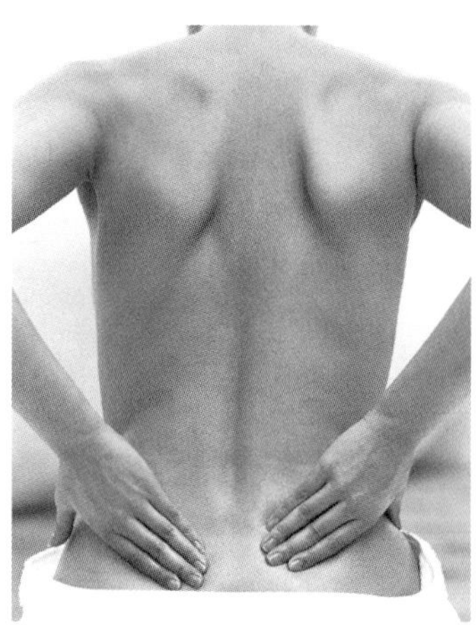

△ Physical and emotional stresses and strains all too commonly gather in the neck and back.

preventative measures

The best way to avoid back pain is by exercising regularly and improving your posture. Alexander technique, yoga and Pilates may all be of great help. Osteopathy and chiropractic can be excellent therapies for dealing with back pain and spinal misalignments. Reflexology is another good way to treat general back pain, and it is one of the easiest therapies to practise at home.

releasing upper back pain

This treatment helps to relieve discomfort and tension in the upper back and neck. It combines simple reflexology with massage techniques, and is very pleasurable to receive. If treating yourself, as shown here, sit on the floor or on a chair with the foot being treated resting in your lap. Do both feet – the right one is shown here.

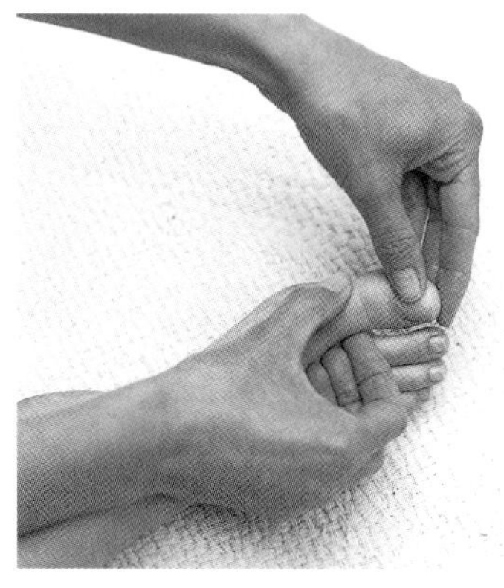

△ **1** Use one hand to support the big toe of the right foot at its base. Hold the big toe with the thumb and index finger of your other hand. Rotate gently three times in a clockwise direction, then three times in an anticlockwise direction.

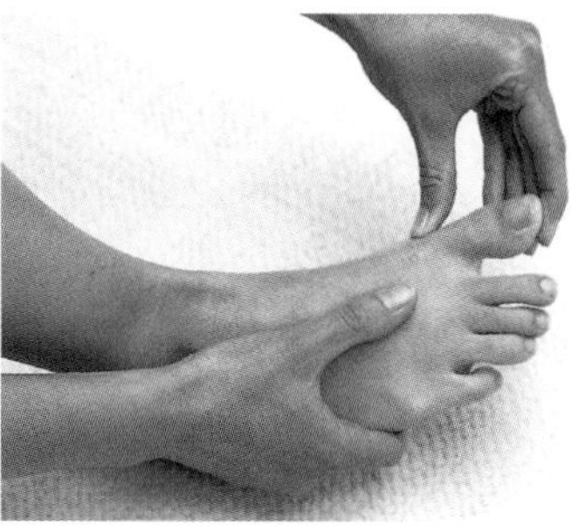

△ **2** Use one hand to support the right foot. With the index finger of the other hand, crawl around the front of the big toe. Start the movement at the edge of your foot, moving around to the webbing in-between the big toe and the second toe (not shown). Then use your thumb to crawl around the base of the toe, from the edge of the foot to between the big toe and toe two (shown here). This helps to mobilize the neck.

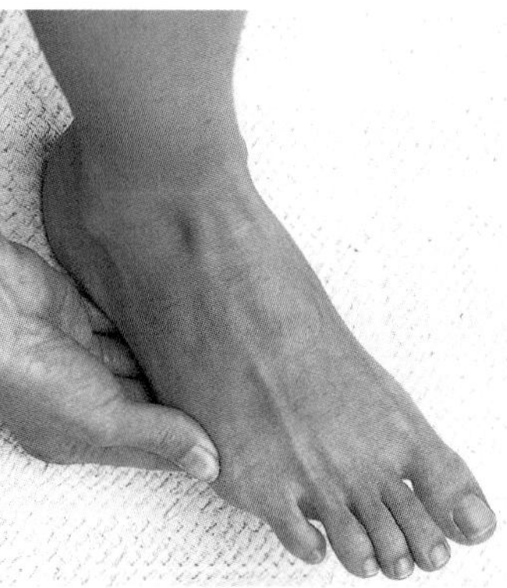

△ **3** Use the thumb-crawling technique to work down the outer edge of the foot, from the base of the little toe to the heel, and back up again. Walk up and down four times (eight walks in total). This helps to release tension from the shoulders.

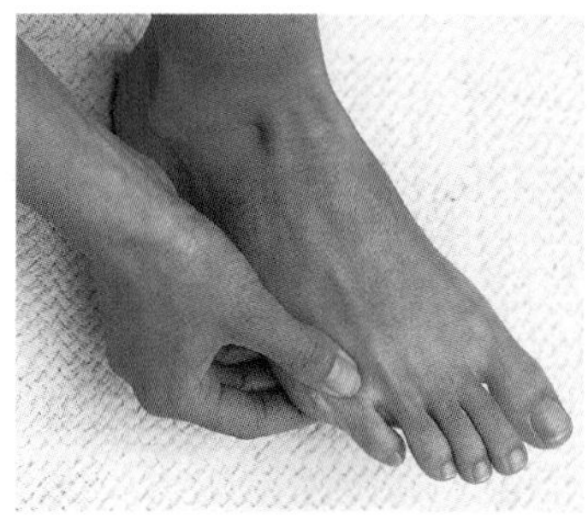

△ **4** Finally, pinch the ball of the foot just under the little toe; your thumb should be on top of the foot and your index finger underneath. Pinch the thumb and finger together, rotating the flesh in a clockwise direction as you do so. Do seven clockwise circles, then seven anticlockwise ones. If it is very painful, work more gently and just do the clockwise circles.

releasing lower back pain

Just a few reflex points are worked in this routine, which can also be done as self-help. They help to improve breathing and relaxation, and also work directly on the spine. It is a good idea to begin these routines with a short, general foot massage, which can make you more receptive to treatment. Make sure that you treat both feet – the right one is shown here.

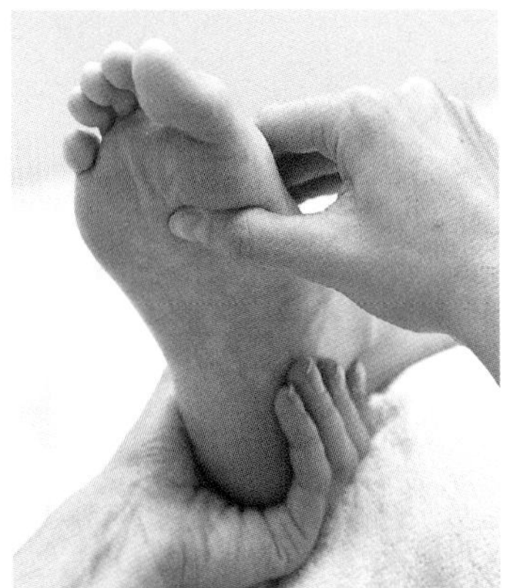

△ **1** Cup the heel of the receiver's foot with your left hand. Now place your right thumb on the edge of their foot, so that the thumb is positioned just below the ball of the foot. It should be pointing across the foot. Walk the thumb in a crawling movement across the sole, remaining just below the ball. Then, repeat once more. This action works on the diaphragm, which helps you to breathe deeply.

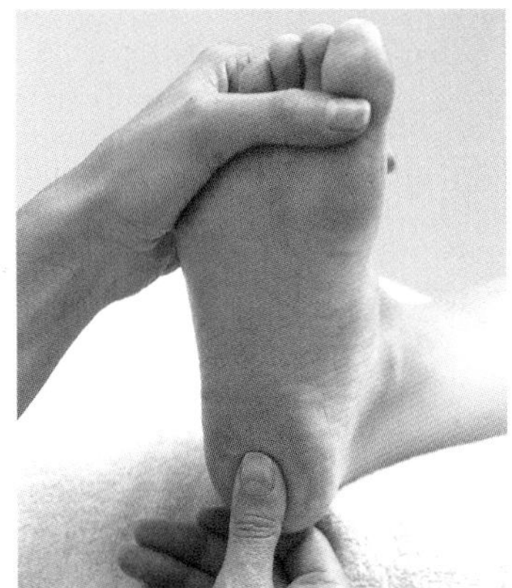

△ **3** Hold the toes with your left hand. Crawl your right thumb from the bottom to the top of the heel pad. Use as many crawls as is needed to cover the whole pad, always working from bottom to top. Now, crawl across the heel pad. Start with your thumb on the inner edge and crawl it to the outer edge. Do this as many times as it takes to cover the area. These movements work on the sciatic nerve, pelvis and lower back.

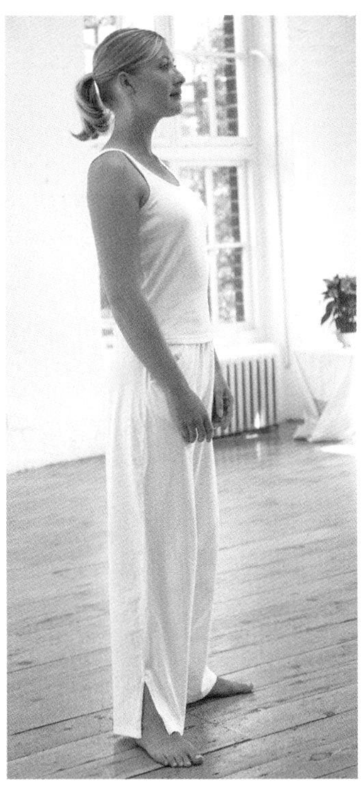

△ **Monitor your posture on a regular basis. Standing and walking tall will help allay countless back problems.**

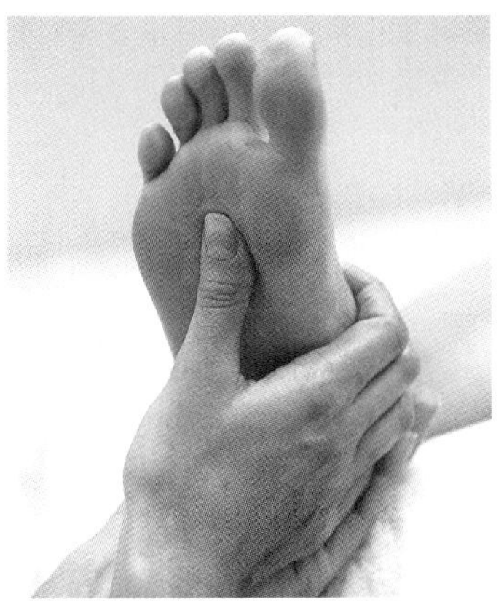

△ **2** Place your thumb in the same position as in step 1, then start to crawl across the foot again. When you are directly in line with toes two and three, turn your thumb to point towards the toes. Press here, on the solar plexus point, three times. Continue the crawl to the outer edge of the foot. Do this movement twice.

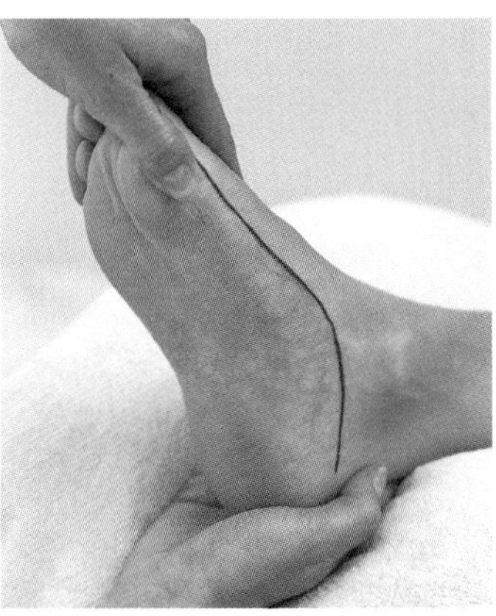

△ **4** Cup the heel in your right hand. Use your left thumb to crawl down the inner edge of the foot. Start from the first joint of the big toe and work to the heel, following the curve of the bone (as marked above). Change hands and crawl back, pressing upwards into the bone as you crawl. Repeat once more. This movement helps to loosen the spine.

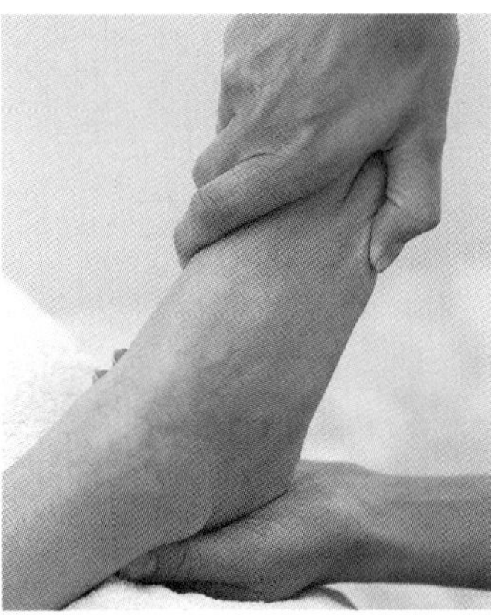

△ **5** Now cup the heel in your left hand. Use your thumb to crawl down the outside edge of the foot from the base of the little toe to the heel, and then work back up to the toe again. Do this once more, then repeat all the steps on the left foot.

Boost your immune system

The immune system is a collection of defences that the body uses to fight infection and disease. Organs such as the liver and kidneys contribute to the immune system, as do whole body systems such as the lymph network. Many illnesses can result from a poorly functioning immune system.

Your body's defences can be depleted by lack of sleep, stress or poor diet. This is why you are more likely to fall ill when you are tired or anxious: your ability to fight infection and to recover from illness is reduced. You can help to keep your immune system functioning efficiently by making sure that you get enough sleep, and that you follow a healthy balanced diet. This should include at least five helpings of fresh fruit and vegetables each day.

Exercising regularly will also help to boost the immune system, because physical exertion helps the circulation. You should also avoid drinking excessively and smoking. Alcoholic drinks and cigarettes introduce toxins into the body and put pressure on the organs that deal with waste.

Complementary therapies such as massage, reflexology and acupressure can all help the immune system. Like exercise, they aid the circulation and they also encourage relaxation, which in turn helps all the organs of the body to function well. Regular treatments are the best way to maintain good health, but you can also use reflexology and acupressure as quick fixes. These are particularly good to do if you feel depleted or as if you are catching a cold.

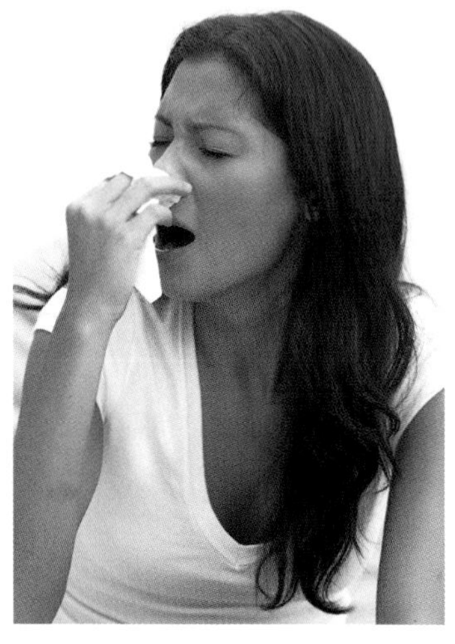

△ **Try the quick immune-boosting acupressure treatments on these pages whenever you feel that you are succumbing to a cold due to stress or overtiredness. They may help to stave it off, or reduce the severity of your symptoms. It can also be helpful to use these routines on a preventive basis, especially if you know you have had a number of late nights or are under a lot of pressure at work.**

useful essentials

Essential oils can enhance the effects of an immune-strengthening treatment. Eucalyptus oil is a good oil to use here. It has antibiotic qualities, and can be added to a steam inhalation to clear a cough or cold, as well as being used in a footbath or in massage. The oil is very strong, so use it sparingly – one drop per 10ml/2 tsp carrier.

Uplifting frankincense is another good oil for the immune system. It has anti-inflammatory properties, so it can help with chest infections, and it is also an antiseptic. If you do not want to use these oils in the foot treatments, try burning them in a vaporizer instead.

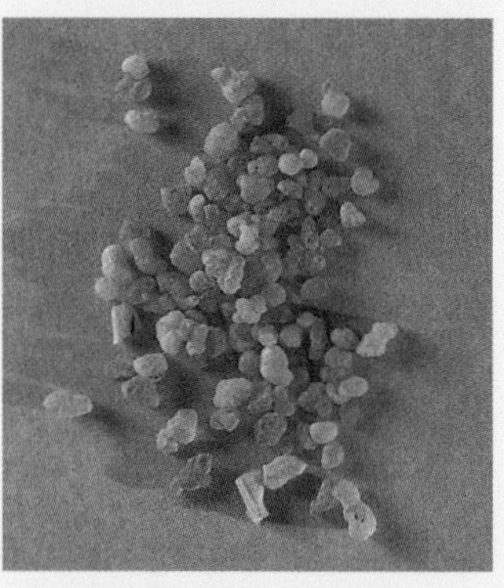

△ **Frankincense oil smells warm and spicy.**

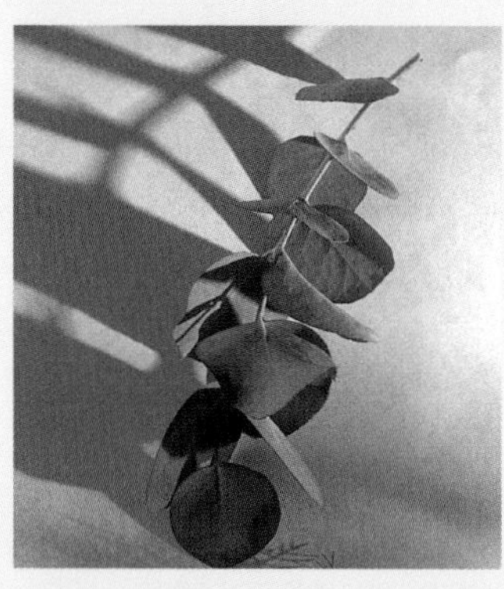

△ **Eucalyptus oil has a strong, lemony aroma.**

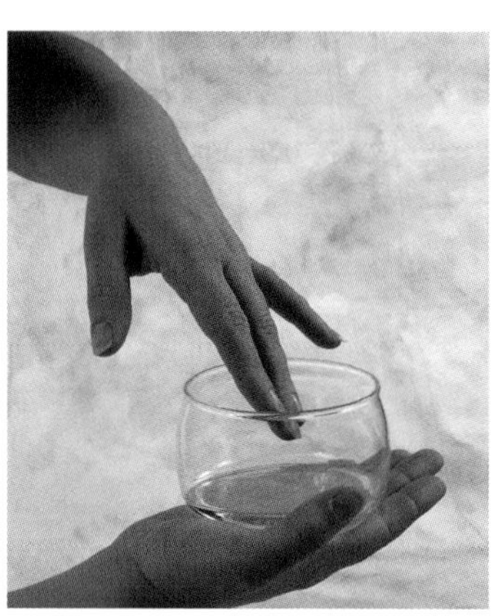

△ **Massaging essential oil into the feet enhances the effects of acupressure. Let the oil sink in.**

fighting infection with acupressure

This self-treatment uses several acupressure points. Acupressure works on the same principles as acupuncture; by pressing certain points you can direct healing energy to wherever it is needed. If you like, you can start the routine by giving a gentle foot massage. This helps to relax and open the foot, making it more receptive to treatment.

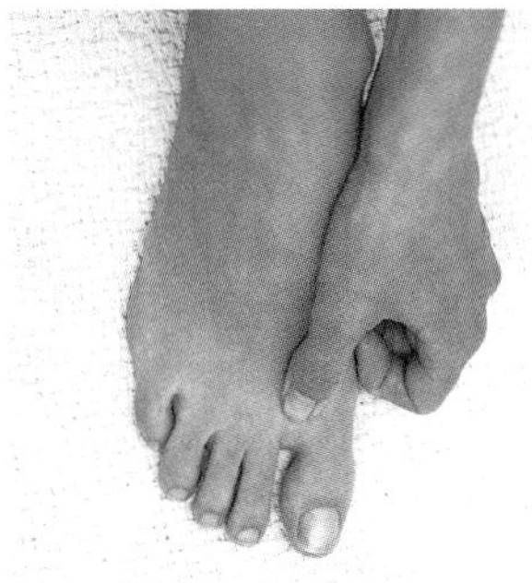

△ **1** Put your right foot flat on the floor. Place your thumb in the groove between the big and second toes. Slide the thumb up along this groove, then back down towards the base of the toe. Repeat a few times, applying firm pressure. This works on the acupressure point Liver 3, which helps to counteract the results of stress.

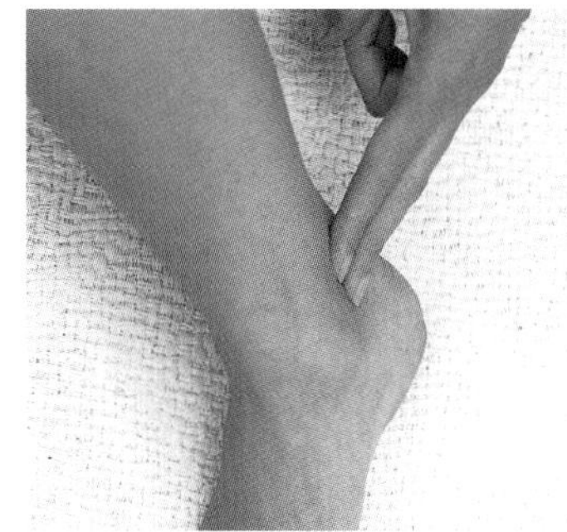

△ **2** Place your index and middle fingers between the inner ankle bone and the Achilles tendon. This is Kidney 3, which is good for when you are feeling depleted or have been overdoing things. Press for a count of 20, then release for a count of 30. Repeat twice more, so that you press the point three times in total. Now, repeat Steps 1 and 2 on the left foot. **Do not work these points during the first three months of pregnancy.**

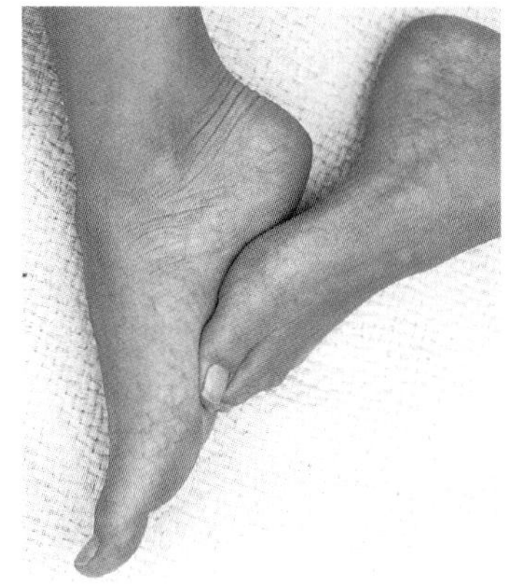

△ **3** Turn the right foot on its side, so that the inner edge points upwards. Use the toes of the left foot to massage along the edge, working from heel to toe. Now do the same on the left foot. This works on the liver and spleen; the spleen produces some of the body's natural antibodies, which fight infection.

reflexology strengthening treatment

When the immune system is functioning correctly, the body is able to fend off infections before they become established. This treatment uses several reflexoxlogy points to boost the immune system. Start on the right foot and repeat on the left.

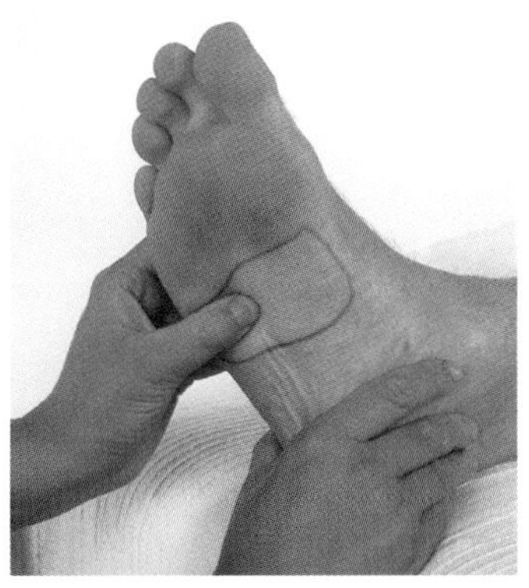

△ **1** Supporting the right foot with one hand, use the other thumb to crawl across the sole from the inner to outer edge. Repeat as needed to cover the area from the base of the ball to the centre of the arch (as marked above). Do this again. Now, crawl to the liver reflex area, where the thumb is positioned in the picture, and do three pressure circles.

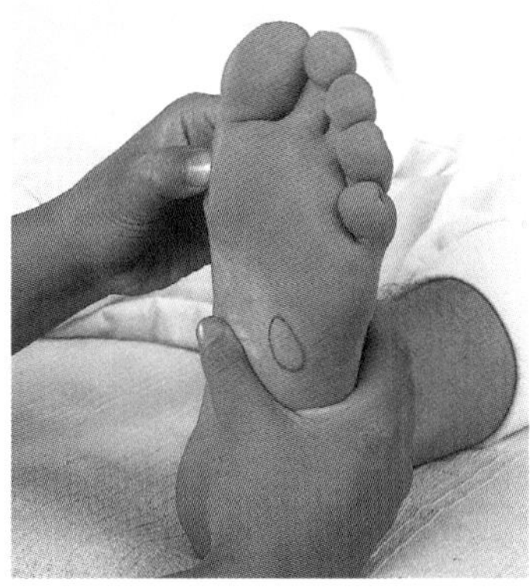

△ **2** Work the area in the same way as in step 1, but this time pause on the thymus point, where the left-hand thumb is positioned in the picture, and do three pressure circles before continuing. When you come to do the left foot, which is the one shown here, work both the thymus point and the spleen point (marked with a circle) in the same way.

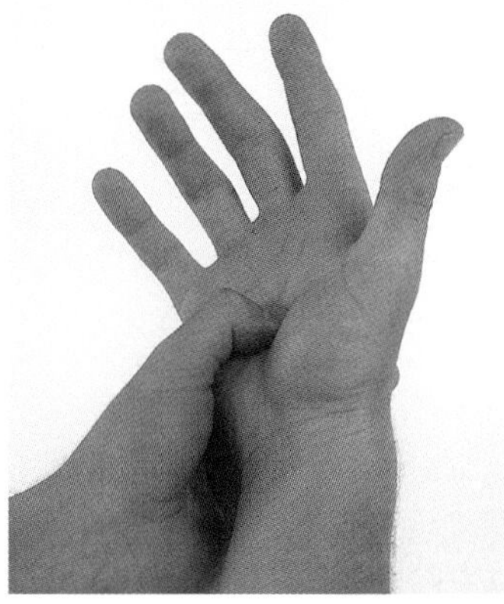

△ **Try a quick treatment on the hand if you are in a public place or cannot easily access the foot. Use thumb-walking to cover the area between the diaphragm and waist lines, which both run across the palm. The diaphragm line is a quarter of the way down; the waist line halfway down.**

Anxiety and insomnia

Everyone gets nervous, particularly before an important event. Knowing a few "emergency" treatments will enable you to soothe feelings of panic or nervousness as they arise. Stopping what you are doing and focusing on breathing deeply for a few minutes can also be very helpful.

Anxiety often affects people's sleep. Most of us will experience some kind of sleep problem at some stage in our lives. Often, this can be caused by changes in lifestyle – such as an increase of stress at work. Most people can cope well with one or two bad nights. However, if you are regularly having disturbed sleep, your general physical and mental health can suffer. If disturbed sleep continues longer than a few weeks, you should talk to your doctor about it.

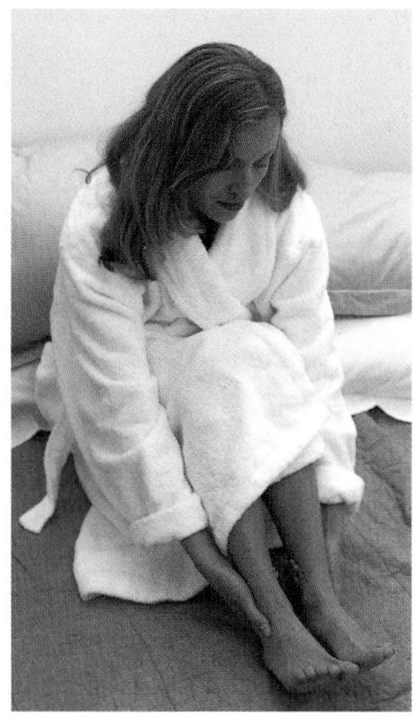

△ **Learning a few acupressure and reflexology points will give you access to immediate treatments for anxiety, exhaustion and insomnia. Breathe deeply when pressing any acupressure or reflexology point. This will help to make you receptive to the treatment, and also has a relaxing effect in itself.**

insomnia relief treatment

Acupressure can be very helpful for temporary sleeping problems. The two points used in this routine are excellent for promoting restful sleep and relieving stress-related insomnia. Sit on a low chair or the floor to work these points, or do the routine sitting up in bed.

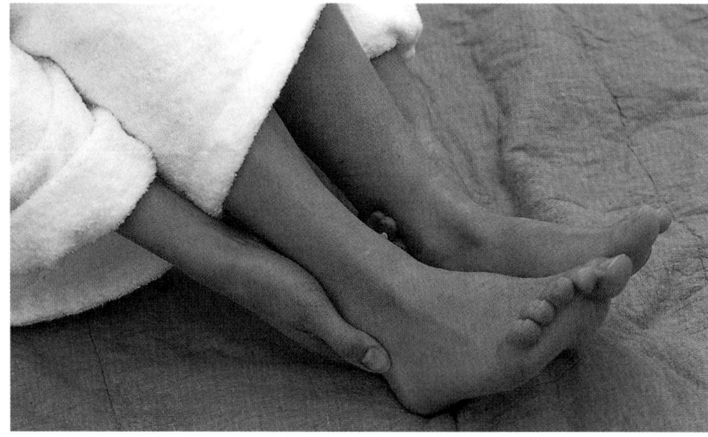

1 Put your feet close together on the floor. Place your thumbs directly below the inner ankle bones of both feet. This is Kidney 6, which is good for sleep problems. Press into the area and hold to a slow count of 30. Release the pressure for one minute, then repeat.

△ **2** Next, place your thumbs directly under the outer ankle bones. Press for the count of 30, release for a minute, then press again. Breathe deeply while your thumbs are pressing into the acupressure point. This point is Bladder 62 – also known as Joyful Sleep – and it has a very soothing effect on the spirit.

working the hand

When you feel anxious, press the solar plexus reflex in the centre of your hand. It encourages good deep breathing and also helps to calm feelings of panic or nervousness.

The solar plexus reflex is right in the centre of the hand, so it is easy to find. Working on a hand point is also much easier to do wherever you are, than working on your foot. To work the solar plexus point, press firmly (but not painfully) and then rotate your thumb in an anticlockwise direction. As you press, breathe deeply and relax your shoulders.

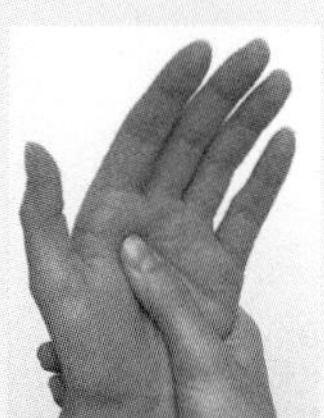

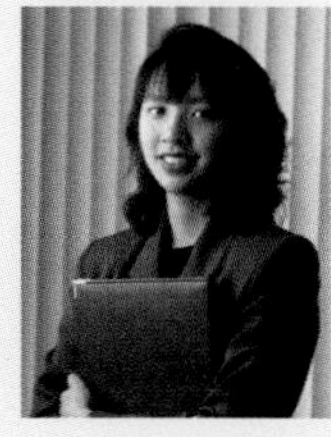

▷ **The solar plexus reflex is an excellent point to work before an interview, exam, big meeting or journey – or when you are doing anything that makes you feel nervous.**

getting a good night's sleep

The following steps may help to ensure a sleep-filled night.

- Establish a regular sleep routine: go to bed and get up at the same time each day. Avoid afternoon napping.
- Don't work late into the evening.
- Spend the last hour or two before bedtime calmly and quietly. In particular, do not do any vigorous exercise, watch TV or have difficult discussions during this time.
- Make sure that your bedroom is clear of anything to do with work, exercise or other activities – keep it for sleeping.
- Open the window a little, to get fresh air circulating.
- Have a warm bath and a hot milky drink before you go to bed.
- Make sure that you have enough bedcovers to keep you warm, but not so many that you become overheated.
- If you do not get to sleep within 20 minutes of turning out the light, get up and go into another room. Return to bed when you feel sleepy.
- Essential oils can assist sleep: add a few drops of chamomile or lavender into a night-time bath, or drop them on to a cotton-wool ball and slip this between the pillow and pillow cover.
- Try meditation or visualization: a short routine will help to ease you into a relaxed sleeping mode.

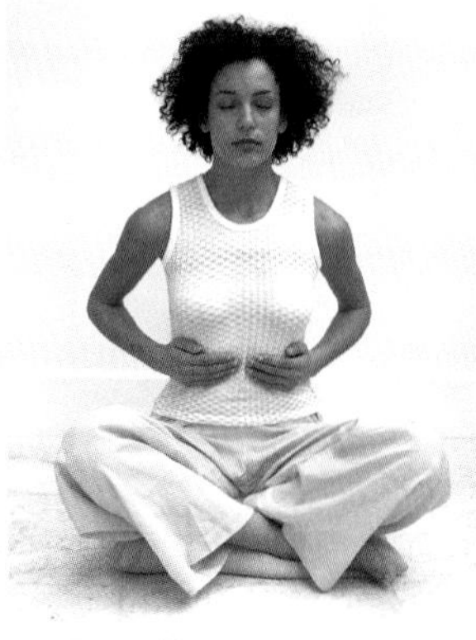

△ **Meditating before you retire will help you to unwind and sleep more peacefully.**

easing anxiety

This is a good routine to do before an important event. It uses two important acupressure points, which are calming and balancing. Working on the feet is an excellent way of combating anxiety because it has a grounding effect on you. Breathing deeply as you work will also be very helpful. Do each point on both feet.

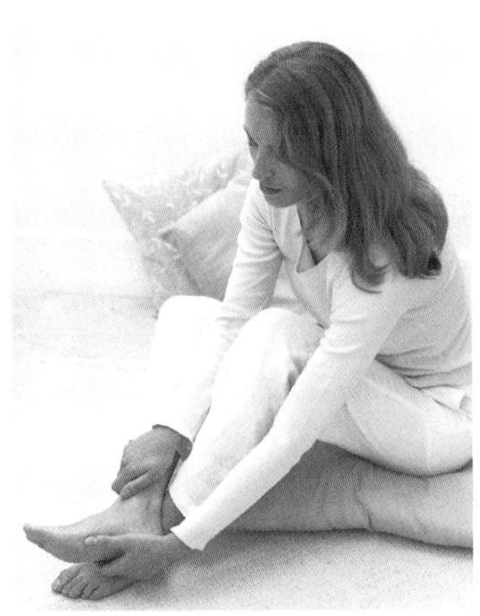

◁ **1** Put the thumb of your left hand on the inner side of the right foot, about one thumb-width below the ball. Press and hold for 30 seconds, breathing deeply. Release the point slowly, breathe for a count of 20, then press again for another 30 seconds. Do the left foot in the same way. This point is Spleen 4, which calms and balances.

▷ **2** Place the two middle fingers of your right hand on the outside of the right lower leg. The fingers should be four finger-widths down from the kneecap and one finger-width towards the outside of the shinbone. This is Stomach 36, which is a good balancing point. Rub up and down briskly to the count of 50, breathing as you work. Rest for one minute, then repeat. Do the same points on the left leg.

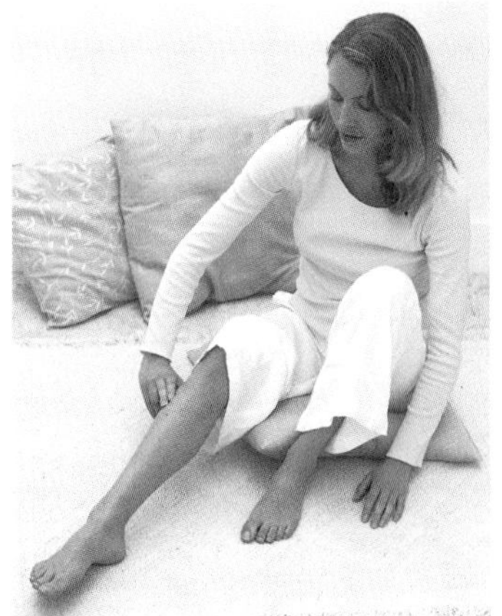

aromatic assistance

Essential oils can be useful addition to the anxiety treatment above. Many oils have a calming, soothing effect. You may like to try chamomile and lavender, diluted in a grapeseed or almond oil carrier. Basil is a good nerve tonic and its aroma combines well with neroli. Clary sage is a good oil to use if you feel very stressed, and sandalwood and rose are other useful oils for anxiety. Massage the oil blend into the ankles, using a circular motion, and allow it to disappear into the skin before working on the acupressure points.

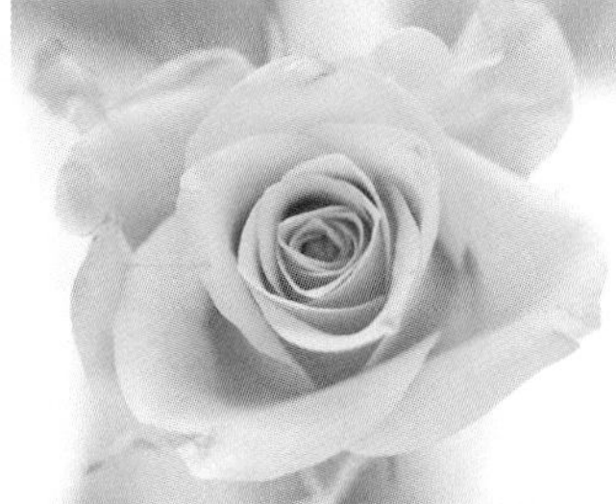

▷ **Rose essential oil is a most effective calmer. It is also very soothing if you are distressed.**

Menstrual problems

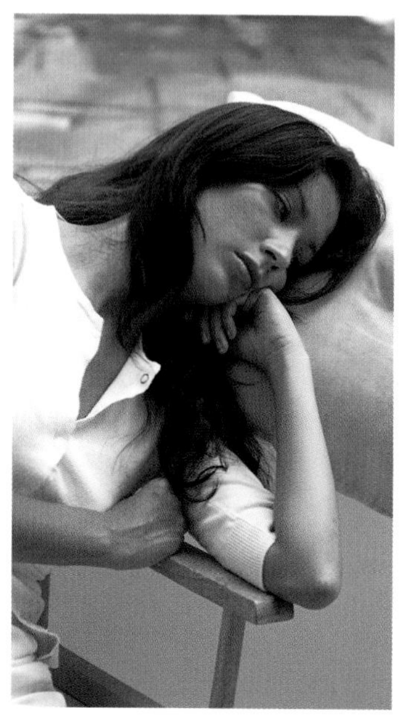

If you suffer from pre-menstrual tension or period pain, it is a good idea to be gentle on yourself at this time of the month. Look at all aspects of your lifestyle, and cut back where you can. For example, reduce the level of exercise that you do, so that you do not place excess demands on your body. Have warm baths in the evening and go to bed a little earlier, and make sure that you are eat soothing foods such as silky mashed potato or pasta.

Most women find that their pain threshold is lower at this time, so don't plan dental appointments or have your legs waxed until after your period. You should also avoid anything that makes you overheated such as saunas or sunbeds.

◁ **You may feel more tired and run-down just before and during your period. If so, make this a time to look after yourself: eat well, sleep well and rest as much as you can.**

hot water bottle help for menstrual aches

Treat your feet with this uplifting rose spray, then rest them on a warming hot water bottle.

ingredients

- 15ml/1 tbsp vodka
- 20ml/ 4 tsp rosewater
- 5ml/1 tsp orangeflower water
- 4 drops rose essential oil
- 5 drops clary sage essential oil
- 3 drops jasmine essential oil

Blend all ingredients together in a 30ml (1fl oz) spray bottle. To use, spray your feet all over, then spray a small hand towel and wrap this around a hot water bottle. Place the wrapped hot water bottle on the floor and rest your feet on it while you relax.

a monthly treat

How women experience menstruation varies widely. You may simply need to rest more at this time, or you may feel a surge of energy in the days before your period. These acupressure points will help to relieve pain and bloating. They can be done at regular intervals during the day.

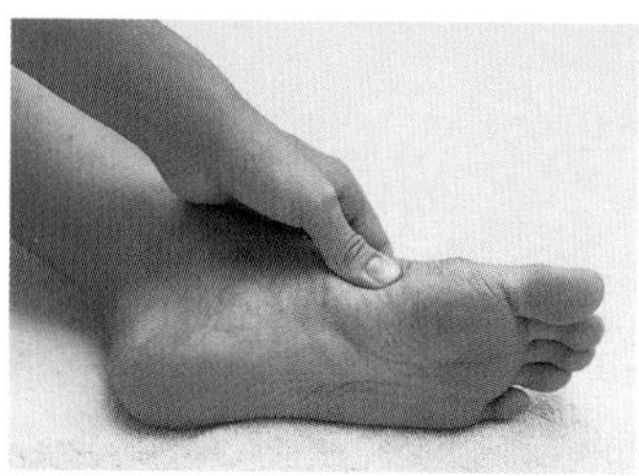

△ **For cramps and digestive problems**
Turn your right foot on its side. Use your right thumb to locate the pressure point one thumb-width down from the ball of the foot, close to the inner edge. This is Spleen 4. Press firmly (but not painfully) and hold for one minute. Release the pressure and pause for another minute, then repeat. Remember to breathe deeply while pressing the point. Repeat the movement on the other foot.

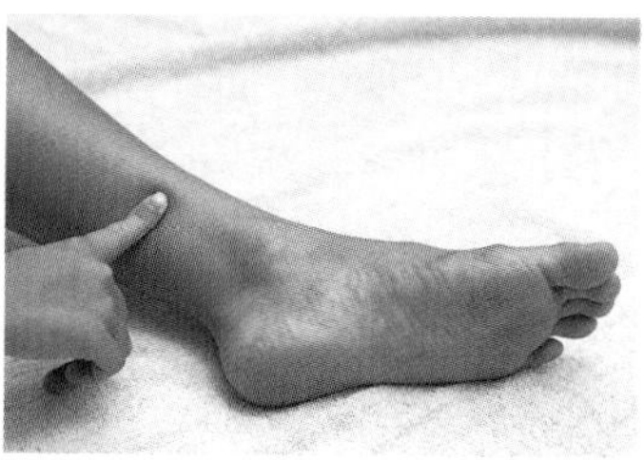

△ **For PMS, irregular periods and water retention**
Turn your right lower leg on its side. Now use the index finger of the right hand to find a pressure point four finger-widths up from the inner ankle bone, keeping close to the side of the shinbone. Press this point, which is called Spleen 6, for one minute and wait. Release for a few moments, then press again for another minute. Keep breathing as you press. Repeat the action on the left foot.

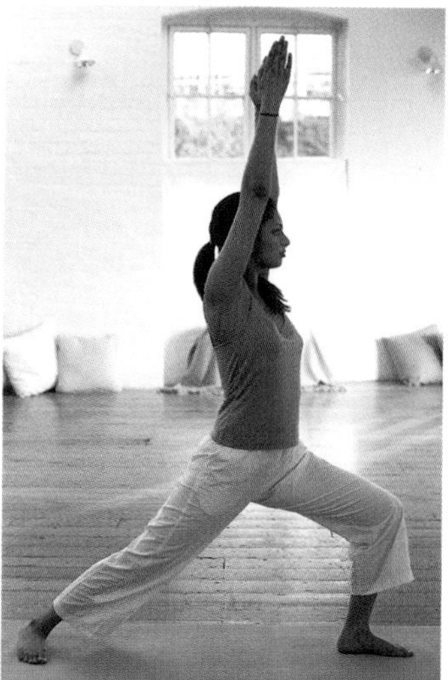

△ **Do not overdo your exercise regime when you are menstruating. Gentle stretches and yoga can be of enormous benefit, but avoid inverted (upside-down) poses.**

Digestive difficulties

The digestive system is essential to good health. It is the means by which we get our energy and nutrients, and it also carries away waste and toxins. An efficient digestion system will help to ensure good general health, clear skin and shining hair.

Many of us experience minor problems such as indigestion, heartburn, food allergies and constipation on a regular basis. Reflexology can be helpful for digestion problems, but you should also eat a healthy diet and adopt good eating habits, to avoid placing undue strain on the system.

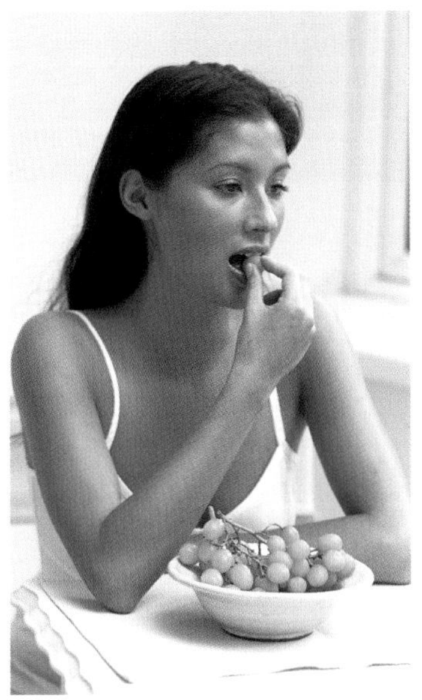

△ Include plenty of fruits and vegetables in your daily diet. As well as being packed with nutrients, these foods contain plenty of fibre. This is needed to aid the elimination of waste from the body.

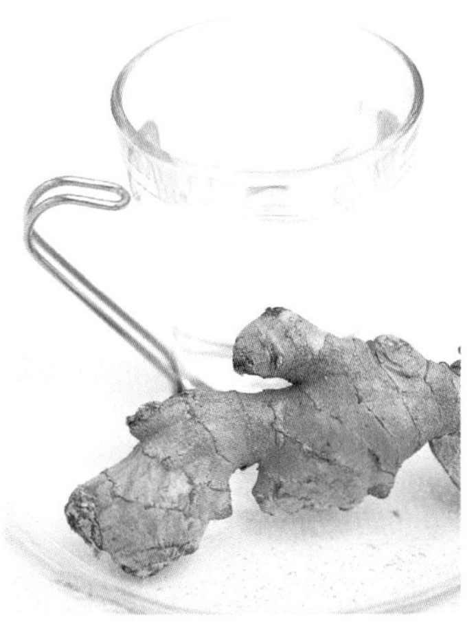

◁ Ginger helps to soothe nausea, morning sickness and indigestion. A ginger tea infusion is comfortingly warming and simple to make.

healthy eating habits

Following a healthy diet will keep your digestion system functioning well. For a healthy system, you should also:

- Eat little and often, rather than having one or two large meals a day.
- Always sit down to eat. Do not eat when you are feeling stressed or anxious.
- Drink plenty of water and keep your coffee, tea and fizzy drink intake to a minimum.
- Eat plenty of fibre-rich foods, such as fruits and vegetables and whole grains (wholemeal bread, brown rice, wholewheat pasta).

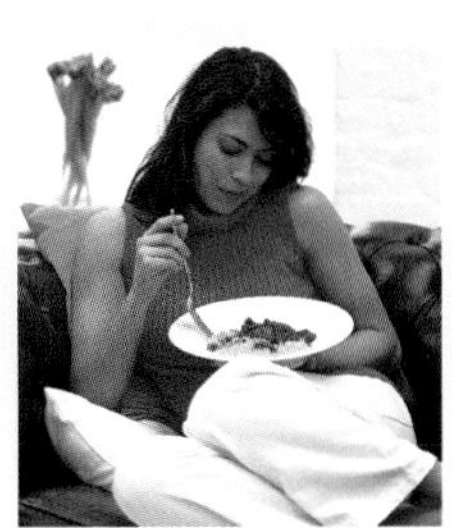

△ Take time to enjoy food. Avoid slumping or awkward postures like this one, as they put pressure on the digestion.

soothing the digestion

These acupressure points direct healing energy to soothe particular digestion problems – choose the one that is most suitable for you. You can massage an essential oil diluted in a carrier oil into the foot first if you like: fennel and sweet ginger are the most suitable oils for digestion problems. Breathe regularly and rhythmically throughout the exercise.

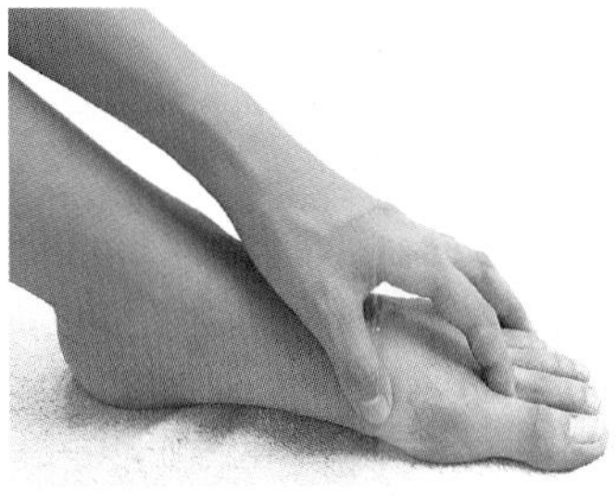

△ **Abdominal cramps**
Place both feet flat on the floor. Place the middle finger of each hand on the corresponding foot. Press into the webbing between the big and second toes, angling the finger towards the big toe. Hold the pressure for a count of 30, release for one minute, then repeat. Rest for five minutes, then press twice more in the same way.

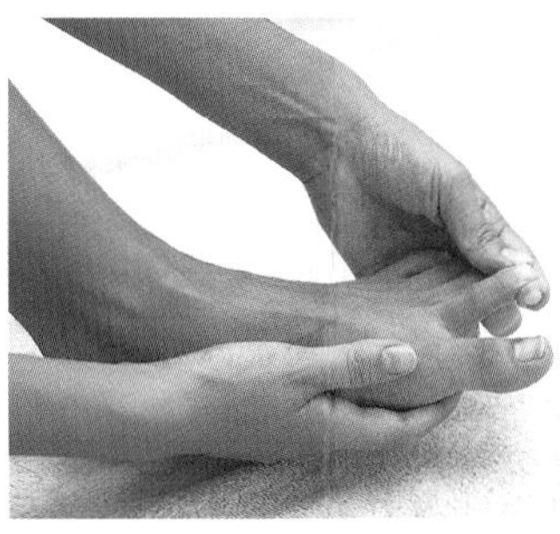

△ **For indigestion, abdominal pain and bloating**
Steady the right foot in your right hand. Place your left thumb and index finger either side of the second toe nail. Squeeze to a count of 60, breathing deeply. Do the same on the left foot.

Feet treat for mothers-to-be

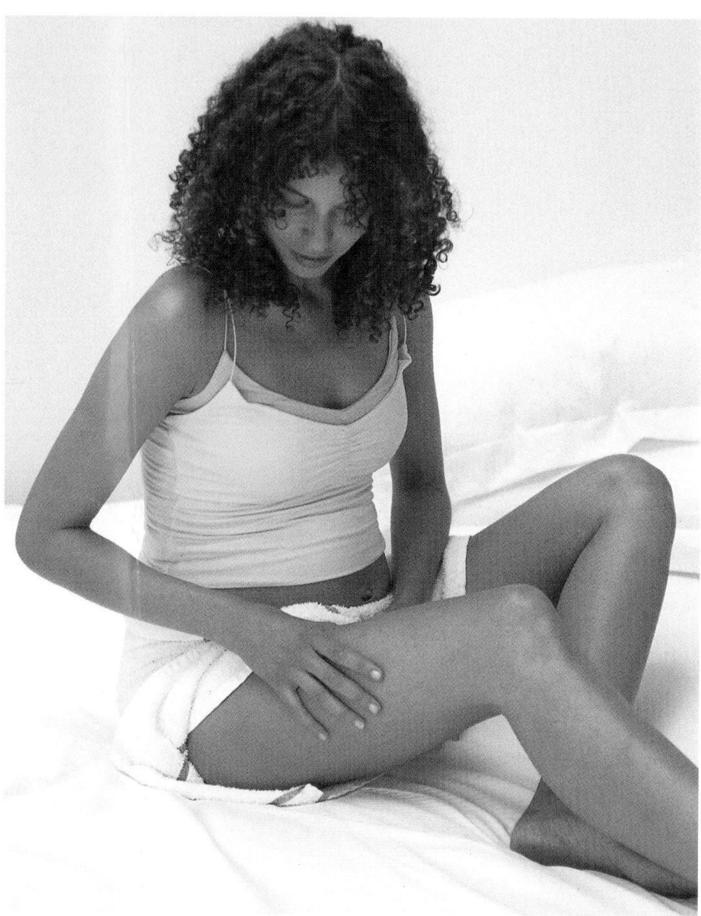

△ In early pregnancy, it is easy to self-massage your legs and feet, and it is extremely helpful for the circulation. However as your pregnancy advances, and the baby grows larger, you are likely to need props, such as marbles in a bowl, or a long-handled brush.

Some women sail through pregnancy with ease, but most will experience minor discomforts of one kind or another. Almost all women feel uncomfortable in the weeks before the birth, and may need some extra support at this time.

Massage has a feel-good factor, which may be particularly welcome in late pregnancy when the woman is likely to feel heavy and tired. Massage is also a good way of oiling the skin, which can get very dry in pregnancy. Working on the feet and lower legs will also help to shift the fluid that tends to collect in these areas during pregnancy. In addition, putting your feet up above heart level regularly will encourage fluid to drain out of the legs, which may prevent varicose veins and reduce feelings of heaviness and aching in the area.

soothing pregnancy routine

This is a gentle and calming routine for pregnant women, which can be adapted for self-treatment (see box). Let the feet soak in the aromatic water for at least five minutes. It's a good idea to put your feet up for 15 minutes after receiving this treatment; enjoy a cup of herbal tea at the same time.

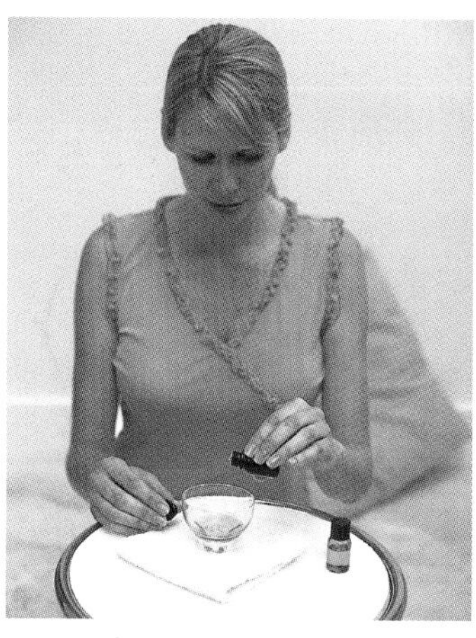

△ **1** Mix 2 drops of essential oil such as mandarin in 20ml/4 tsp of carrier oil – you need a lighter dilution than normal when treating in pregnancy.

safe oils in pregnancy

You should be careful about the essential oils that you use in pregnancy; many are not suitable because they may have an adverse effect. It is best not to use any essential oils other than citrus oils such as mandarin and tangerine during the first three months of pregnancy. Thereafter, always check that any oil is safe for use during pregnancy: chamomile, geranium, lavender and sandalwood are good oils for most women, but should only be used well-diluted.

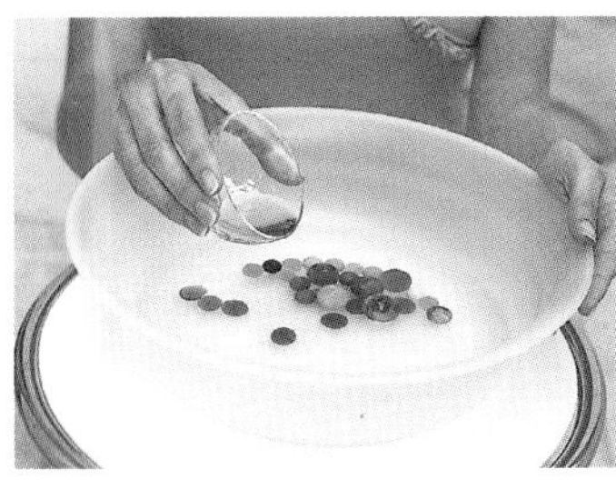

△ **2** Half-fill a foot bowl with warm water, then add a layer of marbles of different sizes. Pour in 5ml/1 tsp of the blended oil.

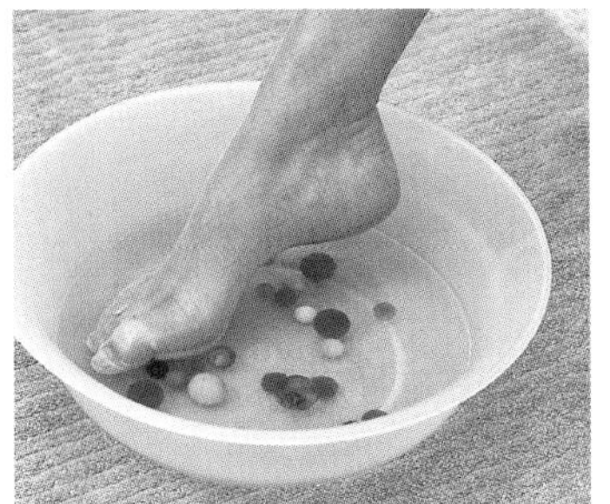

△ **3** Place the feet in the bowl, and push them backwards and forwards over the marbles: this gives a massage-like effect. Move the toes between the marbles. Stretch the feet by lifting up the heels and then placing them flat on the base of the bowl. Now raise up the toes. All these movements will help to open up the feet and to stimulate the circulation in the feet and lower legs. Remove the feet from the bowl and dry thoroughly.

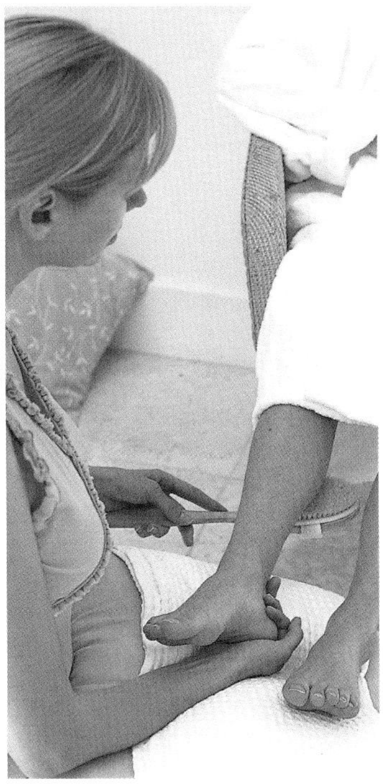

△ **4** Dampen a soft-bristled brush with warm water. Then pour about 5ml (1 tsp) of the oil over the bristles. Rub the brush over the top of the foot, using upward strokes. Cover the area three times, adding more oil if necessary. Rub up the heel and around the ankle area, followed by the front, and then the back, of the lower leg, using upward strokes. Again, cover the area three times. This helps to remove dead skin cells and will also stimulate the circulation.

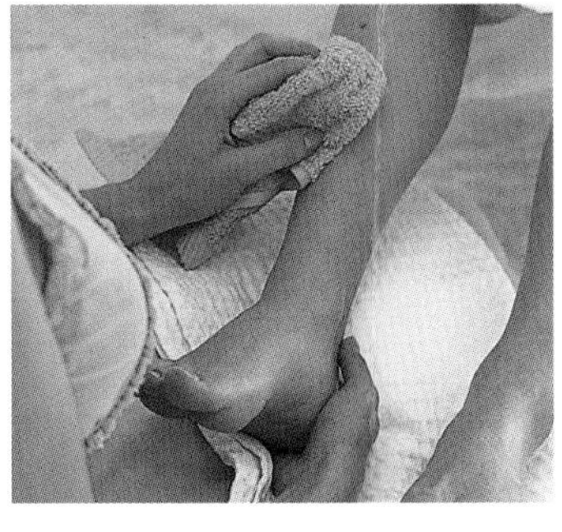

△ **5** Wipe off any excess oil with a cloth. Then use the cloth to stroke gently all over the top of the foot and the front of the lower leg. Once this area feels dry and comfortable, wipe the back of the leg.

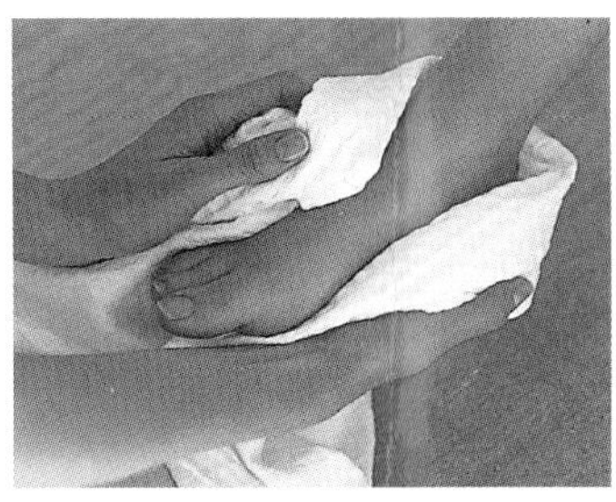

△ **6** Take a small hand towel and fold into a long strip. Holding either end, pass the towel backwards and forwards across the back of the leg. Start just above the ankle and work up the leg to just below the knee. As in step 4, this helps to activate the circulatory system. Now repeat steps 4 to 6 on the left foot and leg.

adapting the routine

Ideally, you should receive this treatment from someone else. However, if this is not possible, the routine works almost as well as a self-treatment. First of all, enjoy soaking your feet, rolling them backwards and forwards on the marbles and lifting the toes up and down – you may wish to spend longer than five minutes doing this. If so, have a kettle filled with boiled water nearby, so that you can top up the footbath when it starts to cool (take care near hot kettles).

It should be easy to apply the oil to your feet using a long-handled brush, as in step 4. To wipe off the excess oil (step 5), simply wrap a soft flannel around the brush, tucking in the edges at the top. Using this means that you do not have to bend down, which can be very uncomfortable in pregnancy. You can try step 6 using a longer towel. However, if this is too difficult for you to manage, simply skip this step. After the massage, make sure that you put your feet up and enjoy at least 15 minutes of peaceful and enjoyable relaxation.

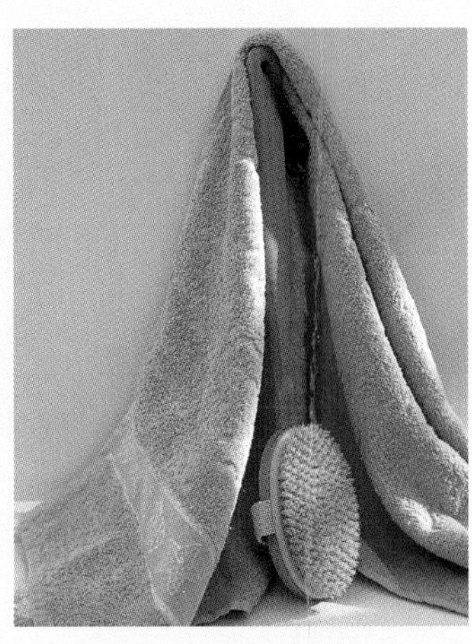

▷ **If you are treating yourself, wrap the head of the brush in a flannel or small towel so that you can remove oil from your feet easily.**

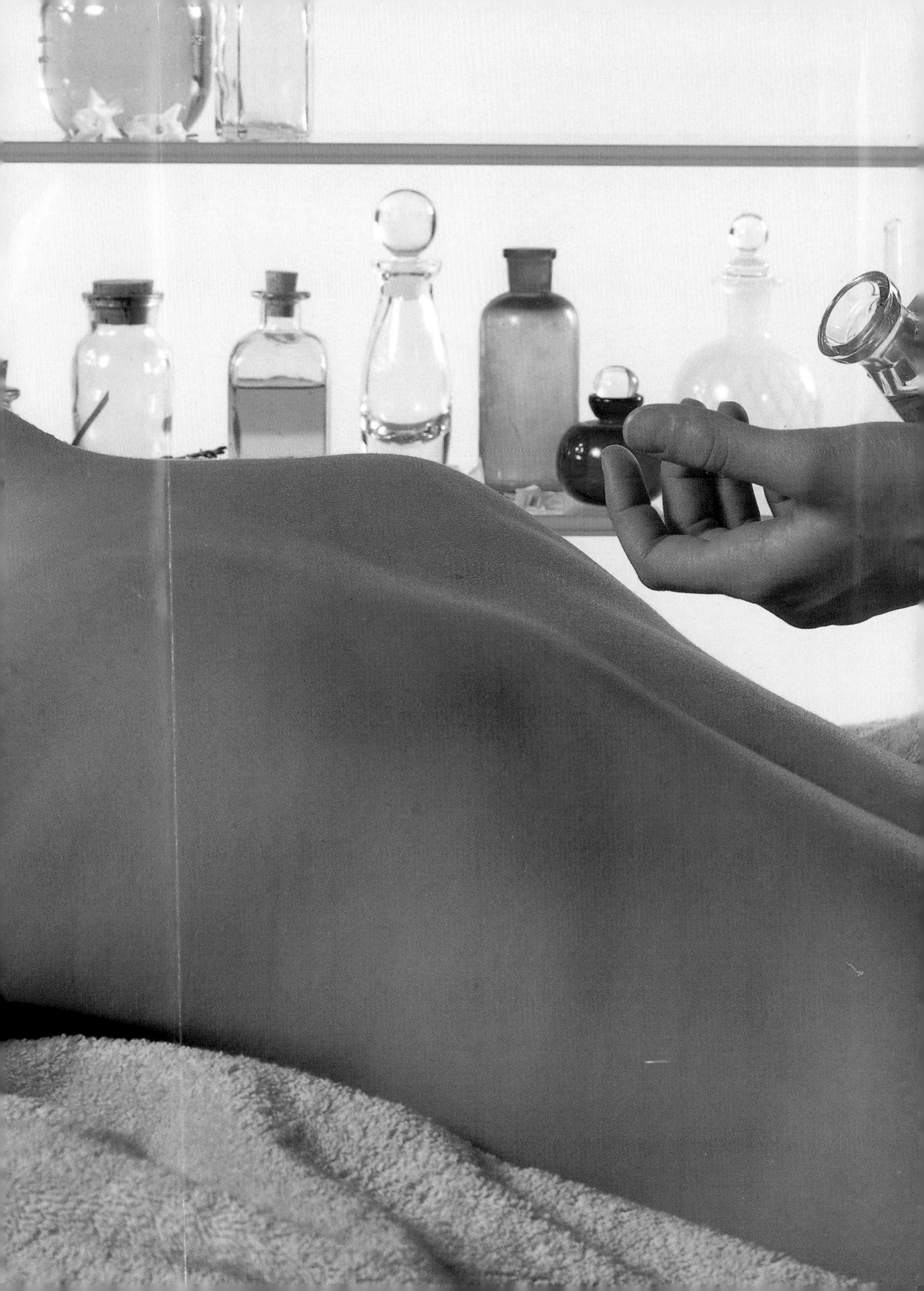

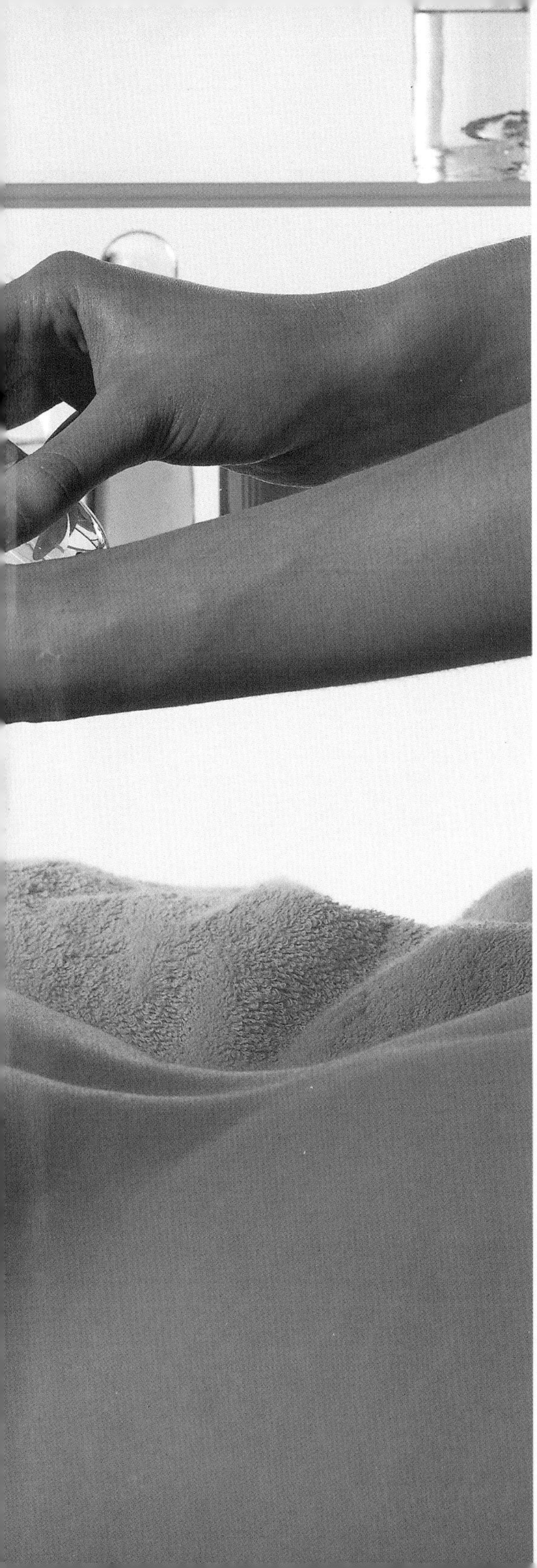

Appendix Massage Oils

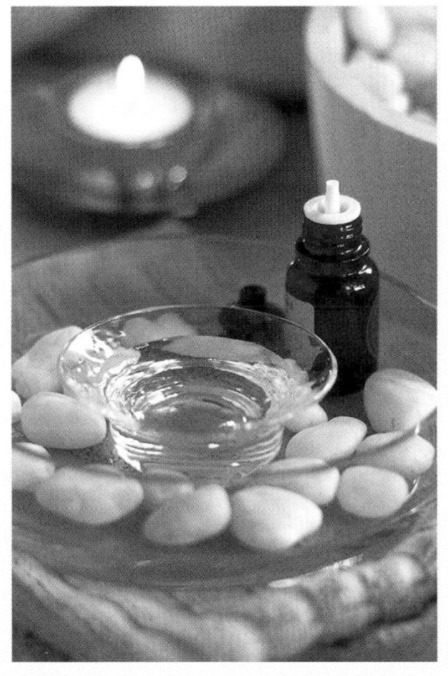

The essential oils

An essential oil is the essence of a plant, the plant's life force distilled for use. The fragrance and character of each oil are as unique as a finger print, as are its therapeutic properties.

Essential oils are natural, volatile substances that evaporate, quickly releasing their aroma into the air, as often happens when someone brushes against an aromatic plant. Approximately 300 essential oils are commercially available, but of these only 50 to 100 have health-giving properties and are suitable for home use and for the aromatherapist.

sources and properties of essential oils

Not all plants contain essential oils. In those that do, the oil, or essence, is contained in specialized glands in the foliage, flower, or other material. The oil helps prevent water loss in the plant. As the oils evaporate they create a barrier around the leaf or other plant part, and so reduce water loss through evaporation in the plant itself. Essential oils may also provide some defence against infection, and attract insects that are vital to pollination.

The plants that contain essential oils are found mainly in hot, dry habitats. In some plants, such as marjoram, the essential oil glands are present in the minute hairs on the leaves, but in woody plants such as rosewood they are embedded in the fibrous bark or wood. In others the oil glands can be seen clearly as shiny, coloured discs on the surface of the leaf or flower.

Most essential oils are lighter than water, although benzoin is an example of an essence that is heavier. All of them differ from vegetable oils in that they are not greasy. Most are colourless; the exceptions include: bergamot, which is green; lemon oil, which is yellow; and chamomile, blue.

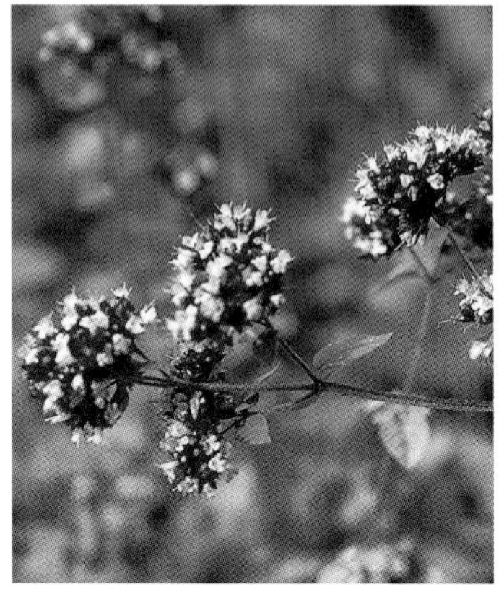

◁ **The essential oil of marjoram is contained in tiny hairs on the surface of the leaves.**

chemical constituents

A particular oil may contain between 50–500 different chemicals. Rose oil contains the greatest number, some of which are found in such minute quantities that they have not yet been identified. This has made it impossible to reproduce accurately the most exquisite of the essential oils.

The chemicals in essential oils unlock the body's ability to heal. They enter the body through the skin and are carried to all parts in the blood, after which they are excreted through the lungs and in urine. After a treatment the essential oil remains in the body for three to four hours, activating the healing process, which can continue for two to three weeks.

extracting essential oils

Most essential oils are extracted by distillation or expression, and given the fragile nature of the raw material, this process usually takes place in the country of origin. The commonest method of extraction is steam distillation, where the

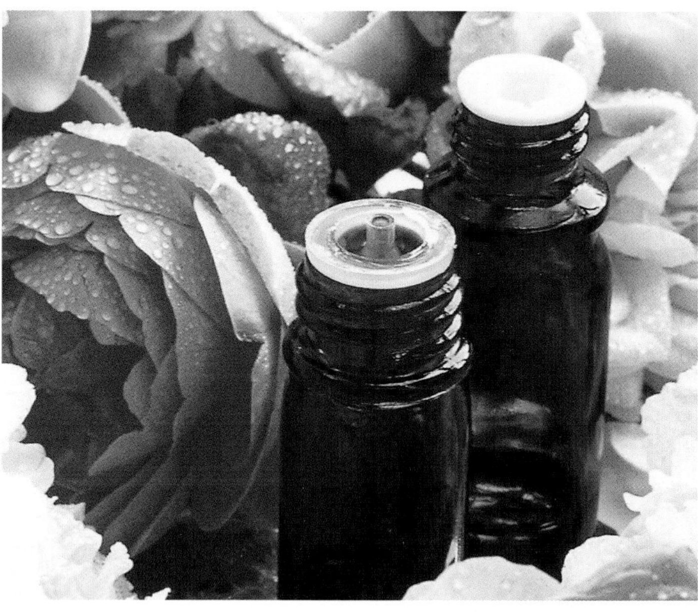

▷ **Rose oil contains the greatest number of different chemical constituents. This complexity makes it impossible to reproduce accurately, and explains its reputation as one of the most exquisite essential oils.**

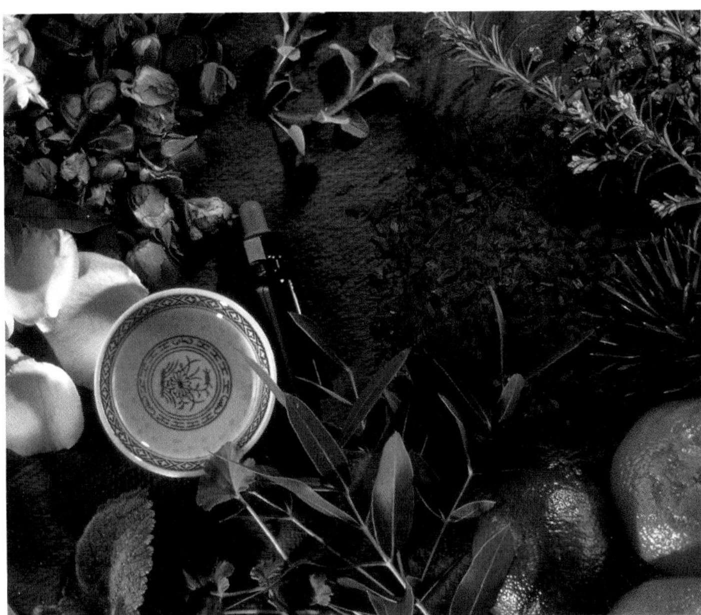

◁ Essential oils are extracted from many different parts of a plant – leaves, flowers, fruits or other material. Each oil contains healing properties, to be enjoyed but also respected.

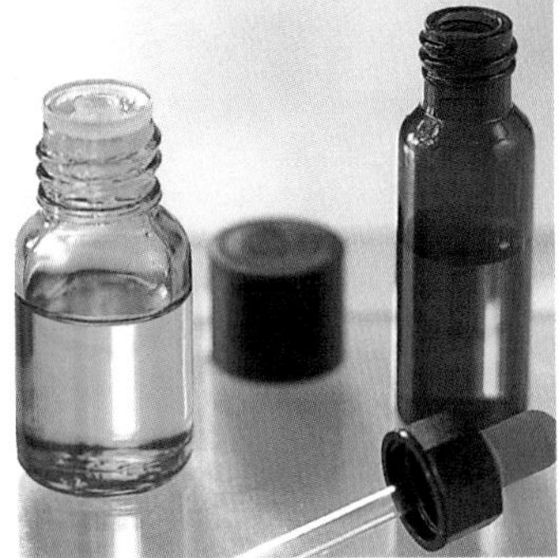

△ Most bottles of essential oil are sold with a built-in dropper. This is very useful given that only a small amount of each oil is usually required.

volatile and water-soluble parts are separated from the rest of the plant. The resulting mixture may need to be distilled a second time to remove non-volatile matter.

In the distillation process the plant is placed in a sealed container. Water in a second container is heated to produce steam, which is passed under pressure through the plant material. The steam causes the essence glands to burst, and the volatile chemicals dissolve in the steam. This rises and is taken into a condensing chamber, where it is cooled. As it cools the oil is separated from the water. Floral water is a by-product of distilling, and like essential oil has therapeutic and commercial uses.

Another process, solvent extraction, is favoured for releasing oil from delicate material, such as jasmine flowers. Plant material is washed with a solvent until the essence dissolves. The resulting material is distilled at a precise temperature to separate the solvent and the aromatic oil. Oil made by this process is known as an absolute.

the mechanics of smelling

When the scent of something is inhaled, the odour molecules float to the back of the nasal cavity. Here they dissolve in the moist environment, and in this form unite with receptor, or olfactory cells. The olfactory cells then trigger electrical signals via nerve pathways to the olfactory bulb in the brain. Most of the essential oil molecules that have triggered the system are breathed out, although some will enter the blood stream via the lungs. Only eight molecules of an aromatic substance are needed to trigger the smell mechanism.

Messages concerning smell are sent to areas of the brain called the cerebral cortex and limbic system. The limbic system controls many vital activities, such as sleep, sexual drive, hunger, and thirst, as well as smell. This is also the area of the brain that relates to emotion and memory, and thereby gives the clue to the link between smell, emotion, and memory. Odours also connect with the part of the brain called the hypothalamus, which controls the endocrine system and nervous system. Through this mechanism the brain comes into direct contact with the outside world.

The fading of a scent occurs when all the receptor cells are full, but after ten minutes or so they are vacated and can be reoccupied, causing the scent to "come back". This explains why we may fail to register a scent after a while, but a person just entering the same area may notice it.

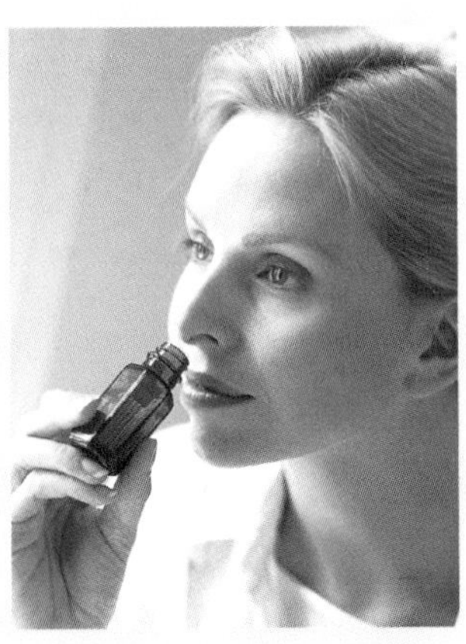

△ Each of us reacts to scents differently, so it is important to develop our own personal aromatic blends, and to be aware that tastes differ.

Properties of oils

Essential oils are powerful agents, and all of them – even those nominated as safe – must be used in the correct amounts and for the conditions to which they are best suited. Essential oils should not be applied undiluted to the skin, but should be mixed first, in the right proportions, in a vegetable carrier oil. Choosing the right carrier oil is also crucial for a good blend.

Citrus oils are photosensitive and should not be used before sunbathing. If you are unsure about the suitability of an oil, always seek the advice of a qualified aromatherapist.

Useful essential oils

bergamot *Citrus bergamia*

Properties: antibacterial, anti-infectious, antiseptic, antispasmodic, antiviral, calming and sedative, cicatrizant, tonic, stomachic.

This pale green essential oil has a refreshing aroma. It is useful both for digestive problems, such as colic, spasm and sluggish digestion, and for calming emotional states, such as agitation and severe mood swings. It must be used with extreme caution if in strong sunlight.

cedarwood *Cedrus atlantica*

Properties: antibacterial, antiseptic, cicatrizant, lipolytic, lymph tonic, mucolytic, stimulant.

Cedarwood has a sweet, woody aroma and is effective for oily skin and scalp disorders. Its antiseptic properties and cleansing aroma are beneficial to bronchial problems. It is unsuitable for pregnant women and children.

clary sage *Salvia sclarea*

Properties: antifungal, anti-infectious, antispasmodic, antisudorofic, decongestant, detoxicant, oestrogen-like, neurotonic, phlebotonic, regenerative.

This strong-smelling oil is distilled from the dried clary sage plant. It should not be confused with sage oil and is not a substitute for it. Clary sage is excellent for all menstrual complications as its oestrogen-like qualities make it good for hormonal problems. It encourages menstruation and is useful for the hot flushes of the menopause. Clary sage is useful for depression and fear, and during convalescence.

cypress *Cupressus sempervirens*

Properties: antibacterial, anti-infectious, antispasmodic, antisudorific, antitussive, astringent, calming, deodorant, diuretic, hormone-like, neurotonic, phlebotonic, styptic.

The astringent action of cypress oil helps to regulate the production of sebum, reduce perspiration (even of the feet) and to staunch bleeding. It is reputed to help calm the mind, and to induce sleep.

eucalyptus *Eucalyptus smithii*

Properties: analgesic, anticatarrhal, anti-infectious, antiviral, balancing, decongestant, digestive, stimulant, expectorant, prophylactic.

Known as gully gum, this tree is native to Australia. The oil is as beneficial, but much gentler, than the more common *Eucalyptus globulus*, or blue gum, which requires care to use. Its gentle action makes it ideal for children. Eucalyptus oil is good for muscular pain and is effective against coughs and colds, both as a preventive and as a remedy.

fennel *Foeniculum vulgare*

Properties: analgesic, antibacterial, antifungal, anti-inflammatory, antiseptic, antispasmodic, cardiotonic, carminative, decongestant, digestive, diuretic, emmenagogic, lactogenic, laxative, litholytic, oestrogen-like, respiratory tonic.

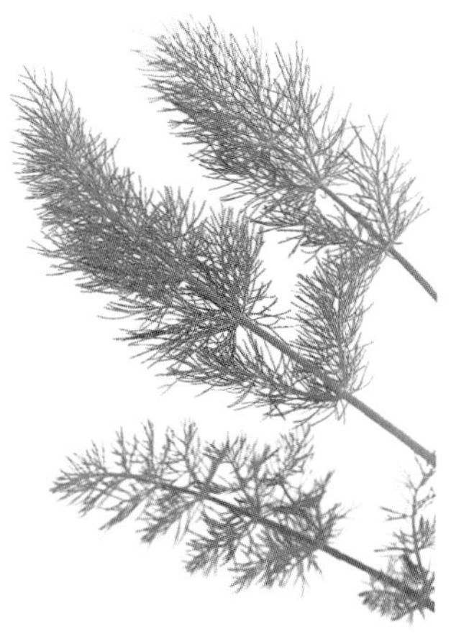

Fennel is recommended for lack of breast milk and, as it is oestrogen-like, it can be valuable for PMS, menopause and ovary problems. It will also work efficiently as a diuretic. It should not be used in pregnancy before the seventh month.

frankincense *Boswellia carteri*

Properties: analgesic, anti-infectious, antioxidant, anticatarrhal, antidepressive, anti-inflammatory, cicatrizant, energizing, expectorant, immunostimulant.

A pale amber-green essential oil, it is an ancient aromatic product once considered as precious as gold. It is a gentle oil that is particularly useful for emotional problems, where it allays anger and irritability and soothes grief.

geranium *Pelargonium graveolens*

Properties: analgesic, antibacterial, antidiabetic, antifungal, anti-infectious, anti-inflammatory, antiseptic, antispasmodic, astringent, cicatrizant, decongestant, digestive stimulant, haemostatic, styptic, insect repellent, phlebotonic, relaxant.

Some geranium oils have a definite rose-like smell and are often referred to as rose geranium. More correctly, rose geranium is when a tiny percentage of rose otto is added to the geranium oil. Geranium will reduce inflammation and is good for acne, herpes, diarrhoea and varicose veins. It is also a relaxant, and will help grief and anger. It is useful for moodiness and to balance the mood swings of PMS.

german chamomile *Matricaria recutica*

Properties: anti-allergic, antifungal, anti-inflammatory, antispasmodic, cicatrizant, decongestant, digestive tonic, hormone-like.

This oil gets its blue colour from a component called Chamazulene. This, in synergy with the other components of the oil, is a strong anti-inflammatory agent. This makes it especially useful for skin problems (particularly irritated skin) and rheumatism, when a compress is most effective. The oil is recommended for PMS, and for calming anger and agitated emotional states.

ginger *Zingiber officinale*

Properties: analgesic, anticatarrhal, carminative, digestive stimulant, expectorant, general tonic, sexual tonic, stomachic.

A yellow oil with a spicy aroma. Ginger essential oil has properties that alleviate most digestive problems, including flatulence, constipation, nausea and loss of appetite. Its ability to dull pain is beneficial to muscular pain and sciatica, while its tonic properties are useful for emotions like fear and apathy, and will also help to draw out a reticent, withdrawn personality.

juniper *Juniperus communis*

Properties: analgesic, antidiabetic, antiseptic, depurative, digestive tonic, diuretic, litholytic, sleep-inducing.

This oil has a sweet, fragrant aroma. Take care when buying it because the berries are used to flavour gin and the residue is often distilled to produce a poor quality essential oil. Even genuine juniper oil is frequently adulterated.

Juniper oil has a strong diuretic action that is useful for treating cystitis, water retention and cellulite. It has a cleansing, detoxifying action on the skin, and is useful for oily skin problems, such as acne. It is especially good for feelings of guilt and jealousy, and for giving strength when feeling emotionally drained.

lavender *Lavandula angustifolia*

Properties: analgesic, antibacterial, antifungal, anti-inflammatory, antiseptic, antispasmodic, calming and sedative, cardiotonic, carminative, cicatrizant, emmenagogic, hypotensive, tonic.

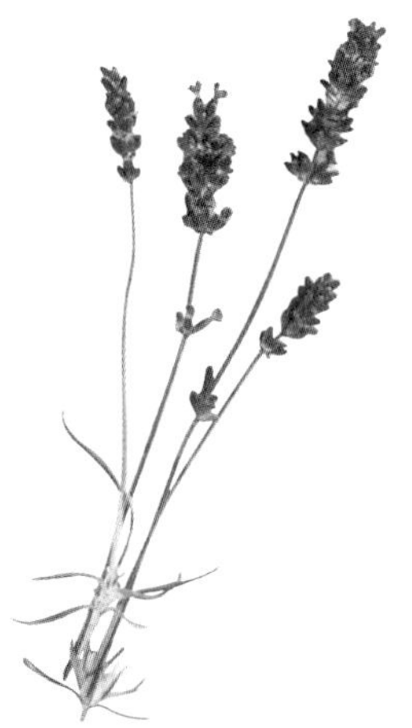

Lavender is the most widely used essential oil and is cultivated worldwide, but in spite of this, it is not easy to find a quality oil. It is a skin rejuvenator, and helps to normalize both dry and greasy skin. It works in combination with other oils to alleviate arthritis and rheumatism, psoriasis and eczema. It aids sleep, relieves tension headaches, and is good for calming nerves, lifting depression, relieving anger and soothing fear and grief.

lemon *Citrus limon*

Properties: anti-anaemic, antibacterial, anticoagulant, antifungal, anti-infectious, anti-inflammatory, antisclerotic, antiseptic, antispasmodic, antiviral, calming, carminative, digestive, diuretic, expectorant, immunostimulant, litholytic, phlebotonic, stomachic.

The clean, lively scent of lemon can lift the spirits, dispel sluggishness and indecision and relieve depression. It is an underestimated and very useful oil. It has an anti-infectious and expectorant effect on the respiratory airways and can help to eliminate the toxins that cause arthritic pain. It is good for greasy skin.

mandarin *Citrus reticulata*

Properties: antifungal, antispasmodic, calming, digestive.

Mandarin oil has digestive properties, and is excellent for treating both adults and children with indigestion, stomach pains and constipation. It can be useful for over-excitement, stress and insomnia. It is often popular with children because of its gentle action and familiar aroma.

melissa *Melissa officinalis*

Properties: anti-inflammatory, antispasmodic, antiviral, calming, choleretic, digestive, hypotensive, sedative, capillary dilator.

Melissa's sedative action relieves headaches and insomnia and is particularly beneficial for a problematic menstrual cycle. It is also a tonic for the heart, calming the turbulent emotions of grief and anger and helping to relieve fear.

neroli (orange blossom) *Citrus aurantium*

Properties: antidepressant, aphrodisiac, sedative, uplifting.

Neroli has a soft, floral fragrance and is the most costly of the orange oils.
It is beneficial for the skin and helps improve elasticity. It is good for scars, thread veins, and pregnancy stretch marks. It has a sedative and calming effect.

orange (bitter) *Citrus aurantium*

Properties: anti-inflammatory, anticoagulant, calming, digestive, sedative, tonic.

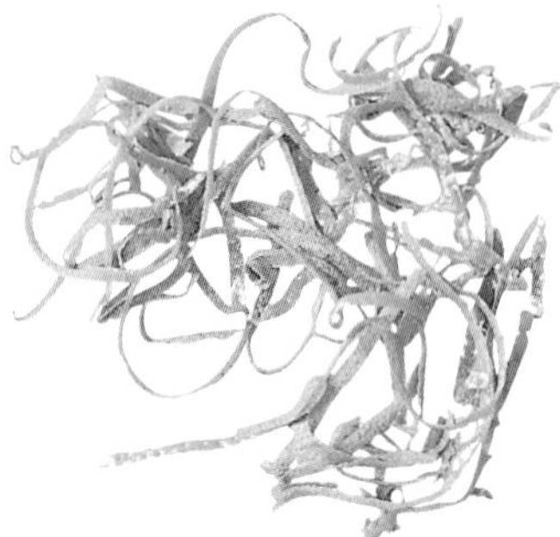

Bitter orange can be helpful for poor circulation, digestive problems and constipation. It has antidepressant qualities, and will promote positive thinking.

patchouli *Pogostemon patchouli*

Properties: antifungal, anti-infectious, anti-inflammatory, aphrodisiac, cicatrizant, decongestant, immunostimulant, insect repellent, phlebotonic.

Patchouli is particularly valuable for broken, chapped and cracked skin, as well as inflamed skin, eczema and acne. It promotes new skin cells, which makes it useful for reducing scar tissue. It is beneficial against haemorrhoids and varicose veins. It has a sedative effect and is said to soothe an overactive mind.

peppermint *Mentha piperata*

Properties: analgesic, antibacterial, antifungal, anti-inflammatory, antimigraine, antilactogenic, antipyretic, antispasmodic, antiviral, carminative, decongestant, digestive, expectorant, liver stimulant, hormone-like, hypotensive, insect repellent, mucolytic, neurotonic, reproductive stimulant, soothing uterotonic.

It has a strong refreshing aroma. Renowned for its beneficial effect on digestive problems, such as indigestion and nausea, but also for respiratory problems. It is useful for congestion or catarrh, bronchitis, sinsusitis and colds. Clears the mind, aids concentration and can overcome mental fatigue and depression.

pine *Pinus sylvestris*

Properties: analgesic, antibacterial, antifungal, anti-infectious, anti-inflammatory, antisudorific, balsamic, decongestant, expectorant, hormone-like, hypotensive, litholytic, neurotonic, rubefacient.

Pine is an excellent disinfectant and air freshener: when dispersed in the air, its antiseptic qualities help to prevent the spread of infections. It is recommended for respiratory tract infections and hay fever, while its anti-inflammatory action makes it useful for cystitis and rheumatism. Pine is an excellent pick-me-up for general lack of energy.

roman chamomile *Chamaemelum nobile*

Properties: anti-anaemic, anti-inflammatory, antineuralgic, antiparasitic, antispasmodic, calming and sedative, carminative, cicatrizant, digestive, emmenagogic, menstrual, vulnerary, stimulant, sudorific

A gentle, soothing and calming oil, it is suitable for children and babies for irritability, inability to sleep, hyperactivity and tantrums. It is also useful for rheumatic inflammation, indigestion and headaches.

rose otto *Rosa damascena*

Properties: antibacterial, anti-infectious, anti-inflammatory, astringent, cicatrizant, neurotonic, sexual tonic, styptic.

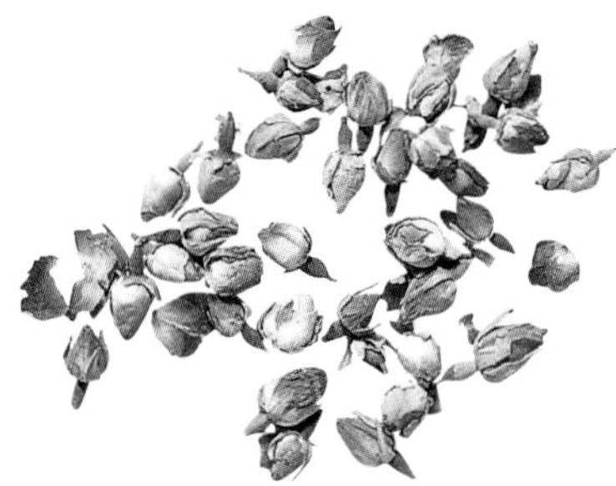

Rose otto has been favoured by women through the ages for its gentle action and fragrant aroma. It is thought to balance the hormones and is helpful for irregular periods. Rose soothes the skin, lifts depression and promotes well-being.

rosemary *Rosmarinus officinalis*

Properties: analgesic, antibacterial, antifungal, anti-infectious, anti-inflammatory, antispasmodic, antitussive, antiviral, cardiotonic, carminative, choleretic, cicatrizant, venous decongestant, detoxicant, digestive, diuretic, emmenagogic, hyperglycaemic, blood pressure regulator, litholytic, cholesterol-reducing, mucolytic, neuromuscular effect, neurotonic, sexual tonic, stimulant.

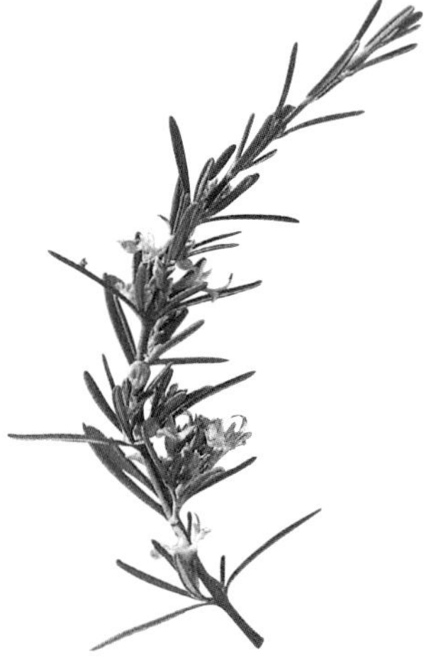

Rosemary is helpful for respiratory problems, arthritis, congestive headaches and constipation. It is also a tonic for the liver. This oil stimulates both body and mind, and is thought to be a good memory aid.

sandalwood *Santalum album*

Properties: anti-infectious, astringent, cardiotonic, decongestant, diuretic, moisturizing, nerve relaxant, sedative, tonic.

Sandalwood is a gentle oil that is important in the treatment of genito-urinary infections, especially cystitis. It is used for its effect on the digestive system, relieving heartburn and nausea, including morning sickness. It has been found to benefit both acne and dry skin (including dry eczema), as well as being useful for haemorrhoids and varicose veins. Its tonic properties are thought to be helpful in impotence.

sweet marjoram *Origanum majorana*

Properties: analgesic, antibacterial, anti-infectious, antispasmodic, calming, digestive stimulant, diuretic, expectorant, hormone-like, hypotensive, neurotonic, respiratory tonic, stomachic, vasodilator.

Sweet marjoram has been shown to be antiviral and is useful for cold sores. It can ease tension and irritability, lift headaches (especially those connected with menstruation) and promote sleep. It is useful for grief and anger, and its ability to calm and uplift makes it useful to combat moodiness.

tea tree *Melaleuca alternifolia*

Properties: analgesic, antibacterial, antifungal, anti-infectious, anti-inflammatory, antiparasitic, antiviral, immunostimulant, neurotonic, phlebotonic.

This oil has strong antiseptic properties with a matching aroma. It has excellent antimicrobial and antifungal action. It is a powerful stimulant to the immune system. It is one of the few essential oils that can be applied directly and undiluted to the skin.

ylang ylang *Cananga odorata*

Properties: antidiabetic, antiseptic, antispasmodic, aphrodisiac, calming and sedative, hypotensive, general tonic, reproductive tonic.

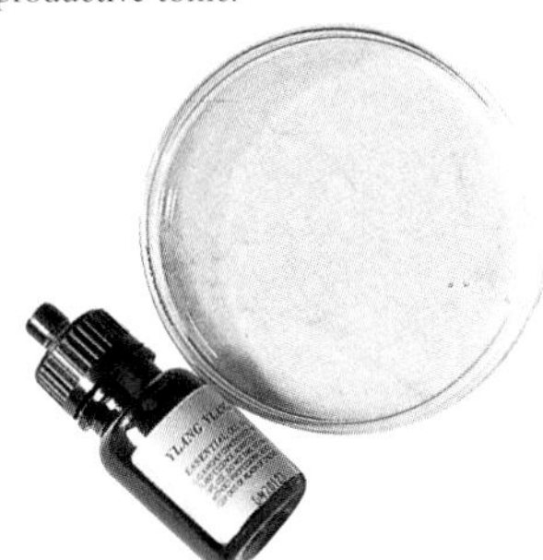

It has an exotic and heady aroma. Widely reputed for its aphrodisiac qualities, ylang ylang is said to counter impotence and frigidity. It can help emotional problems such as irritability and fear. It also helps regulate cardiac and respiratory rhythm.

▷ **Choose a carrier oil to suit the type of skin you are massaging. From left: almond for all skin types, sesame for dry and sunflower for oily.**

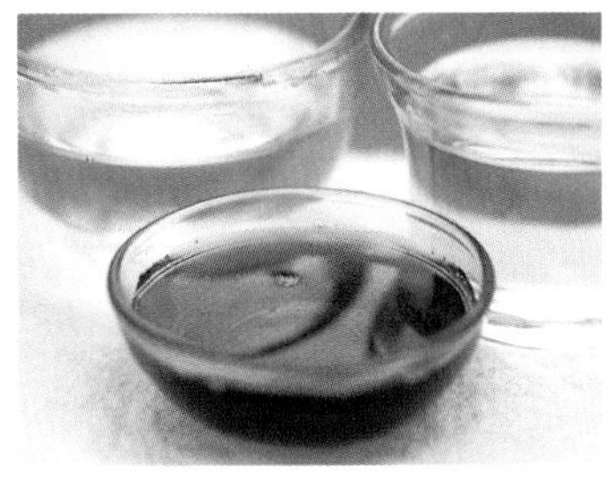

vegetable carrier oils

These oils often have their own health-giving qualities, so choosing an appropriate oil will heighten the dynamic nature of a massage and can have specific benefits, such as helping to guard against heart disease or inflammatory diseases such as arthritis. They can also help to boost the immune system.

Vegetable oils are made up of essential fatty acids and contain the fat-soluble vitamins A, D, and E. Some oils also contain large amounts of gamma linoleic acid (GLA), useful for the treatment of PMS. The fatty acid compounds help to reduce blood cholesterol levels and strengthen cell membranes, slowing down the formation of fine lines and wrinkles and helping the body to resist attack from free radicals.

Heat-treated oils lose nutritional value, so always use a cold pressed, unrefined vegetable oil as a carrier oil for essential oils. Likewise, use a certified organic vegetable oil, as this guarantees that no chemical fertilizers, pesticides, or fungicides have been used in its production. The darker the colour and stronger the odour, the less refined the oil, so it will be richer in health-giving properties. The following oils can be used alone, or as a carrier oil for essential oils. Once opened, store in the refrigerator.

almond oil A good source of vitamin D. It is suitable for all skin types, but is especially good for dry or irritated skin.
avocado oil Easily absorbed into the deep tissues, it is excellent for mature skin. It can help to relieve the dryness and itching of psoriasis and eczema. It blends well with other oils, and its fruity smell may influence which essential oils you choose.
borage oil One of the richest sources of GLA and useful for eczema and psoriasis, as well as for the symptoms of PMS.
carrot oil A valuable source of beta carotene, and useful for healing scar tissue and soothing acne and irritated skin.
evening primrose oil Rich in GLA, it is useful for the relief of eczema, psoriasis, dry skin, PMS, and tender breasts. It is also suitable for face treatments, but is a sticky oil and should be mixed with a lighter oil, such as grapeseed, soya, peanut, or peachnut.
grapeseed oil A non-greasy oil that suits all skin types. It is widely available in a refined state and is best enriched with almond oil.
hazelnut oil Its astringent qualities make it useful for oily and combination skins.
jojoba oil Good for all skin types and penetrates more easily than other oils. Rich in vitamin E, it is excellent for massaging faces with sensitive or oily complexions. It also has anti-bacterial properties, making it a useful oil for treating acne.
olive oil Too sticky for massage, but excellent in a blend for mature or dry skin.
peachnut oil A fine oil, rich in vitamin E and good for delicate skin, and ideal for face massage.
peanut oil Highly nutritious if unrefined, but rarely available. Its refined form makes a good base oil for massage, but is best enriched with a more nutritious oil if you require more than just a slippage medium.
safflower oil It is light and penetrates the skin well. Cheap and readily available in an unrefined state, it is a useful base oil.
sesame oil Made from untoasted seeds, it is good for skin conditions. It has sunscreen properties and is used in many suncare products. Use commercial preparations with a stated SPF number.
sunflower oil A light oil rich in vitamins and minerals. It can be enriched by the addition of more exotic oils.
walnut oil Contains small amounts of GLA and has a pleasant, nutty aroma.
wheatgerm oil Rich in vitamin E and useful for dry and mature skin. It is well known for its ability to heal scar tissue, smooth stretch marks, and soothe burns. It is too sticky as a massage oil, so add small amounts of it to a lighter oil. It should not be used on people with wheat intolerance.

Glossary

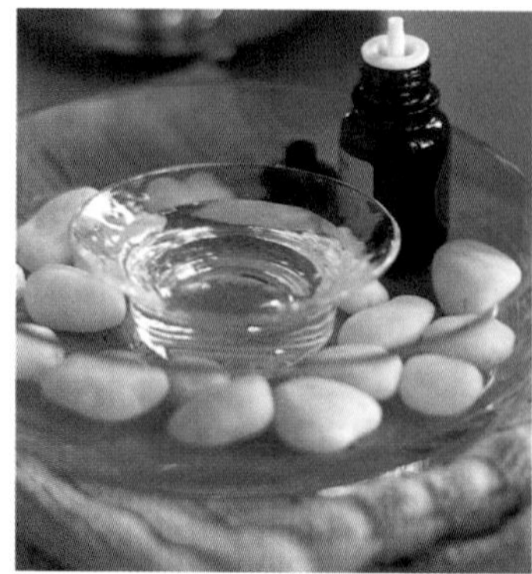

analgesic reduces sensitivity to pain.
anti-allergic acts to reduce sensitivity to various substances.
antibacterial agent that kills bacteria.
anticoagulant stops blood from clotting.
antidiabetic prevents the development of diabetes.
antifungal prevents the development of fungus.
anti-inflammatory reduces inflammation.
antilactogenic prevents or slows down the secretion of milk in nursing mothers.
antimigraine reduces or helps to prevent migraines.
antiparasitic prevents the development of parasites.
antipruritis relieves itching.
antipyretic counteracts inflammation or fever.
antisclerotic anti-ageing; prevents the hardening of tissues.
antiseptic prevents the development of bacteria.
antispasmodic prevents muscle spasm, convulsion.
antitussive relieves or prevents coughing.
antiviral agent that prevents the development of viruses.
aphrodisiac arouses sexual desire.
astringent causes the contraction of living tissue.
balsamic fragrant substance that softens phlegm.
capillary dilator dilates the capillaries, and so aids circulation.
cardiotonic has a tonic effect on the heart.
carminative relieves flatulence (wind).
choleretic stimulates the production of bile in the liver.
cicatrizant healing; promotes scar tissue.
decongestant relieves congestion in the skin, digestive, circulatory and respiratory systems.
depurative purifying or cleansing.
diaphoretic see *sudorific*.
digestive stimulant stimulates a sluggish digestion.
emmenagogic induces or regularizes menstruation.
essential oil volatile plant oil obtained only by distillation (exception: oil obtained by expression of the peel of citrus fruits).
febrifuge reduces temperature; antipyretic.
hypertensor increases blood pressure in hypotensive person.
hypotensor reduces blood pressure in hypertensive person
lactogen promotes the secretion of milk.
laxative loosens the bowel content.
lipolytic breaks down fat.
litholytic breaks down sand or small kidney or urinary stones.
mucolytic breaks down mucus and catarrh.
neurotonic stimulates and tones the nervous system.
oestrogenic stimulates the action of the female hormone, oestrogen.
phlebotonic improves or stimulates lymph circulation; lymph tonic.
prophylactic prevents disease.
rubefacient increases local blood circulation, causing redness of the skin.
stomachic stimulates secretory activity in the stomach.
styptic arrests haemorrhage by means of astringent quality; haemostatic.
sudorific induces or increases perspiration.
synergy the working together that occurs when two or more substances used together give a more effective result than the same substances used alone.
utertonic agent that improves the tone of the uterus (womb).
vasodilator causes blood vessels to increase in lumen (the hollow inside of the blood vessel).
vulnerary speeds up the healing process of wounds.

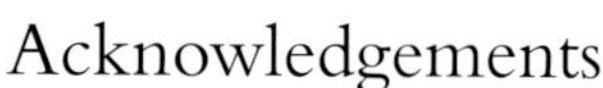

Acknowledgements

Head Massage – Francesca Rinaldi

I am grateful to my children Sam, Joe and Ben for inspiring me and for their generosity in putting up with me while writing this book. I have valued Sam's realism, Joe's clarity and patient computer support, and Ben's enthusiasm.

Thanks to therapists Karine Buchart, Jocelyn Ford Beazley, Susie Berkeley, Liz, Sulia Rose, Ibrahim Lingwood, Susan Harwood and Amanda Lindsey, for their professional input, and to Joanne of Anness Publishing for her incisive clarity and direction. Thanks also to Amanda Relph for her encouragement and the use of her beautiful home for photo shoots. Thank you to my parents and friends, especially Diane, for encouragement and to all the other helpers, seen and unseen.

picture acknowledgements

Thanks to the following agencies for permission to use their images:

The Bridgeman Art Library: p10 bottom left, p11, p32 bottom left. **Corbis**: p33, p35 top right & top left, p46 top. **Sylvia Cordaiy**: p32 top right, p34 bottom left.

Body Massage – Nitya Lacroix and Sharon Seager

Special thanks to Josette Bishop, Kim Brown, Laura Ciammarughi, Paul Farquharson, Richard Good, Audrey Graham, Sandra Hadfield, Annie Heap, Syreeta Kumar, Isabelle Massé, Christian Monsoy, Maria Morris, Nikki Reading, M W Smith, Gillian Lewis, Warwick Powell.

picture acknowledgements

Materials and equipment from The Body Shop, Crabtree and Evelyn, Descampes, The Futon Shop, Neal's Yard Remedies, Nice Irma's and the Tisserand Institute.

Foot Massage – Renée Tanner

Thanks and appreciation go to my husband and my family for their constant support; to my PA, Jane, for her endless patience; to copy editor, Kim Davies; to Michelle Garrett and her assistant Lisa Shalet for the excellent photography; to the models who interpreted my directions so expertly; and finally to my editor, Ann Kay, for her advice, technical guidance and support.

picture acknowledgements

Many thanks to all involved, including MOT Models agency; Sam Elmhurst for the illustrations on pages 182–3; and Pat Coward for the index.

Thanks to the following picture agency for permission to reproduce: p225 centre right: Man wearing bead bracelets, © Cat Gwynn/Corbis.

Index

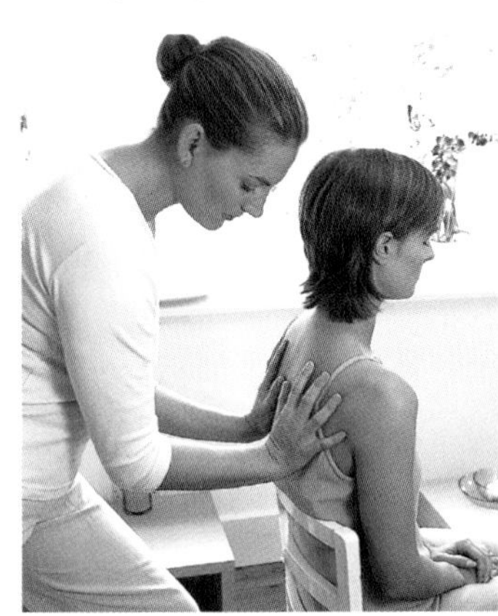

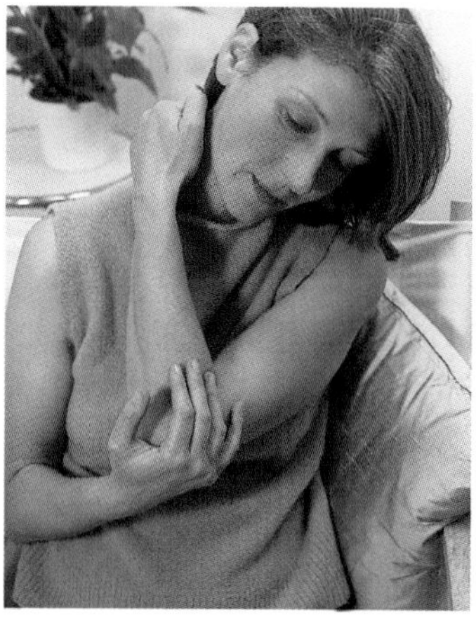

Notes

NOTES

Notes

Notes

Notes

NOTES